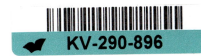

Handbook of Intensive Care

Handbook of
Intensive Care

Edited by

W. H. Bain MD, FRCS(Edin), FRCS(Glas)
Titular Professor of Cardiac Surgery
University of Glasgow
Consultant Cardiac Surgeon, Western Infirmary,
Royal Infirmary and Stobhill Hospital, Glasgow

and

K. M. Taylor MD, FRCS, FSA(Scot)
Senior Lecturer in Cardiac Surgery
University of Glasgow
Consultant Cardiac Surgeon
Western Infirmary and Royal Infirmary, Glasgow

WRIGHT · PSG
BRISTOL · LONDON · BOSTON
1983

Published by:
John Wright & Sons Ltd, 823–825 Bath Road, Bristol BS4 5NU, England.
John Wright PSG Inc, 545 Great Road, Littleton, Massachusetts 01460, USA.

British Library Cataloguing in Publication Data
Handbook of intensive care.
  I. Critical care medicine
  I. Bain, W. H.   II. Taylor, K. M.
  616'.028   RC86.7

ISBN 0 7236 0597 1

Library of Congress Catalog Card Number: 82–50759

Printed in Great Britain by
John Wright & Sons (Printing) Ltd, at The Stonebridge Press, Bristol BS4 5NU

Preface

We believe that this is an appropriate time to produce a handbook of intensive therapy practice. The initial phase of development in intensive therapy, as with all developing specialties, has brought with it a variety of opinion and practice and a somewhat alarming rate of growth. Most authorities would agree that the pioneering phase of intensive therapy has now given way to a longer period in which a broad consensus has appeared. This is not to say that controversy has ceased to flourish, for there is more than a grain of truth in the idea that when an issue ceases to be controversial it ceases to be interesting. Rather, the picture now is of continual refinement of well-established techniques and lines of therapy, in which increasing inroads are being made not only in terms of mortality figures but even more so in terms of reducing the morbidity associated with life-threatening illness.

No textbook may claim to be sufficiently comprehensive or authoritative in the vast area of intensive therapy practice. However, the multi-disciplinary approach to intensive therapy is reflected in the choice of authors in this handbook. They have been selected not only for their expertise and knowledge of a particular aspect of intensive therapy, but because their experience has been gained over many years as clinicians actively involved in general intensive therapy units.

The handbook has been compiled with an emphasis on practical patient care. Where management régimes are proposed, details of the author's preference and dosage are included as well as a discussion of alternative management régimes. Each author has been encouraged to discuss in some detail the broad principles of pathophysiology and of therapy, since an appreciation of these foundation stones of intensive therapy practice allows for the assimilation and integration of future developments.

The editors are grateful to the contributing authors for their efforts to keep to the systematic style suggested to them.

Mr Roy Baker has, on behalf of the publishers, maintained a keen and valued interest in the textbook as it has materialised. Mrs Jane Sugarman's expertise in reviewing and organising the original manuscripts has been invaluable.

The editors wish to thank Mrs Jean Kennedy for secretarial assistance, and the medical photographic departments in the Royal and Western Infirmaries, Glasgow, for their help with the illustrations.

Finally, our thanks must go to our medical, nursing and technical colleagues, with whose help and in whose company intensive therapy practice continues to progress.

WHB
KT

List of Contributors

M. E. M. Allison MD, FRCP(Edin and Glas) Senior Lecturer in Medicine, University of Glasgow, Consultant in Renal Medicine, Royal Infirmary, Glasgow, UK

The Renal System   Chapter 19

J. Askanazi MD Assistant Professor of Anesthesia, College of Physicians and Surgeons of Columbia University, New York, USA

Fluid Therapy of Surgical Patients   Chapter 6

W. H. Bain MD, FRCS(Edin), FRCS(Glas) Titular Professor of Cardiac Surgery, University of Glasgow, Department of Cardiac Surgery, Level 9, Western Infirmary, Glasgow, UK

Principles of Intensive Therapy   Chapter 1
The Cardiovascular System   Chapter 15

J. A. Bradley FRCS Lecturer in Surgery, Department of Surgery, Intensive Care Unit, Western Infirmary, Glasgow, UK

Infection and Septic Shock   Chapter 9

D. Campbell FRCS, DA Professor of Anaesthesia, University of Glasgow, Consultant Anaesthetist, Royal Infirmary, Glasgow, UK

The Respiratory System   Chapter 14

D. C. Carter MD, FRCS(Edin), FRCS(Glas)   Professor of Surgery, University of Glasgow; Consultant Surgeon, Royal Infirmary, Glasgow, UK

The Alimentary System   Chapter 13

Cecil T. G. Flear MD, FRCPath   Senior Lecturer and Honorary Consultant, Department of Clinical Biochemistry and Metabolic Medicine, The Royal Victoria Infirmary, Newcastle upon Tyne

The Sick-cell Concept and Hyponatraemia   Chapter 8

J. Graham FRCS   Consultant Orthopaedic Surgeon, Western Infirmary, Glasgow, UK

Major Orthopaedic Trauma   Chapter 21

J. M. Hood FRCS   Consultant Surgeon, Royal Victoria Hospital, Belfast, Northern Ireland

The Hepatic System   Chapter 18

D. Hopkins MD   Consultant, Glasgow and West of Scotland Blood Transfusion Service, Law Hospital, Lanark, UK

Blood Transfusion and Haematology   Chapter 10

I. Hutton MD, FRCP(Glas)   Senior Lecturer in Cardiology, University of Glasgow; Consultant Cardiologist, Royal Infirmary, Glasgow, UK

Cardiac Arrhythmias   Chapter 16

A. C. Kennedy MD(Glas), FRCP   Muirhead Professor of Medicine, University of Glasgow, Department of Medicine, Royal Infirmary, Glasgow, UK

The Renal System   Chapter 19

J. M. Kinney MD   Professor of Surgery and Director of the Surgical Metabolism Program, College of Physicians and Surgeons of Columbia University, New York, USA

Fluid Therapy of Surgical Patients   Chapter 6

Iain McA. Ledingham MD(Glas), FRCS(Edin), MRCP(Glas), FRSE   Professor of Intensive Care, University of Glasgow; Consultant, Intensive Therapy Unit, Western Infirmary, Glasgow, UK

Infection and Septic Shock   Chapter 9

Christine McCartney BSc, PhD   Lecturer in Bacteriology and Immunology, Department of Bacteriology and Immunology, Intensive Therapy Unit, Western Infirmary, Glasgow, UK

Infection and Septic Shock   Chapter 9

A. J. McKay FRCS(Glas)   Senior Registrar, Department of Surgery, Royal Infirmary, Glasgow, UK

The Peripheral Vascular System   Chapter 20

K. J. Maxted BSc   Senior Physicist, University Department of Cardiac Surgery, Royal Infirmary, Glasgow, UK

Haemodynamic Monitoring   Chapter 3

J. Douglas Miller MD, PhD, FRCS(Edin), FRCS(Glas), FACS   Professor and Chairman, University Department of Surgical Neurology, The Royal Infirmary, Edinburgh, UK

The Nervous System   Chapter 17

B. Moule DMRD, FFR   Consultant Radiologist, Royal Infirmary, Glasgow, UK

Radiology   Chapter 11

D. H. Osborne FRCS(Ire)   Lecturer in Surgery, University Department of Surgery, Royal Infirmary, Glasgow, UK

The Alimentary System   Chapter 13

J. G. Pollock FRCS(Edin), FRCS(Glas)   Consultant Surgeon, Royal Infirmary, Glasgow, UK

The Peripheral Vascular System   Chapter 20

Penelope J. Redding MBBS   Senior Registrar in Bacteriology and Immunology, University Department of Bacteriology and Immunology, Intensive Therapy Unit, Western Infirmary, Glasgow, UK

Infection and Septic Shock   Chapter 9

W. H. Reid FRCS(Edin, Eng and Glas)   Consultant Plastic Surgeon, Canniesburn Hospital, Glasgow, UK

Burns   Chapter 12

A. Shenkin BSc, MB, ChB, PhD   Consultant Biochemist, Royal Infirmary, Glasgow, UK

Nutritional Support   Chapter 7

C. M. Singh PhD, MD   Professor of Cardiothoracic Surgery, Christian Medical College, Ludhiana, Punjab, India

The Sick-cell Concept and Hyponatraemia   Chapter 8

K. M. Taylor MD, FRCS, F.S.A.(Scot)   Senior Lecturer in Cardiac Surgery, University of Glasgow; Consultant Surgeon, Department of Cardiac Surgery, Royal Infirmary, Glasgow, UK

Principles of Intensive Therapy   Chapter 1
The Cardiovascular System   Chapter 15

A. B. M. Telfer FFARCS   Consultant Anaesthetist, Division of Anaesthesia, Royal Infirmary, Glasgow, UK

Logistics of Intensive Care   Chapter 2

W. S. T. Thomson PhD, FRCS(Glas), FRCPath   Consultant Biochemist, Southern General Hospital, Glasgow, UK

Disorders of Water and Electrolyte Balance   Chapter 4
Disorders of Acid–base Regulation   Chapter 5

D. G. Young FRCS(Edin), FRCS(Glas)   Senior Lecturer in Paediatric Surgery, University of Glasgow; Consultant Surgeon, Royal Hospital for Sick Children, Yorkhill, Glasgow, UK

Paediatrics   Chapter 22

Contents

Chapter 1

Principles of Intensive Therapy

W. H. Bain and K. M. Taylor

The word 'intensive' implies a concentration of effort. This emphasizes the important point that intensive therapy is not an alternative type of medical care, but merely a concentration of existing techniques of diagnosis, measurement and treatment, in the presence of life-threatening, but potentially curable, pathology.

Intensive therapy units have evolved over the past 30 years as the logical result of the concept of 'progressive patient care'. Even before this label was applied, progressive care was seen, in practice, in the 'Nightingale' wards. Those patients requiring most care, either as a result of their illness itself or of necessary therapeutic intervention, would be sited nearest to the nurses' station. The degree of recovery could be traced accurately thereafter, progress up the ward being directly proportional to improving health. In the 1960s, patient care areas within a ward became designated as Intensive, Intermediate or Convalescent. Also at this time, certain specialties, e.g. cardiac surgery, cardiology and renal medicine, found it more efficient and expedient to train their staff to apply newly available techniques in purpose-built units.

Recognition of the value of such concentration of expertise and necessary equipment, both in terms of patient care and of economics, led to the inclusion of the provision of specially designated Intensive Therapy Units in the Department of Health and Social Security's 1970 recommendations for new hospital buildings.

We have previously indicated that intensive therapy units are primarily concerned with patients suffering from life-threatening, but potentially curable, pathology. The life-threatening or critical nature of the pathology may be actual or potential, and is often associated with secondary pathological effects on other organs or systems. In addition, the critically ill patient frequently exhibits disorders of essential homeostatic mechanisms,

1

for example water and electrolyte imbalance, acid-base disorders and haematological disturbance. The multisystem pathophysiology associated with critical illness is reflected in the awareness of the need for a multidisciplinary approach in intensive therapy. Unfortunately, the early emphasis on artificial ventilation as the major feature of intensive therapy led to an unwarranted assumption by others that intensive therapy units were the proper domain of anaesthetists and that anything more than a short visit every day was tantamount to territorial invasion. Thankfully, the determined efforts of the early intensive therapy clinicians to break down these artificial barriers have largely been successful, and a multidiscipline approach to intensive therapy is now widespread with inevitable mutual benefit. Incorporation of intensive therapy experience in training schemes for general medical, surgical, anaesthetic and laboratory medical staff has done a great deal to encourage familiarity with, and continued involvement in, intensive therapy practice.

Progress in intensive therapy over the past 10–15 years has been considerable. The critical nature of the illness or pathology inevitably present results in relatively high mortality figures. These mortality statistics have, however, greatly improved during this period, and continue to fall. Furthermore, increasing attention is being paid towards reducing the high morbidity associated with critical illness or trauma. Intensive therapy practice has, commendably, been accompanied by continual evaluation of results of therapy, and a constant search for improved methods of selection of patients likely to benefit from intensive therapy. Such self-assessment has allowed the definition, however arbitrary, of principles of intensive therapy practice. These include the following:

1. Selection of patients requiring intensive therapy.
2. Initial resuscitation and transfer to the intensive therapy unit.
3. Establishment of measurement and monitoring techniques.
4. Assessment of priorities in therapy.
5. Application and monitoring of primary and secondary therapy.
6. Use of system support or system replacement techniques where indicated.
7. Transfer and rehabilitation of convalescent patients.

At the present time, selection of patients for admission to an intensive therapy unit (ITU) is usually based on clinical judgement and experience. Recognition of the presence or potential development of a critical illness associated with severe physiological disturbance must be accompanied by the expectation of amenability to appropriate therapy and the possibility of a successful outcome. The search continues for an objective, quantitative method for accurate selection of patients most likely to benefit from intensive therapy admission. Several multivariant predictive indices are currently under investigation, and may be helpful to the clinician in quantitating and even predicting the likely overall effect of the primary pathology and secondary complications present in any patient.

In the acutely ill patient, initial resuscitation is of vital importance in restoring some degree of physiological stability in order to 'buy time' for a full assessment of the patient's condition. The shocked patient is an excellent example, where restoration of optimal perfusion and empirical correction of perfusion-related acid–base disturbance must take precedence over detailed investigation. Resuscitation techniques have developed in parallel with intensive therapy, not only in relation to initial presentation, but also in the course of the intensive therapy stay where acute episodes may occur. Successful initial resuscitation should be associated with rapid but controlled transfer of the patient to the ITU. Recent reports have drawn attention to the importance of the transfer phase in critically ill patients, whether within the confines of a particular hospital, or over much greater distances requiring the use of specially equipped and manned transfer ambulances or 'mobile intensive therapy units'.

The establishing of appropriate monitoring and measurement is of fundamental importance in intensive therapy. Lord Kelvin observed in 1889 'when you can measure what you are speaking about and express it in numbers, you know something about it; but when you cannot measure it, when you cannot express it in numbers, your knowledge is of a meagre and unsatisfactory kind'. Selectivity in the choice of parameters to be monitored and measured should be practised, since 'blanket-measurement' of every conceivable measurable index is wasteful, confusing and may impair patient management. Such selectivity requires clinical awareness of the values and limitations of the indices chosen, and is best achieved by continual communication and co-operation between ITU clinicians and laboratory staffs. The biochemist, haematologist, bacteriologist and radiologist should be integral members of the intensive therapy team. In addition, many of the ITU monitoring techniques presently used require sophisticated electronic equipment, and accurate calibration and regular maintenance are necessary in order to ensure optimal sensitivity and reproducibility of desired information. Though current monitoring techniques may appear complex, requiring considerable expertise on the part of physicists and technical staff, there is a continual search for non-invasive monitoring techniques of increased simplicity.

When the critically ill patient has been resuscitated and transferred to the ITU, the initial presumptive diagnosis may be confirmed and the patient's overall clinical status assessed by clinical examination and the information gained from measurement and monitoring. It is then necessary to set out priorities in therapy, to identify and if possible anticipate and prevent the development of complications secondary to the primary pathology. For example, the patient with acute peripheral circulatory failure due to low cardiac output requires immediate optimalization and maintenance of cardiovascular status, while the secondary effects of the low output on brain and kidney, while of significance, are of less immediate priority. Assessment of priorities in therapy and appreciation of the pathophysiological effects of particular pathological conditions demand a high degree of clinical judgement, and considerable experience.

Despite the apparent emphasis on measurement, monitoring and on an awareness of pathophysiology, intensive therapy remains an exercise in therapy. Treatment is, or should always be, what is concentrated upon in the ITU. Furthermore, such treatment is not necessarily of a complex nature, rather that in the presence of a life-threatening situation, the treatment should be appropriate to the condition, adequate in terms of effective dosage at the pathological site, and administered at the optimal time in relation to the time-course of the underlying pathological process. Ideally, the treatment chosen should not be associated with the development of, or aggravation of, secondary complications. This last point is not possible to achieve in every situation.

We believe it to be important to differentiate primary from secondary therapies.

Primary therapy is that directed towards the treatment of the underlying, primary pathology.

Secondary therapy is that directed towards the protection of other vital organs or systems which are secondarily affected by the malfunction of the organ or system affected by the primary pathology. (For example, in acute low cardiac output, adrenaline may be given as a primary therapy, and mannitol infused as a secondary therapy designed to give some degree of renal protection from hypo-perfusion.) The terms primary and secondary do not imply that one is more important than the other, or even that one should be administered before the other in terms of time. It is of great importance, however, that there should be maximal understanding of the nature and anticipated benefits of every treatment given. In addition, the effects of therapy should be carefully monitored, as should meaningful assessments of their biological activity and hence adequacy of dosage.

The application of appropriate therapy may produce the expected improvement in the patient's condition. However, the progress or even the initial severity of the pathology may produce life-threatening malfunction of a vital organ or bodily system, for example respiratory insufficiency in the presence of severe pneumonia. In such a situation, mechanical system support may be necessary until a sufficient improvement in the patient's own system function has occurred. Techniques for respiratory support, circulatory support (the intra-aortic balloon pump), renal dialysis and haemo-perfusion in hepatic failure, are presently available and in widespread use in intensive therapy practice. Where recovery of the patient's failing system is anticipated, such system support techniques are of immense value in the critical phase of the patient's illness. Where the patient's own system fails completely, or where recovery does not occur, system replacement techniques may be feasible. Homotransplantation techniques continue to develop, and mechanical prostheses, e.g. artificial heart, are also being developed, though such devices are at present largely experimental.

The final principle of intensive care practice concerns the transfer and rehabilitation of successfully treated, convalescent patients. The timing of discharge from the ITU is perhaps of similar importance to the selection of patients for admission. Most ITU patients are transferred back to a general medical or surgical ward, where the nature of medical and nursing care, though no less valuable, must of necessity be less concentrated. The difficulty in discharge timing is indicated by many series reporting the death of several patients after discharge from the ITU, and emphasizes that the provision of 'intermediate' care may be necessary in certain patients.

As previously indicated, principles of intensive therapy practice tend to reflect the personal experience and prejudice of those who propound them. We have, in this textbook, attempted to reflect our appreciation of these broad principles in the choice of authors, subjects and in the overall presentation of the text. The multidisciplinary nature of intensive therapy is reflected in the wide-ranging experience of the authors. The importance given to measurement and monitoring is seen in those chapters devoted to general aspects of haemodynamics, biochemistry, haematology, bacteriology and radiology. In addition, specific mention of appropriate tests and measurements is included in the systematic chapters, where their particular value in the context of particular bodily systems is emphasized. Multiauthor textbooks suffer inevitably from the different textual styles of the various authors. While not enforcing a rigid discipline of style, we have suggested to contributing authors of the systematic Chapters 12–22, a rough framework in order to produce some uniformity in the 'systematic approach'. The principal syndromes necessitating intensive therapy are outlined; techniques of measurement and monitoring appropriate to that system are described; pathophysiological mechanisms are discussed in relation to the primary pathology and to the development of secondary complications; therapy is described and classified where appropriate as primary or secondary; finally system support or replacement techniques are detailed where such techniques exist.

The dictionary offers as one definition of principle 'fundamental truth'. This is clearly unsatisfactory in relation to the constantly evolving nature of intensive therapy. We prefer to take the dictionary's alternative of 'a general law as a guide to action, as a basis of reasoning'. For inherent in that definition are thought and action, and the suggestion of forward movement.

Chapter 2

Logistics of Intensive Care

A. B. M. Telfer

INTRODUCTION

Progressive Patient Care

With the advent of intensive care units in the 1960s the concept of progressive patient care was complete. For many years it has been accepted that patients require going through a period of less intensive care, known as convalescence, *following* illness or operation; the increasing complexity of surgical procedures and the availability of complex life support systems made it necessary to manage the most severely ill patients in special units during the acute phase of their illness. Thus intensive care units (ICU) were developed and patients progress from these to intermediate care wards and finally to convalescent wards offering little more than hotel care.

A number of patients inevitably need long-term care, such as those who remain unconscious following a head injury, or who require long-term respiratory support. The Scandinavian poliomyelitis epidemic of 1952 was probably one of the earliest examples of this, with patients continuing to require mechanical assistance to ventilation for many years after their initial illness. The provision of facilities for this type of care has a direct bearing on the work of the acute intensive care unit, since their absence can lead to patients having to remain in the acute unit for much longer than is desirable.

Mobile Intensive Care

Events prior to admission to intensive care obviously have a profound effect, not only on the patient's eventual recovery, but also on the quality of recovery. Periods of hypotension, or hypoxia, whether associated with surgery and anaesthesia, myocardial infarction, drug overdose, or a road traffic accident, can profoundly influence the quality of recovery especially with regard to renal and cerebral function. Depending on local arrangements, the staff of the ICU may be able to influence these events, either in association with the Accident and Emergency Department of their own hospital or perhaps in consultation with the staff of another hospital without an ICU to which the patient has initially been admitted. It is for this latter situation that the concept of mobile intensive care has been developed; the principle is that the patient is adequately resuscitated and the cardiovascular and respiratory systems stabilized before transfer, which then takes place in a specially equipped vehicle in which it is possible to continue all the monitoring and life support procedures until arrival at the ICU [1]. The same principle applies to transfer within the hospital[2].

Location

Fig. 2.1 shows the possible flow pathways of progressive patient care. It will be apparent that there are advantages in having the intensive therapy unit physically adjacent to the emergency admissions area and to the operating theatres and recovery room. There are also advantages in having the various intensive care disciplines adjacent to each other, and sharing

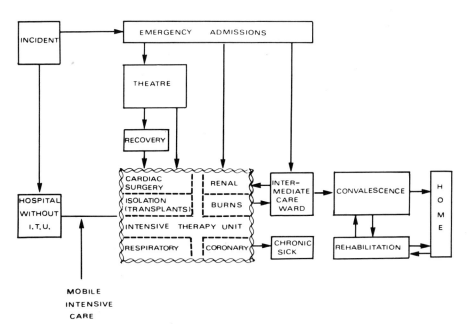

Fig. 2.1. Progressive patient care.

common services, although there are many reasons why they should be physically separate, one of the most important being to reduce the risk of cross-infection.

STRUCTURAL DESIGN

Size of ICU

It is generally accepted that for efficient management an ICU should not exceed eight beds, or at the very most ten, and that the minimum number should be four[3]. A unit with less than four beds does not merit its own medical staff. This is essential and will be discussed later in this chapter. If there are more than about eight beds it becomes very difficult for the staff to have the detailed knowledge of each patient which is so necessary in intensive care. If more than ten beds are required then another unit should be opened. This should seldom be necessary with the division of the intensive therapy facility into specialties as shown on the flow diagram. The Department of Health and Social Security has recommended that 1% of the beds in a large general hospital should be for intensive care[4].

Many of the earlier units were conversions of existing wards and this inevitably imposed a number of design limitations, particularly with regard to space. As a general rule at least as much floor area is required for *non-patient* use, e.g. storage, cleaning, maintenance, staff and visitors' accommodation, as is required for the patient areas. It is in the provision of non-patient space that the older units are particularly lacking.

Patient Areas

The British Medical Association[3] recommendation is for 200–300 ft^2 (18·9–28·4 m^2) per bed in the open areas and the DHSS[4] recommends 195 ft^2 (18·5 m^2). These sizes need to include a space of about 3 ft 3 in (1·0 m) between the head of the bed and the wall, as well as a similar space at the foot of the bed. The minimum distance between bed centres should be 11 ft 6 in (3·6 m) in the open areas. Thus a bed in an ICU requires approximately twice the floor area of a bed in an intermediate care ward, and circulation space has to be added as well.

The patient accommodation should be divided into an open area with, say, six beds, and two cubicles, or single rooms. These should be separately ventilated so that not only may they be either warmer or cooler than the main ward, but they may also be maintained at a higher or lower pressure, for the reduction of air-borne cross-infection. A unit which is entirely composed of single rooms is not desirable. It is particularly demanding of the nursing staff and it is more difficult to deal with emergency situations.

Treatment Room

There should be a special procedures room, or treatment room, which as the name implies may be used for such special procedures as tracheostomy, insertion of shunts for renal dialysis or burr holes for intracranial pressure monitoring.

Research Room

It should be possible to have an additional room, or perhaps one of the patient cubicles, more intensively monitored than the other beds, and equipped particularly from the point of view of clinical research. A convenient arrangement is to have the unit laboratory next to this room with connections to physiological measurement equipment taken through the wall.

Nursing Station

The nursing station should be slightly elevated and so sited within the unit that all beds are visible from it. It is the 'nerve centre' of the unit and should accommodate the communications equipment (preferably out of earshot of the patient), controls for heating, lighting and ventilation, and the controlled drugs cupboards. It will have monitoring displays if a central monitoring system is installed, and also recording facilities. It should additionally have a visual display unit and keyboard for any data-handling equipment which may be installed.

NON-PATIENT AREAS

Equipment Accommodation

Considerable space is required for the storage of presterilized disposable items, such as endotracheal and tracheostomy tubes, airways, intravenous cannulae, dressings, etc., as well as infusion and dialysis fluids.

Non-disposable equipment, including ventilators and monitors, must be cleaned, sterilized and then stored, and also have first-line maintenance carried out in the unit. There is therefore a requirement for a mechanical/electronic workshop, in addition to cleaning and sterilizing areas.

Clean bed linen occupies a considerable space and the amount required is proportionately greater than in an ordinary ward. There should also be special arrangements for disposing of soiled linen, and other infected materials, through a disposal room with separate exit. Conversely, the clean storage accommodation should be near the entrance to the unit so that it can be serviced by staff without entering the patient area.

Space must be provided for the cleaning and preparation of bedside trolleys adjacent to the storage areas. These trolleys, if suitably designed, can conveniently act as bed dividers[5] and, as such, may be of considerable size.

If there is no special treatment room then space must also be available for setting up special procedures trolleys, e.g. for thoracentesis.

Laboratory Accommodation

There should be a laboratory for the performance of the simpler or more urgent biochemical and haematological tests, such as blood gases, serum potassium, blood sugar or packed cell volume. In certain instances this may be staffed by technicians but, more usually, the equipment is maintained by the technical staff and the medical staff are trained to use it.

Staff and Relatives' Accommodation

The staff accommodation should include offices for the senior and junior medical staff and for the senior nursing staff. There must be an office for the secretary which should be large enough to accommodate data-link terminals and other computer equipment.

The importance of regular staff meetings will be emphasized later and suitable accommodation should be provided. This can also be used for teaching and be additional to the normal staff rest room, with beverage bay, which should be available to all grades of medical, nursing and paramedical staff.

The resident doctor must have a bedroom in the unit, preferably with its own toilet and shower, and there should also be overnight facilities for patients' relatives, to include a sitting room, bedroom and toilet accommodation. There should be an interview room and waiting area for both professional visitors and relatives.

Ancillary Accommodation

This includes rooms for the air-conditioning equipment, switchgear, storage of gas cylinders, a small kitchen, and adequate toilet and changing accommodation for all grades of staff, as well as the usual requirements for storage of cleaning equipment and materials.

SERVICES

Electrical

Power points—a *minimum* of eight, and preferably ten, 13 amp power points should be provided at each bed, arranged so that they are accessible from both sides of the bed. They should preferably not be all on the same circuit so that should a fault develop some of the points at the bed will remain live.

Lighting: Daylight

The importance of daylight, and windows with a view, cannot be over-emphasized. A number of earlier units were built in basements and therefore had no windows. There have been several papers pointing out the serious psychological consequences both for staff[6] and patients,[7] of working and being treated in a windowless environment. It is particularly important that the rest room should have windows with a view so that the medical and nursing staff can maintain visual contact with the outside world at least during their rest periods.

Lighting: Artificial

The artificial lighting of the bed areas should be so arranged that it cannot shine into the eyes of a horizontal paralysed patient. It is usually fluorescent and should be of an appropriate daylight colour rendering. Localized tungsten bedhead lighting of variable intensity is also useful and portable high intensity spotlights for minor operative procedures are required. Separate diffused lighting of variable intensity should be available for night-time.

All electrical supplies to the unit should be connected to the essential electrical service with an automatic no-break changeover to the emergency supply if the main supply should fail.

Medical Gas Supplies

Each bed should have a minimum of two oxygen points and two suction points. In addition there should be an outlet for respirable compressed air to supply ventilators and other respiratory apparatus and consideration should be given to providing nitrous oxide and/or Entonox.

Scavenging

Expired gas scavenging systems have not generally been installed in ICUs up to the present time. However, increasing awareness of pollution hazards and the more widespread use of nitrous oxide in the postoperative period may increase the need for such systems.

In addition, many patients on intermittent positive-pressure ventilation (IPPV) may have a respiratory tract infection and a case can undoubtedly be made for the direct ducting of their expired gas to the exterior[8].

Cable Ducting

The extent and physical arrangement of physiological monitoring will vary depending on the type of unit, but facilities must be provided for cable ducting to accommodate all present and anticipated needs. A future development may be the inclusion of narrow bore gas-sampling tubes within the cable ducting, for example, to a mass spectrometer in the laboratory. The ducting will normally extend from each bed to the nursing station, treatment room, research room and doctors' office.

Since it may be required to carry cables for data-handling equipment it should also extend to the secretary's office and to the computer room.

Plumbing

There should be a wash-basin at each bed or between each pair of beds and one in each cubicle. The waste-traps should be fitted with heaters[9].

Facilities should also be installed (in particular appropriate drainage) to facilitate haemodialysis in at least one of the cubicles.

Ventilation

The unit should be fully air conditioned with no recirculation of air. The system should provide fifteen air changes per hour in the patient area and should be so arranged that air does not flow from one bed over another to reach its outlet. Indicators should be available at the nursing station to confirm that the system is functioning normally but the actual adjustment of temperature and humidity is best left to the engineers. The unit should be slightly pressurized with respect to the corridor outside to prevent the ingress of contaminated air from other parts of the hospital; reference has already been made to the desirability of maintaining the cubicles at a higher or lower temperature and pressure than the main unit, if required.

Siting of Services

There are several options for the siting of services at the bedside. The most usual is to have the various gas and electrical outlets positioned on the wall behind the head of the bed. This is the simplest and cheapest arrangement and is often combined with a system of wall rails for mounting the associated flowmeters, suction bottles, etc. It has the disadvantage that it impedes easy access to the head of the bed since there is inevitably a number of tubes and wires crossing the intervening space. An expensive alternative is to provide the services from some form of overhead boom, or, more practically, to use a 'parking meter' or bollard system. In this system each bed space has a bollard approximately $0.5 \times 0.5 \times 1.0$ m positioned 1 m out from the wall, which contains the electrical points, medical gas and suction outlets and patient monitoring inputs, as well as the nurse call panel and lighting switches. The head of the bed is positioned adjacent to the bollard and is thus at least one metre out from the wall, with no tubes or wires crossing the space. Suction bottles, sphygmomanometers, etc. are mounted on lengths of rail on the head of the bed and on the bollard.

Communications

Telephonic communication to all parts of the hospital and beyond is obviously essential. The instruments should be out of earshot of the patients and should have a suitably modulated ringing tone. The standard British Telecom 'Trimphone' with its warble tone which increases in volume from very quiet to adequately loud has been found to be satisfactory at the nursing station. Direct lines on a separate system to Accident and Emergency, Theatre Suite and Recovery Areas will be found useful, as will a second British Telecom line for outgoing calls only.

'Intercom' systems may be useful between the offices, rest room, laboratory, secretary, nursing station and doctor's bedroom, and it is usual to have some form of call system from the cubicles to the nursing station. Any such system should be unobtrusive and confidential.

A data-link terminal for the main hospital computer should be provided in the unit, usually in the secretary's office.

EQUIPMENT

A great deal of expensive equipment has to be bought for an ICU and the choice will be dictated by the type of unit, by financial considerations and by the personal preferences of the staff.

The particular requirements of neonatal intensive care units have been reviewed by Milner et al.[10] and the *British Journal of Clinical Equipment* devoted an entire issue to equipment for intensive care.[11]

I. Resuscitation Equipment

All ICUs require basic resuscitation equipment which will take the form of a portable resuscitator (e.g. AMBU bag) at every bed and intubation equipment on the bedside trolley. There should be a 'crash trolley' conveniently situated within the unit containing all the usual emergency equipment and drugs including a battery-powered defibrillator with a built-in oscilloscope. This trolley should ideally never leave the unit.

In some cases, unit staff may operate the hospital 'crash call' system and indeed may be despatched as part of the flying squad to accidents throughout the hospital. For these occasions there must be separate portable resuscitation equipment available in the unit.

II. Equipment for Transfer

Reference has already been made to the transfer of patients to the ICU using a mobile intensive care unit. There may also frequently be a need to move patients within the hospital, e.g. to other departments for special investigations, and this must be done without interruption to their monitoring or therapy. A portable battery-operated oscilloscope with a minimum of two channels for ECG and arterial pressure is required and a small portable ventilator with a suitable oxygen supply should also be available. It should be possible to maintain positive end-expiratory pressure (PEEP) during transport and PEEP valves are available for attachment to the familiar AMBU bag if hand ventilation is to be employed.[12]

III. General Equipment

The type of unit will have a considerable bearing on the equipment required, for example lung ventilators will be found in respiratory and cardiac surgery units, and renal dialysis and haemo-perfusion equipment will be in many 'general' units as well as in renal units, but an intra-aortic balloon pump is only likely to be found in relation to the cardiac surgery unit.[13] Facilities for pulmonary artery catheterization should be generally available but the need for an extracorporeal membrane oxygenator (ECMO) will be extremely limited.

1. *Ventilators*

Ventilators are available in all shapes and sizes, from the very expensive to the relatively cheap, offering either a wide variety of facilities, such as intermittent mandatory ventilation (IMV), PEEP, continuous positive airways pressure (CPAP), etc., or very few facilities. It has to be decided whether all the ventilators in a unit should be the same, or whether some should be complex and some simple, or some electrically powered and some gas powered to cope with electrical failures. There are advantages in having a variety from the point of view of teaching, but the prime requirements are that they should be easy to sterilize, volume-cycled, quiet and reliable, and be as simple to operate as possible in relation to the facilities which they offer. All ventilators should be fitted with some form of alarm.[14] This is usually a pressure detecting device and the more expensive machines have these built-in.

In units handling complex respiratory problems most of the ventilators should be of the more expensive variety offering a wide range of facilities; units dealing with cardiac surgery where the need is mostly for overnight postoperative ventilation can perhaps use less complex machines. With the greater throughput of patients in these units, there are advantages in having all the ventilators the same and an adequate supply of interchangeable patient circuits.

2. *Monitoring*

The philosophy of patient monitoring has changed considerably in the past decade and the development of the silicon chip and the microprocessor has enabled more and more facilities to be incorporated into an ever smaller package.

In the early days 'central monitoring' was popular in many units; these systems always presented their information at the nursing station but not always also at the bedside. It is now accepted that information should primarily be displayed at the bedside, though it may be repeated at the nursing station if desired.

The need for recording facilities will depend on the type of unit. Cardiac surgery and coronary care units need this most and the latter generally use a central display console to observe the ECG of several patients simultaneously; this is because the principle of 'one nurse beside each patient at all times' is less essential in coronary care units. These units also use arrhythmia detectors and automatic pacing equipment.

The 'general' intensive care unit will include direct blood pressure and two-channel temperature measurements in its basic monitoring package. The intra-arterial cannula has been described as a 'highway for information', since it provides easy access to arterial blood for biochemical and blood gas analysis as well as revealing haemodynamic details such as systolic and diastolic blood pressure, heart rate and rhythm, etc. The two-channel temperature facility is to monitor both central and peripheral temperature simultaneously as an indication of peripheral perfusion.

In addition to these basic parameters, facilities should be available for measurement of pulmonary artery and pulmonary artery wedge pressures with a flow-directed catheter, and also for cardiac output by the thermal dilution technique. A popular arrangement is to consider this as 'second line' monitoring and have the equipment mounted on a separate trolley to be brought to the bedside when required. Alternatively, if the basic monitoring package has two pressure channels, then it can display both arterial and pulmonary artery pressure and only the cardiac output computer need be provided additionally. Equipment of modular design has the advantage that an extra pressure module or perhaps a cardiac output module can be added to adapt the basic package to the immediate requirement.

Bedside monitoring equipment should be sited so that it is easily visible to the staff, but not seen by the patient. It is thus usually above and behind the bed and there is again the problem of trailing cables. Some units have a pendant hanging over the bed to take monitoring inputs which then pass overhead in the ceiling and down to the display units.

Future developments are likely to be in the field of intravascular electrodes for the continuous monitoring of blood gases and perhaps also of potassium, and in the further development of non-invasive methods of monitoring. The application of microprocessors will continue to increase. Already oscilloscopes can display trend graphs over several hours and in the longer term on-line physiological data can be stored, recalled and hard-copied. The collection and presentation of the vast amount of laboratory data which accumulates about patients in ICUs can also be greatly facilitated by modern computer techniques, and can be displayed at the bedside on the same screen as the on-line physiological data. The calculation of fluid balance and the on-line derivation of the more complex respiratory parameters from basic ventilator data are tasks which are currently being demanded of microprocessors and small bedside computers. The ultimate application of this type of technology is in the automatic control of therapy in response to on-line physiological input data—the 'feed back' system. Examples of this include the administration of fluids in response to drainage and urinary output, vasodilators or inotropic agents in response to haemodynamic changes, and anticonvulsants in response to EEG changes in status epilepticus. It is also possible to adjust automatically the minute ventilation in response to changes in, for example, end-tidal CO_2 in patients on IPPV.[15]

It should be remembered that while a monitoring system can in many cases replace an educated forefinger, it cannot as yet replace eyes and ears, or the sixth sense of the experienced nurse, whom many would regard as the best monitor of all.

3. *Humidifiers*

Humidifiers will be provided on all the ventilators but there must also be humidifiers for spontaneously breathing patients. These can be electrically powered or operate from pipeline oxygen or respirable air. In either case there should be a facility to vary the inspired oxygen concentration from 21 to 100%.

Every unit should have one ultrasonic humidifier for particularly difficult cases where maximum humidification is required. Humidifiers, being warm and wet, harbour organisms and special attention must be paid to cleanliness and sterility.

4. *Bronchoscopes*

A set of rigid bronchoscopes with fibreoptic illumination, and facilities for oxygen injection, is required. These are relatively inexpensive and can accept a rubber or plastic suction catheter for the rapid clearance of secretions from the larger airways. They have now been complemented by the fibreoptic bronchoscope, a very expensive flexible instrument which gives good access to the smaller bronchi but which has a rather small suction channel. It can also be used for difficult intubations and has the great merit that IPPV can be continued during bronchoscopy.[16] No respiratory intensive care unit should be without one of these instruments.

5. *Infusion pumps*

There is an increasing demand for the continuous intravenous infusion of powerful drugs, either in small volumes of strong solutions, using infusion pumps, or in larger volumes of weaker solutions using infusion controllers. Continuous development has led to pumps and controllers which are reliable and easy to use and drugs such as morphine, dopamine, insulin, heparin and Althesin (alphadolone, alphaxalone), are now regularly administered by this method. Provision of at least two, and preferably four pumps for each bed, would not be excessive.

IV. Equipment for Patient Well-being

Patients with tracheostomies or who are on ventilators cannot speak and frequently cannot write, and this inability to communicate is a source of intense frustration both to themselves and the staff. Cards with photographs of objects such as bedpans, etc., and letters of the alphabet to be pointed at have been in use for many years. Electronic word games are an improvement on this but only display one word at a time. Better still is a small keyboard which allows a whole message to be printed and retained on a visual display unit. For paralysed patients, a modification allows the equipment to be operated by a micro-switch controlled by a finger or even by blowing. Television is a most important and useful aid to the recovery of many patients who have passed the most acute phase of their illness; the main problem is usually in convincing the administrators of the need for it.

ANCILLARY SERVICES

Intensive care units make a heavy demand on many of the laboratory and paramedical services in the hospital. Unless this is appreciated and the priority needs of the unit discussed fully, the unit cannot function efficiently. Biochemistry, haematology, bacteriology, radiology and physiotherapy are most affected. If possible it is desirable that someone in each of these departments is designated to oversee samples from the ICU and in the case of radiology and physiotherapy, the department should have its own nucleus of experienced staff who service the ICU. Regular visits to the unit by consultants from these disciplines makes for closer co-operation and understanding and frequent unannounced bacteriological surveys are particularly important.

STAFFING

The staffing of ICUs has been reviewed[17] and further reference is made in this chapter, *see* Operational policy.

Medical Staffing

There is at present in this country no definite career structure for intensive therapists, and indeed very few permanent appointments devoted solely to intensive therapy. The Joint Conference of Surgical Colleges in 1979 resolved that the development of intensive care as a specialty in its own right should be avoided[18] but Tinker,[17] in his review, took the opposite view, pointing out that intensive therapy is now as much concerned with circulatory and metabolic issues as with respiratory care, and advocated a rotational training appointment at senior registrar level through coronary care, renal dialysis, cardiac surgery and medical instrumentation and electronics.

There is undoubtedly a need for a clinician in administrative charge, a position for which anaesthetists by their training are well suited, and in this country most general ICUs are administered by an anaesthetist who also shares, to a greater or lesser extent, the clinical care with the admitting consultant. Other specialists are called in to advise, when by mutual agreement this will be to the patient's benefit.

The junior medical staff must provide continuous resident cover in the unit. In 'general' units they are frequently trainee anaesthetists, or there may be some junior house officer posts allocated to the unit. In cardiac surgery, coronary care and renal units, the junior staff of the parent unit usually provide the cover. Continuous cover can be achieved with two or three junior staff. The maximum period of continuous duty should be 24 hours, and a compromise has to be reached to satisfy the conflicting requirements of continuity of patient care, and rest and leisure time.

There may also be other grades of medical staff working in the unit. These include anaesthetists of senior registrar grade on secondment for higher professional training as well as visitors from home and overseas on clinical attachments. Too many staff means that the opportunities for acquiring experience in the technical skills may be limited and this is a situation to be avoided.

Nurse Staffing

The basic principle of 'one trained nurse per patient at all times' is still the ideal to be aimed at but most units cannot achieve this at the present time. Allowing for sickness and holidays this requires 4·25 nurses per bed,[17] plus a sufficient number of sisters, so that at least one is on duty on each shift. In a hospital with several specialist intensive care units it is convenient to have a nursing officer in overall charge; this facilitates the interchange of staff between the units to suit the varying workload.

Ideally there should be an adequate nucleus of trained staff but suitably experienced enrolled or senior enrolled nurses have a significant place in ICUs and can do a great deal to compensate for shortages of trained staff. Likewise, there is a place for nursing orderlies and they may also very well act as storekeepers and, under supervision, clean and sterilize much of the equipment. For these tasks they may be better than male orderlies and they also come under the direct supervision of the nursing administration which is an advantage.

The place of pupil or student nurses in ICUs is more controversial. On the one hand if they never see these units during their training they miss a significant part of acute medicine; on the other hand they tend to be too immature and inexperienced to do a useful job if they are seconded to the unit.

Intensive care nursing is essentially for postgraduates and a properly constituted course is the best way to learn it. The Joint Board of Clinical Nursing Studies has approved a number of 6-month courses at centres throughout the United Kingdom, and the steady stream of applicants testifies to the interest in the subject as well as making a significant contribution to the maintenance of staffing levels.

There can be a high price to pay for insufficient nursing staff in a busy intensive care unit. Even when fully staffed the work can be stressful and, in times of shortage, it is much more so. Psychological problems can occur and the rate of staff turnover may be increased. However, it is the patient who will suffer most because shortage of staff leads to a reduction in nursing standards and discipline with a consequent increase in the infection rate, and in morbidity and mortality, producing even more stress on the already overworked staff. It is an accepted fact that the workload of intensive therapy units is extremely variable and staff should not be transferred to work elsewhere when the load is light—it will not be light for long!

Technical Staff

Much of the equipment necessary for intensive care is of a complex technical nature, and unless skilled technical assistance is available within the ICU it cannot be used with maximum effectiveness.[19]

Local arrangements will vary, but whether the technical staff are members of a larger department, or work full-time in the unit, they are an essential part of the intensive care team. Nothing is more frustrating or less cost effective than equipment which will not work when it is most needed, and faulty apparatus is frequently a potential hazard to the patient. The technicians must therefore carry out routine maintenance and safety checks as well as instructing all grades of staff in the technical aspects of the operation of a wide variety of equipment including blood gas analysers, ventilators, monitors, infusion pumps, etc.

Secretarial Staff

Every unit must have access to secretarial assistance, or preferably its own secretary. Even in a unit of only eight beds there are case-sheets to be kept up-to-date, laboratory results to be filed, letters to be typed, telephone calls to be made and visitors to be looked after. In addition, many units will have some form of data storage system either on feature cards or a computer, and the accuracy of the data retrieved from such systems is entirely proportional to the accuracy of the input—another task for the secretary.

OPERATIONAL POLICY

The purpose of an ICU is to provide a high level of individual medical and nursing care, using all available forms of monitoring and life-support, to those patients who may reasonably be expected to benefit. To achieve this there must be a clearly-defined operational policy, with the day-to-day running based on mutually agreed arrangements which will depend greatly on local circumstances.

Staffing

The resident junior medical staff should be the final common pathway for all therapeutic decisions; these should be agreed between the senior staff of the unit and the referring clinician.

Staffing of the unit has been dealt with elsewhere but it is important to re-emphasize that the unit must have its own medical staff. Any arrangement in which the only permanent staff are nurses and where individual clinicians admit patients and then order and carry out their own treatment is quite unsatisfactory. Ideally there should be three or four consultants who share the management of the unit. They are frequently from one discipline, often anaesthesia, though this is not essential and will of course vary depending on the type of unit, e.g. respiratory, coronary care or postoperative cardiac surgery. At all times one of these consultants should be immediately available and at least during normal working hours should preferably be physically in the unit with no other commitments. This implies the allocation of 'sessions' for the work—an arrangement which may not always be possible.

Each patient will already be under the care of a consultant whose willingness to hand over the patient to the care of the ICU staff may vary enormously, and whose desire to take an active part in clinical management will also vary enormously. Much depends on personalities and on the local reputation of the unit.

Clinical

Routine management such as fluid therapy, oxygen therapy, ventilator therapy, antibiotics, etc., would normally be supervised entirely by the unit staff, and they would call on the services of other disciplines, e.g. bacteriology, haematology, biochemistry and radiology to provide basic information.

More specific decisions, e.g. removal of drains in a surgical patient or use of specific drug therapy, e.g. anticonvulsants, in a medical patient, would normally be taken in consultation with the referring clinician. This can be done either when he visits the unit, almost inevitably at a time of *his* choosing, or by active communication by unit staff when a decision is required.

It is unrealistic to expect clinicians to always visit their patients at fixed times for the convenience of the unit. Some may prefer to come before their own ward rounds, some after, and interruption of ward rounds in the unit is a constant problem which has to be accepted. On the other hand, visitors should be welcome on routine rounds (minimum twice daily) and the concept of a weekly 'grand round' has much to commend it provided the numbers attending are not excessive.

Uniform Therapeutic Policies

It is desirable that for any given clinical situation a uniform therapeutic policy should be adopted, e.g. a forced alkaline diuresis should be carried out in the same prescribed manner in all patients unless there is a particular reason for not doing so. Similarly the technical details of the administration of agents such as dopamine should be consistent; whatever method is used to provide an accurate dose minute by minute, e.g. infusion controller with a dilute solution or a continuous infusion pump with a strong solution, it should be consistent, otherwise confusion and mistakes can occur and patient safety will be compromised.

Admission and Discharge Policy

There must be an agreed arrangement for admission of patients from both the clinical and administrative points of view.

Even if the situation is an acute emergency, which has responded to active resuscitation, a decision to admit the patient should only be taken after consultation with the consultant in charge of the unit at the time. It should not be possible for non-unit staff, no matter how senior, to 'mandate' patients into the unit.

The clinical criteria to be applied to a request for admission is an important and developing subject. In a time of increasing staff shortage and financial restraint, the provision of this most expensive form of treatment for patients in whom it will be of doubtful benefit has to be most carefully considered. The unit must never be allowed to become a 'dumping ground' for patients who will surely die. Every case must be considered on its merits and the selection of patients suitable for admission is considered to be of such importance as to merit an entire chapter in *Recent Advances in Intensive Therapy*.[20] Ideally the patient should be seen by a senior member of the unit staff before admission, even if this means travelling to another hospital some distance away. In addition to confirming (or more importantly refuting) the clinical condition as initially described, fitness for transfer can also be assessed (e.g. secure airway, stable circulation) and any special transport requirements arranged.

Discharge of patients should not present clinical problems, but it is frequently associated with administrative difficulties, the usual one being that 'there are no beds'. This is especially true when transfer is required for long-term care, e.g. patients who remain unconscious following head injuries. It must be clearly understood that whereas patients cannot be 'mandated' into the unit they can be 'mandated' out, and their original unit must find a bed for them. However, only in exceptional circumstances should patients whose death is imminent be transferred out of the unit.

Laboratory Investigations

It is commonly thought that much of the therapy practised in an ICU is of an obscure and complicated nature, but this is not always so and a very large part of its function is to ensure that relatively straightforward therapy is managed more efficiently and reliably than is possible in an ordinary ward. This involves the gathering of a great deal of information on a daily basis, or more frequently, and arrangements have to be made for this to be done. For example, daily electrolyte and haematology specimens should be available by 0900 hours, be given priority in the laboratory, and the results returned to the unit by 1030 or 1100 hours. The radiology and bacteriology departments must accord a similar degree of priority to the unit and the latter is particularly important in monitoring the overall infection situation.

An accurate record must be kept of all laboratory estimations requested, and of the results, and these must be readily available for consultation. The increasing application of computer and data-handling techniques promises to improve greatly this aspect of unit organization.

Most units have their own laboratory for the estimation of variables most frequently and urgently required, in particular blood gases and packed cell volume, and reference has already been made to this. There is the additional advantage that the unit may be more self-sufficient in times of industrial dispute in the main laboratories.

Staff Meetings

All of this implies the need for regular meetings and discussions amongst the unit medical, nursing and technical staff. These will not normally involve other clinicians and are to deal primarily with management problems and policy in the day-to-day running of the unit. For example, departures from standard procedures for purposes of clinical research should be carefully assessed since many patients in ICUs are unable to give informed consent. The assessment of new equipment, especially in proto-type form, is frequently requested. Such apparatus should be most carefully inspected by the technical staff to ensure that it complies with safety standards before it is put into use in the unit.

REFERENCES

1. Hothersall A. P., Waddell G., Smith H. C. et al. (1977) Mobile intensive care II—secondary transport. In: Ledingham I. McA., ed., *Recent Advances in Intensive Therapy*, pp. 239–250. Edinburgh, Churchill-Livingstone.
2. Hanning C. D., Gilmour D. G., Hothersall A. P. et al. (1978) Movement of the critically ill within hospital. *Int. Care Med.* **4**, 137–143.
3. British Medical Assocaition Planning Unit (1967) *Intensive Care*, Report No. 1.
4. Department of Health and Social Security (1970) *Intensive Therapy Unit No. 27.* Health Building Note.
5. *British Health Care and Technology—Intensive Care* (1974) Newcastle upon Tyne, The Royal Victoria Infirmary Intensive Care Unit.
6. Vairub S. (1972) Windows for the soul. *Arch. Intern. Med.* **130**, 297.
7. Keep P., James J. and Inman M. (1980) Windows in the intensive therapy unit. *Anaesthesia* **35**, 257–262.
8. English I. C. W. and Manley R. E. W. (1970) The Brompton system of artificial ventilation (a scheme for the intensive care unit). *Anaesthesia* **25**, 541–547.
9. Ayliffe G. A. J., Babb J. R., Collins B. J. et al. (1974) *Pseudomonas aeruginosa* in hospital sinks. *Lancet* **2**, 578.
10. Milner A. D., Robertson N. C. R. and Hale P. (1977) Neonatal intensive therapy equipment. *Br. J. Clin. Equip.* **2**, 93–126.
11. (1978) Equipment for intensive therapy. *Br. J. Clin. Equip.* **3**, 93–126.
12. Telfer A. B. M. (1979) *Acute respiratory distress and positive end-expiratory pressure.* INFO 79, Issue No 44. Abbott Laboratories Ltd.
13. Tobias M. A., Challen P. D., Franklin C. B., et al. (1979) Intra-aortic balloon counter-pulsation. *Anaesthesia* **34**, 844–854.
14. Seed R. F. (1979) Alarms for lung ventilators. *Br. J. Clin. Equip.* **4**, 114–121.
15. Slee I. P. and Stewart J. (1980) Experiences with infra-red carbon dioxide analysis related to servo-controlled ventilation. *Int. Care Med.* **6**, 38.
16. Lindholm C. E. and Grenvik A. (1979) Flexible fibre-optic bronchoscopy and intubation in intensive care. In: Ledingham I. McA., ed., *Recent Advances in Intensive Therapy.* pp. 47–66. Edinburgh, Churchill-Livingstone.
17. Tinker J. (1976) Intensive therapy: the staffing and management of intensive therapy units. *Br. J. Hosp. Med.* **16**, 399–406.
18. Vickers M. D. (1980) Medicine and books. *Br. Med. J.* **280**, 292.
19. Hayes B. (1974) Equipping the intensive care unit. In: Wise A. R. J., ed., *British Health Care and Technology—Intensive Care*, p. 25. London Health & Social Service Journal/Hospital International.
20. Civetta J. M. (1977) Selection of patients for intensive care. In: Ledingham I. McA., ed., *Recent Advances in Intensive Therapy*, pp. 9–18. Edinburgh, Churchill-Livingstone.

Chapter 3

Haemodynamic Monitoring

K. J. Maxted

Haemodynamic measurement in operating theatres and intensive care units has developed from a laboratory science to clinical practice during the past two decades. A great deal of sophisticated pioneering work has been performed for more than a hundred years but the realization of practical methods is principally due to the advances in materials science, providing the modern clinical unit with an armoury of catheters, cannulae, taps and infusion sets that can be used safely and effectively to connect measuring equipment into the central circulation.

The foundations of haemodynamic measurement were laid in the last century when researchers discovered means by which the pulsatile pressure and flow of blood could be recorded graphically. Soon these waveshapes were being related to the pumping action of the ventricles of the heart. Improvements in equipment design led away from simple mechanical and pneumatic–mechanical devices to transducers with low mechanical intertia and low volume compliance, which optically amplified the pressure pulses by means of mirrors mounted on the sensing diaphragm, the resultant light beam deflection being recorded on photographic paper. These devices were complicated pieces of laboratory equipment, not well adapted to use in the clinical environment but used none the less in advanced clinical centres and instrumental in the development of modern haemodynamic measurement.

Modern transducer design, advanced electronics and the use of disposable cannulae and catheters has virtually eliminated the problem of assembling a pressure measurement system. Electromagnetic and ultrasonic flowmeters can conveniently be used in today's vascular operating theatres. However, a widespread lack of understanding of the basic principles of haemodynamics often casts doubt and suspicion on the results obtained using this equipment and a general preference exists for measurements which are intuitively felt to be correct, such as those using the simple non-invasive technology of the sphygmomanometer.

In the following sections the principles of measurement will be explained simply and the relative merits and drawbacks of different techniques discussed. A deeper study of these principles may be made with reference to the works listed.

HAEMODYNAMIC PRINCIPLES

Fluid mechanics is the study of fluid behaviour and, if a standard text on the subject is consulted, the reader will be confronted with theory of hydraulic steps, flow in weirs and canals and possibly, if it is an advanced text, pulsatile flow in rigid pipes may be discussed. When the behaviour of blood flow in the circulation was first studied, it was apparent that classic fluid mechanic theory was not adequate to describe what was being observed. The human circulation consists of a branched network of elastic vessels, the cross-sectional area of which increases from about $6\,cm^2$ at the ascending aorta to about $32\,m^2$ at the level of the capillary bed, an area ratio of about $1 : 50\,000$. The elasticity of blood vessel walls depends on the relative content of smooth muscle, collagen and elastin and varies throughout the circulation. The elasticity of the vessel wall changes passively with distending pressure variations and can be affected actively by the tone of smooth muscle in the wall structure.

The importance of the elastic behaviour of blood vessels can be illustrated by an observation which seems to contradict our preconceived notions of fluid behaviour. In general, we accept that fluid flows from a region of high pressure to a region of low pressure: if we consider a human, supine, and were to measure systolic pressure at intervals along the aorta and its major branches, we would encounter the surprising phenomenon that the systolic pressure actually increases as measurements progress towards the periphery. Further investigation would show that diastolic pressure decreases correspondingly. If the mean pressure were computed at each location then indeed a progressive fall in mean pressure would be observed towards the periphery.

With this in mind we can consider basic hydrodynamics and then observe the differences we must be aware of when extending the study to the circulation of blood in elastic vessels.

HYDROSTATIC PRESSURE

Consider a vertical column of fluid under the action of gravitational force; the fluid column tries to fall but is constrained by the bottom of the containing cylinder. The cylinder bottom is exerting an upward force on the bottom of the fluid column equal to the downward force exerted by the mass of the fluid column itself, so we have a physical stalemate and nothing moves. The pressure, or force per unit area, is being exerted over the area of the bottom of the cylinder. This pressure is proportional to the height of the fluid column, h, irrespective of what shape the fluid column takes: the pressure is numerically equal to the height of the column, multiplied by the density of the fluid, and the acceleration due to gravity. Thus, it can be seen that the area of cross-section of the fluid at the cylinder bottom or, indeed, at any point in the fluid column is of no consequence to the pressure measured at that point. Pressure due to a static head of fluid is often referred to as a hydrostatic pressure. Another way of storing energy in a fluid (a hydrostatic pressure being a source of potential energy) is to contain it under pressure in an elastic container; one good example is a balloon. In fact all the blood vessels in the body are elastic to some extent and, when stretched, exert a pressure on the contained blood; this is again a hydrostatic pressure but it must be remembered that the net pressure at a point in a closed fluid system will be a combination of pressure due to the height of fluid above that point plus the elastic container exerting a pressure due to the stretch of the containing walls. The pressure in an elastic vessel can be related to the tension in the wall of the vessel. The mathematical relationship in the case of very thin-walled vessels is a simple one and can be calculated from a simple equilibrium of forces.

PRESSURE IN A CYLINDER

In a cylinder, considered to be infinitely long so that the effect of the ends is not of significance, the equilibrium is demonstrated by slicing the cylinder axially into two parts. When the cylinder is under pressure, tension is generated in the wall which would tend to pull the cylinder apart across the line of the cut. This tension, T, is usually in equilibrium with tension T on the opposite side of the cut. So the forces holding the two cylinder halves together must be T at the top and the bottom, a total of 2T for each half; the total force acting is 2T per unit length of cylinder. Pressure acts on each half producing the tension but the pressure acts on the normal area presented by each cylinder half: that is the projected area in this case $2r \times l$ where l is the cylinder length and $2r$ is the area per unit length. The force exerted by the pressure on each half is:

Pressure $\times$ Area or $P \times 2r$ per unit length

This force is equal to the tension in each half, i.e.

$$P \times 2r = 2T$$
$$P \times r = T$$
$$P = \frac{T}{r} \text{ for a cylinder}$$

this is independent of length as both P and T were per unit length and this factor cancels out.

PRESSURE IN A SPHERE

By a similar argument the total tension in each half is $T \times$ length of cut, i.e.

$$T \times 2\pi r$$

The pressure gives a force on each half:

$$\text{Force} = P \times \pi r^2$$

so

$$T \times 2\pi r = P \times \pi r^2$$

therefore

$$P = 2T/r$$

This last equation is known as the 'Laplace relationship' and is widely used in haemodynamics to describe the relationship between muscle fibre tension and developed pressure in the heart at different radii. It is easily seen that if r is large, i.e. the heart distended, then the tension required to develop a given pressure is higher than at a normal filling volume. However, the greater the initial tension in the muscle fibres, the higher the developed tension when the heart contracts, but this is so only until the peak of Starling's curve is arrived at. Beyond this, tension development rapidly falls, and the heart fails.[1]

DYNAMIC PRESSURE

When any moving body is made to slow down, a force is exerted on the external agent causing the braking effect; this may seem a back-to-front way of looking at the problem, but the reacting force between bodies is equal and opposite and this action and reaction is equally valid when applied to fluids. A moving fluid possesses kinetic energy, energy of movement and, if a moving body of fluid is made to slow down, for instance a wave breaking on a sea wall, a pressure is exerted and as this pressure results from movement it is known as dynamic pressure.

We now have three sources of pressure in a moving column of fluid in an elastic tube: a hydrostatic pressure proportional to column height plus the pressure due to strain in the tube walls in a closed system, and a dynamic component due to the forward motion of liquid being progressively arrested by resistance to flow and impingement of the moving liquid onto surfaces in the flow channel.

FLUID FLOW

A moving mass of liquid whether flowing in a pipe or falling freely to the ground possesses kinetic energy: to start such a mass of fluid into motion requires a source of energy, which may be derived from a pump or may be the potential energy of liquid contained in a high storage tank. Chemical energy, in the form of a fuel for the pump or potential energy due to position, has been converted directly into kinetic energy of motion and this in turn may be converted to heat energy, the energy of sound waves and potential energy. Whatever happens the total energy is conserved but may exist in several forms: heat, strain energy, potential energy, chemical energy, etc.

The Steady Flow of Liquids in Cylindrical Tubes

To accelerate a column of liquid and to maintain velocity against the effect of the internal resistance or viscosity, energy must constantly be fed into the fluid system in the form of a pressure difference between the region the fluid is flowing from and the region it is flowing to. The greater the pressure difference, the greater the velocity, thus the potential energy of the pressure source is converted to the kinetic energy of fluid flow. Due to the frictional effect between the moving fluid and the walls of the tube, a braking force is experienced both proportional to the length of the tube (l) and to the inverse of the fourth power of the radius (R). If the fluid is flowing at a constant rate then the pressure drop ($P_1 - P_2$) along the tube of length L, radius R is:

$$(P_1 - P_2) = \frac{KQL}{R^4} \text{ where } K \text{ is a constant}$$

or rearranged in terms of flow (Q):

$$Q = \frac{(P_1 - P_2)}{KL} \cdot R^4$$

i.e. flow is proportional to pressure, the fourth power of the radius and is inversely proportional to the length of the pipe.

In the Poiseuille equation we have quoted, we have included viscosity in the constant K. The more usual form of the equation is:

$$Q = \frac{(P_1 - P_2)R^4}{8\mu l}$$

where μ is the viscosity of the fluid.

In the derivation of Poiseuille's law from first principles, laminar flow is assumed. If we were to look at the velocity of fluid at different distances from the wall of the tube conducting a steady flow, we would find that the velocity at the wall is zero rising to a maximum on the tube axis. The profile of velocities across the tube assumes a parabolic form and if we were able to introduce a plan front of dye into the tube we would find this distorted into a parabola downstream in the direction of flow.

The Poiseuille law does not accurately describe pulsatile flow and, in describing circulatory blood flow, is only a poor approximation. It can be used, however, to give a qualitative feel as to what would happen to flow and pressure at stenoses and the coarctations. The approximations made in the application of this law to physiology are immense but the more accurate Womersly equations, which describe pulsatile flow in elastic vessels, are very complex.[2]

Haemodynamics

One very good reason for not delving into the mathematics of fluid flow is that, when we apply basic fluid mechanics to the blood circulation, we find that the sweeping assumptions we must make to accommodate classical fluid dynamic theory render the results virtually meaningless.

Several factors contribute to this. Perhaps the most obvious, the fact that blood is really a suspension and not a true Newtonian fluid, is the least important because in the major vessels of the body its non-Newtonian behaviour is barely significant. The principal difficulty arises from the compliance of the blood vessels and the interaction with the pulsatile output of the heart. In simplistic terms, pressure waves are being generated and the velocity at which they propagate through the system is not necessarily the same as the velocity of the fluid flow and will be dependent, amongst other things, on the frequency of the pulsation, the density of the fluid, and the size, compliance and structure of the containing blood vessel.

The mathematics become indigestibly complicated and we will simply look at the causes and effects of this phenomenon. A full mathematical treatment of all aspects of fluid flow and haemodynamics can be found in the book *Blood Flow in Arteries* by McDonald.[2]

Pulsatile Flow

We consider the heart in isolation as an organ capable of imparting kinetic energy to a volume of blood over a short period of time—the ejection time. Outside this time interval, the heart is effectively out of circulation as far as the aorta is concerned because the aortic valve is shut. Much of the kinetic energy, perhaps in excess of 60%, is stored as potential energy in the stretched walls of the aorta and its communicating vessels; the walls stretch during ejection or systole and release their energy during diastole when the aortic valve is closed. This energy release is simply due to potential energy stored in the stretched elastic walls being converted into kinetic energy of movement of blood flowing out of the system.

Reflections, Harmonics and Dispersion

In addition to this gentle expansion–contraction process, we must add the effect of the travelling pressure waves moving rapidly along the fluid column and undergoing reflections and phase shifts. In exactly the same way in which if one was to shout out in a subway and hear a garbled echo by reflection from the many bends in the passage, every change in diameter, branching or partial obstruction of the blood vessel will cause a part of the incident wave to be reflected. As a consequence, the shape of the produced wave which, at any point, is a sum of direct and reflected components, will vary from position to position in the circulation.

Any waveshape that is not an isolated event but a continuous repetitive wave chain can be represented mathematically by a series of sine waves composed of the fundamental at the cycle frequency and many harmonics added together with the appropriate amplitude and phase angles. This mathematical fact has a practical significance. If we extract harmonics from a waveform we influence the shape of the wave. With electrical waves and sound waves, it is relatively easy to absorb the energy of some components of the wave and leave the other components intact; this can be achieved with tuned filters. The resultant waveform lacks the filtered component and may look or sound quite different from the original wave. If we wish to record a waveform with great fidelity, we must be sure to record it on equipment capable of responding to the full spectrum of the frequencies involved or else the waveform will be distorted. If a waveshape has parts with very rapidly rising or falling edges, the harmonic components may extend to very high frequencies and to accurately record the shape of pressure or flow waves, particularly in or near the left ventricle of the heart, we need a system capable of responding to beyond the 20th harmonic—which if the heart rate is 80 beats/min is at about 27 Hz. In the Introduction, the observation was made that the pressure pulse recorded at sites along the aorta and major vessels leading from it varied considerably in amplitude, but the mean pressure dropped progressively at points progressively further from the heart. Several factors contribute to the amplitude change, for example dispersion. In this sense, dispersion is referring to the different wave velocities at which the harmonic components of the pressure pulse travel. When the fundamental and harmonic frequencies are summated at some distant point in the circulation, the faster-moving harmonics will add out of phase and the original waveform will be altered. By far the largest effect on waveshape is due to the reflected components of the wave, the degree of reflection varying significantly with changes in the vasoactive state of the periphery.

These alterations in waveshape can make it very difficult to make a determination of the normalized wave velocity or the transit time of a pulse wave from the heart to a point in the peripheral circulation, such as the site of an arterial pressure cannula in the radial artery. The time delays involved are quite significant (*Fig.* 3.1) and can be of vital importance if the pressure tracing is being used to control the operation of a piece of equipment synchronized with cardiac activity, such as an intra-aortic balloon pump.

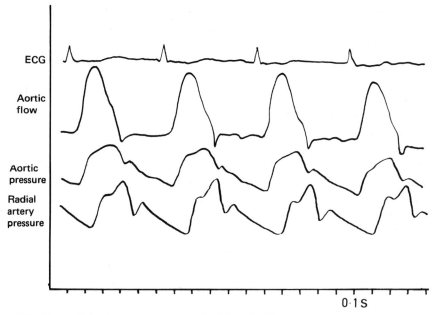

Fig. 3.1. The radial artery pressure wave is delayed with respect to aortic pressure.

DETERMINATION OF BLOOD PRESSURE

We can divide all physiological measurements into two broad groups: invasive and non-invasive. An invasive measurement requires some instrument to penetrate the skin or other surface membrane to make direct contact with some internal vessel or organ; non-invasive techniques can be applied without breaking into the organism. As soon as the external protective barrier of the organism is breached, a route for infection is created and problems, such as biological reaction to the transducer or probe materials, are encountered.

Generally speaking, a non-invasive measurement being indirect inevitably suffers some loss of accuracy.

Blood pressure measurement is a good example to demonstrate the merits and demerits of the two concepts.[3]

Indirect Blood Pressure Measurement

Sphygmomanometry, or the indirect non-invasive measurement of blood pressure using inflatable occluding cuffs, is one of the most familiar of medical measurements. The principle on which it works is as follows: if a pressure is applied externally to an artery, the artery will collapse and blood flow cease when the surrounding tissue pressure exceeds, by a small factor, the intraluminal pressure. When an inflatable cuff exerts pressure, the tissue it encircles is displaced both radially and longitudinally away from the cuff. At all times, the forces exerted by the cuff on the tissue must equal the force exerted by the tissue on the cuff and, at the interface between cuff and tissue, cuff pressure equals tissue pressure. Often the occluding cuff is not long enough to encircle a limb and it is desirable that the inflatable portion can sandwich the vessel it is wished to occlude between displaced tissue on the one side and a bone on the other. When cuff pressure is released, there will come a pressure at which only the peaks of systolic blood pressure exceed the occluding pressure sufficiently to allow a small spurt of blood to move in the vessel. This will cause a small distal pulse which will increase in amplitude until cuff pressure drops below diastolic pressure. Concurrent with the pressure flow pulse is a sound wave generated probably by a combination of vessel wall movement at the point of occlusion and the sound of a flow jet at this point. The sounds heard are called the Korotkoff sounds and may be heard by placing a stethoscope over the brachial artery at the antecubital fossa distal to the occluding cuff.

The Korotkoff sounds are documented as having five stages and there is some controversy in the literature as to which of the final stages 4 and 5 corresponds most closely to the diastolic pressure. The stages are:
1. Appearance of faint tapping sounds which gradually increase in amplitude. The first appearance of this sound corresponds closely to systolic pressure.
2. Sounds soften and resemble a 'swish'.
3. Sharper sounds return although not as intense as in stage 1.
4. Abrupt muffling—sounds become soft and blowing.
5. Complete disappearance of all sounds.

General opinion favours the fifth stage as being the closest to intra-arterial diastolic pressure and there can be as much as 10 mmHg between stage 4 and stage 5. The recommendation of the World Health Organization is that both stage 4 and 5 should be recorded.

The technique is open to a number of errors both of technical and observer origin. It is important that the cuff is correctly applied and, if a short cuff is used, it should be centred over the brachial artery. Observer bias may unwittingly be applied in favour of the anticipated result and rarely is enough time taken to identify the onset of the systolic sounds.

In general, the systolic pressure determined by sphygmomanometry is lower than that recorded by intra-arterial means. When the peripheral vasculature is shut down and a peaky systolic pressure waveform is present, an intra-arterial systolic pressure will be consistently higher than the cuff-derived pressure.

The sphygmomanometric method has been incorporated as the basis of rather more complicated instruments which have been developed to ease the burdens of the observer, but would seem to have succeeded in introducing further errors. The simplest of these is the device incorporating a microphone in the blood pressure cuff to sense the Korotkoff sounds. At best this instrument will sense systolic sounds, but the accuracy and reproducibility will vary from patient to patient and the instrument is hopelessly inadequate for diastolic pressure determinations. More sophist-icated versions sense other phenomena, such as the distal blood flow, with ultrasonic transducers or the pressure pulse by oscillotonometric methods employing a transducer connected to the cuff. These devices eliminate observer bias but are still prone to inaccuracies due to cuff and transducer positioning; they are very much more reliable than the cheaper microphone instruments but are no more accurate or reproducible than a skilled observer using a simple standard sphygmomanometer.

Whereas it is reasonably easy for the unaided observer to palpate a pulse in a young healthy person, a stethoscope is essential for determination of diastolic sounds in most subjects and enables a more accurate deter-mination of the systolic sounds. There will be circumstances in which it is impossible to hear the pulse using only a stethoscope and it becomes necessary to use a Doppler flowmeter to sense flow in the distal vessel. This technique is widely used with premature neonates, but requires some training to manipulate the sensing device.

For shocked patients, neonates and the atherosclerotic, a form of pulse sensor becomes essential and probably the most versatile is the non-invasive Doppler ultrasound probe. The pencil-sized probe generates and detects an ultrasonic signal reflected from moving blood in a vessel. Currently a new device of fountain pen size is available incorporating the ultrasonic transducer, generator and amplifier and is used in conjunction with a standard stethoscope ear tube assembly.

Direct Blood Pressure Measurement

A more accurate measurement of blood pressure (*Fig.* 3.2) can be achieved by inserting the measuring device into the circulation directly. A blood pressure transducer, an electrical device which converts pressure to voltage,

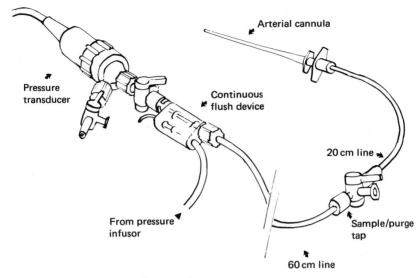

Fig. 3.2. A typical transducer for intensive care use.

is connected via a cannula or catheter into a blood vessel, the amplified electrical output is displayed on a monitor. Pressure waveform, systolic, diastolic and mean pressure can be recorded. Using this technique, pressure can be measured in the heart and central circulation. The principal disadvantage of the direct method is that the circulation is exposed to the risk of embolism and infection. For these reasons, the technique is used primarily in major surgical procedures and in intensive care. The most common site for introduction of the cannula for arterial pressure measurement is at the radial artery, although other peripheral arteries can be used. The same type of transducer system can be used for venous pressure determination, there being a wide choice of veins for the purpose.

The method has several complications:

1. Dissection, false aneurysm.
2. Ischaemic damage to the periphery caused by plaque dislodgement, emboli and vessel obstruction.
3. Infection.

The transducer may be connected to the measurement site by a manometer line filled with heparinized saline. To prevent the vessel cannula becoming obstructed by clot, a constant flush device is used to provide a small, but steady, flow of heparinized saline into the cannula. The practice of intermittent flushing by syringe is dangerous. The transducer should be supported at the level of the right atrium, on an adjustable stand. Wrist-mounted transducers introduce a static negative pressure that varies with posture. Most modern blood pressure monitors have only a limited zero range and such an offset cannot be eliminated.

The display format is of great importance in practical use. Non-fade trace oscilloscopes are easier to read than the older bouncing ball types, but it is still desirable to have some metered display, either analogue or digital. Analogue displays such as meters and light columns tend to be regarded as being old fashioned; however, they do have some advantages over digital types and are particularly well suited for use when rapid changes in pressure are possible. This is because they respond rapidly to a change and the rate of rise and fall of a meter is easier to interpret than a blur of rapidly changing figures. Most digital displays are set to change slowly to avoid this problem and thus reflect a filtered version of the dynamic situation, which is suitable for most purposes.

THE PERFORMANCE OF CATHETER TRANSDUCER SYSTEMS

The fidelity of the recorded signal and the accuracy of parameters such as systolic and diastolic pressure are determined by the dynamic characteristics of the transducer and catheter system.

It is essential from both the point of view of safety and that of accuracy that the manometer line, catheter/cannula and transducer dome are completely free of air bubbles. The implications of air entrainment on performance are outlined below; it is a hazard particularly with a left heart measurement, such as left atrial pressure. Vessel spasm and cannula malpositioning can also cause a damped tracing and, under these conditions, only the mean pressure has any significance. The use of end-hole cannulae and catheters may cause an elevation in monitored systolic pressure because of the dynamic pressure due to flow impinging on the catheter end; however, this is not likely to exceed 10 mmHg under normal conditions but can introduce an error of 20–30 mm in conditions of extreme vasoconstriction.

Standardization and Testing of BP Transducer Systems

For general monitoring requirements in the operating theatre and ICU, modern blood pressure transducers, disposable taps, manometer lines and cannulae provide reasonably accurate results. This statement applies particularly to the measurement of mean blood pressure, but when it is necessary to record systolic or diastolic values or to compute indices of cardiac performance, the demands on the measuring system become greater.

The single biggest enemy to the transducing system is compliance. As discussed previously, compliance is the tendency of a system to expand in volume when pressure within the system is increased. We have already met this concept when looking at the haemodynamics of the circulation.

A blood pressure transducer is a compliant device. When connected at the end of a long thin catheter or manometer line and subjected to an elevated pressure transmitted from the distant end of the line, this tiny volume displacement must be filled by a flow of fluid along the line which then returns as the pressure is released. Of course the flow is microscopic and any pressure measurement error resulting is under ideal circumstances equally microscopic and beyond the resolution of the system. However, if a tiny volume of air is introduced, not only is there an appreciable flow as the bubble contracts under high pressure, but the effect of the long fluid column springing against the compliant bubble is rather like suspending a weight from a spring—when the weight is released the spring stretches then contracts and the weight oscillates up and down. In the fluid-filled catheter system this effect introduces an undesirable artefact on the leading and trailing edges of the blood pressure waveform, elevating systolic peaks and deepening diastolic troughs. An even greater quantity of air or equally, and this is very important, a length of soft catheter, can absorb so much of the pulse pressure energy that the pressure waveform becomes flattened or damped out.

Any catheter system will be compliant and the longer the catheter or the greater its diameter, the larger the compliance effect. As a general rule, the more demanding the measurement the shorter is the length of catheter and manometer line between the measurement site and the transducer. Taps in the system should be reduced to the practical minimum, a continuous flushing device of low compliance such as the Sorens 'Intraflo' should be used to maintain patency of the catheter or cannula, and all air excluded, preferably by using de-aerated water to fill the measurement system; pyrogen-free saline or water is suitable for the purpose.

For a measurement system assembled from commercially available components, it is difficult to give a recipe that will give an adequate dynamic performance in all circumstances. The compliance of modern transducers varies widely from manufacturer to manufacturer, as does the range of characteristics of manometer lines; similar looking systems can have performance characteristics ranging from the very poor to the very good. There are several methods available for testing the dynamic response of systems: probably the most widely used is the transient or 'pop' test which subjects the manometer line and transducer to a rapidly falling pressure resulting from the puncture of a balloon connected at the 'patient end' of the transducing system; dynamic swept-frequency testing equipment can be constructed to perform a test very similar to that used to determine the frequency response of an audio amplifier system. One advantage of this form of testing is that both amplitude and phase characteristics can be plotted (*Fig.* 3.3).[4]

It is impossible to control the damping characteristics of a resonant catheter system, using special needle valves and restrictor sections to achieve what is known as critical damping, i.e. there is no overshoot on a transient test. This expedient is impractical in clinical practice (*Fig.* 3.4).

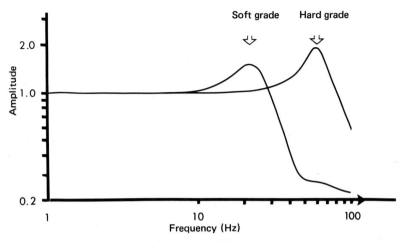

Fig. 3.3. The frequency response of a neonatal blood pressure measurement system. The selection of a hard grade catheter gave a high resonant frequency. Resonance should occur at a frequency at least ten times that of the heart if the results are critical.

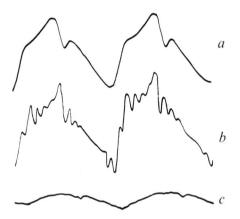

Fig. 3.4 The distortion on good waveform (a) introduced by (b) resonant and (c) overdamped pressure systems. Resonance is often caused by bubbles in the transducer dome. Overdamping is usually due to a clotted cannula.

If measurement requirements are very stringent, it is advisable that catheter tip transducers are utilized whenever the situation and budget allows. These transducers are not subject to the defects of low frequency resonance, changing characteristics and the risk of air embolus. They do, however, suffer the disadvantage that they can neither be zeroed or calibrated in situ and, in this respect, must be very stable in use or there will be offset and calibration errors.[5]

FLOTATION CATHETERS—THE SWAN–GANZ CATHETER

One area of great interest in cardiovascular monitoring is the measurement of pulmonary artery and pulmonary wedge pressures. The latter is of particular value as it reflects the left ventricular filling pressure. Normally a right heart catheterization is a procedure for the catheter laboratory equipped with X-ray screening, but the use of a catheter which has a balloon at its tip makes it possible to float the catheter into position blindly. Confirmation of its position is given by the monitored pressure waveform.[6]

Flotation catheters are available for most thermodilution cardiac output monitors and are generally introduced using the Seldinger technique.[7] The vein of choice is the right internal jugular as it affords a straight route into the superior vena cava. The catheter tends to soften a little as it warms and its manipulation characteristics will change somewhat. As it should be fluid filled before insertion, it is possible to cool and gain a little rigidity by injecting cold saline through the pressure lumen. No fluid should enter the balloon lumen and only carbon dioxide should be used for balloon inflation (*Fig.* 3.5).

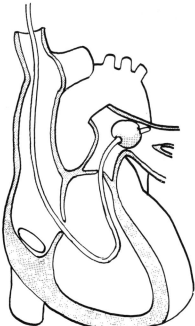

Fig. 3.5. Swan–Ganz catheter with balloon inflated floating in the right pulmonary artery.

ULTRASONIC FLOWMETRY

Doppler ultrasound flowmetry has proved very valuable in the assessment of peripheral vascular disease, but is still considered to be mainly a qualitative technique. Compact Doppler devices are available that permit the localization of stenotic segments of vessels running close to the skin and allow evaluation of the flow pulse at many points of the anatomy. Flowmetry in the true sense is rather more difficult, as the device measures velocity of flow and the received Doppler signal requires complex processing to produce an analogue output. Calibration is difficult because the angle the probe presents to the vessel may change the Doppler-shifted frequencies and measurement of volume flow is dependent on a knowledge of the vessel lumen diameter. Doppler flow instruments that measure vessel diameter by a ranging technique have been developed and an instrument has been constructed to measure cardiac output by beaming a time-gated Doppler beam across the top of the aortic arch. This time-gated beam will provide, in addition to the Doppler frequency shift arising from reflection of ultrasound from moving corpuscles, a depth sounding function that measures the diameter of the blood vessels and a measurement of velocity at several points across the lumen of the vessel. From these different velocities, which of course vary within each cardiac cycle, the overall flow profile can be built up and volume flow calculated. The presence of turbulence can upset the Doppler readings, but it is reported that the flow resumes a reasonably laminar pattern only a short distance downstream from the aortic valve. It is possible that, with developments in microcomputer technology, such techniques will find a place in the intensive care unit; however, at present these are devices for the dedicated enthusiast.

ELECTROMAGNETIC FLOWMETRY

The electromagnetic flowmeter is used to measure flow in an exposed and accessible artery or vein. For most clinical applications, a perivascular probe is used, although it is possible to use cannulating flow heads and intraluminal catheter tip devices. Most clinical applications are found in the operating theatre for the determination of blood flow in venous and arterial grafts. Catheter tip devices are used in some catheterization procedures when there is particular interest in computing parameters such as stroke power and stroke work.

In the intensive care unit, these flowmeters have found only restricted application using withdrawable flowmeter probes in position around the aorta to measure cardiac stroke volume. These probes are looped around the aorta during a cardiac operative procedure and exteriorized through a stab incision in the chest wall. By cutting a suture which holds the probe in its encircling form, gentle traction will remove the probe, it is claimed, without damage. There are several drawbacks to the technique whose only real merit is that it provides a beat-by-beat measurement.[8]

The accuracy of a flowmeter working on the electromagnetic principle depends very much on the geometry and construction of the probe. The way in which the probe operates is as follows: an electromagnet in the probe head produces a uniform magnetic field diametrically across the vessel encircled by the probe. Blood flowing perpendicularly through the magnetic field, cuts through the magnetic flux. In the same way that a dynamo produces an electro-motive force (e.m.f.) by moving a conductor through a magnetic field, so the conductive blood also produces an e.m.f. in a direction mutually perpendicular to the field and the direction of motion. The e.m.f. produced is very small, of the order of $10\,\mu V$, but it is proportional to velocity of flow and, by a fortuitous mathematical relationship, if the flow is axisymmetric, the induced voltage is directly proportional to the average flow velocity. Hence a flow probe can be calibrated in terms of volume flow rate, as its diameter is defined by its construction. To avoid electrochemical potentials developed between the sensing electrodes and the vessel wall and to virtually eliminate sensitivity to bioelectric potentials such as ECG and EMG, an alternating current is used to excite the flow probe magnet. The flowmeter demodulates the signal picked up from the vessel to give a time varying d.c. output to a meter or recorder. As the potential produced by the moving blood is picked up through the vessel wall, the wall must be conductive; veins and arteries are reasonably conductive and so are most well-wetted vascular graft materials, but solid plastics will not permit a perivascular probe to function.

The variable geometry of a flexible flow probe (*see above*) compromises magnet and electrode construction and make it a difficult device to calibrate and it should be standardized against an indicator dilution method in situ, if an absolute value is to be used.

Most of the probes used for operative measurement can have reproducibility and accuracy of around 10% of the reading on a normal vessel, but thickening of the vessel wall can considerably distort the flow symmetry, alter the vessel wall conductivity and hence destroy much of the method's inherent accuracy.

INDICATOR DILUTION TECHNIQUES

Indicator dilution methods have become established as routine for the determination of cardiac output and the subsequent derivation of circulatory indices in intensive care units. Historically, these methods have evolved from two fundamental principles: the Fick principle and the Stewart–Hamilton indicator dilution method.[9]

The Fick Principle

The Fick principle is based on the fact that, if the uptake of a suitable indicator is measured and its arterial and mixed venous concentrations are determined, cardiac output can be calculated by dividing the rate of uptake by the difference in concentration between the arterial and venous compartments. In practical terms oxygen is the indicator of choice. Although carbon dioxide can be used, it is less suitable as changes in pH may affect results. The method is theoretically sound, but to obtain accurate results venous blood must be sampled from the right ventricle or the pulmonary artery. The use of a Swan–Ganz catheter greatly simplifies the right heart catheterization, but it should be pointed out that the trauma of catheterization and arterial puncture may influence cardiac output and give a falsely high value.

$$\text{Cardiac output} = \frac{\text{Oxygen uptake}}{a\text{–}v \text{ concentration difference}}$$

where oxygen uptake is measured in l/min; a–v concentration difference is the difference in oxygen concentration measured in l/l and cardiac output is then in l/min.

The Stewart–Hamilton Method

The method which has almost displaced the Fick method as a standard of cardiac output measurement uses indocyanine green dye as the indicator. The dye is injected as a bolus into a central vein and the concentration is measured by a cuvette through which blood is withdrawn from a peripheral artery. The concentration time curve will, after coming to a peak, decay exponentially until recirculating dye appears in the sample (*Fig.* 3.6). Most modern instruments for cardiac output determination will compute the value taking into account the recirculation. It is absolutely essential that the dye is injected as a bolus; if this is not achieved the output curve will be distorted, and the passage time increased, with consequent errors.[10,11]

The Thermal Dilution Method

The thermal dilution method[12] is more prone to systematic errors than the dye method but has the advantage that serial determinations can be made without the risk of overloading the liver with indicator dye. In some instruments operator skills are largely eliminated by having automatic injection and refrigeration of the injectate (saline or dextrose). In using manual injection, care must be taken not to warm the injectate above the temperature the instrument is set for and to inject as a reproducible bolus. A further source of error in the method arises from the proximity of the airway to the pulmonary artery in which the sensing thermistor lies. Changing patterns of ventilation can cause an extravascular warming effect

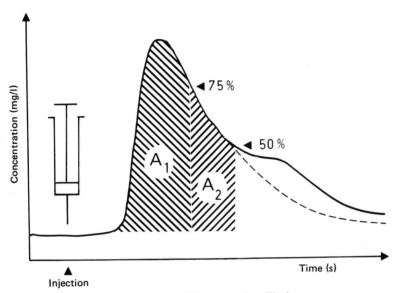

Fig. 3.6. Calculation of cardiac output (CO) from a dye-dilution curve.

$$CO = 60 \times \frac{\text{amount of indicator injected, } I \text{ (mg)}}{\text{mean concentration} \times \text{passage time, } A \text{ (mg} \cdot \text{l}^{-1} \cdot \text{s)}}$$

where A = area under extrapolated curve

$$= A_1 + 3A_2.$$

and result in causing errors of reproducibility. This is most likely when the patient is breathing spontaneously. The simplicity of the Swan–Ganz catheter makes this a very attractive method of cardiac output determination, particularly as pulmonary artery and pulmonary wedge pressures can also be monitored to provide a fairly comprehensive picture of the patient's cardiovascular status.

INDICES DERIVED FROM PRESSURE AND FLOW

Pressures and flows can be combined together in various ways to produce other physical quantities such as work and power, systolic pressure–time index (SPTI) and endocardial viability ratio (EVR), which can be used as guides to the patient's well-being.

Time indices were derived to provide a means of indirectly monitoring the oxygen demands of the left ventricle. The indices are the product of mean pressure in systole and diastole with the duration of the respective part of the cardiac cycle. This gives, respectively, systolic pressure–time index and diastolic pressure–time index (SPTI and DPTI). The SPTI closely follows changes in ventricular work and hence oxygen demand, while DPTI reflects coronary blood flow (since coronary blood flow occurs during diastole) and is thus related to oxygen supply. The ratio of supply to demand

$$\frac{DPTI}{SPTI}$$

has been dubbed 'endocardial viability ratio' or EVR. Correlation of this ratio with the incidence of subendocardial ischaemia suggests that, to avoid the latter, patient management should endeavour to keep the EVR value above unity.[13]

As the ratio relies on true systolic and diastolic waveshapes, it is not adequate to use peripheral arterial pressure lines as the pressure waveform is considerably modified in transmission. Further, it is necessary to subtract from the aortic pressure waveform the mean right atrial pressure, as the effective perfusion pressure is the difference between arterial and venous pressure. Whilst right atrial pressure is relatively easily measured using a Swan–Ganz catheter, the provison of a central arterial line is a difficult and potentially hazardous procedure. These indices are not widely used but can be of value when extracorporeal circulatory support, such as an intra-aortic balloon pump, is being used.

Vascular Resistance

Informed interpretation of the blood pressure should take into account the effect of changes in vascular resistance. This derivative is also used as a yardstick by which the effect of vasoactive drugs can be compared and evaluated. The length of a vascular channel is only slightly variable in comparison to the diameter, which can change sometimes over a remarkable range. Vascular resistance changes observed are primarily determined by radius changes in the vasculature. Most of the peripheral resistance is found at the level of the arterioles and pre-capillaries and about 60% of the total drop from arterial pressure to venous pressure occurs at this level of the circulation. It is clear that any measurement that can reflect the change in diameter of these peripheral vessels would be a very useful tool for patient management.

Considering Poiseuille's law in its simple form ($P_1 - P_2 = KQ$), we find that pressure drop is proportional to flow and the constant of proportionality, K, is a direct analogue of the term 'resistance' in Ohm's law which describes the voltage and current in electrical circuits: voltage = resistance × current.

The use of vascular resistance has its critics and it can be agreed that only part of the pressure drop occurs at the periphery albeit a large part. Also we have used an equation, Poiseuille's law (derived for steady flow), inappropriately to describe a pulsatile phenomenon. Nevertheless, if considered more as an index than as an absolute physical quantity, vascular resistance changes with various changes in physiological state and pharmacological intervention have a great deal of relevance.

Vascular resistance is simply measured by subtracting the mean pressures at the inlet and outlet of the vascular beds in question and dividing by the mean flow into the vascular bed.

The units of measurement are thus

$$\frac{\text{pressure}}{\text{flow}}$$

in SI terms this is in $Pa/m^3/S$ or $kPa/l/S$, but in more practical terms mmHG/l/min, known as the 'peripheral vascular resistance' unit (PRU).

The last set of units is most appropriate to the measurement of total peripheral vascular resistance, that is the resistance summated of all vascular beds in the circulation. Note that as these vascular beds are effectively in parallel, the peripheral vascular resistance as seen from the heart is less than that of most of the individual vascular beds.

Total peripheral vascular resistance

$$= \frac{(\text{Mean aortic pressure} - \text{Mean right atrial pressure})}{\text{Cardiac output}}$$

i.e.

$$\text{PVR (total)} = \frac{(\text{MAP} - \text{MRAP})}{\text{CO}}$$

(Cardiac output is calculated in l/min for the answer in PRU. To convert to the dyne-cm-s, CGS system, multiply by 79·968:

$$\text{dyne} \cdot s \cdot cm^{-5} = \text{PRU} \times 79 \cdot 968$$

The peripheral vascular resistance index (PVRI) is calculated by dividing PVR by body surface area (BSA):

$$\text{PVRI} = \frac{\text{PVR}}{\text{BSA}}$$

Stroke Work

Stroke work is the product of mean left ventricular ejection pressure minus ventricular end diastolic pressure and stroke volume. For an accurate calculation it is essential that left ventricular cavity pressure is measured and averaged over the ejection period. If the inaccuracy is permissible, a peripheral arterial pressure trace may be used; the mean value of systolic pressure is computed for the duration of the ejection phase. This value will omit work losses in the ventricular outflow tract and aortic valve and will be to some extent, dependent on vascular compliance.

Stroke work = mean left ventricular pressure during ejection × stroke volume (SV)

In the more commonly used systems of units, normal values are:

Clinical units
  5000–10 000 mmHg · ml
  (Pressure: mmHg; SV: ml)

SI units
  6665–13335 N · m
  (Pressure: kPa; SV: l)

Dyne second centimetre system (CGS system)
  6665–13 335 dyne · cm
  (Pressure: dyne/cm^2; SV: cm^3 *or* clinical units × 1·3336).

STARLING CURVE

It is possible to use a combination of wedge pressure and cardiac output to optimize 'preloads' and 'afterload' to give maximum pumping efficiency. If a graph is plotted using cardiac output as the abscissa and mean pulmonary wedge pressure as the ordinate, a Starling curve can be drawn by entering pairs of measurements taken at different load levels. Load can be varied by volume infusion and vasodilators. It should be possible to keep the patient on the ascending limb of the curve just below the peak by monitoring the pulmonary wedge pressure.

This intervention should, however, be done in conjunction with other clinical evaluation and recognition of the possibility that oxygen delivery to the myocardium may not be adequate to support the level of afterload required.

SUMMARY

This chapter has outlined the methods used to measure pressure and flow. Although these variables are in themselves valuable indicators of the circulatory condition they are only of value if a knowledge of their inter-relationship and their correlation with external physical signs has been developed. A blood pressure measurement is only of value if related to pulse rate and the state of peripheral perfusion of the patient; a flow measurement in isolation is equally difficult to interpret.

The availability of compact and powerful computing equipment makes possible the inter-relation and correlation of variables giving a clinical management tool hitherto only acquired after long experience. Use of computing demands high standards of measurement, in which the quality of the patient–machine interface is of paramount importance; no amount of sophisticated programming will correct poor data.

Derived haemodynamic data will become more easily obtainable with the newer generations of monitor but skills, such as sphygmomanometry, will always find application in patient management and deserve good training and careful application.

REFERENCES

1. Katz A. M. (1977) *Physiology of the Heart*. New York, Raven Press.
2. McDonald D. A. (1974) *Blood Flow in Arteries*, 2nd ed. London, Edward Arnold.
3. Geddes L. A. (1970) *The Direct and Indirect Measurement of Blood Pressure*. Chicago, Year Book Medical Publishers.
4. Shelton C. D. and Watson B. W. (1968) A pressure generator for testing the frequency response of catheter transducer used for physiological pressure measurements. *Phys. Med. Biol.* **13**, 523–528.
5. Millar H. D. and Baker L. E. (1972) A stable ultra-miniature catheter-tip pressure transducer. *Med. Biol. Eng.* **11**, 86.
6. Swan H. J. C. and Ganz W. (1975) Use of balloon flotation catheters in critically ill patients. *Surg. Clin. North Am.* **55**, 501–520.
7. Seldinger S. I. (1953) Catheter replacement of the needle in percutaneous arteriography. *Acta Radiol. (Stockh.)* **39**, 368.
8. Williams B. T., Sancho-Forres S., Clark D. B. et al. (1972) The Williams–Barefoot extractable blood flow probe. *J. Thorac. Cardiovasc. Surg.* **63**, 917–921.
9. Folkow B. and Neil E. (1971) *Circulation*. Oxford University Press, Oxford Medical Publications.
10. Zierler K. L. (1962) Theoretical basis of indicator dilution methods for measuring flow and volume. *Circ. Res.* **10**, Pt 2, 393–407.
11. Hetzel P. S., Swan G. J. C., De Arellano A. A. R. et al. (1958) Estimation of cardiac output from first part of arterial dye-dilution curves. *J. Appl. Physiol.* **13**, 92–96.
12. Ganz W. and Swan H. J. C. (1972) Measurement of blood flow by thermodilution. *Am. J. Cardiol.* **29**, 241–246.
13. Philips P. A., Marty A. T., Miyamoto A. M. et al. (1975) A clinical method for detecting sub-endocardial ischaemia after cardiopulmonary bypass. *J. Thorac. Cardiovasc. Surg.* **69**, 30–39.

Chapter 4

Disorders of Water and Electrolyte Balance

W. S. T. Thomson

The investigation and assessment of disorders of water, electrolyte and acid–base balance depend on the integration of clinical history, clinical observations and the results of laboratory investigations. In the majority of cases, if properly applied, this permits a fluid replacement regime to be drawn up, the objectives of which may be defined as:

1. The restoration of extracellular fluid (ECF) volume; an adequate intravascular volume must be maintained without overloading the interstitial compartment.

2. Sufficient water must be provided to maintain normal osmolality in the ECF and intracellular fluid (ICF) and to allow secretion of an optimal volume of urine. It must be emphasized that osmolality is a function of body water content whereas ECF volume is a function of body sodium content.

3. The maintenance of total body potassium with a normal distribution between cells and ECF.

4. The restoration of normal acid–base status.

The successful implementation of these fundamental principles requires knowledge of basic facts relating to volume, electrolyte composition, osmolality and distribution of body fluids and also a clear grasp of the pathophysiological features which characterize and distinguish the common disorders of electrolyte, water and acid–base metabolism.

This chapter will consider the systematic approach to such disorders, as they may present in seriously ill patients, under the following sections:

  I. Disorders of water balance.
 II. Disorders of sodium balance.
III. Disorders of potassium balance.

Total Body Water

This is normally 60% of the body weight in kilograms (42 l in a 70-kg man) and varies with age, sex and adiposity. It is distributed into two main compartments. Intracellular (40% of the body weight—28 l) and extracellular (20% body weight—14 l), the latter being further subdivided into interstitial fluid (15% of body weight—10·5 l) and plasma (5% of body weight—3·5 l).

Electrolyte Composition of Body Fluids

Sodium is by far the major cation in the ECF and potassium assumes that role within the cell. The sodium concentration in the ECF is 140 mmol/l and in ICF is 10 mmol/l, whereas the ECF potassium concentration is 4·0 mmol/l and in the ICF is 150 mmol/l. In the ECF the main anions balancing sodium are chloride and bicarbonate. In the cell the principal anions are protein and organic phosphate. The maintenance of this striking gradient of sodium and potassium across the cell membrane depends on the integrity of ion pumps.

Osmolality, Volume and Distribution of Body Fluids

1. *ECF and ICF*

Despite the differing electrolyte composition of the ECF and ICF, their osmolalities are identical because water freely distributes itself across the cell membrane and dissipates any existing osmotic gradient. The prinicipal osmotically active particles are sodium and potassium with their accompanying anions. ECF osmolality is, therefore, proportional to its sodium concentration and ICF osmolality to its potassium concentration. Plasma osmolality and, therefore, ICF osmolality approximates to twice the plasma sodium concentration but this must be qualified in the presence of uraemia and hyperglycaemia where urea and glucose make a significant contribution to the total osmolality. As osmolality is held constant across the total body water, the ECF volume must be a function of its sodium content whilst that of the ICF relates to its potassium content. Moreover, total body water (TBW) must be proportional to total body sodium plus total body potassium. Sodium loss leads to loss of extracellular water and potassium loss to a reduction of intracellular water. Loss or gain of isotonic saline is confined exclusively to the ECF and a proportionate contraction or expansion results. On the other hand, because of the total body distribution of water, only one-third of a pure water excess or deficit expands or contracts the ECF. Thus, the loss of a given volume of isotonic saline leads to a far greater circulatory disturbance than does the loss of an equal volume of water.

2. *Plasma and Interstitial Fluid*

ECF osmolality is approximately 285 mosmol/kg due, principally, to sodium salts which readily penetrate the capillary wall. The distribution of fluid between the plasma and interstitial fluid, therefore, largely depends on the balance between the hydrostatic capillary pressure and the oncotic pressure of the plasma proteins, particularly albumin. Thus the protein content of the plasma by its osmotic effect plays a principal part in determining its volume.

I. DISORDERS OF WATER METABOLISM—OSMOLALITY DISORDERS

Water Balance

Normal water balance is detailed in *Table* 4.1. Water is obtained by drinking, from that present in the diet and from the oxidation of food to carbon dioxide and water, 'water of metabolism'. Water intake is regulated by the thirst mechanism in which cerebral angiotensin has recently been implicated.

Table 4.1. Water balance

	Intake, ml			Output, ml
Water as fluid	1200	Urine		1500
Water as food	1000	Insensible loss		900
Water of oxidation	300	Respiration	400	
		Skin	500	
		Faeces		100
	2500			2500

Although water is lost from the body in urine and faeces and in evaporation from the lungs and skin, only renal losses may be regulated to maintain balance.

Regulation of Water Balance

This is mediated through osmoreceptors in the hypothalamus which respond to changes in plasma osmolality and its principal determinant

Thirst—Neurohypophyseal—Renal system

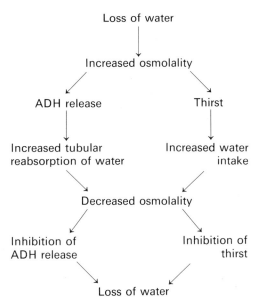

Fig. 4.1 A schematic representation of water balance regulation. Water balance is normally regulated through osmolality mechanisms.

plasma sodium, by either stimulating or inhibiting thirst and the secretion of antidiuretic hormone (ADH) (*Fig.* 4.1). In health the lowest plasma osmolality encountered is 280 mosmol/kg. At this level ADH secretion is completely suppressed and urine osmolality is minimal at around 50 mosmol/kg. Rising plasma osmolality is then accompanied by proportional increases in plasma ADH levels and, when a plasma osmolality of 295 mosmol/kg is attained, there is maximum antidiuresis with a urine osmolality in excess of 1000 mosmol/kg. At this stage thirst is experienced.[1] Thus the osmotic control of thirst and ADH release normally maintain plasma osmolality in the range of 280–295 mosmol/kg.

However, as can be seen from *Table* 4.2, factors other than increased plasma osmolality may induce thirst and ADH secretion. ADH may be released by volume depletion, pain, trauma, nausea and various drugs[2] and thirst may be stimulated by volume depletion and angiotensin.[3] Though

Table **4.2. Factors affecting ADH release and thirst**

ADH release	*Thirst stimulation*
1. Increased osmolality	1. Increased osmolality
2. Hypovolaemia	2. Hypovolaemia
3. Pain, trauma, nausea, drugs	3. Renin–angiotensin

water balance is normally regulated through osmolality mechanisms, these non-osmotic stimuli (particularly to ADH, but also to thirst), are often sustained and persistent and can over-ride the normal inhibitory effect of hypotonicity and thus lead to the water retention which characterizes the various hyponatraemic states.

Water Depletion

The obligatory loss of water from the lungs and skin is increased by hyperventilation and fever, and excessive urinary loss of water occurs when there is a defect in renal concentration, for example cranial diabetes insipidus and nephrogenic diabetes insipidus of hypercalcaemia and potassium depletion. It must be emphasized, however, that these losses will not result in water depletion if water is freely available and the thirst mechanism which is extremely sensitive to hyperosmolality, remains intact.[4]

Body Fluid Changes

As cell membranes are freely permeable to water, a water deficit is shared equally between the ECF and ICF and is accompanied by a rise in total body water osmolality. This increased osmolality leads first to ADH secretion. Water is conserved as a concentrated high osmolality urine is secreted. As the plasma osmolality approaches 295 mosmol/kg, thirst is stimulated. This is a more important protective measure than ADH as obligatory water losses of up to 1 l/24 h continue via skin, lungs and urine and can only be restored by drinking water. However, if water is unavailable or the patient is too ill to respond to the thirst stimulus, then water depletion becomes established (*Fig.* 4.2). When water loss approaches 3 l the reduction in ECF volume stimulates aldosterone secretion resulting in sodium retention and potassium excretion. Osmotic equilibrium is again restored by further transfer of water from the cells, thus maintaining ECF volume at the expense of intracellular volume (*Fig.* 4.3). Vascular collapse and shock are only encountered in very severe degrees of water depletion, as only one-twelfth of the total deficit is derived from the plasma whose volume is further protected by the increased oncotic pressure of the plasma proteins which accompanies dehydration and to some extent by the sodium retention of secondary aldosteronism.

Water Excess

In health the normal response to a water-load is the excretion of a large volume of dilute urine with an osmolality of less than 100 mosmol/kg

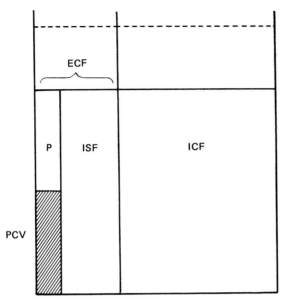

Fig. 4.2. Mild water depletion. Only one-third of total water deficit lost from ECF. Signs of ECF volume depletion are, therefore, absent unless losses are massive. In this and subsequent Marriott diagrams: ECF, extracellular fluid; ISF, interstitial fluid; ICF, intracellular fluid; P, plasma; PCV, packed cell volume; dotted line represents the normal volume.

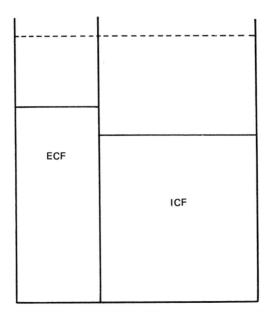

Fig. 4.3. Severe water depletion. Secondary aldosteronism present due to ECF volume depletion. Leads to sodium retention and potassium loss which results in preservation of ECF volume at the expense of intracellular volume.

water. This water diuresis prevents the development of sustained hypo-natraemia and is due to the suppression of ADH secretion by the reduced plasma osmolality. However, in many types of illness there is a restricted ability to deal adequately with a water-load and hyponatraemia results. Acute and chronic renal failure with a reduction in functional renal mass are fairly obvious examples. But hyponatraemia occurs much more commonly in conditions where renal function is not primarily affected and where the water retention is due either to a secondary intra-renal defect in urinary dilution (e.g. reduced GFR) or to the persistence of excess circulating ADH which has been released by non-osmotic stimuli and is, therefore, not suppressed by the accompanying hypo-osmolality.[5]

The three components of the urinary diluting mechanism, each of which must function normally to ensure the secretion of a dilute urine, are detailed in *Table* 4.3. Also listed are possible defects in the mechanism together with commonly associated clinical conditions.

Table **4.3. The renal diluting mechanism**

Normal function	*Abnormal function*	*Clinical disorder*

1. Adequate volume of isotonic fluid from proximal tubule must reach distal diluting sites	Reduction in volume due to:
	 a. Fall in GFR
	 b. Increased proximal tubular reabsorption of sodium and water
		Sodium depletion
		 Oedematous states:
		   Congestive cardiac
		     failure
		   Cirrhosis
		   Nephrosis
		 Hypothyroidism
		 Hypopituitarism
		   (cortisol lack)

2. Dilution of tubular fluid occurs in ascending loop of Henlé as sodium is reabsorbed without water	Sodium reabsorption reduced	Diuretic therapy
3. Collecting duct impermeable to water as ADH is absent. As sodium reabsorption continues further dilution of tubular fluid occurs	Collecting duct permeable to water	ADH* Hypopituitarism (cortisol lack)

*ADH released by non-osmotic stimuli, e.g. volume depletion, pain, trauma, nausea, drugs, syndrome of inappropriate ADH secretion. These stimuli are often sustained and persistent and over-ride the normal inhibitory effect of hypotonicity.

Body Fluid Changes in Water Excess Syndromes

The excess water first results in expansion of the ECF with a fall in plasma sodium concentration and osmolality. Water then passes into the ICF until the osmolality of the two compartments again becomes equal but at a lower

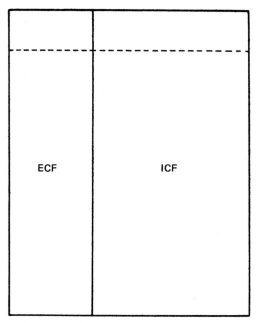

Fig. 4.4. Water excess. Only one-third of excess water retained in ECF. Therefore, clinical oedema absent.

level than normal. Two-thirds of the retained water is contained within the ICF. The one-third which expands the ECF cannot be detected clinically and does not cause oedema (*Fig.* 4.4).

II. DISORDERS OF SODIUM METABOLISM—ECF VOLUME DISORDERS

Sodium Balance

Normal sodium balance is detailed in *Fig.* 4.5. The body sodium content is approximately 4000 mmol, the bulk of which is shared between the ECF and bone, a small amount, about 300 mmol, lying within the cells of the soft tissues. In contrast to the urgency of thirst in water depletion, there is no craving for salt in sodium depletion and intake normally varies between

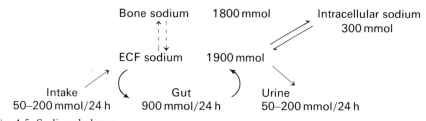

Fig. 4.5. Sodium balance.

50–200 mmol/24 h. As extra renal losses of salt in sweat and faeces are generally very small (10 mmol/24 h), balance is achieved by alteration in renal excretion.

Regulation of Sodium Balance

Detailed knowledge of the renal response is limited. Changes in GFR and aldosterone secretion via the renin–angiotensin mechanism are obviously important. Recent evidence suggests that other very potent mechanisms regulate proximal tubular reabsorption; these include oncotic and hydrostatic forces in the peri-tubular circulation and, possibly, a hormonal inhibitor to tubular reabsorption (natriuretic hormone). How these factors are integrated is incompletely understood, but they are thought to function through volume receptors, a fall in plasma or ECF volume leading to sodium retention and vice versa.

Sodium Depletion

Reduced sodium intake is not a cause. On a salt-free diet, the kidney actively conserves sodium and urinary sodium falls to 1 mmol/24 h in a few days. Therefore for depletion to develop, excessive losses must occur via the gut, skin or kidney.

Body Fluid Changes in Sodium Depletion

The concurrent loss of sodium and water causes ECF volume depletion which induces thirst probably via renin–angiotensin activation. The patient, therefore, ingests water and initially renal excretion of water is adjusted so that the overall losses of sodium and water are in isotonic proportions. Thus, in the early stages of sodium depletion (deficit less than 400 mmol), there is ECF reduction with a normal plasma sodium concentration, i.e. osmolality is preserved at the expense of volume (*Fig.* 4.6). The packed cell volume (PVC), increases and the concentration of plasma proteins rise. If renal function is intact, the urine sodium falls to negligible levels probably due to aldosterone secretion. As sodium depletion advances and the total deficit approaches 400 mmol, renal water retention occurs. Water loss now no longer keeps pace with that of sodium and the plasma sodium concentration falls.[6] The volume of the ECF is now being maintained at the expense of osmolality. Water moves from the ECF to ICF along the osmotic gradient leading to intracellular overhydration (*Fig.* 4.7). The renal retention of water is due to the fall in ECF volume. This leads to reduced delivery of isotonic fluid from the proximal tubules to the

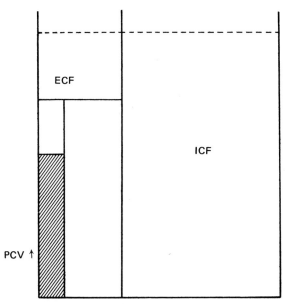

Fig. 4.6. Mild sodium depletion: isotonic ECF volume contraction. Na deficit <400 mmol. Equal loss of sodium and water. Therefore, low ECF volume with normal plasma sodium concentration and osmolality.

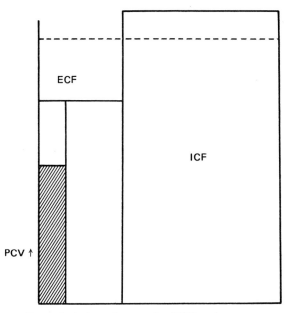

Fig. 4.7. Severe sodium depletion: hypotonic ECF volume contraction. Na deficit >400 mmol. Sodium loss continues, but low ECF volume now induces renal water retention. Ingested water retained and hyponatraemia results with consequent water shift between ECF and ICF. Therefore, reduced ECF volume with hypotonicity.

distal diluting sites and, together with volume mediated ADH release, results in the secretion of an inappropriately concentrated urine and hence to water retention with hyponatraemia.

Sodium Excess

Sodium excess has different clinical presentations; one with and one without ECF expansion.

1. *Sodium Excess with ECF Expansion*

a. *Isotonic expansion*

Following injury there is an obligatory retention of sodium and water with a consequent expansion of ECF volume (*see Fig.* 4.8). After major trauma or surgery this fluid retention may result in weight gains of up to 15% of the body weight and its distribution between the intravascular and interstitial compartments is such that clinical oedema does not occur (*see* Chapter 6). Its aetiology remains controversial. Recent studies suggest that aldosterone

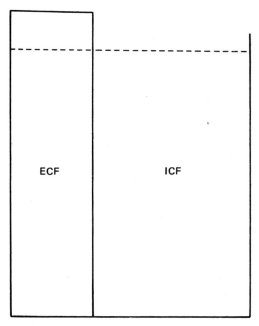

Fig. 4.8. Sodium excess: isotonic ECF volume expansion. Equal amounts of sodium and water retained. Therefore, increased ECF volume with normal plasma sodium concentration and osmolality. Encountered clinically in: (1) postoperative or post-traumatic states if replacement therapy optimal and (2) early oedematous states.

is not the principal factor and the possibility of glycogen-obligated water retention has been raised.

Certain oedematous states, congestive cardiac failure, cirrhosis and nephrosis, are also included in this category. In each case, several factors are responsible for the sodium retention, but the final common path is increased tubular reabsorption of sodium by the kidney due to excess secretion of aldosterone secondary to inadequate renal perfusion. The end result is that sodium and water are retained in equivalent amounts leading to an isotonic expansion of the ECF, particularly that of the interstitial compartment which results in clinical oedema.

b. *Hypotonic expansion*

In their advanced stages, these oedematous states are associated with a decrease in the plasma sodium concentration. Such patients have an increase in the total body sodium but now have a disproportionately greater increase in total body water which has occurred because of renal water retention (*Fig.* 4.9). Paradoxically, the mechanism is similar to that occurring in sodium depletion. Because of the inadequate effective arterial

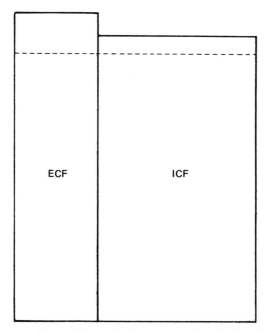

Fig. 4.9. Sodium excess: hypotonic ECF volume expansion. In the advanced oedematous states, water is retained in excess of sodium because of renal water retention induced by decrease in 'Effective Arterial Plasma Volume'. Hence, plasma sodium concentration and osmolality fall.

plasma volume which occurs in the oedematous states, the GFR is reduced and the proximal tubular reabsorption of sodium and water enhanced. The result is decreased delivery of isotonic fluid to the distal diluting sites which, in conjuction with volume-mediated ADH release, leads to the secretion of an inappropriately concentrated urine of high osmolality with consequent renal retention of water and hyponatraemia.[2]

2. *Sodium Excess without ECF Expansion (Hypernatraemia)*

This is classically encountered in intravenous overload with hypertonic saline or sodium bicarbonate. It also occurs with salt poisoning in children. The increased ECF osmolality induces a water shift from the ICF to the ECF, but the resulting ECF expansion is small and does not lead to systemic oedema (*Fig.* 4.10).

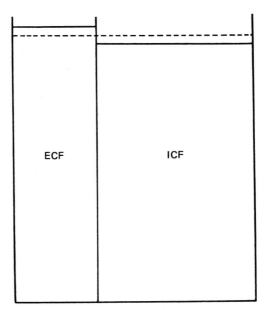

Fig. 4.10. Sodium excess: hypertonicity with normal ECF volume (solute excess). Encountered clinically in acute intravenous sodium overload. Sodium retained in excess of water. Therefore, increased osmolality and hypernatraemia, but systemic oedema absent.

In clinical practice mixed disturbances of sodium and water are the rule and are much more commonly encountered than the isolated deficits or excesses which have been described. They present as disturbances of both ECF volume and osmolality, the contracted or expanded ECF volume being due to sodium depletion or excess and the hyper- or hyponatraemia to associated water depletion or excess. It is logical and clinically useful to

classify these disorders as:
1. Hyponatraemia with contracted, normal or expanded ECF volume.
2. Hypernatraemia with contracted, normal or expanded ECF volume.

1. Clinical Approach to the Hyponatraemic Patient

The finding of hyponatraemia is generally the first clue to the presence of water excess due to a defect in urinary dilution. Unfortunately hypo-natraemia and hypo-osmolality cannot always be equated and before embarking on further investigations the presence of a true hypo-osmolal state must be established. The following conditions must therefore be excluded:

i. *Pseudo-hyponatraemia.* Displacement of plasma water by excess lipid or protein leads to a low plasma sodium value when expressed in mmol/l plasma but a normal result when expressed per litre of plasma water. The measured plasma osmolality in mosmol/kg water is, of course, normal.

ii. *Excess extracellular solute.* Excess impermeable solute, such as glucose which is largely confined to the ECF, exerts an osmotic effect withdrawing water from the ICF to the ECF and leading to hyponatraemia.

iii. Laboratory error and dilution of the blood sample by withdrawal at a site proximal to a hypotonic intravenous infusion must also be excluded.

a. *Hyponatraemia with Contracted ECF Volume*

The underlying pathophysiology has been previously dealt with in detail under sodium depletion (p. 56). Initially there is an isotonic contraction of the ECF but, as the total sodium deficit approaches 400 mmol, water retention supervenes culminating in hyponatraemic contraction of the ECF with cellular over-hydration.

Clinical presentation

The signs and symptoms are those of ECF depletion and not of hypo-osmolality. The major effects are in circulatory and renal function and *Table* 4.4 relates the severity of the symptoms to the degree of sodium deficit. The plasma sodium concentration may be normal but in severe cases it falls particularly if the water intake has been maintained. Poor renal perfusion leads to pre-renal uraemia and a diagnostic feature is a plasma urea rising at a greater rate than creatinine. This is due to back diffusion of urea at low urinary flow rates. If losses are extra-renal, the urine is small in volume with a high urea concentration and osmolality and

Table 4.4. **Symptoms of sodium depletion**

	Sodium deficit, mmol	Signs and symptoms
Mild	300	Lassitude, fainting Postural hypotension may be present
Moderate	300–600	Loss of tissue turgor Tachycardia Marked postural hypotension GFR depressed Plasma urea elevated
Severe	600–1300	Shock, very low BP Uraemia, confusion, coma, plasma sodium low

Table 4.5. **Hyponatraemia with contracted ECF volume**

Urinary sodium < 20 mmol/l Extra-renal loss	Urinary sodium > 20 mmol/l Renal loss

Gastrointestinal losses
  Vomiting*
  Diarrhoea
  Fistula
Excess sweating
Third space effect
  burns, peritonitis,
  muscle trauma, ileus
	Diuretic excess†
	Osmotic diuresis:
	  urea, glucose, mannitol
	Primary adrenal insufficiency
	Sodium wasting renal disease
	Proximal renal tubular acidosis

* If vomiting severe and continuous, urine sodium > 20 mmol/l as urinary bicarbonate excretion increases.
† When diuretic therapy discontinued, urine sodium < 20 mmol/l.

is practically sodium free. A random urine sodium estimation is therefore an extremely useful diagnostic aid and allows the classification outlined in (*Table* 4.5).

Treatment

The sheet anchor of therapy (in hyponatraemia) is undoubtedly 0·9% isotonic saline which replaces the sodium deficit and, by expanding the ECF volume, improves renal perfusion and allows the excess water to be excreted thus correcting the hyponatraemia. Severe depletion may require as much as 9 l of intravenous isotonic saline. The first 2 l should be infused rapidly within 1–2 h to expand the ECF volume. If shock is severe, plasma may be preferred, as it is imperative that adequate blood volume and pressure be restored. Thereafter, treatment can follow a more leisurely course taking some 24–36 h to replace the total deficit. Formulae exist for calculating sodium deficits but are of limited value. It is far better to start treating the patient and to rely on continued clinical observation of, in particular, the lung bases, tissue turgor, jugular venous pressure, central venous pressure, blood pressure, urine output and by monitoring plasma electrolytes if the sodium has been very low. This programme will be modified according to the results of these measurements and may require potassium chloride and sodium bicarbonate supplements depending on the prevailing potassium and acid–base status.

b. *Hyponatraemia with Expanded ECF Volume*

The common clinical causes are listed in *Table* 4.6. The pathophysiology of the oedematous states has previously been considered under sodium excess (p. 58). The diluting defect which leads to hyponatreamia is mediated by the reduced effective arterial plasma volume which stimulates ADH release and decreases fluid delivery to the distal nephron. The signs and symptoms are related to the underlying disease and to the ECF volume expansion, but occasionally inappropriate intravenous therapy may lead to severe hypo-osmolality necessitating intravenous hypertonic saline. More commonly the treatment consists of water restriction plus appropriate therapy for the primary illness.

Table 4.6. Hyponatraemia with expanded ECF volume

Urinary sodium < 20 mmol/l	Urinary sodium > 20 mmol/l
Cardiac failure	Acute renal failure
Cirrhosis	Chronic renal failure
Nephrosis	

c. *Hyponatraemia with Normal ECF Volume*

This category of hyponatraemia is due to pure water excess, occurring in patients whose sodium balance is normal with urinary sodium excretion reflecting intake and generally in excess of 20 mmol/l. *Table* 4.7 lists the common clinical causes. There is obviously a slight increase in ECF volume as it holds one-third of the retained water, but clinically this is undetectable and oedema is absent. Biochemically there is a fall in plasma osmolality and in the plasma sodium and plasma protein concentrations. The PCV is not altered as the excess water is shared equally between the red cell water and plasma water. The urine is generally hypertonic with respect to plasma, but, in a patient with hyponatraemia due to water excess, a urine

Table 4.7. **Hyponatraemia with normal ECF volume**

Cortisol deficiency   *a.* Hypopituitarism
                       b. Abrupt cessation of steroid therapy
Hypothyroidsim
Postoperative
Potassium depletion—may be diuretic induced
Antidiuretic drugs
Reset osmostat
Syndrome of inappropriate ADH secretion

osmolality greater than 100 mosmol/kg is physiologically inappropriate and implies a defect in urinary dilution.

Clinical presentation

Signs and symptoms, if present, are due to hypotonicity and not to increased ECF volume and may be attributed to overhydration of cells of the gastrointestinal tract and muscle but particularly of the central nervous system. They include anorexia, nausea, vomiting, muscle cramps, head-ache, lethargy, disorientation, convulsions and coma. Papilloedema and other signs of increased intracranial pressure may be present. The severity of the symptoms depends both on the rate of development and the degree of hyponatraemia and are not usually encountered unless the plasma sodium has fallen acutely (within hours) to less than 125 mmol/l. A patient with a plasma sodium of 110 mmol/l may be virtually symptomless, but here the rate of fall of the plasma sodium can be measured in days or weeks rather than hours. It is probable that in chronic hyponatraemia, cerebral oedema is minimized by the loss of intracellular solute.

Acute Water Intoxication—Acute Symptomatic Hyponatraemia

The clinical setting is the rapid administration of an excessive water-load either orally or intravenously to a patient who had impaired water excretion from any of the causes listed in *Table* 4.7. If the plasma sodium concentration falls abruptly to less than 125 mmol/l, then the symptoms of acute hypotonicity described above declare themselves.

Treatment

This is a medical emergency as it carries a mortality of 50%.[2]
i. Intravenous hypertonic saline (5%, 855 mmol Na$^+$/l) should be infused in an attempt to withdraw the excess water from the brain cells. The plasma

sodium should not be restored to normal as there is a risk of acute ECF over-expansion with pulmonary oedema. Marked clinical improvement, however, can result if the plasma sodium is raised slowly to 130 mmol/l. Millilitres of 5% saline required to achieve this can be calculated thus:

$$\frac{(130 - \text{estimated sodium}) \times \text{total body water in litres}}{855} \times 1000$$

and this volume should be infused over a period of 6 hours thus avoiding the too rapid correction of cerebral oedema which may precipitate brain haemorrhage. The plasma sodium should be estimated hourly and therapy ceased when the value reaches 130 mmol/l.

ii. An alternative treatment, which avoids over-expansion of the ECF and hence is very useful in hypervolaemic patients, consists of hourly administration of a loop diuretic to initiate a diuresis. The urine is analysed hourly for its sodium and potassium content which is then replaced by intravenous 5% saline with added KCl. The plasma sodium should be restored at the same rate and to the same level as recommended above.

Chronic Hyponatraemia

Here hyponatraemia has developed slowly and has not been exacerbated by a massive water overload. Symptoms, if present, are much less severe than with water intoxication and the mortality from hypotonicity is very low. There is no question of therapy with intravenous 5% saline. This is reserved solely for acute cerebral oedema. Treatment consists of water restriction and therapy directed towards the underlying disorder.

2. The Clinical Approach to the Hypernatraemic Patient

If solute overload can be excluded, then all cases of hypernatraemia may be considered due to a relative or absolute deficit of water. However, the thirst mechanism is so sensitive to hyperosmolality that severe persistent hypernatraemia only occurs in patients who cannot respond to thirst by the voluntary ingestion of water. It is, therefore, generally encountered in extremely ill patients or in comatose states.

a. Hypernatraemia with Contracted ECF Volume

This occurs in patients who sustain losses of both sodium and water, but with water loss predominating, and is due to hypotonic fluid losses through the gut, skin or kidney (*Table* 4.8). This leads to hypernatraemia which is accentuated and maintained by failure to ingest water.

Table 4.8. Hypernatraemia with contracted ECF volume

Urinary sodium < 20 mmol/l *Extra-renal loss*	*Urinary sodium > 20 mmol/l* *Renal loss*

Gastrointestinal losses:
  particularly gastroenteritis
  in children
Excess sweating
	Osmotic diuresis:
	  glucose, urea

Clinical presentation

The symptoms are generally those of ECF volume depletion, the tendency to hypernatraemia having been blunted by the accompanying sodium loss.

Treatment

As ECF contraction is more dangerous to life than hypertonicity initial therapy is, therefore, directed towards ECF expansion with 0·9% isotonic saline. When this has been achieved, the hypertonicity is gradually corrected by intravenous 5% glucose.

b. *Hypernatraemia with Normal ECF Volume*

The pathophysiology has been discussed under pure water depletion (p. 52). On theoretical grounds, because of body water distribution, only one-twelfth of the total deficit should be lost from the intravascular volume but, in practice, this compartment is afforded further protection by the accompanying rise in plasma protein oncotic pressure and by the sodium retention of secondary aldosteronism. Signs of hypovolaemia are, therefore, rare unless losses are massive. The usual causes are listed in *Fig.* 4.11 but it must be re-emphasized that water losses do not lead to hypernatraemia if the patient is capable of responding normally to thirst.

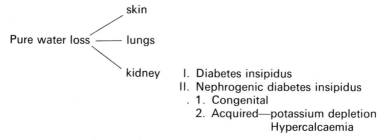

Fig. 4.11. Hypernatraemia with normal ECF volume.

Clinical presentation

The symptoms are those of increased osmolality and relate to cellular dehydration particularly of cerebral cells, viz. thirst, lethargy, confusion, convulsions and coma. The plasma sodium and osmolality are increased as is the plasma protein concentration. Initially the PCV is normal as the water deficit is shared equally between red cell water and plasma water. Oliguria is present with a high urea concentration and increased osmolality unless the primary fault is renal, for example in diabetes insipidus.

Treatment

A useful formula for calculating a pure water deficit can be derived as follows:

$$\text{Normal TBW} \times \text{Normal plasma Na}^+$$

$$= \text{Patient's TBW} \times \text{Patient's plasma Na}^+$$

Assuming

$$\text{Body water content} = 60\% \text{ Body weight}$$

and

$$\text{Normal plasma Na}^+ = 140 \text{ mmol/l}$$

Then in a 70-kg male

$$\text{Water deficit (Normal TBW} - \text{Patient's TBW)}$$

$$= 0.6 \times \text{Body weight (kg)} \times \left[1 - \frac{140}{\text{Patient's Na}^+} \right]$$

Water should be given orally if possible, otherwise as 5% glucose intravenously. Hypernatraemia must be corrected slowly as the brain cells appear to adapt to chronic hyperosmolality by accumulating intracellular solute (idiogenic osmoles), the identity of which is unknown but which protects the brain from undue shrinkage. If treatment is too energetic the increase in intracellular solute may promote cerebral oedema (isotonic water intoxication) and it is suggested that half the calculated deficit should be replaced in 12 h, full correction taking two days or more.[1] If possible, the underlying disorder which has contributed to the water depletion should be treated, for example the administration of vasopressin for diabetes insipidus.

c. *Hypernatraemia with Increased Total Body Sodium*

This has already been discussed under sodium excess without ECF expansion. It is an uncommon type of hypernatraemia, as the normal kidney can readily excrete a sodium load having the capacity to attain a urinary sodium concentration of 300 mmol/l. It occurs with intravenous overload of hypertonic saline or sodium bicarbonate and also with salt poisoning in children. The osmolality induced ECF expansion due to the water shift from the ICF to the ECF is minimal and does not lead to systemic oedema. There is, however, a danger of pulmonary oedema due to acute circulatory overload.

Treatment

The excess sodium can be removed by diuretics or, if renal function is impaired, by dialysis. Simultaneously, 5% glucose should be administered by slow intravenous infusion to alleviate any accompanying neurological symptoms.

The Hyperosmolar State

It is now appropriate to consider the hyperosmolar state which has aroused increasing interest over the past decade. A clinically important distinction must be made between hyperosmolality occurring with and without hypertonicity (*Fig.* 4.12). In both, measured osmolality is high but

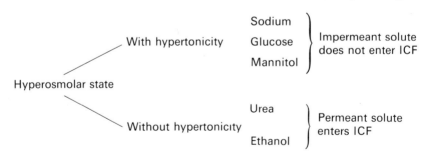

Fig. 4.12. Hyperosmolar states.

hyperosmolality with hypertonicity is characterized by increased plasma concentration of sodium salts or other solutes which are osmotically effective and, therefore, create an osmotic gradient between the ECF and ICF with a resulting fluid shift. On the other hand, in hyperosmolality without hypertonicity, the plasma contains excess solute which can readily penetrate the cell membrane. Such solute is, therefore, not osmotically effective and thus no fluid shift occurs between the ICF and ECF.[7] There is no evidence that hyperosmolality per se is harmful; it makes no contribution to the symptomatology of alcohol excess or to the uraemic syndrome and clinical interest centres exclusively on hyperosmolality with hypertonicity where the appreciable fluid shift that occurs leads to many of the clinical features. Hypernatraemia has already been discussed. It now remains to consider hypertonicity due to glucose and to mannitol.

Hyperglycaemia

This leads to the fairly rapid development of an extremely involved and complex type of hypertonic state.[8]
i. The increased osmolality due to the hyperglycaemia induces a water shift from the ICF to the ECF. The ECF expands and the plasma sodium falls by approximately 1·6 mmol/l for each 5·5 mmol/l increment in glucose.[9]
ii. Simultaneously, the profound osmotic diuresis due to glucose results in a loss of large volumes of hypotonic urine with a sodium concentration of approximately 50 mmol/l in addition to appreciable quantities of potassium.[10] The urinary water loss may be aggravated because the hypertonicity due to hyperglycaemia does not stimulate ADH release and thirst to the same extent as hypernatraemia.[1] There is, therefore, a tendency to hypernatraemia which may be offset in the initial stages at least by the water shift induced by glucose. To assess external water balance it is, therefore, necessary to calculate a corrected plasma sodium figure:

$$\text{Corrected Na}^+ = \text{Measured Na}^+ + \left[\frac{\text{Measured Blood glucose} - 5 \cdot 5}{5 \cdot 5} \times 1 \cdot 6 \right]$$

This is the plasma sodium concentration that would obtain in the absence of hyperglycaemia (*Table* 4.9). Volume depletion ensues because of the continuing urinary sodium loss but the accompanying hyperglycaemia exerts a temporary protective effect by holding fluid within the ECF. If this is undone by rapid therapeutic correction of the blood glucose level before sufficient ECF expansion has been achieved by saline infusion, then a catastrophic fall in blood pressure may result. Volume depletion leads to a reduction in GFR which maintains the plasma glucose at its characteristically high level and also accounts for the marked pre-renal rise in the blood urea. The osmotic diuretic loss of potassium is accentuated by secondary aldosteronism due to volume depletion. However, the resulting potassium depletion does not usually result in hypokalaemia as the hypertonicity due to hypernatraemia and hyperglycaemia lead to a shift of potassium from the cells to the plasma.[11]
iii. The final composite picture (*Table* 4.9) is that of volume depletion with hypernatraemia denoting marked water depletion, hyperglycaemia,

Table **4.9. Hypertonicity due to hyperglycaemia**

	Normal	*Mild hyperglycaemia*	*Severe hyperglycaemia with ECF volume contraction and water depletion*
Glucose (mmol/l)	5·5	30·2	60·4
Sodium (mmol/l)	140	130	155
Corrected sodium (mmol/l)	140	140	175
		(External water balance normal)	(Water depleted)
ECF volume	N	↑ (Not clinically detectable)	↓↓↓ (Volume depleted)
Osmolality (mosmol/kg)	285	300	390

elevated urea, normal plasma potassium despite total body potassium depletion and grossly elevated osmolality, findings characteristic of hyperosmolar, non-ketotic diabetic coma.

Mannitol

This is used as an osmotic diuretic in the treatment of cerebral oedema and diagnostically in acute renal failure. The usual dose is 20 g intravenously which will elevate plasma osmolality by 3 mosmol/kg in a 70-kg male. Severe hypertonicity will, therefore, only result when repeated doses are used in anuric patients. Hypertonicity following mannitol is generally due, not to the mannitol itself, but to hypernatraemia resulting from the water loss of the osmotic diuresis.

III. DISORDERS OF POTASSIUM HOMEOSTASIS

Disorders of potassium homeostasis are due either to alterations in internal or external balance or both (*Fig.* 4.13). The factors affecting internal potassium balance (potassium distribution) are summarized in *Fig.* 4.14.

Factors affecting External Potassium Balance (Body Potassium Content)

Potassium intake is approximately 50–150 mmol/24 h of which only 5–10 mmol/24 h are excreted in the faeces, the remainder being lost in the urine. Potassium balance, therefore, is achieved by regulation of urinary potassium excretion. Essentially all filtered potassium is re-absorbed in the

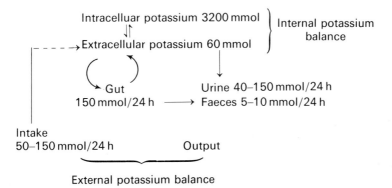

Fig. 4.13. Potassium homeostasis. Total body potassium is 3500 mmol of which 98% is intracellular. The intracellular potassium concentration is 150 mmol/l and extracellular is 4·0 mmol/l.

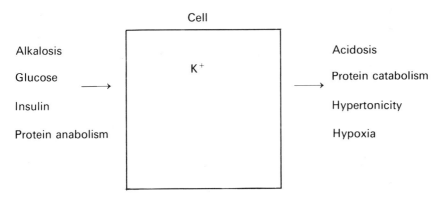

Fig. 4.14. Factors affecting internal potassium balance.

proximal tubule. The major factors which control its secretion by the distal tubule are as follows:

1. *Dietary Potassium and Aldosterone*

Increased potassium intake leads to an elevation in the plasma potassium level which in turn stimulates aldosterone secretion. Both aldosterone and increased plasma potassium enhance peritubular potassium uptake,[12] resulting in an increase in intracellular potassium concentration which favours potassium secretion into the lumen. In addition, aldosterone accelerates potassium secretion by increasing the permeability of the luminal membrane to potassium.[12] The converse occurs with a reduction in dietary potassium and aldosterone.

2. Sodium Intake and Distal Tubular Flow Rate

Increased distal tubular flow rate leads to a kaliuresis if cell potassium concentration is high, but has little effect on the rate of potassium secretion if the cellular potassium concentration is low.[13] The well-documented effect of diminished potassium excretion with sodium depletion and increased excretion with sodium excess can be attributed principally to alterations in tubular flow rate.

3. Acid–base Status

Acute acidosis decreases and alkalosis increases potassium secretion, probably through inhibition and stimulation of peritubular potassium uptake. The mechanisms of chronic acid–base disturbances are less well understood. Apart from respiratory alkalosis, which has no demonstrable effect on potassium secretion, all lead to kaliuresis, possibly due to increased distal tubular flow rate.[14]

All the factors detailed as influencing the internal or external balance of potassium are of course implicated in the genesis of the hypo- and hyperkalaemic states.[15]

Hypokalaemia

This is defined as a plasma potassium of less than 3·5 mmol/l resulting from a redistribution of potassium into cells or a reduction in total body potassium.

Redistribution Hypokalaemia Syndromes

1. Alkalosis

The fall in plasma potassium which occurs in both respiratory and metabolic alkalosis is in part due to increased cellular uptake, potassium entering the cells in exchange for hydrogen ions.

2. Hypokalaemic Periodic Paralyses

This is a rare familial condition characterized by intermittent episodes of flaccid paralysis of limbs and trunk lasting up to 24 h. Plasma potassium remains low during the attack and rises with recovery.

3. *Increased Protein Anabolism*

In the treatment of megaloblastic anaemias with vitamin B_{12} plasma potassium falls due to the high rate of incorporation of potassium into the newly synthesized red blood cells.[16]

4. *Insulin*

Potassium uptake by muscle and liver is accelerated[17] following high intravenous glucose loads, for example, in parenteral nutrition. The increase in insulin secretion often leads to hypokalaemia.

Potassium Deficiency Syndromes

1. *Inadequate Intake*

Starvation can lead to potassium depletion as there is a continuing obligatory loss of up to 10 mmol of potassium per 24 h in urine and faeces. Note that the kidney does not conserve potassium as efficiently as it does sodium.

2. *Excess Urinary Loss*

DIURETIC THERAPY. Thiazide and loop diuretics inhibit sodium and water reabsorption in the ascending loop of Henlé and the resulting increased delivery of solute and water to the distal nephron leads to a kaliuresis.[18]

A diuretic-induced metabolic alkalosis may also enhance potassium secretion by increasing distal tubular flow rate.

Finally, diuretics often lead to ECF volume depletion with consequent secondary aldosteronism which again augments potassium loss.

OSMOTIC DIURESIS. Irrespective of the nature of the loading solute (glucose, mannitol, sodium bicarbonate) a marked kaliuresis ensues, possibly due to decreased proximal reabsorption of potassium in combination with increased distal delivery of solute and water.

EXCESS MINERALOCORTICOID PRODUCTION. Increased potassium excretion is characteristic of primary and secondary aldosteronism, Cushing's syndrome, steroid therapy, ectopic ACTH production and Bartter's syndrome, but the kaliuresis is closely linked to the maintenance of distal tubular flow rate. For example in Conn's syndrome, hypokalaemia may not declare itself if the sodium intake is low and, in the secondary aldosteronism of congestive cardiac failure, hypokalaemia may only occur after diuretic therapy has lead to an increase in distal tubular flow rate.[11]

RENAL TUBULAR ACIDOSIS. In proximal renal tubular acidosis, the defect in the proximal reabsorption of bicarbonate leads to distal delivery of bicarbonate-rich fluid with consequent increased potassium secretion. In distal renal tubular acidosis, the kaliuresis is probably associated with sodium depletion and secondary aldosteronism. In both types, the metabolic acidosis itself will lead to potassium depletion.

3. Gastrointestinal Loss

The hypokalaemia of severe vomiting is partly due to direct potassium loss in the vomit and to redistribution into cells as a result of the accompanying metabolic alkalosis. The principal cause of potassium depletion, however, is the high urinary potassium excretion due both to the metabolic alkalosis and to the secondary aldosteronism of sodium depletion.

Severe potassium losses can also occur with diarrhoea or laxative abuse.

Symptoms of Hypokalaemia

Hypokalaemia and potassium depletion lead to profound effects on cellular metabolism. A number of enzymes are known to be affected by changes in intracellular potassium concentration and ICF volume itself is determined by total body potassium. In addition, alterations in plasma potassium lead to changes in cell membrane potential which present clinically as impaired neuromuscular function. Renal function may also be adversely affected.

From skeletal muscle effects, the symptoms range from fatigue and weakness to paralysis and tend to appear as plasma potassium falls below 2·5 mmol/l. The ECG is abnormal and hypokalaemia predisposes to digitalis toxicity. Smooth muscle is also paralysed. Constipation, intestinal dilatation and ileus, are fairly common manifestations.

Potassium depletion affects renal function in a number of ways. For some inexplicable reason the GFR is reduced. Vacuolation and necrosis are often seen in the cells of the proximal tubules. There is inability to secrete a concentrated urine as the tubules are no longer responsive to ADH, thus thirst and polyuria are frequent symptoms. There is a defect in urinary acidification. Hypokalaemia increases ammonia synthesis by tubular cells but titratable acidity production is impaired.

Treatment of Hypokalaemia

Estimation of the degree of depletion can be extremely difficult because no definite correlation exists between the plasma potassium level and body potassium content. Rough guide lines are as follows.

In the absence of any acid–base disturbance, a deficit of 100–200 mmol potassium results in a reduction in plasma level of about 1·0 mmol/l. After the plasma potassium reaches 3·0 mmol/l, a further fall to 2·0 mmol/l is associated with an additional potassium deficit of 200–400 mmol. Continuing potassium loss then has little further effect on the plasma potassium level which appears to stabilize around 2·0 mmol/l.[19]

Many different potassium salts are available for oral or intravenous use: chloride, bicarbonate, citrate and gluconate. Oral (e.g. 'Slow K', 8 mmol potassium chloride per tablet) or intravenous potassium chloride 2 mmol/ml, should be used for hypokalaemia associated with metabolic alkalosis. On the other hand, potassium bicarbonate or intravenous citrate should be administered in the potassium depletion associated with the hyperchloraemia of renal tubular acidosis.

In general, the concentration of potassium in intravenous fluids should not exceed 40 mmol/l and the rate should not usually be greater than 10 mmol/h. It is generally unwise to administer more than 240 mmol/24 h. If fast administration is desired, for example 40 mmol/h to patients with muscular paralyses or serious arrhythmias, then a close watch must be kept on the plasma potassium level, the urine output and the ECG, (see Chapter 16).

Hyperkalaemia

This is defined as a plasma potassium above 5·5 mmol/l resulting from redistribution of potassium or an increase in total body potassium. It must be emphasized, however, that hyperkalaemia can occur with a total body potassium deficit.

Redistribution Hyperkalaemia Syndromes

Acidosis

The elevation in plasma potassium encountered in both metabolic and respiratory acidosis is generally attributed to exchange of cellular potassium ions for hydrogen ions. However, it has recently been shown that changes in plasma bicarbonate can affect potassium distribution independently of pH change.[20] Moreover, in metabolic acidosis the nature of the acid plays a key role, excess mineral acids producing a greater rise in plasma potassium than organic acids.[21,22]

Hypertonicity

The resulting increase in intracellular potassium concentration is thought to contribute to net efflux from the cells but an alteration in cell permeability may also be involved. The effect is independent of the nature of the solute.[11]

Insulin lack

This is an important feature of the hyperkalaemia of diabetic coma though other factors, such as hypertonicity and acidosis, are obviously involved.

Increased Protein Catabolism

This is encountered in the catabolic phase of severe injury, and with the cell necrosis that follows destruction of tumour tissue with chemotherapy. Severe hyperkalaemia can occur particularly if renal failure is associated.

Hypoxia

Oxygen lack curtails the synthesis of ATP whose high energy bonds are necessary to maintain potassium within the cell (sodium potassium pump). Moreover, under hypoxic conditions, lactic acid is formed and as it is buffered by intracellular protein, potassium is released into the extra-cellular fluid.

Total Body Potassium Excess

Excess Intake

When renal function is normal, this is an extremely uncommon cause of hyperkalaemia and is only encountered when the rate of an intravenous potassium infusion exceeds 40 mmol/h. However, in patients with renal impairment, administration of exogenous potassium is fraught with risk, particularly when urine flow rate is low since potassium excretion is flow dependent.

Decreased Renal Excretion

Hyperkalaemia commonly occurs in acute renal failure because of the reduction in urinary output and the associated metabolic acidosis. Increased catabolism often coexists.

On the other hand, in chronic renal failure potassium balance is maintained until late in the course of the disease unless potassium intake is excessive or increased protein breakdown is present. Potassium homeostasis is generally preserved until the GFR falls to approximately 20 ml/min. This is due to an ill-understood compensatory increase in both colonic and tubular potassium secretion which may be related to a secondary increase in aldosterone secretion. If, however, flow rate falls and oliguria supervenes, hyperkalaemia is inevitable.

Aldosterone lack is associated with urinary potassium retention and sodium loss, but hyperkalaemia is generally not encountered until sodium depletion develops. This further depresses potassium secretion because of the consequent reduction in distal tubular flow rate.

The potassium sparing diuretics, such as spironolactone, triamterene and amiloride, block potassium secretion at the distal tubule and may result in hyperkalaemia. Extreme care must be exercised when prescribing potassium supplements in conjuction with these diuretics.

Symptoms of Hyperkalaemia

These are related to the neuromuscular, gastrointestinal and cardiovascular systems.

Common skeletal muscle symptoms are weakness, paraesthesia and ascending paralysis, whilst those of gastrointestinal tract involvement range from nausea and vomiting to abdominal pain and ileus. Its effects on cardiac conduction can present as heart block, tachycardia, fibrillation or asystole. A plasma potassium greater than 7·5 mmol/l is dangerous and demands immediate treatment.

Treatment

Initially 100 ml of 50% glucose containing 20 units of soluble insulin is administered followed by the intravenous injection of 10–20 ml of 10% calcium gluconate. Calcium antagonizes the potassium effect on the myocardium. Glucose and insulin promote potassium uptake by the cells. Any metabolic acidosis present should be neutralized by sodium bicarbonate thus further promoting cellular potassium uptake.

If necessary, total body potassium can be reduced by resonium A or by haemo- or peritoneal dialysis.

REFERENCES

1. Feig P. U. and McCurdy D. K. (1977) The hypertonic state. *N. Engl. J. Med.* **297**, 1444.
2. Goldberg M. (1981) Hyponatraemia. *Med. Clin. North Am.* **65**, 251.
3. Anderson R. J. and Linas S. L. (1978) Sodium depletion states. In: Brenner B. M. and Stein J. H., ed., *Sodium and Water Homeostasis*, p. 154. New York, Churchill Livingstone.

4. Berl T., Anderson R. J., McDonald K. M. et al. (1976) Clinical disorders of water metabolism. *Kidney Int.* **10**, 117.
5. Berl T. and Shrier R. W. (1978) Water metabolism and the hypo-osmolar syndromes. In: Brenner B. M. and Stein J. H., ed., *Sodium and Water Homeostasis*, p. 1. New York, Churchill Livingstone.
6. McCance R. A. (1936) Experimental sodium chloride deficiency in man. *Proc. R. Soc. Lond. (Biol.)* **119**, 245.
7. Loeb J. N. (1974) The hyperosmolar state. *N. Engl. J. Med.* **290**, 1184.
8. Feig P. U. (1981) Hypernatraemia and hypertonic syndromes. *Med. Clin. North Am.* **65**, 271.
9. Katz M. A. (1973) Hyperglycaemia-induced hyponatraemia: calculation of expected serum sodium depressions. *N. Engl. J. Med.* **289**, 843.
10. Gennari F. J. and Kassirer J. P. (1974) Osmotic diuresis. *N. Engl. J. Med.* **291**, 714.
11. Cox M. (1981) Potassium homeostasis. *Med. Clin, North Am.* **65**, 363.
12. Hierholzer K. and Wiederholt M. (1976) Some aspects of distal tubular solute and water transport. *Kidney Int.* **9**, 198.
13. Khuri R. M., Wiederholt M., Strieder N. et al. (1975) Effect of flow rate and potassium intake on distal tubular potassium transfer. *Am. J. Physiol.* **228**, 1249.
14. Gennari F. J. and Cohen J. J. (1975) Role of the kidney in potassium homeostasis: lessons from acid base disturbances. *Kidney Int.* **8**, 1.
15. Kliger A. S. and Hayslet J. P. (1978) Disorders of potassium balance. In: Brenner B. M. and Stein J. H., ed., *Acid Base and Potassium Homeostasis*, p. 168. New York, Churchill Livingstone.
16. Lawson D. H., Murray R. M. and Parker J. L. W. (1972) Early mortality in the megaloblastic anaemias. *Q. J. Med.* **41**, 1.
17. Zierler K. L. and Rabinowitz D. (1964) Effect of very small concentrations of insulin on forearm metabolism. Persistence of its action on potassium and free fatty acids without its effect on glucose. *J. Clin. Invest.* **43**, 950.
18. Morgan T. and Berliner R. W. (1969) A study by continuous microperfusion of water and electrolyte movements in the loops of Henlé and distal tubule of the rat. *Nephron* **6**, 388.
19. Scribner B. H. and Burnell J. M. (1956) Interpretation of the serum potassium concentration. *Metabolism* **5**, 468.
20. Fraley D. S. and Adler S. (1976) Isohydric regulation of plasma potassium by bicarbonate in the rat. *Kidney Int.* **9**, 333.
21. Orringer C. E., Eustace J. C., Wunsch C. D. et al. (1977) Natural history of lactic acidosis after grand mal seizures. A model for the study of an anion gap acidosis not associated with hyperkalaemia. *N. Engl. J. Med.* **297**, 746.
22. Oster J. R., Perez G. O. and Vaamonde C. A. (1978) Relationship between blood pH and potassium and phosphorus during acute metabolic acidosis. *Am. J. Physiol.* **235**, F345.

Chapter 5

Disorders of Acid–base Regulation

W. S. T. Thomson

PHYSIOLOGY OF ACID–BASE REGULATION

Acid Production

Each day tissue metabolism generates carbon dioxide equivalent to 13 000 mmol hydrogen ions. In addition about 70 mmol of fixed acid (non-volatile) are produced. This consists principally of sulphuric and phosphoric acid derived from oxidation of sulphur and phosphorus in tissue proteins and may also include large quantities of lactic and acetoacetic acid from incomplete oxidation of carbohydrate and fat. These acids must be excreted and changes in body fluid pH minimized. This is accomplished by the following three mechanisms:

1. Buffering.
2. Pulmonary excretion of carbon dioxide.
3. Renal excretion of fixed acids.

Buffer Systems

Body Fluid Buffers

Bicarbonate is the principal buffer in the ECF (plasma and interstitial fluid); protein predominates in red blood cells (haemoglobin), tissue cells and plasma; phosphate is low in the ECF but is more important in tissue cells. A hydrogen ion load is shared between these buffers and a linked equilibrium is soon established between these systems. As blood is readily accessible for analysis its buffering systems have been studied and evaluated in detail. The changes occurring in the blood buffer systems are, therefore, used to characterize clinical disorders of acid–base balance.

Blood Buffers

For simplicity they can be divided into two types, the bicarbonate and the non-bicarbonate buffer systems, principally haemoglobin.

Buffering and transport of carbon dioxide

$$H_2CO_3 + Buffer^- \rightarrow HBuffer + HCO_3^-$$

(i.e. non-bicarbonate buffer system)
Carbon dioxide is conveyed from the tissues to the lung mainly in the form of plasma bicarbonate formed inside the red cell by the buffering of carbonic acid by haemoglobin, the remainder being carried as carbamino compounds and dissolved carbon dioxide. These reactions are reversed at the lung capillaries and carbon dioxide is excreted at a rate determined by the product of alveolar ventilation and alveolar carbon dioxide concentration.

Buffering of fixed acids

$$H^+ + HCO_3^- \longrightarrow H_2CO_3 \quad \text{(bicarbonate buffer)}$$

$$\frac{H^+ + Buffer^-}{Buffer\ base} \longrightarrow \frac{HBuffer}{Buffer\ acid} \quad \text{(non-bicarbonate buffer)}$$

Endogenous hydrogen ion production (fixed acid) is buffered by both bicarbonate and non-bicarbonate buffer systems and the buffer bases are converted to their respective buffer acids. The reconstitution of the depleted buffer bases is directly dependent on the ability of the distal renal tubule to synthesize bicarbonate, and this is inextricably linked to the renal secretion of hydrogen ions.

In the buffering of fixed acids, the bicarbonate system is quantitatively the more important.

$$pH = pK + \log \frac{[HCO_3^-]}{[H_2CO_3]}$$

$[H_2CO_3]$ can be replaced by $0.03 \times P_{CO_2}$ as H_2CO_3 is in equilibrium with dissolved CO_2 which in turn is in equilibrium with the alveolar and arterial P_{CO_2}. 0.03 is the solubility coefficient of CO_2 in plasma at $37\,^\circ C$. Thus

$$pH = pK + \log \frac{[HCO_3^-]}{0.03 \times P_{CO_2}}$$

The pK (log dissociation constant) $= 6.10$ and normal values for

$HCO_3^- = 25 \, mmol/l$ and for $P_{CO_2} = 40 \, mm \, Hg$. Thus

$$pH = 6 \cdot 1 + \log \frac{25}{1 \cdot 2} = 6 \cdot 10 + \log 20 = 7 \cdot 40$$

Physicochemically this represents a poor buffer system as its pK of $6 \cdot 1$ is too far removed from the pH of blood, but it is unique in that it is the only buffer system capable of physiological adjustment, the P_{CO_2} being regulated by the respiratory system and the bicarbonate concentration by the kidney. Moreover, pathophysiological disturbances alter pH by inducing primary changes in either the P_{CO_2} or the bicarbonate. Thus, this buffer system directly links chemical buffering with pathophysiological disturbances and physiological adjustments and is, therefore, chosen to characterize all disorders of acid–base balance.

Respiratory Role

The primary role of the lung in acid–base homeostasis is the excretion of CO_2 and the stabilization of arterial P_{CO_2} at around $40 \, mmHg$. The rate of CO_2 excretion equals alveolar ventilation × alveolar P_{CO_2}. As alveolar P_{CO_2} and arterial P_{CO_2} are virtually identical and in steady state, CO_2 excretion = CO_2 production. Therefore

$$\text{Arterial } P_{CO_2} = \frac{CO_2 \text{ production}}{\text{Alveolar ventilation}}$$

Because the respiratory centre responds rapidly to very small alterations in arterial P_{CO_2}, any change in CO_2 production rate is swiftly followed by appropriate changes in the rate of alveolar ventilation.

Renal Role

The kidney participates in acid–base homeostasis by stabilizing the plasma bicarbonate concentration at 22–26 mmol/l. The basic mechanism is the exchange of a hydrogen ion generated from carbonic acid within the renal tubular cell (see Table 5.1) with a sodium ion in the tubular fluid. The end result depends on the nature of the buffer in the tubular urine at the site of exchange. For every millimole of hydrogen ion excreted in the form of titratable acidity and ammonium, 1 mmol of bicarbonate is added to the plasma. So hydrogen ion excretion is inextricably linked to bicarbonate synthesis. Sufficient bicarbonate is synthesized to back titrate non-bicarbonate buffer acids to bases and to replenish the bicarbonate used up in buffering endogenous hydrogen ion production. In acid–base disorders the kidneys can regulate net hydrogen ion excretion to correct or to

Table 5.1. **Bicarbonate reabsorption and regeneration**

Buffer in tubular lumen accepting H^+	Process		Site
HCO_3^-	Reabsorption of filtered bicarbonate		90% in proximal tubule 10% in distal tubule
HPO_4^- NH_3	Titratable acidity Ammonium formation	Regeneration of bicarbonate	Distal tubule

compensate for any hydrogen ion imbalance in the extracellular fluid. Renal regulation is slow, requiring days to achieve full compensation, but is the only final way of eliminating acid from the body.

ACID–BASE DISORDERS

General Classification

There are four principal acid–base disorders: respiratory acidosis and alkalosis; metabolic acidosis and alkalosis (*Table* 5.2).

Table 5.2. **Simple acid–base disorders**

Disorder	Primary change	Secondary and compensatory change
Respiratory acidosis	P_{CO_2} ↑↑	HCO_3^- ↑
Respiratory alkalosis	P_{CO_2} ↓↓	HCO_3^- ↓
Metabolic acidosis	HCO_3^- ↓↓	P_{CO_2} ↓
Metabolic alkalosis	HCO_3^- ↑↑	P_{CO_2} ↑

Respiratory disorders are initiated by a change in P_{CO_2}. This elicits a buffer and renal response which results in a secondary and compensatory change in plasma bicarbonate which returns the blood pH towards, but not to, normal.

Metabolic disorders are initiated by a change in plasma bicarbonate. This elicits a ventilatory response that results in a secondary and compensatory change in the P_{CO_2} which returns the blood pH towards, but not to, normal.

The compensatory response is not an independent abnormality but an essential and integral part of the whole acid–base disorder. It pursues a characteristic time course and its magnitude is directly proportional to the extent of the initiating disturbance but it fails to restore the blood pH completely to normal.

Acid–base Measurements

Arterial Blood pH

This is the index of overall acid–base state. It normally lies in the range 7·36–7·44, values below 7·36 (acidaemia) indicating the presence of an acidosis either metabolic or respiratory, and values above 7·44 (alkalaemia) indicating the presence of an alkalosis either metabolic or respiratory. The pH range compatible with life is 6·80–7·70, i.e. a H^+ concentration from a half to four times the normal (*Table* 5.3). This is far in excess of the tolerable variation range for sodium and potassium.

Table **5.3. Blood acidity**

pH	$H^+ nmol/l$
6·80	158
7·00	100
7·20	63
7·40	40
7·70	20

Arterial $P\text{CO}_2$

This is an excellent index of the adequacy of alveolar ventilation and is, therefore, the index of the respiratory component of the acid–base equilibrium. The normal range is from 35–45 mmHg. Values below 35 indicate the presence of a primary respiratory alkalosis or the compensatory response to a primary metabolic acidosis. Values above 45 mmHg indicate the presence of a primary respiratory acidosis· or the compensatory response to a primary metabolic alkalosis.

Base Excess and Bicarbonate

Although bicarbonate does vary with the concentration of fixed acid and base, as in metabolic disorders, it is also influenced by the $P\text{CO}_2$ level. In an attempt to circumvent this an index termed the 'base excess' was introduced,[1] which, in vitro, is independent of $P\text{CO}_2$ (*Table* 5.4) but, in vivo, as the $P\text{CO}_2$ rises above 50 mmHg, the base excess value falls due to bicarbonate synthesized within the red cell diffusing into the interstitial fluid (ISF) (*see* Acute respiratory acidosis). Thus both base excess and bicarbonate vary with acute changes in $P\text{CO}_2$. At present two systems are in current use for characterizing the blood acid–base status. In the United States, plasma bicarbonate is used to represent the metabolic component, whereas in Western Europe base excess is generally preferred. Both indices

Table 5.4. **Buffering of carbonic acid in vitro**

Concept of buffer base and base excess

$$Buffer\ acid \rightleftharpoons H^+ + Buffer\ base$$
$$H_2CO_3 \rightleftharpoons H^+ + HCO_3^- \text{ (bicarbonate buffer)}$$
$$HBuffer \rightleftharpoons H^+ + Buffer^- \text{ (non-bicarbonate buffer)}$$

1. With excess or deficit of fixed acid total buffer base falls or rises and hence base excess (observed buffer base − normal buffer base) assumes a negative or positive value

2. $H_2CO_3 + Buffer^- \downarrow \rightarrow HBuffer + HCO_3^- \uparrow$

   but with excess or deficit of H_2CO_3, HCO_3^- and $Buffer^-$ vary reciprocally and hence buffer base and base excess remain unchanged

will be used throughout this text. The reference range for base excess is $0 \pm 2 \cdot 5$ mmol/l and for bicarbonate 22–26 mmol/l. In general terms, low values for the metabolic component indicate the presence of a primary metabolic acidosis or the compensatory response to a primary respiratory alkalosis. High values for the metabolic component indicate the presence of a primary metabolic alkalosis or the compensatory response to a primary respiratory acidosis.

SIMPLE ACID–BASE DISTURBANCES

Metabolic Acidosis

This disorder is initiated by a reduction in the plasma bicarbonate level which can be attributed to:
1. Bicarbonate loss via the gut or kidney, e.g. diarrhoea, fistula, proximal renal tubular acidosis and carbonic anhydrase inhibitors.
2. Increased organic acid production, e.g. ketoacidosis, lactic acidosis and organic acid excess with poisons.
3. Impaired renal excretion of hydrogen ions, e.g. renal failure and distal renal tubular acidosis.
4. Excessive intake of acid (ammonium chloride, the hydrochlorides of lysine or arginine).
   However the final bicarbonate concentration depends, not only on the rate and severity of the acid gain or bicarbonate loss, but also on the renal response to the metabolic acidosis. With normal renal function, after a delay of 2–4 days net hydrogen ion excretion (and hence bicarbonate synthesis) can rise to ten times normal.

Respiratory Compensation

The low blood pH stimulates medullary respiratory centres leading to an increase in alveolar ventilation. This results in a secondary and compensatory fall in the P_{CO_2} which returns the blood pH towards, but not to, normal. This adaptive response takes some 12–24 h to reach a maximum because the blood brain barrier delays the equilibration of bicarbonate between the plasma and cerebral interstitial fluid. Clinical studies have shown that in stable uncomplicated metabolic acidosis the P_{CO_2} is linked to the plasma bicarbonate as follows[2]:

$$P_{CO_2} = 1 \cdot 5 \, [HCO_3^-] + 8 \pm 2$$

If the observed P_{CO_2} falls outside these predicted limits then an independent respiratory acid–base disturbance is present.

The Anion Gap

The metabolic acidotic states are associated with well-defined changes in the plasma electrolyte pattern particularly in chloride and bicarbonate levels which are compared in *Table* 5.5 with those occurring in the other acid–base disturbances. It can be seen that the anion gap[3] i.e. the difference between the concentration of sodium and the sum of chloride and bicarbonate levels, remains unchanged when bicarbonate and chloride vary reciprocally. This occurs in all acid–base disturbances, the only exception being that group of metabolic acidoses associated with excess organic acid production and with renal failure, where the fall in bicarbonate is offset not by the chloride but by the anions of the acid causing the acidosis. The plasma chloride concentration now remains static and it is the anion gap that varies reciprocally with the bicarbonate. Thus metabolic acidosis may be divided into two groups, one characterized by a high and the other by a normal anion gap, and this considerably narrows the diagnostic possibilities (*Table* 5.6).

Clinical Manifestations of Metabolic Acidosis

Hyperventilation may dominate the clinical picture (e.g. the Kussmaul breathing of diabetic coma) and central nervous system symptoms, if present, can range from stupor to coma. Gastrointestinal dysfunction may be manifested in nausea and vomiting, but the most dangerous effects are cardiovascular including depressed cardiac contractility and peripheral vasodilation, changes which may lead to pulmonary hypotension and oedema.

   In metabolic acidosis, the intracellular buffering of hydrogen ions favours movement of potassium from the intra- to the extracellular fluid and thus hyperkalaemia is a fairly common finding particularly if there is associated oliguria. Hyperkalaemia is more likely to complicate the inorganic rather than the organic acidoses and often masks a considerable

Table 5.5. **Plasma chloride, bicarbonate and anion gap in acid–base disorders**

Disorder		Bicarbonate	Chloride	Anion gap	Excess unmeasured anions
Metabolic acidosis	1. Diabetic	↓	NC	↑	Ketones
	2. Lactic acid	↓	NC	↑	Lactate
	3. Renal failure	↓	NC	↑	Sulphate, phosphate
	4. Poisons	↓	NC	↑	Other organic acids
Metabolic acidosis	1. Bicarbonate loss	↓	↑	NC	Nil
	2. HCl gain (NH₄Cl)	↓	↑	NC	Nil
Metabolic alkalosis		↑	↓	NC	Nil
Chronic respiratory acidosis		↑	↓	NC	Nil
Chronic respiratory alkalosis		↓	↑	NC	Nil

Sodium concentration is assumed to remain unchanged throughout.
Chloride and bicarbonate change reciprocally apart from metabolic acidosis with excess organic acids and with renal failure.
NC = No change.

Table 5.6. **Differential diagnosis of metabolic acidosis**

Normal anion gap	*High anion gap*
Bicarbonate loss	Ketoacidosis
A. Gastrointestinal tract	Lactic acidosis
Diarrhoea	Renal failure
Fistulae	Ingestions
Ureteral diversions	Salicylate
	Methyl alcohol
B. Renal	Ethylene glycol
Proximal renal tubular acidosis	
Carbonic anhydrase inhibitors	
Renal	
Early renal failure	
Distal renal tubular acidosis	
Ingestions	
Ammonium chloride	

degree of potassium depletion which only becomes evident when severe hypokalaemia develops during corrective therapy.

Treatment of Acute Metabolic Acidosis

A blood pH less than 7·10 is generally considered to be dangerously low as cardiovascular symptoms are liable to supervene. Clinically this is most likely to be encountered in the organic acidoses (ketoacidosis, lactic acidosis, other organic acids in some types of poisoning). Therapy consists of intravenous infusion of 50 ml 8·4% sodium bicarbonate (50 mmol) over 30 min. The arterial pH should be checked and sodium bicarbonate therapy repeated half-hourly until the blood pH reaches 7·10.[4] On average, a severe ketoacidotic patient will require 100–150 mmol sodium bicarbonate but in lactic acid acidosis the dose can vary from 500 to 2000 mmol.

Complications of Bicarbonate Therapy

Hypernatraemia and volume overload

This can occur in the treatment of severe lactic acidosis when large volumes of hypertonic sodium bicarbonate solution (8·4%) are infused. The hypernatraemia can be avoided by switching to isotonic sodium bicarbonate once the diagnosis is established. The danger of volume overload can be lessened by commencing hourly intravenous diuretic therapy and replacing the urinary losses of sodium chloride and water with intravenous isotonic sodium bicarbonate. If renal function is impaired dialysis may be required.

Hypokalaemia

As acidosis is corrected rapidly, there is intracellular movement of potassium. It is, therefore, essential that potassium be given in adequate amounts during high dose bicarbonate therapy.

Hypocalcaemia

The total serum calcium is low in chronic renal failure. If bicarbonate therapy is excessive there is a danger of tetany as the relative alkalosis will tend to increase protein binding and reduce the ionized calcium fraction.

Alkalosis

There is both a respiratory and metabolic element to the alkalosis that can occur during the repair of an acute organic metabolic acidosis. As bicarbonate steadily rises, respiratory compensation lags behind because of the delay in bicarbonate equilibration between the plasma and the cerebral interstitial fluid. The P_{CO_2} is now inappropriately low for the prevailing bicarbonate level and a respiratory alkalosis therefore develops.

With therapy, the sodium salts of organic acids are oxidized to sodium bicarbonate and, if urinary losses have been minimal, then the plasma bicarbonate will revert completely to normal but if, in addition, sodium bicarbonate has been administered, some may be retained and lead to a metabolic alkalosis.[5] This tendency to alkalosis can be minimized by administering sodium bicarbonate in small doses as recommended above; this is very effective because the plasma bicarbonate concentration is very low in severe acidosis and, as the blood pH is proportional to the ratio of bicarbonate over P_{CO_2}, very small changes in bicarbonate can produce relatively large changes in pH. It is important to discontinue bicarbonate therapy as soon as the blood pH reaches 7·10 allowing further bicarbonate rise to occur from endogenous synthesis from the sodium salts of the organic acid. Finally, attention must be directed towards correction of factors, such as ECF volume contraction and potassium depletion, which by increasing proximal tubular reabsorption of bicarbonate can maintain any existing metabolic alkalotic state.

Paradoxical cerebrospinal fluid pH

Following bicarbonate therapy to ketoacidotic patients, the rise in blood pH depresses ventilation, probably via the peripheral chemoreceptors and the arterial P_{CO_2} rises. CO_2 unlike bicarbonate, diffuses rapidly into the cerebrospinal fluid (CSF) and produces a paradoxical fall in pH which has been held responsible for various cerebral nervous system symptoms.[6] However, it has recently been demonstrated that in ketoacidotic patients, CSF pH falls irrespective of bicarbonate administration and, therefore, the occurrence of so-called paradoxical CSF acidity should not be used as an argument against bicarbonate therapy.[7]

Impairment of tissue oxygenation

In chronic acidosis the Bohr effect facilitates tissue oxygen release, but this is nullified by the suppressive effect of the low concentration of 2,3-diphosphoglycerate. Following bicarbonate therapy, as the pH rises the Bohr effect is immediately reversed but it takes some considerable time for the resynthesis of new 2,3-diphosphoglycerate molecules and it is during this period that tissue oxygenation may be impaired. However, this complication appears to be largely theoretical and there is little concrete evidence that, in clinical practice, it impairs tissue oxygenation.[7]

Management of Chronic Metabolic Acidosis

This is managed in a much more conservative fashion. In chronic renal failure and renal tubular acidosis, where acid production is not increased, alkali is given orally and the daily dose adjusted until plasma bicarbonate reaches the desired level. Oral sodium bicarbonate often leads to gastric discomfort because of evolution of CO_2 and Shohls solution, a mixture of sodium and potassium citrate, is a very acceptable alternative. It should be noted that the alkalizing effects of sodium citrate and sodium lactate are dependent on their metabolic conversion to sodium bicarbonate in the liver, but in severe acidotic states the liver cannot metabolize lactate and its administration, therefore, is contra-indicated in severe acidosis, hypotension and liver failure. Finally, calcium salts cannot be mixed with bicarbonate as precipitation occurs. The only alternative is to use lactate, citrate or acetate.

Metabolic Alkalosis

This disorder is initiated by an elevation in the plasma bicarbonate level and is typically accompanied by a parallel fall in the plasma chloride concentration. Thus all types of metabolic alkalosis have a similar electrolyte pattern which contrasts with metabolic acidosis where the two distinctive electrolyte patterns (normal and high anion gap) often provide considerable diagnostic help.

The underlying pathophysiology is best appreciated if considered in terms of the two key processes involved. First, there must be loss of acid by kidney or gut or gain of exogenous alkali to generate the alkalosis but as the kidney can normally excrete enormous quantities of bicarbonate, up to 1000 mmol/day[8] then clearly, if the alkalosis is to be maintained, the excess bicarbonate must be retained either through reduced glomerular filtration (renal failure) or, more commonly, by increased tubular reabsorption.

The Generation and Maintenance of Metabolic Alkalosis

Gastric alkalosis

The hydrogen ions in gastric juice are derived from intracellular dissociation of carbonic acid. As hydrogen and chloride ions are lost in the vomit, bicarbonate is immediately generated and, as its plasma level rises, that of chloride falls. In a rapidly developing metabolic alkalosis, the increased filtered bicarbonate load temporarily exceeds the reabsorptive capacity of the renal tubules and the urine contains abundant bicarbonate, sodium and potassium but little chloride. Sodium and potassium depletion therefore develop because of the loss of these ions in the vomit and urine (*Fig.* 5.1).

Both ECF volume and potassium status affect bicarbonate reabsorption by the proximal tubule (*Table* 5.7).[9] When the ECF is contracted sodium reabsorption is, of course, increased and this secondarily increases bicarbonate reabsorption. Potassium depletion by increasing intracellular hydrogen ion concentration accelerates sodium/hydrogen ion exchange which also increases bicarbonate reabsorption.

Table **5.7. Factors increasing bicarbonate re-absorption in proximal tubule**

ECF volume contraction
Potassium depletion
Hypercapnia
Hypercalcaemia ⎫
Hypoparathyroidism ⎭ Parathyroid hormone ↓

Note that bicarbonate is not synthesized in proximal tubule so above factors can maintain but not initiate a metabolic alkalosis.

Thus, as vomiting ceases or becomes less severe, the alkalosis is maintained by increased proximal tubular reabsorption of bicarbonate induced by ECF volume contraction and potassium depletion. The bicarbonate diuresis diminishes and sodium and potassium excretion fall. The urine gradually becomes acid as net hydrogen ion excretion rises to

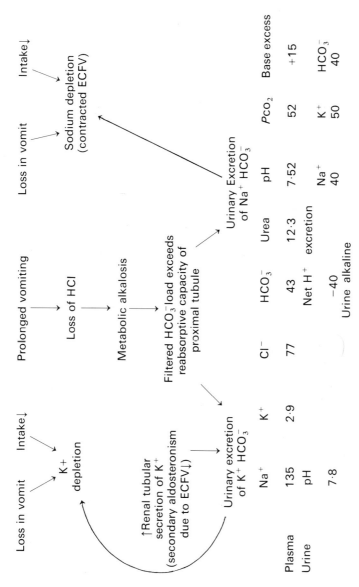

Fig. 5.1. Generation of gastric alkalosis. Schematic representation of the development of alkalosis with sodium and potassium depletion. ECFV = ECF volume. Net H^+ excretion and urine Na^+, K^+ and HCO_3^- were measured in mmol/24 h.

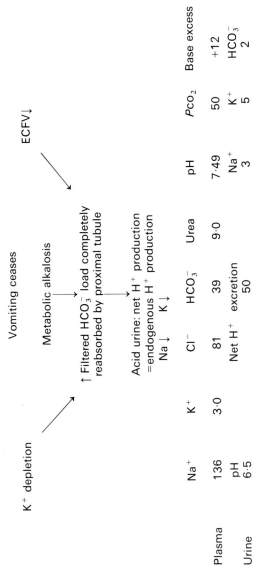

K⁺ depletion

Vomiting ceases

Metabolic alkalosis

ECFV↓

↑ Filtered HCO₃⁻ load completely reabsorbed by proximal tubule

Acid urine: net H⁺ production
=endogenous H⁺ production
Na ↓   K ↓

	Na⁺	K⁺	Cl⁻	HCO₃⁻	Urea	pH	$P\text{CO}_2$	Base excess
Plasma	136	3·0	81	39	9·0	7·49	50	+12
Urine	pH 6·5		Net H⁺ excretion 50			Na⁺ 3	K⁺ 5	HCO₃⁻ 2

Fig. 5.2. Maintenance of gastric alkalosis. An acid urine (paradoxical aciduria) with H⁺ ion excretion equal to endogenous H⁺ ion production, i.e. in external H⁺ ion balance but with an alkaline blood pH. To maintain the alkalosis, the kidney must: (1) reabsorb all filtered bicarbonate (by ECF contraction and K⁺ depletion); (2) excrete all H⁺ ions produced by tissue metabolism. Net H⁺ excretion and urine Na⁺, K⁺ and HCO₃⁻ were measured as mmol/24 h.

balance endogenous hydrogen ion production, thus preventing dissipation of the alkalosis. The patient is now in external hydrogen ion balance with an acid urine (paradoxical aciduria) and an alkaline plasma: a state of chronic stable metabolic alkalosis exists (*Fig.* 5.2).

Renal alkalosis

To generate a renal metabolic alkalosis, net hydrogen ion excretion (titratable acidity + ammonium − bicarbonate) must exceed endogenous hydrogen ion production. This can only occur with a combination of aldosterone excess and potassium depletion which act synergistically to increase distal hydrogen ion secretion. Additional requirements are enhanced ammonia synthesis to accept the newly generated hydrogen ions and increase ammonium production (this occurs in potassium depletion) and an adequate distal delivery of sodium salts so that accelerated exchange with hydrogen can occur (*Table* 5.8).[10]

Table **5.8 Factors increasing net H$^+$ excretion (bicarbonate synthesis) in distal tubule**

Mineralocorticoid excess ⎫
Potassium depletion ⎟
Increased distal sodium delivery ⎬
Increased ammonia synthesis ⎭

Hypercalcaemia ⎫
Hypoparathyroidism ⎬ Parathyroid hormone ↓

These factors can both initiate and maintain a metabolic alkalosis.

Conn's syndrome

This is a classic example of a renal alkalosis. The excess aldosterone leads to increased sodium reabsorption and enhanced potassium excretion. Potassium depletion quickly ensues unless dietary potassium intake is extremely high. Sodium retention occurs and the ECF volume expands but aldosterone escape eventually supervenes with increased distal delivery of sodium salts. Thus the combination of excess aldosterone, potassium depletion, increased ammonia synthesis and increased distal delivery of sodium salts leads to the rate of net urinary hydrogen ion excretion exceeding the rate of endogenous hydrogen ion production and a metabolic alkalosis is, therefore, generated.

The contrasting effects of potassium depletion and ECF volume expansion on the proximal tubule are self-cancelling. The alkalosis is, therefore, maintained by the same distal mechanism which generated it, i.e. increased distal bicarbonate reabsorption from excess aldosterone and potassium depletion.

Diuretic therapy

OEDEMATOUS PATIENTS. Chronic contraction of effective arterial volume leads to secondary aldosteronism. Diuretic therapy increases distal sodium delivery and will aggravate any tendency to potassium depletion. Thus the metabolic alkalosis is generated by a distal mechanism but maintained by increased proximal reabsorption of bicarbonate due to ineffective arterial volume and potassium depletion.

NON-OEDEMATOUS PATIENTS. Diuretic therapy leads to increased distal sodium delivery and sodium depletion may eventually develop with contracted extracellular fluid volume and secondary aldosteronism. Thus as above, the alkalosis is generated by a distal but maintained by a proximal mechanism: contracted ECF volume and potassium depletion.

Exogenous bicarbonate

The kidney has an enormous capacity to deal with excess sodium bicarbonate and can excrete up to 1000 mmol/24 h without appreciable alkalosis developing.[8] The excess sodium ion expands the ECF, proximal tubular reabsorption of bicarbonate is suppressed and a bicarbonate diuresis results.

In renal failure, the reduced glomerular filtration rate (GFR) does not permit excretion of an excessive bicarbonate load.

Sodium bicarbonate is often administered intravenously in the treatment of organic acid acidoses with the subsequent development of a metabolic alkalosis (*see* p. 58). The bicarbonate is retained by increased proximal tubular reabsorption due to a combination of volume and potassium depletion. Attention to these factors should allow a bicarbonate diuresis.

The role of potassium

There is no evidence that pure potassium depletion can increase net hydrogen ion excretion and so generate a metabolic alkalosis.[11] It can only do so in combination with excess aldosterone (renal alkalosis).

It has, however, been shown that potassium depletion can increase proximal tubular reabsorption of bicarbonate and, therefore, assist in maintaining an alkalosis but, in metabolic alkalosis due to vomiting, the potassium depletion (which is generally less than 500 mmol) plays only a minor role in perpetuating the alkalosis as volume repletion with saline without added potassium leads to the complete elimination of the alkalosis. However, cases have been reported where potassium deficits in excess of 1000 mmol have ocurred in the absence of volume depletion and excess aldosterone. Here the alkalosis is refractory to saline and requires potassium repletion for its eradication.[12] So, if of sufficient severity, potassium depletion may itself maintain an alkalosis.

Respiratory Compensation

The high blood pH depresses the respiratory centre and the resulting fall in alveolar ventilation leads to a secondary and compensatory rise in the arterial P_{CO_2} which returns the blood pH towards normal. Because the blood brain barrier delays bicarbonate equilibration between the plasma and cerebral interstitial fluid, a steady state P_{CO_2} level is not attained for some 12–24 hours. The respiratory response is not so predictable as in metabolic acidosis, but in general terms the P_{CO_2} increases by 6 mmHg for each 10 mmol/l rise in bicarbonate[13] with an upper limit of 55–60 mmHg[14] as higher values would lead to increasingly severe hypoxaemia (*see* Alveolar air equation, p. 102).

Clinical Manifestations

Symptoms relate mainly to volume depletion, e.g. postural hypotension and muscle cramps and to potassium depletion, e.g. polyuria, polydipsia and muscle weakness. Alkalotic tetany may occur due to increased protein binding and reduction in the ionized calcium fraction. The plasma potassium is often very low because, in addition to the presence of potassium depletion, the alkalosis leads to intracellular migration of potassium in exchange for hydrogen ions.

Differential Diagnosis and Treatment

As metabolic alkalosis is invariably associated with high plasma bicarbonate and low chloride values, calculation of the anion gap does not help in differential diagnosis, but patients can be divided into two groups depending on their response to administered saline (*Table* 5.9). As a general rule, the saline-responsive group has a contracted ECF volume and a low urinary excretion of sodium and chloride (less than 10 mmol/l), whereas the saline-resistant group has a normal or expanded ECF with a high urinary excretion of sodium and chloride (greater than 20 mmol/l).

Saline responsive

Vomiting, nasogastric suction and diuretics, are the common causes of alkalosis maintained by ECF volume contraction. Exogenous bicarbonate

Table 5.9. **Metabolic alkalosis**

Saline responsive		Saline resistant	
Gastric generation of bicarbonate	Naso-gastric suction Vomiting	Renal generation of bicarbonate	A. Excess mineralocorticoid activity Conn's syndrome Cushing's syndrome Bartter's syndrome Liquorice Carbenoxolone
Renal generation of bicarbonate	Diuretics: no oedema Post hypercapnic		B. Severe potassium depletion C. Diuretics: oedema D. Hypoparathyroidism Hypercalcaemia
Exogenous Bicarbonate	Sodium bicarbonate Sodium lactate citrate Massive blood transfusion	Exogenous bicarbonate	Sodium bicarbonate Sodium lactate citrate Massive blood transfusion

therapy is also included in this category as intravenous sodium bicarbonate or massive blood transfusions are often administered in a clinical situation when accompanying ECF contraction does not permit an appropriate bicarbonate diuresis. Saline administration expands the ECF, the stimulus to sodium reabsorption is removed and excess bicarbonate excreted. Note that the correction of the alkalosis and the hypochloraemia requires the provision of both sodium and chloride ions, sodium to expand the ECF volume and chloride to replenish the accompanying chloride depletion.

Saline resistant

MINERALOCORTICOID EXCESS. This type of alkalosis is generated and maintained by excess aldosterone and potassium depletion. ECF volume is moderately increased, is not stimulating sodium reabsorption and, therefore, the alkalosis does not respond to saline. It can be corrected with massive doses of potassium chloride or by antagonizing the aldosterone excess with aldactone or by the surgical removal of an adrenal tumour where implicated.

SEVERE POTASSIUM DEPLETION. The alkalosis in volume-depleted patients may be resistant to saline in the presence of severe potassium depletion (>1000 mmol). In these cases the plasma potassium is generally less than

$2\cdot0$ mmol/l. As potassium depletion is corrected, sensitivity to saline is restored.

OEDEMATOUS PATIENTS. As already described, patients with congestive cardiac failure, cirrhosis or nephrosis often develop alkalosis due to diuretic therapy. Saline is contra-indicated as it would increase the oedema. Treatment centres around acetazolamide, which corrects both the alkalosis and the oedema, hydrochloric acid or dialysis. Ammonium chloride is contra-indicated as it releases both ammonia and hydrochloric acid. The increased ammonia formation may precipitate hepatic coma and it also results in high blood urea levels.

RENAL FAILURE. Because of the low glomerular filtration rate (GFR), patients in renal failure may develop alkalosis after bicarbonate admini-stration. Saline is obviously contra-indicated and, if treatment is required, it is restricted to hydrochloric acid and/or dialysis.

Respiratory Acidosis

This disorder is initiated by an increase in the arterial $P\text{CO}_2$ which, in turn, can be attributed to alveolar hypoventilation. Some of the commoner causes are listed in *Table* 5.10.

Table **5.10. Causes of respiratory acidosis**

Respiratory centre depression	Drugs: Morphine, barbiturates, anaesthetics
	CNS: Trauma, infections
Neuromuscular disease and rib cage deformity	Myasthenia gravis, poliomyelitis, kyphoscoliosis
Lung disease	Chronic obstructive lung disease
	Severe asthma
	Pulmonary oedema

Compensatory Mechanisms

The resulting fall in blood pH is minimized by a secondary and com-pensatory rise in the plasma bicarbonate concentration. This occurs in two stages the first being related to the blood buffering of carbonic acid, the second to increased bicarbonate synthesis by the kidney (*Table* 5.11).

Table 5.11. **Respiratory acidosis**

		pH	P_{CO_2}	HCO_3^-	Base excess	Na^+	K^+	Cl^-
Start		7·40	40	25	Zero	138	3·9	103
Blood buffering (immediate) Acute respiratory acidosis		7·18	80	29	−5	138	5·2	99
	Compensatory mechanisms							
Renal response (2–4 days to attain steady state) Chronic respiratory acidosis		7·30	80	39	+5	138	4·8	89

Acute respiratory acidosis

$$H_2CO_3 + Buffer^- \quad \rightarrow \quad HBuffer + HCO_3^-$$

(i.e. non-bicarbonate buffer system, mainly haemoglobin)
The non-bicarbonate blood buffers react immediately with the excess carbonic acid. Bicarbonate is generated and its plasma level increases by approximately 1 mmol/l per 10 mmHg rise in P_{CO_2}.[13] Thus even with a P_{CO_2} of 80 mmHg the bicarbonate increment is restricted to 3–4 mmol/l, with an upper limit of 28–30 mmol/l.[15] This contrasts sharply with the very large increase observed in vitro and is attributable to bicarbonate synthesized in the red cells diffusing into the ISF.

Chronic respiratory acidosis

Following the acute stage of hydrogen ion buffering, the bicarbonate level remains unchanged for a few hours until renal compensation gets underway and results in a further gradual rise in the plasma bicarbonate concentration. This is due to the high P_{CO_2} accelerating distal sodium hydrogen exchange and increasing the net hydrogen ion excretion (mainly in the form of ammonium) above that of endogenous hydrogen ion production. New bicarbonate is, therefore, synthesized. The rate of bicarbonate reabsorption in both proximal and distal tubules is also increased during hypercapnia and this ensures that all the newly generated bicarbonate is retained. This process takes some 2–4 days to reach a maximum when a state of chronic stable respiratory acidosis is said to exist. The plasma bicarbonate increases by approximately $3 \cdot 5$ mmol/l per 10 mmHg rise in P_{CO_2}[13] with an upper limit of 45 mmol/l.[16] As the plasma bicarbonate rises chloride falls due to the enhanced renal excretion of chloride mainly in the form of the ammonium salt.

Symptoms

Clinical manifestations appear to be related to the increase in intracranial pressure which is due to the cerebral vasodilating effect of an increased P_{CO_2} and range from stupor and confusion to coma. Papilloedema may also be present. When breathing room air, hypercapnia is invariably associated with a fall in alveolar and arterial P_{O_2} and hypoxic symptoms many well be super-added.

Treatment

The treatment is that of the underlying illness accompanied by efforts to improve alveolar ventilation. Two avoidable complications can occur in the treatment of respiratory acidosis associated with chronic obstructive airways disease.

If the patient is hypoxic, controlled oxygen therapy must be given (28% oxygen) otherwise there is a danger of CO_2 narcosis due to a reduction in the hypoxic drive.

Again, if assisted ventilation is contemplated, the P_{CO_2} must be reduced slowly. If not, a post-hypercapnic metabolic alkalosis ensues with central nervous system symptoms, such as confusion and convulsions due to the rapid development of a CSF alkalosis. Even in the presence of normal ECF volume and potassium status it takes 1–2 days for the resulting alkaline diuresis to normalize the plasma bicarbonate level.

Respiratory Alkalosis

This disorder is initiated by a decrease in the arterial P_{CO_2} which in turn can be attributed to alveolar hyperventilation. Some common causes are detailed in *Table* 5.12.

Compensatory Mechanisms

The resulting increase in blood pH is ameliorated by a secondary adaptive reduction in the plasma bicarbonate concentration. Again this occurs in

Table 5.12. Causes of respiratory alkalosis

| Respiratory centre stimulation: | Anxiety, hysteria
Metabolic: Liver failure, Gram-negative sepsis, salicylate, fever
CNS: Vascular, trauma, infections, neoplasia
Hypoxia |
| Intrathoracic processes: | Pneumonia
Asthma
Pulmonary emboli
Congestive cardiac failure } In absence of hypoxaemia |

two steps, the first being related to the immediate response of the blood buffers to carbonic acid reduction, the second to the more prolonged response of the renal compensatory mechanisms (*Table* 5.13).

Acute respiratory alkalosis

$$HCO_3^- + HBuffer \quad \rightarrow \quad H_2CO_3 + Buffer^-$$

(i.e. non-bicarbonate buffer system, mainly haemoglobin)
As P_{CO_2} falls, the non-bicarbonate buffer system reacts immediately by consuming bicarbonate, the plasma concentration falling by approximately 2·5 mmol/l for each 10 mmHg decrease in P_{CO_2}.[13] The decrement is restricted to 3–4 mmol/l with a lower limit of 18–20 mmol/l.[17]

Table 5.13. Respiratory alkalosis

		pH	P_{CO_2}	HCO_3^-	*Base excess*	Na^+	K^+	Cl^-
Start		7·40	40	25	Zero	138	3·9	103
Blood buffering (immediate) Acute respiratory alkalosis	} Compensatory mechanisms	7·63	20	21	+4	138	3·0	107
Renal response (2–4 days to attain steady state) Chronic respiratory alkalosis		7·49	20	15	−4	138	3·3	113

Chronic respiratory alkalosis

The bicarbonate level remains stable for several hours, then a further fall occurs as the renal adaptive mechanism comes into action. This is mediated by the low $P\text{CO}_2$ which suppresses distal sodium hydrogen ion exchange and thus the rate of net hydrogen ion excretion diminishes. Eventually both ammonium and titratable acidity production fall to zero and no bicarbonate is synthesized. The tubular reabsorption of bicarbonate is also decreased by the low $P\text{CO}_2$ level, hence bicarbonate is lost in the urine and the plasma level falls by approximately 5 mmol/l for each 10 mmHg decrease in the $P\text{CO}_2$, with a lower limit of 15 mmol/l.[13] This renal response is complete within 2–4 days. It should be noted that this is the only acid–base disturbance where the compensatory mechanism can return the pH completely to normal.

Symptoms

Symptoms occur predominantly in the acute rather than the chronic type of respiratory alkalosis and are obviously related to its associated alkalaemia. Paraesthesia of the extremities and circum-oral area and carpopedal spasm are fairly frequently encountered. In addition, central nervous system symptoms, such as light-headedness and states of altered consciousness, are not uncommon and may be due to the decrease in cerebral blood flow which accompanies hypocapnia.

Treatment

This should be directed towards the underlying cause. In hysterical hyperventilation rebreathing into a paper bag may be effective and relieve the symptoms by raising the $P\text{CO}_2$.

RESPIRATORY FAILURE

Acid–base disturbances are a common feature of respiratory failure. The primary function of the respiratory system is to maintain optimal levels of oxygen and carbon dioxide in the arterial blood ($P\text{O}_2$ 80–100 mmHg; $P\text{CO}_2$ 35–45 mmHg) and this is achieved by the integration of two key processes, ventilation and gas exchange. Impairment of either may lead to frank respiratory failure which is defined as an arterial $P\text{O}_2$ <60 mmHg in a patient breathing air at rest. The arterial $P\text{CO}_2$ may be normal, low or high.[18]

Alveolar Ventilation

Alveolar P_{CO_2}

This is related to the rate of alveolar ventilation and to the metabolic rate.

$$\text{Alveolar } P_{CO_2} = \frac{CO_2 \text{ produced}}{\text{Alveolar ventilation}}$$

Alveolar P_{O_2}

This depends on the rate of alveolar ventilation, the metabolic rate and the inspired oxygen concentration. These relationships are best expressed in the *alveolar air equation.*

$$\text{Alveolar } P_{O_2} = \text{Inspired } P_{O_2} - \frac{\text{Arterial } P_{CO_2}}{0.8}$$

$$= \text{Inspired } P_{O_2} - (1.25 \times \text{Arterial } P_{CO_2})$$

It follows that in alveolar hypoventilation as alveolar and arterial P_{CO_2} rise, alveolar and arterial P_{O_2} must fall. Ventilatory failure is, therefore, characterized by a reduction in arterial P_{O_2} and an increase in arterial P_{CO_2}.

The assessment of alveolar ventilation

Arterial P_{CO_2} is the criterion of the adequacy of alveolar ventilation.

Gas Exchange

This is the matching of ventilation with perfusion. The key to effective gas exchange is the ventilation perfusion ratio (V/Q) of the individual alveoli. Exchange is optimal when the ratio is 0.8. Diffuse lung disease is invariably associated with the presence of both low and high ratios which interfere with the exchange of both oxygen and carbon dioxide. The areas of low V/Q are perfused with a large volume of pulmonary capillary blood whose gas composition approximates to mixed venous blood, i.e. a low P_{O_2} (approximately 40 mmHg) and high P_{CO_2} (approximately 45 mmHg). This mixes in the systemic circulation with (1) an extremely small volume of blood with high P_{O_2} and low P_{CO_2} from the high ratio areas and (2) blood of normal gas content from the unaffected areas of the lung.

The meagre volume of blood that issues from the high V/Q areas makes little impact on the gas concentrations in the mixed systemic blood whose gas values are dictated mainly by the composition and contribution from the low ratio areas. Therefore, in mixed systemic arterial blood, the Po_2 is low and the Pco_2 high.

The high systemic Pco_2 then stimulates the central chemoreceptors. Total ventilation is increased and is distributed as follows:
1. To the high V/Q areas where it serves no useful purpose and merely increases dead space ventilation.
2. No distribution to the low V/Q areas where lung disease prohibits air entry.
3. To the unaffected areas of the lung where the arterial Po_2 is increased and the arterial Pco_2 is decreased. The relatively straight shape of the CO_2 dissociation curve in the physiological range allows the low arterial Pco_2 to be accompanied by a parallel reduction in CO_2 content which is sufficient to offset the CO_2 retention of the low ratio areas, but a similar compensation cannot occur for the hypoxaemia because the flat top to the oxyhaemoglobin dissociation curve only permits the elevated Po_2 to be accompanied by a trivial increase in the oxygen content.

Therefore, in gas exchange failure due to ventilation perfusion imbalance, the arterial Po_2 is reduced and the arterial Pco_2 is normal or low.

The assessment of gas exchange

This is assessed by measurement of the alveolar–arterial Po_2 difference (normal $< 20\,\text{mmHg}$). The arterial Po_2 and Pco_2 are measured from an arterial blood sample and alveolar Po_2 is calculated from the alveolar air equation.

The development of respiratory failure in lung disease

Generally hyperventilation reduces the Pco_2 and the blood gas pattern is that of hypoxaemia with normal or low Pco_2. This is encountered clinically in pneumonia, pulmonary oedema, pulmonary fibrosis, contusion, asthma, emphysema, myocardial infarction and shock. These are undoubtedly the commonest causes of hypoxaemia in clinical practice (*see Table* 5.14).[19]

If lung disease is chronic and progressive and perhaps exacerbated by acute infection, increasing V/Q mismatch occurs. Moreover, the energy demands of increased ventilation are so high that eventually a compromise is reached and the Pco_2 is allowed to rise. This manoeuvre allows the same volume of CO_2 to be excreted (CO_2 balance is maintained) and can be regarded as a compensatory mechanism though a highly perilous one, as

Table **5.14. The development of respiratory failure in lung disease**

	Progressive lung disease leads to increasing V/Q mismatch with slight rise in P_{CO_2} but large fall in P_{O_2}		*High P_{CO_2} stimulates chemoreceptors, Hyperventilation restores P_{CO_2} but not P_{O_2} to normal*
pH	7·40	7·37	7·40
P_{CO_2} (mmHg)	40	48	40
P_{O_2} (mmHg)	95 $\longrightarrow$	40 $\longrightarrow$	50
Bicarbonate (mmol/l)	25	28	25
Base excess (mmol/l)	Zero	+1	Zero
	Normal	Hypoxaemia with high P_{CO_2}	Hypoxaemia with normal P_{CO_2}

hypoxaemia is intensified and there is increased risk of CO_2 narcosis and respiratory acidosis.

The classification of respiratory failure in *Table* 5.15 is based on the two characteristic arterial blood gas patterns and on the alveolar–arterial P_{O_2} difference.

Table **5.15. Classification of respiratory failure**

Type of respiratory failure	*Lung disease*	*Arterial gases*	*Alveolar–arterial P_{O_2} difference mmHg*
Gas exchange	Present	$P_{O_2} \downarrow$ P_{CO_2} N or $\downarrow$	>20
Ventilatory ——— Present		$P_{O_2} \downarrow\downarrow P_{CO_2} \uparrow$	>20
Absent		$P_{O_2} \downarrow$ $P_{CO_2} \uparrow$	<20
	a. Respiratory centre depression		
	b. Neuromuscular disease		
	c. Rib cage deformity		

A simple clinical approach to patients with lung disease is to assess their respiratory function in terms of ventilation and gas exchange. This merely requires a blood gas estimation, knowledge of the inspired oxygen concentration, and calculation of the alveolar P_{O_2} from the alveolar air equation. Some representative clinical samples will now be discussed.

Clinical Examples of Respiratory Failure

Hypoxaemia with normal P_{CO_2}

This occurs in emphysema, pneumonia, pulmonary oedema, etc.

Arterial blood gases breathing air:

pH	HCO$_3^-$	Base excess	Po_2	Pco_2
7·47	24	+1	35	32

$$\text{Alveolar } Po_2 = \text{Inspired } Po_2 - (1·25 \times \text{Arterial } Pco_2)$$
$$= 150 - 40$$
$$= 110$$

As Arterial $Po_2 = 35$
Then Alveolar–arterial Po_2 difference $= 75\,\text{mmHg}$

TREATMENT. Respiratory control is normal in these patients and oxygen therapy will not result in alveolar hypoventilation. Oxygen may therefore be given in any concentration necessary to achieve a satisfactory arterial Po_2.

Hypoxaemia with raised Pco_2

This occurs typically in an acute exacerbation of chronic bronchitis where progressive lung disease has led to both V/Q mismatch and ventilatory failure.
Arterial blood gases breathing air:

pH	HCO$_3^-$	Base excess	Po_2	Pco_2
7·20	31	−2	20	80

$$\text{Alveolar } Po_2 = \text{Inspired } Po_2 - (1·25 \times \text{Arterial } Pco_2)$$
$$= 150 - 100$$
$$= 50$$

As Arterial $Po_2 = 20$
Then Alveolar–arterial Po_2 difference $= 30\,\text{mmHg}$
   When breathing air the arterial Pco_2 rarely exceeds 80 mmHg as higher Pco_2 levels would obviously lead to fatal hypoxaemia (arterial $Po_2 < 20\,\text{mmHg}$). Death therefore occurs from hypoxia, not from CO_2 narcosis or respiratory acidosis.

TREATMENT. Therapy with high concentrations of oxygen often results in the following blood gas values:

	pH	HCO$_3^-$	Base excess	Po_2	Pco_2
Start	7·20	31	−2	20	80
Finish	7·10	37	−2	60	120

   In these patients the respiratory drive stems principally from hypoxia, not from CO_2, and thus the relief of hypoxaemia with high inspired oxygen concentration leads to a further fall in alveolar ventilation with arterial P_{CO_2} rising to narcotic levels and the development of a severe respiratory acidosis.

INTERMITTENT OXYGEN THERAPY. Arterial blood gases breathing 50% oxygen: P_{O_2} 60 mmHg; P_{CO_2} 120 mmHg,

$$\text{Alveolar } P_{O_2} = \text{Inspired } P_{O_2} - (1.25 \times \text{Arterial } P_{CO_2})$$
$$= 355 - 150$$
$$= 205$$

As Arterial $P_{O_2} = 60$
Then Alveolar–arterial P_{O_2} difference $= 145$ mmHg
   If oxygen therapy is misguidedly discontinued then the arterial P_{CO_2} still remains at 120 mmHg but the inspired P_{O_2} falls to 150 mmHg.

$$\text{Alveolar } P_{O_2} = \text{Inspired } P_{O_2} - (1.25 \times \text{Arterial } P_{CO_2})$$
$$= 150 - 150$$
$$= 0$$

The patient must possess considerable powers of hyperventilation to blow off CO_2 and so raise alveolar P_{O_2} to obtain a viable arterial P_{O_2}. Oxygen therapy if commenced must NOT be discontinued in acute phase of illness particularly if arterial P_{CO_2} is very high.

CONTROLLED OXYGEN THERAPY—28% OXYGEN. As the patient's arterial P_{O_2} lies on the steep part of the oxyhaemoglobin dissociation curve a very small rise in P_{O_2} will result in a relatively large increase in oxygen content. Thus controlled oxygen therapy permits an acceptable rise in P_{O_2} to be attained without the P_{CO_2} rising to narcotic levels.[20]
   Arterial blood gases breathing 28% oxygen:

	P_{O_2}	P_{CO_2}	
Start	20	80	Best response
Finish	40	80	

$$\text{Alveolar } P_{O_2} = \text{Inspired } P_{O_2} - (1.25 \times \text{Arterial } P_{CO_2})$$
$$= 200 - 100$$
$$= 100$$

As Arterial $P_{O_2} = 40$
Then Alveolar–arterial P_{O_2} difference $= 60$ mmHg
   Twenty-eight per cent oxygen increases the inspired P_{O_2} by 50 mmHg (200–150).
   However, because of the accompanying failure in gas exchange the maximum increment in arterial P_{O_2}, ventilation remaining unchanged, is only of the order of 20 mmHg.

Arterial blood gases breathing 28% oxygen:

	P_{O_2}	P_{CO_2}	
Start	20	80 ⎫	Worst response
Finish	20	96 ⎭	

$$\text{Alveolar } P_{O_2} = \text{Inspired } P_{O_2} - (1\cdot25 \times \text{Arterial } P_{CO_2})$$

$$= 200 - 120$$

$$= 80$$

An Arterial $P_{O_2} = 20$,

Then Alveolar–arterial P_{O_2} difference $= 60\,\text{mmHg}$

At worst the patient hypoventilates because of reduction in hypoxic drive and the arterial P_{CO_2} keeps rising until the arterial P_{O_2} falls back to its starting level of 20 mmHg and the hypoxic drive to ventilation is restored. Note, however, that the rise in the arterial P_{CO_2} is limited and will not cause CO_2 narcosis nor greatly intensify the respiratory acidosis.

The respiratory centre generally retains some sensitivity to CO_2. It is not working solely on an hypoxic drive. It is, therefore, uncommon for the P_{CO_2} to rise to the theoretical limits and the usual response lies somewhere between these two extremes, e.g. $P_{O_2} = 30\,\text{mmHg}$; $P_{CO_2} = 88\,\text{mmHg}$ where the P_{O_2} increment is sufficient to relieve the hypoxia.

MIXED ACID–BASE DISORDERS

In the intensive care unit cardiac, renal, liver and respiratory failure are relatively common. Sepsis and shock are frequently encountered. Diuretics, blood and intravenous bicarbonate are regularly administered. Contracted and expanded ECF volume, hypo- and hypercapnia and hypo- and hyperkalaemia are everyday occurrences. All these factors can induce, exacerbate, modify or maintain acid–base disturbances. Therefore, it is not surprising that mixed acid–base disorders[13,21] are the rule rather than the exception. Correct interpretation of their development is mandatory as it can have a considerable bearing on diagnosis and therapy. This can only be achieved by careful appraisal of the clinical history, the therapy and drugs already administered, physical examination and laboratory findings. With regard to the latter, particular attention should be paid to the values for plasma chloride, bicarbonate and the anion gap (*Table* 5.5), to plasma potassium as an approximate index of plasma pH and, finally, to a consideration of the acid–base indices themselves. Knowledge of other non-electrolyte chemistries, such as glucose or ketones, is also, invaluable.

A mixed acid–base disturbance is defined as the coexistence of two or more simple acid–base disturbances. Partically every conceivable combination may occur but some of the commoner ones will now be discussed

Table 5.16. Compensatory responses for simple acid–base disorders

Disorder	Component affected	Mechanism	Time to steady state	Predicted value	Limits of compensation
Metabolic acidosis	P_{CO_2}	Respiratory hyperventilation	12–24 h	$1 \cdot 5 (HCO_3^-) + 8 \pm 2$	10 mmHg
Metabolic alkalosis	P_{CO_2}	Respiratory hypoventilation	12–24 h	Increases 6 mmHg for each 10 mmol/l rise in HCO_3^-	55–60 mmHg
Acute respiratory acidosis	HCO_3^-	Non-HCO_3^- Blood buffer	Immediate	Increase of 3–4 mmol	28–30 mmol/l
Chronic respiratory acidosis	HCO_3^-	Renal Net H^+ excretion ↑	2–4 days	Increases by $3 \cdot 5$ mmol/l for each 10 mmHg rise in P_{CO_2}	45 mmol/l
Acute respiratory alkalosis	HCO_3^-	Non-HCO_3^- Blood buffer	Immediate	Decrease of 3–4 mmol/l	18–20 mmol/l
Chronic respiratory alkalosis	HCO_3^-	Renal Net H^+ excretion ↓	2–4 days	Falls by 5 mmol/l for each 10 mmHg fall in P_{CO_2}	15 mmol/l

briefly stressing that the key to the unravelling of these complex disorders lies in knowledge of the magnitude, limits and time course of the compensatory responses that occur in simple acid–base disturbances. These are listed in *Table* 5.16.

Metabolic Acidosis and Respiratory Acidosis

In this situation three distinct blood gas patterns are encountered. Note that CO_2 retention prevents respiratory compensation for the metabolic acidosis and the metabolic disturbance prevents renal compensation for the respiratory acidosis. In *Table* 5.17 under (*A*) as P_{CO_2} is high and

Table **5.17. Metabolic acidosis and respiratory acidosis**

	A	B	C
pH	7·04	7·19	7·25
P_{CO_2}, mmHg	65	40	65
Bicarbonate, mmol/l	17	15	28
Base excess, mmol/l	−19	−14	−3

bicarbonate and base excess low, the diagnosis of a mixed disturbance is self-evident. Under (*B*) in a simple metabolic acidosis with a bicarbonate value of 15 mmol/l, a P_{CO_2} of 40 mmHg is inappropriately high as the predicted value is 30 ± 2 mmHg. A superimposed respiratory acidosis is, therefore, present. Under (*C*) in a simple chronic respiratory acidosis, with a P_{CO_2} of 65 mmHg, a plasma bicarbonate of 28 mmol/l is inappropriately low as the predicted value is 33 mmol/l, and a superimposed metabolic acidosis is, therefore, present. These combinations are frequently encountered in cardiopulmonary arrest, pulmonary oedema, drug overdose, and in chronic obstructive airways disease. In cardiopulmonary arrest simultaneous failure of ventilation and tissue perfusion lead to CO_2 retention and lactic acidosis.

In pulmonary oedema, as the disease advances, ventilation fails and P_{CO_2} rises. The lactic acidosis is due to poor tissue perfusion from the accompanying left heart failure. In drug overdose respiratory centre depression results in elevated P_{CO_2} levels. The lactic acidosis arises from the direct effect of the drug on intermediary metabolism or from circulatory collapse which is a common finding in severe intoxications. In chronic obstructive lung disease an acute exacerbation of the illness often leads to acute hypoxia with the development of lactic acidosis.

Metabolic Acidosis and Respiratory Alkalosis

Table 5.18 lists typical figures. In a simple metabolic acidosis with a bicarbonate value of 13 mmol/l, the predicted P_{CO_2} is 28 ± 2 mmHg. Thus the observed value of 22 mmHg denotes the presence of an independent respiratory alkalosis. This disturbance is met in salicylate intoxication where toxic levels of salicylate directly stimulate the respiratory centre. The metabolic acidosis is due to the uncoupling of oxidative phosphorylation with lactic acid production. In septic shock the metabolic acidosis is due to excess lactic acid production and the respiratory alkalosis to direct stimulation of the respiratory centre by bacterial endotoxins.

Table 5.18. Metabolic acidosis and respiratory alkalosis

pH	7·39
P_{CO_2}, mmHg	22
Bicarbonate, mmol/l	13
Base excess, mmol/l	−9

Metabolic Alkalosis and Respiratory Acidosis

Representative values are listed in *Table* 5.19.
1. In a simple metabolic alkalosis a P_{CO_2} of 65 mmHg is inappropriately high as the P_{CO_2} rise is generally limited to 55–60 mmHg. A superimposed respiratory acidosis is, therefore, present.
2. In a simple chronic respiratory acidosis with a P_{CO_2} of 65 mmHg the predicted bicarbonate is 33 mmol/l. Thus the observed value of 50 mmol/l denotes the presence of an independent metabolic alkalosis. This mixture is encountered in chronic obstructive pulmonary disease where excessive diuretic therapy often results in a metabolic alkalosis. This must be treated with volume, chloride and potassium to ensure an adequate bicarbonate diuresis, otherwise the high blood pH will result in further respiratory depression.

Table 5.19. Metabolic alkalosis and respiratory acidosis

pH	7·48
P_{CO_2}, mmHg	65
Bicarbonate, mmol/l	50
Base excess, mmol/l	+18

To avoid the complication of post-hypercapnic metabolic alkalosis, the P_{CO_2} should be lowered slowly during mechanical ventilation and ECF volume and potassium status normalized to allow the kidney to excrete bicarbonate appropriately.

Metabolic Alkalosis and Respiratory Alkalosis

With this combined disturbance, three distinct blood gas patterns are frequently encountered. Note that the metabolic process prevents compensation for the respiratory alkalosis and hyperventilation prevents compensation for the metabolic alkalosis. In *Table* 5.20, under (*A*), as

Table **5.20. Metabolic alkalosis and respiratory alkalosis**

	A	B	C
pH	7·68	7·55	7·55
P_{CO_2}, mmHg	26	40	25
Bicarbonate, mmol/l	32	36	22
Base excess, mmol/l	+11	+11	+2

P_{CO_2} is low and bicarbonate and base excess high, the diagnosis of a mixed disturbance is obvious. Under (*B*) in a simple metabolic alkalosis with a bicarbonate of 36 mmol/l a P_{CO_2} of 40 mmHg is inappropriately low as the predicted value is 47 mmHg. Thus a superimposed respiratory alkalosis is present. Under (*C*) in a simple chronic respiratory alkalosis with P_{CO_2} of 25 mmHg the predicted bicarbonate is 17 mmol/l. Thus the observed value of 22 mmol/l denotes the presence of an independent metabolic alkalosis.

This combination is encountered in two situations:

1. In hepatic failure diuretic therapy often leads to a metabolic alkalosis. Respiratory alkalosis is common in liver disease and is generally attributed to respiratory stimulation by excess ammonium ions or to hypoxaemia from disturbed ventilation perfusion relationships.

2. In massive blood transfusion sodium citrate used as an anticoagulant in stored blood is oxidized in the body to sodium bicarbonate. This can generally be excreted quite readily but some patients develop metabolic alkalosis. This can be due to a low GFR (acute or chronic renal failure) or to factors such as ECF volume contraction or potassium depletion which retain bicarbonate by increasing its reabsorption in the proximal tubule.

In such critically ill patients, respiratory alkalosis is commonly encountered in association with excessive mechanical ventilation, hypoxaemia, hypotension and sepsis.

Metabolic Acidosis and Metabolic Alkalosis

The two different patterns which are encountered are listed in *Table* 5.21. They occur in the following clinical settings.

I. Normal Anion Gap—Diarrhoea and Vomiting

The metabolic acidosis occurring with diarrhoea is of the normal anion gap variety. Hence when vomiting ensues the resulting electrolytes and blood gas values are as depicted in *Table* 5.21 under (*A*).

II. High Anion Gap Acidoses

1. Chronic renal failure and vomiting.
2. Vomiting with lactic acid acidosis.
3. Treatment of high anion gap acidosis with sodium bicarbonate.

As the acidoses are of the high anion gap variety the resulting electrolyte and blood gas values are as depicted in *Table* 5.21 under (*B*). Note that a high anion gap with a relatively normal bicarbonate should always arouse suspicion of a mixed metabolic acidosis and metabolic alkalosis.[3] In this mixed disorder the final pH depends, of course, on the intensity of each individual disturbance. For simplicity in the examples shown, acidosis and alkalosis precisely neutralize each other.

Table **5.21. Metabolic acidosis and metabolic alkalosis**

	Sodium mmol/l	Potassium mmol/l	Chloride mmol/l	Bicarbonate mmol/l	Anion gap	pH	P_{CO_2} mmHg	Base excess mmol/l
A	138	3·0	103	25	10	7·40	40	Zero
B	138	3·0	88	25	25	7·40	40	Zero

REFERENCES

1. Siggaard-Anderson O. (1963) The acid base status of the blood. *Scand. J. Clin. Lab. Invest.* [Suppl.] **15**, 70.
2. Albert M. D., Dell R. B. and Winters R. W. (1967) Quantitative displacement of acid base equilibrium in metabolic acidosis. *Ann. Intern. Med.* **66**, 312.
3. Emmett M. and Narins R. G. (1977) Clinical use of the anion gap. *Medicine* **56**, 38.
4. Ireland J. T., Thomson W. S. T. and Williamson J. (1980) *Diabetes Today*, p. 102. London, H. M. & M. Publishers Ltd.
5. Addis G. J., Thomson W. S. T. and Welch J. D. (1964) Bicarbonate therapy in diabetic acidosis. *Lancet* **2**, 223.
6. Posner J. B. and Plum F. (1967) Spinal fluid pH and neurologic symptoms in systemic acidosis. *N. Engl. J. Med.* **277**, 605.
7. Narins R. G. and Gardner L. B. (1981) Simple acid base disturbances. *Med. Clin. North Am.* **65**, 321.
8. Van Goidsenhoven G., Gray O. V., Price A. V. et al. (1954) The effect of prolonged administration of large doses of sodium bicarbonate in man. *Clin. Sci.* **13**, 383.

9. O'Connor G. and Kunau R. T. (1978) Renal transport of hydrogen and potassium. In: Brenner B. M. and Stein J. H., ed., *Acid Base and Potassium Homeostasis*, p. 1. New York, Churchill Livingstone.

10. Seldin D. W. and Rector F. C. (1972) The generation and maintenance of metabolic alkalosis. *Kidney Int.* **1**, 306.

11. Sebastian A., Hulter H. N. and Rector F. C. (1978) Metabolic alkalosis. In: Brenner B. M. and Stein J. M., ed., *Acid Base and Potassium Homeostasis*, p. 101. New York, Churchill Livingstone.

12. Garella S., Chazan J. A. and Cohen J. J. (1970) Saline-resistant metabolic alkalosis or 'chloride-wasting nephropathy'. *Ann. Intern. Med.* **73**, 31.

13. Narins R. G. and Emmett M. (1980) Simple and mixed acid base disorders: a practical approach. *Medicine* **59**, 161.

14. Elkington J. R. (1966) Clinical disorders of acid base regulation: a survey of seventeen years of diagnostic experience. *Med. Clin. North Am.* **50**, 1325.

15. Brackett N. C., Cohen J. J. and Schwartz W. B. (1965) Carbon dioxide titration curve of normal man; effect of increasing degrees of acute hypercapnia on acid base equilibrium. *N. Engl. J. Med.* **272**, 6.

16. Schwartz W. B., Brackett N. C. and Cohen J. J. (1965) The response of extracellular hydrogen ion concentration to graded degrees of chronic hypercapnia. The physiological limits of the defense of pH. *J. Clin. Invest.* **44**, 291.

17. Arbus G. S., Herbert L. A., Levesque P. R. et al. (1969) Characterisation and clinical application of the 'significance band' for acute respiratory alkalosis. *N. Engl. J. Med.* **280**, 117.

18. Campbell E. J. M. (1965) Respiratory failure. *Br. Med. J.* **1**, 1451.

19. West J. B. (1977) *Pulmonary Pathophysiology*, p. 36. Baltimore, Williams & Wilkins Company.

20. Sykes M. K., McNicol M. W. and Campbell E. J. M. (1976) *Respiratory Failure*, p.127. Oxford, Blackwell Scientific.

21. Bia M. and Thier S. O. (1981) Mixed acid base disturbances: a clinical approach. *Med. Clin. North Am.* **65**, 347.

Chapter 6

Fluid Therapy of Surgical Patients

J. M. Kinney and J. Askanazi

The evolution of fluid therapy of surgical patients to a large degree reflects changing attitudes towards the handling of sodium in injury. Attention has shifted from plasma and the renal handling of salt and water to the extracellular space and the overall behaviour of sodium. This change in attitude has resulted in marked changes in fluid therapy of acute surgical patients. Isotonic saline, which once was felt to be contra-indicated in the immediate postoperative period, is now regarded as being essential. However, it is clear that excesses can result in complications.

Essential to proper fluid therapy is an understanding of body composition and of the changes which occur in injury. The abnormal body composition of the injured patient after resuscitation is the result of the therapy superimposed upon the body's response to the injury. The daily fluid and electrolyte therapy for such a patient will be the sum of normal requirements and additional needs, which are associated with the particular stage of convalescence after injury.

This review will focus on the fluid therapy of the injured adult surgical patient. For the purpose of this discussion the unique problems of the patient with a major burn will not be considered.

NORMAL BODY COMPOSITION

The adult body is composed of three functional components: body fat, the body cell mass and the extracellular supporting structures. The amount of each varies as a function of age, sex and body size.

Total body water (TBW) is the largest single component of body weight, being greatest in the young muscular adult male (over 60%) and least in the elderly obese female (under 45%).[1] In general, total body water is

114

considered to be distributed into two major fluid spaces: Intracellular fluid (ICF) consisting of 25–30% of average body weight and extracellular fluid (ECF) consisting of 20–25% of normal body weight.

The body content of electrolytes is generally discussed in terms of their exchangeable components, when measured with an isotope dilution technique. Body stores of potassium can be measured by whole body counting of the naturally occurring isotope. Neutron activation has recently been used[2] to measure many tissue components. Minerals which are incorporated into bone, collagen and connective tissue exchange very slowly with plasma and generally are not considered in determining the composition of parenteral fluid therapy needed to achieve daily balance.

The total exchangeable potassium can be considered as equivalent to the body stores of potassium for clinical purposes. The healthy adult male (70 kg) will have a pool of exchangeable potassium of 2700–3400 mmol, while the range for the adult female is 2100–2300 mmol. The major fraction of this pool is intracellular, the small extracellular portion approximating 1–2% of the total.

In contrast to potassium, exchangeable sodium is only 65% of total body sodium. Males contain approximately 2800 mmol (70 kg), while females contain approximately 2600 mmol.[1] The fraction of sodium in the skeleton is only slowly exchangeable.[3] The normal 70-kg adult male contains approximately 2100 mmol of chloride.[1]

NORMAL DAILY BALANCE

Water

The daily amount of water and dilute liquids required by the normal individual varies widely with habit and climate, but in temperate climates the average adult exchanges 2500–4500 ml of water daily with a body pool of 25–45 l. Fluid intake averages 1000–2500 ml/day. Water in foods averages 1000–1500 ml. Water of oxidation adds 200–400 ml/day.

Losses take place by four different routes: urinary output, the water content of stool, and evaporation from the respiratory tract and from the skin. The latter two are termed, 'insensible losses'. In the normal individual, water intake and losses balance each other very closely. Daily body weight usually fluctuates by less that 2%, and often by less than 1% if measured at the same time of day. Insensible losses depend on body size, physical exertion, environmental temperature and humidity. Surface evaporation and sweat together average 600–800 ml/day.[4] Total insensible water loss is between 300 and 500 ml per metre of body surface area per day, with minimal activity in a temperate environment.[5, 6] Sweat volume is small in a temperate climate except with vigorous activity, but may reach several litres a day, with serious losses of both water and sodium chloride, in warm humid environments with exposure to the sun.[7] Markedly obese patients have a much increased water loss which is largely due to sweat. Such patients show marked changes in daily weight consistent with unusually large fluctuations in ECF.

Electrolytes

The daily sodium intake of the normal individual varies between 50 and 100 mmol. Normal body composition is maintained primarily as the result of the renal capacity to excrete any excess intake. When there is a low intake, or extrarenal losses, the kidney has the capability of reducing sodium excretion to as low as 1 mmol per day. As renal function is lost in disease, the capability of this extreme reduction in sodium excretion may be lost and certain renal disorders have a wasting of sodium considerably in excess of the daily intake.

The daily intake of potassium varies from 40 to 80 mmol/day. However, potassium metabolism is strongly influenced by acid–base balance and the normal kidney does not respond to a reduction in intake by prompt conservation of potassium in the way that it does for sodium.

SERUM ELECTROLYTE CONCENTRATIONS

The electrolyte composition of body fluids has been extensively discussed by Gamble.[8] A classic summary of the patterns of water and electrolyte abnormalities seen in disease and injury has been presented by Moore,[9] based upon extensive studies of metabolic balance and body composition in surgical patients. A definite relationship exists between the serum concentration of sodium and potassium and the total exchangeable sodium and potassium, which has been explored by Edelman et al.[10] These studies have demonstrated the poor correlation which often exists between the serum sodium and total body sodium. Edelman et al. has demonstrated that:

Serum sodium =

$$1\cdot1 \times \frac{[\text{Total exchangeable sodium}] + [\text{Total exchangeable potassium}]}{[\text{Total body water}]} - 26$$

Thus, serum sodium can be increased by additional potassium or sodium or restriction of free water. Retention of water in excess of sodium can lead to hyponatraemia even with an excess of total body sodium. Administration of potassium can raise the serum sodium concentration in hyponatraemic patients.[11]

Most potassium is contained in the intracellular fluid, leaving only a small fraction of body potassium in plasma. Thus, the absolute reduction of serum potassium which occurs with depletion can be expected to reflect a very large total body potassium deficit. However, a change in acid–base status may alter the serum potassium levels quite markedly as H^+ is exchanged for K^+, thus, alkalosis may lower serum K^+ markedly, particularly if there is a pre-existing total body deficit.

To maintain electroneutrality:

$$\text{Serum}[Na^+]+[Ca^{2+}]+[Mg^{2+}]+[K^+] = [Cl^-]+[HCO_3^-]$$
$$+[\text{Protein}]+[\text{Sulphate}]+[\text{Phosphate}]+[\text{Organic acids}]$$

Thus:

$$[Na^+]+[K^+] = [HCO_3^-]+[Cl^-]+14$$

The factor of 14 is commonly termed the anion gap. If

$$[\text{sodium}+\text{potassium}]-[\text{bicarbonate}+\text{chloride}]$$

exceeds 18, the substantial addition of an anion must be suspected. These are:

1. HPO_4^{2-} and SO_4^{2-}, as in renal failure.
2. Lactic acid, as in hypoxia, shock states and salicylate intoxication.
3. Keto acids, as in diabetic ketoacidosis.

If the anion gap is less than 5, hypoproteinaemia is the most likely cause.

LOSSES FROM THE GASTROINTESTINAL TRACT

The normal daily volume of secretion into the gastrointestinal tract is not precisely known but has been estimated to be 8000–10 000 ml per day, of which saliva constitutes 1–2 l; gastric juice, including both acid and mucoid secretions, about 2500 ml, bile 500–750 ml, and pancreatic juice in the range of 100 ml. In addition, secretion of the upper small bowel mucosa contributes between 2000 and 3000 ml. All but 100–200 ml of the secretions are normally reabsorbed by the small bowel and the colon.[7]

Abnormal losses from the gastrointestinal tract include water and electrolytes and varying amounts of protein. The electrolyte content of fluid from the gastrointestinal tract varies significantly with the level from which most of the fluid is derived. *Table* 6.1 shows the average value and the range of variation of sodium, potassium, chloride and bicarbonate in fluids from different levels of the intestine. It is important to note that, of all the secretions, only bile and pancreatic juice are approximately isotonic in their electrolyte content. The average calculated osmolality of saliva is about 160 mosmol; of upper small bowel content, 220 mosmol; and of fluid from the distal ileum about 240 mosmol. Other substances including

Table 6.1. Electrolyte content of gastrointestinal secretions, from Randall[5]

Source of fluid	Na^+, mmol/l	K^+, mmol/l	Cl^-, mmol/l	HCO_3^-, mmol/l
Saliva	60	20	16	50
Gastric	30–90	4·0–12	50–155	0
Upper small bowel	70–120	3·0–7·0	70–120	= 10
Ileum	90–140	3·0–8·0	80–125	15–20
Bile	145	4·0–7·0	80–110	= 50
Pancreas	120–140	5–8	60–80	

mucoproteins, other polysaccharides, urea, calcium and phosphate add to these approximations of the total osmolality.

The values shown in *Table* 6.1 may be used for semi-quantitative replacement of gastrointestinal tract losses. When volumes of these losses exceed 2000 ml in 24 hours or, when substantial losses (1 l or more per day) continue for more than a few days, it is wise to send an aliquot of the 24-hour drainage to the laboratory for measurement of electrolytes and protein and to determine the pH of a freshly obtained specimen. More precise replacement can be made with this information. It is important to note that replacement of abnormal losses should be provided in addition to baseline requirements.

Table 6.2. Baseline fluid requirements. Modified from Randall [5]

	Age, years	Fluid, ml per kg per day
Average adults	25–55	35
Young active adults	16–30	40
Older patients	55–65($\pm$)	30
Elderly	> 65	25

Adults—based on 'ideal' weight for height and age

The data listed in *Table* 6.2 are intended only as approximate guidelines in fluid replacement. Fluid therapy should be individualized for a given patient. In general, urinary output serves as a useful guide to fluid therapy and should be maintained at levels of 600 ml/day, or more. If output decreases below 600 ml/day, in association with a decreasing central venous pressure or a decrease in body weight, an increase in fluid requirements is indicated. A decrease in urinary output, associated with a rising central venous pressure and weight gain, may indicate the onset of interstitial pulmonary oedema and diuretic therapy should be instituted.

The common use of the term 'dehydration' can lead to confusion since two different clinical syndromes may each be referred to as dehydration. One syndrome is due to the loss of sodium and chloride with contraction of the extracellular volume, causing decreased skin turgor, a rapid pulse and a lowered blood pressure. Laboratory findings are related to increased haemoglobin and haematocrit with lower sodium and chloride values in the plasma while the urine volume and concentration is not remarkable. Another syndrome is associated with the primary loss of water without loss of electrolytes. Skin turgor, together with circulatory signs and symptoms, are usually normal even though thirst becomes intense. Oliguria with maximal urine concentration is associated with elevated plasma sodium and chloride. When referring to dehydration, sufficient description should be provided to clarify which of these two syndromes is under discussion.

FLUID AND ELECTROLYTE CHANGES IN INJURY

Normal individuals usually tolerate large amounts of intravenously administered sodium chloride. In the immediate postoperative period these same individuals will tend to retain some of the administered fluid and may even develop respiratory symptoms from relatively modest excesses of sodium chloride. This observation of 'postoperative salt tolerance' was recognized as early as 1911.[12] In subsequent years complications, secondary to salt loss, were increasingly recognized and an era of postoperative saline administration ensued.[13–15] The studies which emphasized the dangers of salt deprivation led to a period where many surgeons administered saline whether or not losses had occurred and the manifestations of fluid overload sometimes became evident. Reports soon followed cautioning against excessive salt administration.[16, 17] In 1944, Coller[18] retracted his previously published formula for fluid administration and stated that no salt solution should be given for the first two postoperative days.

In 1950, Ariel and Kremen[19] performed 'salt tolerance tests' prior to and following elective operation. They noted that, postoperatively, a great fraction of the administered salt load shifted into the interstitial space. Lyon et al.[20] determined that postoperative preservation or restoration of blood or plasma volume appeared to be dependent on a state of positive fluid balance. Patients in negative fluid balance following operation had delayed recovery of the 'available fluid' until a state of positive fluid balance was established. In 1953, Aronstam[21] demonstrated an expansion of the extracellular space which followed major thoracic operations.

Wiggers[22] noted that animals which did not survive haemorrhagic shock demonstrated haemoconcentration even though the shed blood was returned. Gilman[23] demonstrated that animals which were deficient in extracellular fluid were sensitive to relatively small degrees of haemorrhage. Reynolds[24] demonstrated that dogs in haemorrhagic shock treated with saline alone could survive with a return of cardiac output.

A series of studies by Shires et al.[25–29] have emphasized that there is a disparate reduction of functional extracellular fluid volume (as measured by the ^{35}S space) induced by haemorrhagic shock. This deficit is not alleviated by return of the shed blood alone or by moderate overexpansion of the intravascular volume with plasma. Rather, the reduction in ECF could be alleviated by use of a balanced salt solution as an adjunct to shed blood replacement. It must be emphasized that these measurements of a reduced functional ECF were made either during, or soon after, the period of injury or shock.

The changes in the ECF following injury and/or shock vary with time. *Table* 6.3, modified from Shires et al.,[30] demonstrates that during shock there is a reduction in the ECF, while following resuscitation the ECF is expanded.

Table 6.3. **Changes in membrane potential and extracellular water following shock. Modified from Shires et al.[27]**

	ECF, % body weight	*Membrane potential, MV*
Control	13·9	−91
Shock	7·7	−65
Resuscitation	18·4	−90

Pluth et al.[31] and Moore et al.[1] demonstrated an expansion of the extracellular space following injury and resuscitation which did not appear to be due to excessive fluid administration. Roth et al.[32] also reported an increase in ECF following injury and suggested moderation in the use of Ringer lactate for resuscitation. Elwyn[33] and Shoemaker[34] reported an expansion of the extracellular space in postoperative patients which was similar to that seen in nutritional depletion. The changes seen in nutritional depletion resolved with adequate nutrition (*Figs.* 6.1 and 6.2).

The weight gain due to fluid administration as immediate treatment for operation or injury is variable and a function of the severity of the injury, as well as the pre-existing clinical state of the patient. Elective operations such as total hip replacement or colon resection are commonly associated with a 3–5% weight gain, while major trauma may be associated with a 10–15% gain in body weight after resuscitation. In our view, such acute weight gains are difficult to avoid. Fluid administration should be guided by parameters such as blood pressure, central venous pressure and urinary output. It is important to note that from the third to the sixth day following injury a diuresis will ordinarily develop.[35] Failure to return to the initial weight by the tenth day after operation or injury should be regarded as a warning of an impending complication (congestive heart failure, sepsis, renal failure, etc).

It has been suggested by Flear et al.[36] that the post-injury changes in ECF and ICF probably reflect a change in permeability of cell membranes and a disturbance in ionic exchange. Thus, injury is thought to lead to an

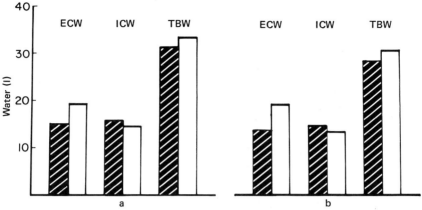

Fig. 6.1. Body composition in (*a*) postoperative and (*b*) depleted patients. Postoperative and depleted patients demonstrate a common response which consists of increases in extracellular water, while the intracellular water is decreased but to a lesser extent. From Elwyn et al.[33] ECW = extracellular water; ICW = intracellular water; TBW = total body water; ▨, experimental; □, observed.

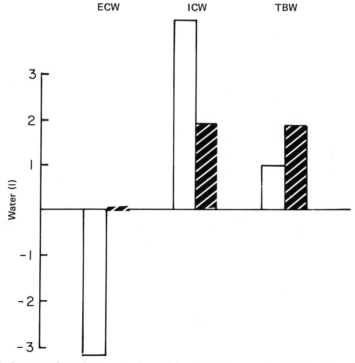

Fig. 6.2. Influence of total parenteral nutrition (TPN) on water distribution of surgical patients. The administration of TPN to depleted patients causes a reduction in the expanded extracellular water while increasing the intracellular water. This is in contrast to the behaviour of postoperative patients where TPN causes a moderate increase in intracellular water. ▨, Postoperative; □, depleted. From Elwyn et al.[33]

increased escape of non-diffusible solutes into the ECF. This causes a decrease in the osmolality of cell fluids, while increasing the osmolality and resultant volume of the ECF. (*See* Chapter 8.)

Skeletal muscle represents the major component of lean body tissue and can be safely sampled by needle biopsy. Studies performed by Bergstrom et al.[37] and Askanazi et al.[38] using the needle biopsy technique have evaluated the role of nutrition and activity level in muscle fluid sequestration. Patients undergoing total hip replacement were assigned to receive a daily intravenous infusion of either 5% dextrose solution or 3·5% amino acid solution (with appropriate electrolytes and vitamins) for the first four postoperative days. Muscle biopsies were performed in the non-operated thigh preoperatively and on the fourth day postoperatively. These studies have demonstrated that an increase in muscle sodium and chloride occurs in non-injured portions of the body (*Fig.* 6.3). These changes are not affected by the form of nutritional support administered. There was an increase in muscle ECF in these patients, which was unaffected by whichever nutrition was administered. In normal subjects on bedrest, receiving either a regular diet or a 5% dextrose solution, there were no comparable changes in muscle composition.

With increasing severity of injury and injury complicated by sepsis, there is a progressive increase in muscle ECF, sodium and chloride (*Fig.* 6.4) while the intracellular space is decreased. Muscle potassium and magnesium tends to decrease with increasing degrees of injury (*Fig.* 6.5).

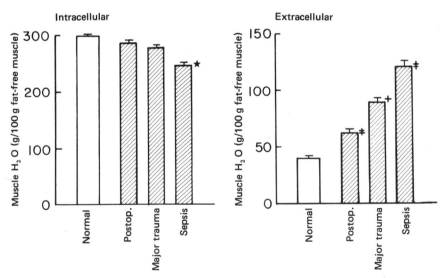

Fig. 6.3. Muscle water (mean ± s.e.). The water content of human muscle (from percutaneous needle biopsies of the vastus lateralis) is presented for various surgical conditions. There is progressive increase in the extracellular water with the severity of injury and/or sepsis. This is associated with a tendency toward a decrease in the intracellular water. *$P < 0.05$, †$P < 0.01$, ‡$P < 0.001$.

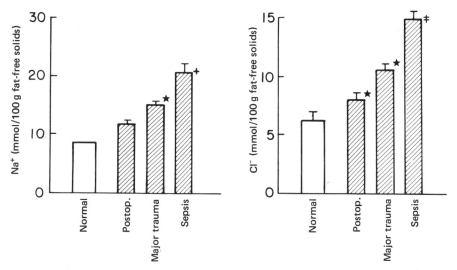

Fig. 6.4. The content of sodium and chloride in the muscle samples referred to in *Fig.* 6.3. is seen to increase with the severity of injury and/or sepsis. *See Fig.* 6.3 for values of *P*.

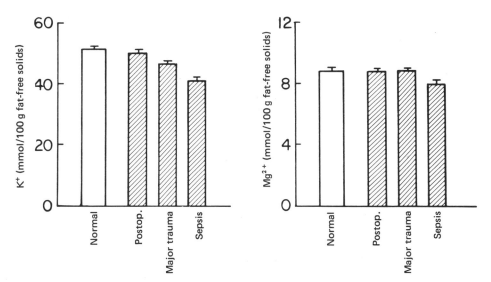

Fig. 6.5. The content of potassium and magnesium in the muscle samples referred to in *Fig.* 6.3 shows no change with moderate injury while modest decreases are seen with severe injury and sepsis.

These studies suggest that there is an obligatory expansion of the ECF following injury. This expansion requires fluid and sodium administration above maintenance levels and results in an increase in body weight. The physiological effect of this weight gain is variable and depends upon the underlying clinical state of the patient. In a young healthy individual a

10–12% weight gain (7l positive fluid balance) may be well tolerated, whereas a much smaller weight gain may be poorly tolerated by the elderly patient with decreased cardiopulmonary system reserve.

USE OF COLLOID IN FLUID RESUSCITATION

The use of albumin in resuscitation of injured patients is a controversial issue.[39] The proponents of the use of colloid as part of fluid therapy argue that resuscitation with crystalloid alone dilutes plasma proteins, thereby reducing plasma oncotic pressure. Reduced oncotic pressure favours fluid movement from the intravascular to the interstitial compartment and, thereby, predisposes the patient to the development of interstitial pulmonary oedema.[41, 43] In contrast to these studies, Lowe et al.,[42] Moss et al.[43] and Virgilio et al.[44] found no advantage to the administration of colloid solutions. Lucas et al.[45, 46] demonstrated that patients receiving large quantities of albumin had a greater dependency on ventilator support with a detrimental effect on renal function.

Our own policy is to utilize a balanced salt solution for resuscitation of postoperative and injured patients together with whole blood. Albumin infusions are generally confined to patients whose serum albumin is below $2 \cdot 5 \, \text{g} \cdot \%$ and who are also receiving nutritional repletion. In the absence of infection, the capillary bed is considered to be intact, therefore, a rise in serum albumin level may be expected with albumin infusion.

FLUID AND ELECTROLYTE REQUIREMENTS IN CONVALESCENCE

The purpose of administering parenteral fluids and electrolytes is to prevent deficiencies that otherwise result from inability of the patient's gastrointestinal tract and kidneys to fulfil their normal function. Also, in acute trauma or when there has been a substantial loss of water, electrolytes or both from the body without adequate replacement, parenteral fluid therapy is required to restore a normal distribution of body fluids.

The requirements for parenteral therapy can be considered in three categories:

I. *Normal requirements*. What does the patient require in water, electrolytes, basic calories and micronutrients to minimize the effects of dehydration and of starvation due to cessation or reduction of oral intake? The calculation of baseline requirements disregards any pre-existing losses, but baseline volumes may require modification in patients with extracellular fluid expansion associated with dilutional hyponatraemia.

II. *Pre-existing deficits or excesses.* What deficits (or excesses) does the patient have in water, electrolytes, blood volume, plasma proteins and micronutrients? What should be done to correct these abnormalities?

III. *Abnormal losses.* What does the patient require in order to replace ongoing abnormal fluid and electrolyte losses resulting from the disease or its treatment. This includes ECF sequestration.

A part of this requirement will be obtained through metabolism of body tissue in a semi-starving state. Endogenous water is derived from the shrinkage or breakdown of protoplasm which is roughly 75% water, as well as the water of oxidation which results from fuel oxidation. Other endogenous water derived from muscle breakdown approximates 800–850 ml for each kg of body cell mass lost. This water is almost completely sodium-free but is rich in potassium, magnesium, phosphate and sulphate.

Oxidation of fat provides approximately 1 ml of water per g of fat oxidized. Moore[1] estimated that about 100 ml of water is available for each 100 kcal which is derived from the burning of body tissues, part of which is fat and part body cells. The daily caloric requirement of the surgical patient depends in part upon sex and age but much more upon the extent and type of trauma, the presence of infection, the degree of immobilization and the amount of energy required to maintain body temperature in the presence of abnormal evaporative water losses, either from hyperventilation or from evaporative cooling which occurs as the result of extensive thermal injury.

The daily caloric requirement of the afebrile patient of average size, at bed rest, will vary from 1300 to 1900 kcal, 400–500 kcal of which are often provided by the administration of isotonic glucose into a peripheral vein. The baseline production of endogenous water of oxidation in this situation will be from 150 to 200 ml, or about 10% of the total daily requirement. However, fever, trauma and infection will increase endogenous water production along with the increased oxidation of tissue fuel.

CLINICAL EVALUATION OF THE PATIENT

External abnormal loss may be in the form of excessive loss of water and electrolytes by normal routes of excretion or secretion, or losses which may occur from intraluminal tubes, drains, fistulae or wounds. The most common source of abnormal external loss in surgical patients is the gastrointestinal tract; next in frequency are the losses from surgical wounds, increased evaporation from the skin and respiratory tract and from direct injury to the skin. Sequestration of extracellular fluids into areas of traumatized or infected tissue produces a decrease in the usual distribution of extracellular fluid without external loss or change in body weight.

Table 6.2 illustrates methods for estimating the parenteral or combined parenteral and oral fluid requirements for surgical patients.

Body Weight

Daily changes in body weight present the most practical index of the changing state of hydration. The daily weight of a patient on conventional fluid therapy by peripheral vein should reveal a loss of approximately 0·2–0·4% of body weight per day until adequate oral nutrition is instituted. Exceptions occur with blood transfusions, or deliberate changes in hydration, as well as during the first 48 hours following trauma or operation when local sequestration of fluid occurs and parenteral fluid is given to compensate for it. The patient who gains weight in other circumstances while on routine fluid therapy is usually being overhydrated or may have developed some complication, most often sepsis. The patient who loses weight at a faster rate, except during a temporary post-traumatic diuresis, is in need of more aggressive fluid therapy. Frequent measurements of body weight are probably the single most important method of recognizing changes in water balance.

Factors modifying Requirements

Factors which increase baseline requirements for fluid intake are essentially those which increase the insensible water loss.

Fever increases the water requirements to a variable degree. Hyperventilation results in increased water loss by evaporation in addition to cutaneous losses. A patient with a fever of 103 °F will require an average of 500 ml of additional water per day.[36] The endogenous water production associated with the hypermetabolism of fever is also increased, but not enough to offset the increased losses.

Sweating will increase the average adult water requirements by 500 ml per day for each degree Fahrenheit of ambient temperature above 85 °F.[7] This is dependent upon the humidity. Sweat is about one-half normal sodium chloride, so that additional salt must be provided in the therapy. The potassium content of sweat is negligible. When the environmental temperature rises above 32 °C, the seriously ill febrile patient should be cooled, preferably by air conditioning, because the insensible loss of water from evaporative cooling becomes very large.

Increased Metabolism

Hyperthyroidism increases the turnover of water substantially, in parallel with increases in caloric requirements. Hyperthyroid patients in the semi-starving state tend to consume massive amounts of lean tissue and fat, producing unusual amounts of endogenous water, and simultaneously losing water both by respiratory evaporation and skin sublimation together with sweating.

REFERENCES

 1. Moore F. D., Olsen K. H., McMurray J. D. et al. (1963) *Body Cell Mass and its Supporting Environment: Body Composition in Health and Disease.* Philadelphia, W. B. Saunders.
 2. Edelman I. S. and Leibman J. (1959) Anatomy of body water and electrolytes. *Am. J. Med.* **17**, 256.
 3. Streeten D. H. P., Rapaport A. and Conn J. W. (1963) Existence of a slowly exchangeable pool of body sodium in normal subjects and its diminution in patients with primary aldosteronism. *J. Clin. Endocrinol. Metab.* **23**, 928.
 4. Gump F. E., Kinney J. M., Lond C. L. et al. (1968) Measurement of water balance—a guide to surgical care. *Surgery* **64**, 154.
 5. Gump F. E. (1977) Fluid and electrolyte management. In: Kinney J. M., Bendixen H. H. and Powers S. R., ed., *Manual of Surgical Intensive Care*, p. 103. Philadelphia, W. B. Saunders.
 6. Shires G. T. (1971) Fluid and electrolyte therapy. In: Kinney J. M., Egdahl R. H. and Zuidema G. D., ed., *Manual of Preoperative and Postoperative Care*, 2nd ed., p. 42. Philadelphia, W. B. Saunders.
 7. Randall H. T. (1976) Fluid, electrolyte and acid base balance. *Surg. Clin. North Am.* **56**, 1019.
 8. Gamble J. L. (1947) *Chemical Anatomy, Physiology, and Pathology of Extracellular Fluid: A Lecture Syllabus*, 5th ed. Cambridge, Harvard University Press.
 9. Moore F. D. (1958) Common patterns of water and electrolyte change in injury, surgery and disease. *N. Engl. J. Med.*, **258**, 277, 377 and 427.
10. Edelman I. S., Leibman J., O'Meara M. P. et al. (1958) Interrelations between serum sodium concentration, serum osmolality and total exchangeable sodium, total exchangeable potassium and total body water. *J. Clin. Invest.* **37**, 1236.
11. Laragh J. (1954) The effect of potassium chloride on hyponatremia. *J. Clin. Invest*, **33**, 807.
12. Evans G. H. (1911) The abuse of normal saline solution. *J. Am. Med. Assoc.* **57**, 2126.
13. Bartlett R. M., Bingham D. C. L. and Pedersen S. (1938) Salt balance in surgical patients. *Surgery* **4**, 441.
14. Coller F. A., Dick V. S. and Maddock W. G. (1936) The maintenance of normal water exchange with intravenous fluids. *JAMA* **107**, 1522.
15. Coller F. A., Bartlett R. M., Bingham D. C. L. et al. (1938) Replacement of sodium chloride in surgical patients. *Ann. Surg.*, **108**, 796.
16. Limbert E. M., Power M. H., Pemberton D. E. F. et al. (1945) Effects of parenteral administration of fluid on the metabolism of electrolytes during postoperative convalescence. *Surg. Gynecol. Obstet.* **80**, 609.
17. White J. C., Sweet W. H. and Hurwitt H. S. (1938) Water balance in neurosurgical patients. *Ann. Surg.* **107**, 438.
18. Coller F. A., Campbell K. N. V. and Vaughan H. H. (1944) Postoperative salt intolerance. *Ann. Surg.* **119**, 533.
19. Ariel I. M. and Kremen A. J. (1950) Compartmental distribution of sodium chloride in surgical patients pre- and post-operatively. *Ann. Surg.* **132**, 1009.

20. Lyon R. P., Stanton J. R., Freis E. D. et al. (1949) Blood and 'available fluid' (thiocyanate) volume studies in surgical patients. Part I, normal patterns of response of the blood volume, available fluid, protein chloride and hematocrit in the postoperative surgical patient. *Surg. Gynecol. Obstet.* **89**, 9.

21. Aronstam E. M., Schmidt C. H. and Jenkins E. (1953) Body fluid shifts, sodium and potassium metabolism in patients undergoing thoracic surgical procedures. *Ann. Surg.* **137**, 316.

22. Wiggars M. D. and Ingraham R. C. (1946) Hemorrhagic shock: definition of criteria for its diagnosis. *J. Clin. Invest.* **25**, 30.

23. Gilman A. (1934) Experimental sodium loss analogous to adrenal insufficiency: the resulting water shift and sensitivity to hemorrhage. *Am. J. Physiol.* **108**, 662.

24. Reynolds M. (1949) Cardiovascular effects of large volumes of isotonic saline infused intravenously in dogs following severe hemorrhage. *Am. J. Physiol.* **158**, 418.

25. Shires T., Carrico C. J. and Cohn D. (1964) Role of the extracellular fluid in shock. *Int. Anesthesiol. Clin.* **2**, 435.

26. Shires T., Williams J. and Brown F. (1960) Simultaneous measurement of plasma volume, extracellular fluid volume, and red blood cell mass in man using ^{131}I, $^{35}SO_4$ and ^{51}Cr. *J. Lab. Clin. Med.* **55**, 776.

27. Shires T., Cohn D., Carrico J. et al. (1964) Fluid therapy in hemorrhagic shock. *Arch. Surg.* **88**, 688.

28. Shires T. (1969) The role of sodium-containing solutions in the treatment of oligenic shock. *Surg. Clin. North Am.* **45**, 365.

29. Carrico C. J., Cohn D., Lightfoot S. A. et al. (1963) Extracellular fluid replacement in hemorrhagic shock. *Surg. Forum* **14**, 10.

30. Shires T., Carrico C. J. and Canizaro P. C. (1973) *Shock*, p. 32. London, W. B. Saunders.

31. Pluth J. R., Clelland J., Meadow C. K. et al. (1967) Effect of surgery on the volume of distribution of extracellular fluid determined by the sulfate and bromide methods. In: Berguer P. E. and Lushbough E. E. (ed.), *Medical Physiology*. Springfield, Ill., USAEC, pp. 217–239.

32. Roth E., Lax L. C. and Maloney J. V. Jr (1967) Changes in extracellular fluid volume during shock and surgical trauma in animals and man. *Surg. Forum,* **18**, 43.

33. Elwyn D. H., Bryan-Brown C. W. and Shoemaker W. C. (1975) Nutritional aspects of body water dislocations in postoperative and depleted patients. *Ann. Surg.* **187**, 76.

34. Shoemaker W. C., Bryan-Brown C. W., Quigley L. et al. (1973) Body fluid shifts in depletion and post stress states and their correction with adequate nutrition. *Surg. Gynecol. Obstet.* **136**, 371.

35. Gump F. E., Kinney J. M., Lond C. L. et al. (1968) Measurement of water balance—a guide to surgical care. *Surgery,* **64**, 154.

36. Flear C. T. G., Bhattacharya S. S. and Singh C. M. (1980) Solute and water exchanges between cells and extracellular fluids in health and disturbances after trauma. *Journal of Parenteral and Enteral Nutrition,* **4**, 98.

37. Bergstrom J., Furst P., Holstram B. et al. (1981) Influence of injury on muscle water and electrolytes: effects of elective operation. (Submitted for publication.)

38. Askanazi J., Gump F. E., Furst P. et al. (1979) Effects of nutrition and activity on muscle water and electrolyte changes following injury. *Journal of Parenteral and Enteral Nutrition* **3**, 24 (abstract).

39. Shoemaker W. C. and Hauser C. J. (1979) Critique of crystalloid versus colloid therapy in shock and shock lung. *Crit. Care Med.* **7**, 117.

40. Skillman J. J. (1976) The role of albumin and oncotically active fluids in shock. *Crit. Care Med.* **4**, 55.

41. Skillman J. J., Retall D. S. and Salzman E. W. (1975) Randomized trial of albumin vs electrolyte solutions during aortic operations. *Surgery* **78**, 291.

42. Lowe R. J., Moss G. S., Jilek J. et al. (1977) Crystalloid vs colloid in the etiology of pulmonary failure after trauma: a randomized trial in man *Surgery* **81**, 676

43. Moss G. S., Siegel D. C., Cochin A. et al. (1971) Effects of saline and colloid solutions in pulmonary function in hemorrhagic shock. *Surg. Gynecol. Obstet.* **133**, 53.
44. Virgilio R. W., Smith D. E. and Zarins C. K. (1979) Balanced electrolyte solutions: experimental and clinical studies. *Crit. Care Med.* **7**, 98.
45. Weaver D. W., Ledgerwood A. M. and Lucas C. E. (1978) Pulmonary effects of albumin resuscitation for severe hypovolemic shock. *Arch. Surg.* **113**, 387.
46. Lucas C. E., Weaver D. W., Higgins R. F. et al. (1978) Effects of albumin vs non-albumin resuscitation on plasma volume and renal excretory function. *J. Trauma* **18**, 564.

Chapter 7

Nutritional Support

A. Shenkin

Until recent years, seriously ill patients would inevitably develop some degree of nutritional depletion whilst in hospital due to their inability to ingest an adequate diet, and the failure of the clinical staff to administer sufficient amounts of nutrients. The rather emotive term 'hospital malnutrition' was introduced to describe this situation. Developments in clinical nutrition have however been rapid, and have covered the areas of both enteral and parenteral nutrition. For the majority of patients, it is now possible to meet the nutritional requirements by one or other route.

In order to understand the current usage of these techniques, it is necessary first to trace some of the historical background to their development.[1]

HISTORICAL BACKGROUND

It has long been recognized that some form of nutritional support is necessary to aid recovery from severe injury. The ultimate objective of research in this field was a system of parenteral nutrition which would meet all the nutritional requirements of the individual.

Despite the early experiments in blood transfusion of Colle (1628) and Denis (1667) who transfused lamb's blood into a youth, and the infusion of wine and ale into a dog by Wren (1656), progress in intravenous nutrition was slow until the end of the nineteenth century. The work of Lister (1870) on asepsis and Pasteur (1877) on microbiological infection provided the basis of safe infusions. Kausch (1911) infused dextrose for nutrition after surgery, and Henriques and Anderson (1913) injected enzymatically hydrolysed protein into animals. Fat was infused experimentally by Murlin and Riche (1916) and was used in man by Yamakawa in 1920. Further progress initially centred on preparation of effective protein hydrolysates and Elman (1937) demonstrated an improvement in nitrogen balance in patients receiving casein hydrolysate. However, it was soon realized that nitrogen (N) equilibrium could only be achieved if an adequate energy intake was also provided.

Attempts to meet the energy requirements by glucose or other water-soluble substances were limited by the problems of hypertonic solutions causing thrombophlebitis, and the large volumes of fluid necessary if less concentrated solutions were used. Early fat emulsions obtained from cotton seed oil had the valuable property of being energy-rich yet isotonic, but they led to a variety of toxic reactions and were withdrawn from use in the United States in 1964.

These problems were overcome in two ways. In the United States, safe infusion of concentrated dextrose directly into the subclavian vein was shown to be possible in both adults and infants.[2] In Scandinavia, a new type of fat emulsion based on soya bean oil with egg yolk phospholipids was developed and proved to be free from toxic reaction.[3] Parenteral nutrition involving the use of fat emulsion for provision of a proportion of the energy was therefore widely used in Europe. However, in the United States, the use of this new generation of fat emulsions has only recently been approved and hence most American clinicians continue to use hypertonic dextrose solutions for provision of energy substrates.

Once the major problems involved in the safe infusion of adequate amounts of energy substrates and nitrogen had been solved, there was a clear incentive for development of preparations of minerals and vitamins suitable for intravenous use. It is, therefore, now possible to meet all the nutritional requirements of the individual by the intravenous route.

Despite the efficacy of total intravenous feeding, it was soon appreciated that major side effects may be associated with its use, in particular complications involving the central venous catheter. It was also realized that many individuals could be fed enterally if a suitable delivery system and appropriate forms of tube feed were available. The clinical benefit which could be derived from intravenous nutrition therefore stimulated a general interest in patient nutrition which, in turn, led to the development of new materials for enteral nutrition. There have recently become available a variety of well-tolerated fine bore feeding tubes and suitable, chemically defined, homogeneous tube feeds. It has been amply proved that such enteral feeding systems can provide adequate nutrition for many patients who would previously have received intravenous nutrition.

The choice of enteral or parenteral nutrition varies in different hospitals, depending largely upon the available experience with the two techniques. As a general rule, intravenous feeding should only be used when an adequate enteral nutrition cannot be achieved. This historical summary may, in part, explain why this is not yet the case and why parenteral nutrition may be used as a first line of nutritional therapy in some patients with a functioning gut. Nevertheless, with greater usage, guidelines for use of enteral/parenteral nutrition will become clearer and thus will ensure appropriate clinical application.

THE NUTRITIONAL REQUIREMENTS OF THE SEVERELY ILL PATIENT

Since the pioneering studies of Cuthbertson (1930),[4] it has been increasingly recognized that trauma and various serious illnesses are associated with marked changes in metabolism. In particular, there is an increase in resting metabolic expenditure (RME) coupled with an increase in net protein catabolism. In a series of studies, Kinney and co-workers[5,6] have clearly demonstrated that the increase in RME depends upon the severity of the illness, ranging from a 10% increase for an elective operation to more than 100% with severe burn injuries. Some of this energy is derived from oxidation of glucose as a result of gluconeogenesis from increased protein catabolism, but most of the energy comes from oxidation of fatty acids released from adipose tissue stores. The RME in health is generally accepted as about 1600 kcal/day. Using this figure, the provision of 1600–3200 kcal is necessary to cover the RME in most patients.

The major objectives of nutritional support are to provide adequate energy substrates and protein precursors to minimize loss of tissue protein and to replete protein in the depleted individual. A close inter-relationship exists between the effects of energy and amino acid provision. Within limits, at a constant nitrogen intake, an increase of energy intake will improve nitrogen balance. A positive nitrogen balance will only be obtained when the energy intake is at least equal to the resting metabolic expenditure. On the other hand, with a constant intake of energy substrates, nitrogen balance will be improved by an increase in amino acid supply. Increased intake of either energy substrates or amino acids eventually leads to a plateau of nitrogen balance, beyond which no further improvement can be obtained.

The ease with which a positive nitrogen balance can be achieved is dependent upon the degree of catabolism and whether the patient is adapted to an inadequate nutritional intake (*Fig.* 7.1). An individual adapted to starvation will readily achieve a positive nitrogen balance if provided with his RME plus about 10 g N per day. The catabolic patient following injury or with sepsis will, however, require not only a higher energy intake to achieve his RME but also a higher intake of nitrogen (15–20 g or more) to achieve positive nitrogen balance. It is widely held that about 200 kcal/g N is required for optimal utilization of the nitrogen provided. In very catabolic patients, however, a ratio as low as 125 kcal/g N might be more appropriate; this can be achieved by increasing the

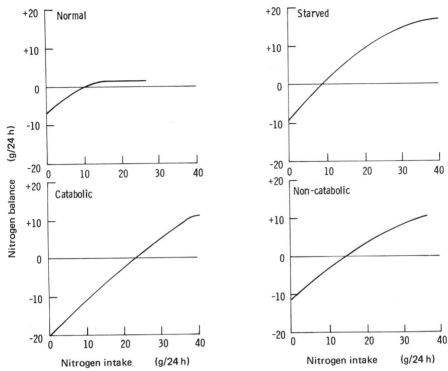

Fig. 7.1. Effects of different clinical situations on the general relationship relating nitrogen intake with nitrogen balance. Total energy intake in each case is equal to metabolic energy expenditure. From Woolfson (1979), with permission of author and publisher.[18]

provision of amino acid nitrogen with a smaller increase in energy substrates necessary to exceed the RME.

A major debate has occurred in recent years as to whether carbohydrate and fat are equivalent in their protein-sparing qualities and in improving nitrogen balance. There is no doubt that high dose glucose therapy, supplemented with insulin, is effective in reducing the high level of urinary nitrogen excretion following severe trauma. Moreover, it has been shown that, in some severely ill patients, protein sparing was a function of glucose intake and was not affected by provision of fat.[7] However, a variety of studies have indicated that following surgical trauma, glucose and fat infusions are almost equivalent in their effect on nitrogen balance, particularly after the first few days of infusions.[8] Although this controversy is not fully resolved, it can be concluded that, in most patients, fat and carbohydrate have a similar effect on nitrogen balance.

Recently, a further factor has been identified as important in the fat or carbohydrate controversy. Oxidation of carbohydrate leads to more CO_2 production than does fat, for the same energy yield.[9] Hence, acutely ill patients with respiratory insufficiency may retain more CO_2 when receiving carbohydrate infusions than when receiving a proportion of their energy from fat. Even if CO_2 is not retained, the increased respiratory rate necessary to remove this extra CO_2 may cause considerable distress. This observation supports the contention that energy provision should be balanced, 30–50% of the energy being provided by fat emulsion. This provision of energy is more physiological, corresponding closely to the normal oral intake.

The metabolic response to trauma or infection is not confined to protein and energy metabolism. Profound changes in minerals can occur, including falls in serum iron and zinc levels, increased excretion of potassium, phosphorus, sulphur and zinc, and decreased excretion of calcium. A rapid fall in plasma ascorbic acid is seen and other vitamins are required in higher amounts to cover the increased provision of energy substrates.

When considering a nutritional support regimen, one major uncertainty is whether to attempt to maintain biochemical 'normality' by aggressive nutritional supplements, or to accept that the metabolic response may, in itself, be beneficial, and that so-called 'normal' biochemical values may not be necessary or even desirable in the post-trauma or septic patient.

Many comparisons of nutritional regimens have suggested different effects on the basis of various biochemical markers. More appropriate end points for clinical studies would be some measure of morbidity and mortality. Until a clear relation is observed between the biochemical markers and clinical outcome, the role of these biochemical measurements must remain in question. They are, however, the only readily available quantitative methods of assessing the adequacy of the nutritional support and hence have an important though limited role.

INTRAVENOUS NUTRITION

Intravenous nutrition is usually given as a substitute for oral intake. One definition of the object of an ideal intravenous nutrition, therefore, is to provide by the intravenous route *all* nutrients in the same amount and chemical form as would normally be absorbed via the gastrointestinal tract from an adequate oral diet. Hence an adequate infusion of all amino acids, energy substrates, minerals and vitamins is necessary. As tentative guidelines only, tables of suggested different levels of requirement are given (*Table* 7.1).

I. Amino Acids

Adequate amounts of the twenty amino acids in human proteins must be present in the cell cytoplasm for protein synthesis. The eight amino acids which cannot be synthesized by the body must be provided in the diet. The

Table 7.1. Tentatively recommended daily allowances of nutrients for patients on complete intravenous nutrition

	Allowances/kg body weight for adults			Allowances/kg body weight for neonates and infants		
	Basal amounts	Moderate amounts	High supply	Basal amounts	Moderate amounts	High supply
Water, ml	30	50	50–100	100–120	125	125–150
Energy	30 kcal = 0·13 MJ	35–40 kcal = 0·15–0·17 MJ	50–60 kcal = 0·21–0·25 MJ	90–120 kcal = 0·38–0·50 MJ	125 kcal = 0·52 MJ	125–150 kcal = 0·52–0·63 MJ
Amino acid	90 mg (0·7 g amino acids)	0·2–0·3 g (1·5–2 g amino acids)	0·4–0·5 g (3–3·5 g amino acids)	0·3 g (2·5 g amino acids)	0·45 g (3·5 g amino acids)	0·5 g (4·0 g amino acids)
Glucose, g	2	5	7	12–18	18–25	25–30
Fat, g	2	3	3–4	4	4–6	6
Sodium, mmol	1–1·4	2–3	3–4	1–2·5	3–4	4–5
Potassium, mmol	0·7–0·9	2	3–4	2	2–3	4–5
Calcium, mmol	0·11	0·15	0·2	0·5	1	1·5–2
Magnesium, mmol	0·04	0·13–0·20	0·3–0·4	0·15	0·15–0·5	1
Iron, µmol	0·25–1·0	1·0	1·0	2		3–4
Manganese, µmol	0·1	0·3	0·6	0·3	0·7	1
Zinc, µmol	0·7	0·7–1·5	1·5–3	0·6	1	1·5
Copper, µmol	0·07	0·3–0·4	0·4–1	0·3		
Chromium, µmol	0·015			0·01		
Selenium, µmol	0·006			0·04		
Molybdenum, µmol	0·003					
Chlorine, mmol	1·3–1·9	2–3	3–4	2–4		4–6
Phosphorus, mmol	0·15	0·4	0·6–1·0	0·4–0·8	1·3–1·5	2·5–3
Fluorine, µmol	0·7	0·7–1·5		3		
Iodine, µmol	0·015			0·04		0·1

The basal allowances will cover resting metabolism, some physical activity and specific dynamic action.
The moderate amounts should be used when the patient has increased losses or is in a depleted status.
The high supply should be used in severe catabolic conditions as burns, after trauma, etc., or during anabolism in a depleted patient.
From Shenkin and Wretlind.[14]

other twelve amino acids can be provided in varying amounts, on the assumption that deficiencies or excesses can be rectified within the body.

It has been shown, however, that amino acids such as cystine and tyrosine, which are normally non-essential, may become essential in certain situations, such as in the postoperative period, or in the premature infant, when normally active metabolic pathways may not be fully operational. Certain amino acids provided in excess, such as glycine, may not be fully utilized and may be excreted in considerable quantities in the urine. This is of particular relevance since glycine is often present in high concentrations in amino acid solutions as a non-specific source of nitrogen, which, it is hoped, will be incorporated into other non-essential amino acids, when required. It has, therefore, been suggested that the most effective way of ensuring that optimal amounts of all non-essential amino acids are present in the cells is to supply a complete mixture of the non-essential amino acids.

The relative amounts of essential and non-essential amino acids should also be considered. Although the proportion of essential amino acids required for maintenance of normal body cell mass is only about 20%, for effective repletion of individuals with some degree of protein depletion, a mixture consisting of 45–50% of essential amino acids is optimal.[10] This type of amino acid mixture corresponds to that most suitable for the growing infant.

Amino acid solutions for use in intravenous nutrition fall into two main classes. Enzymatic hydrolysates of casein and fibrin, proteins of high biological value, have been used fairly satisfactorily for many years. Because of the presence of peptides which could not be metabolized in vivo and which were excreted in the urine, these solutions have been replaced by solutions of pure crystalline amino acids. A wide variety of formulations of such solutions have been developed commercially. These solutions differ in terms of amino acid formulation (total concentration of amino acids, proportion of essential to non-essential amino acids, and the amounts of individual amino acids, particularly non-specific nitrogen sources) as well as electrolyte concentration and, of course, price. The amino acid content of some of these solutions is summarized in *Table* 7.2.

The selection of amino acid solution to be used is a difficult decision. There is a growing tendency for individual hospitals to have a clear policy by using only one or two different amino acid solutions, the choice being made from them for patients with particular clinical problems. This would seem to be a sensible method of obtaining experience and confidence in the use of certain regimens. Not many direct comparisons of individual amino acid solutions have been made and, in only a few cases, have clear differences in effect on nitrogen balance been observed.

Most solutions have been shown to promote a positive nitrogen balance when accompanied by a suitable intake of energy substrates. Nevertheless, in general, a better nitrogen balance is achieved with amino acid solutions which contain a complete well-balanced amino acid profile, and do not contain excesses of individual amino acids. None of the amino acid solutions shown in *Table 7.2* has a profile identical to that in the portal vein after a high quality protein meal. The nearest is probably the Vamin[K] range but this preparation has considerable amounts of glutamic acid, an amino acid usually metabolized initially in the small intestinal cells, which are largely bypassed by intravenous infusions.

In practice, the selection of a particular amino acid will probably depend upon:
1. The amino acid formulation of the preparation, with particular reference to the completeness of the preparation and whether there may be any limitations in a particular patient with regard to synthesis of non-essential amino acids.
2. The total concentration of amino acids, in relation to the total requirement of the patient for amino acid N and the volume of infusion planned.
3. The cost of the preparation. This is often expressed per gN, but a more appropriate calculation might be the cost per g N excluding glycine, since glycine may not be fully utilized.
4. The mineral and/or vitamin content, but this should be a very minor factor, since these additives will generally be made separately.
5. The experience of individual clinicians. In this field, confidence in use of individual preparations is of major importance.

II. Carbohydrate

It has long been considered that one of the main functions of an adequate carbohydrate intake is to prevent ketosis. The minimum amount of carbohydrate intake necessary for this is about 100 g/day. The complete prevention of ketosis is, however, not necessarily beneficial. Some recent studies have indicated that patients who are able to 'ketoadapt', that is develop an increased amount of ketones in blood and urine in response to a hypocaloric input, may have a better prognosis after surgery than those individuals who fail to develop an elevation in ketones. The implication is that individuals who ketoadapt are mobilizing large amounts of fat stores, whereas those who do not ketoadapt have a greater degree of protein catabolism. Complete suppression of the ketone response may, therefore, only be beneficial when the total nutritional intake is adequate.

Nevertheless, in the formulation of a nutritional support regimen, either intravenously or enterally, there is little doubt that an adequate carbohydrate intake is necessary, both to maintain blood glucose concentration and to provide the intermediary metabolites for full metabolism of fat and ketone bodies. In the normal oral diet, the carbohydrate content provides about 40–50% of the total energy intake, although in some societies as much as 90% of the energy may be met from carbohydrate

Table 7.2. Quantity of amino acid in 16 g of nitrogen (equivalent to approximately 100 g amino acid)

L-Amino acids	Egg protein[a]	Aminosol 10%[b]	Aminofusin Forte[c]	Aminoplex 5[d]	Aminoplex 12[d]	Freamine II[e]	Intramin Forte[b]	Synthamin 9[f] 14 17	Vamin N[b] Vamin glucose*
Isoleucine	6·6	6·5	3·3	3·8	4·9	7·5	4·6	4·6	6·6
Leucine	8·8	11·4	4·6	5·4	7·5	9·9	7·2	6·0	9·0
Lysine	6·4	10·1	5·3	10·2	7·0	7·9	5·2	5·6	6·6
Phenylalanine }	5·8	6·4	4·6	5·4	8·9	6·1	7·2	6·0	9·4
Tyrosine	4·2	1·1	—	—	—	—	—	0·4	0·8
Methionine }	3·1	3·7	4·4	7·7	6·2	5·8	7·2	5·6	3·2
Cystine }	2·4	1·8	—	—	—	—	—	—	2·4
Threonine	5·1	5·0	2·1	3·8	4·1	4·4	3·3	4·1	5·1
Tryptophan	1·6	1·3	0·95	1·9	1·8	1·7	1·7	1·8	1·7
Valine	7·3	8·7	3·15	6·4	5·8	7·2	5·2	4·4	7·3
Total essential	51·3	56·0	28·4	44·6	46·2	50·5	41·6	38·5	52·1
Alanine	7·4	4·1	12·6	17·9	12·9	7·7	15·0	20·2	5·1
Arginine	6·1	4·3	8·4	12·8	11·9	4·0	9·4	10·1	5·6
Aspartic acid	9·0	8·6	—	2·4[g]	2·6[g]	—	8·1	—	7·0

Glutamic acid	16·0	27·6	18·9	—	2·6	—	—	—	15·3
Glycine	3·6	2·4	21·0	14·4	5·7	21·8	9·4	20·2	3·6
Histidine	2·4	3·2	2·1	3·5	2·8	3·1	5·6	4·2	4·1
Proline	8·1	13·4	14·7	4·8	15·5	12·2	9·4	4·1	13·8
Serine	8·5	5·6	—	—	3·1	6·4	4·7	—	12·8
Essential, % total	46	45	27	45	45	48	40	40	44
Total N, g/l solution	12·6	12·6	15·2	5·0	12·4	12·5	17·1	9·3 / 14·3 / 16·9	9·4
Carbohydrate/alcohol	—	—	—	Sorbitol 125 g/l Ethanol 50 g/l	—	—	—	—	*Glucose 100 g/l
Electrolytes, mmol/l									
Sodium	136	40	40	35	35	10	<1	73	50
Potassium	—	30	30	15	30	—	<1	60	20
Magnesium	—	5	5	—	2·5	—	<0·1	5	1·5
Calcium	—	—	—	—	—	—	<0·2	—	2·5
Phosphorus	15	—	—	—	—	10	<0·1	30	—

[a] Included for reference purposes.   [b] Vitrum, Stockholm, Sweden.   [c] BDH, Hampshire, England.   [d] Geistlich, Chester, England.   [e] Boots, Nottingham, England.   [f] Travenol, Thetford, England.   [*] As ornithine-L-aspartate.

sources. Hence to substitute for the normal oral intake by intravenous nutrition, approximately 50% of the energy intake should also be provided by carbohydrate. A minimum of 20% of the energy must be provided by carbohydrate to meet essential functions, and up to 100% can be and indeed is still used, particularly in the United States, where other energy sources have not been widely available.

The carbohydrate used most often in intravenous nutrition is glucose. The main benefits of glucose infusions are that glucose can be used by all tissues of the body, and that glucose metabolism can be modulated by insulin infusion. Furthermore, glucose utilization can be monitored by measurement of the blood glucose concentration; no other carbohydrate can be as readily monitored.

In the post-injury period or during an episode of sepsis, glucose intolerance may develop, due to a relative lack of insulin. Although this can usually be controlled by insulin infusions, its occurrence has led to the search for alternative carbohydrates which may be less likely to lead to hyperglycaemia in the post-injury situation. Fructose has been proposed as one such carbohydrate and it has been widely used in intravenous nutrition. Fructose is initially metabolized to glucose in the liver, and its further metabolism is dependent upon insulin for uptake of this glucose into skeletal muscle, for example. Fructose metabolism cannot therefore be considered to be insulin independent. Fructose in the form of sucrose is, of course, a component of the normal oral diet. An intravenous intake of fructose of up to 100 g/day would mimic this. Large fructose infusions have been associated with a variety of metabolic complications, particularly lactic acidosis, hypophosphataemia and hyperuricaemia. Sorbitol has also been frequently used, mainly because it can be autoclaved in the presence of amino acid solutions, but it is metabolized to fructose and suffers the same problems. Urinary losses of sorbitol may be considerable and lead to osmotic diuresis.

Ethanol has also been used as a carbohydrate source. Ethanol is not a glucose precursor and its transient popularity stemmed from its higher calorific value (about 7 kcal/g). An adequate energy intake is, however, associated with excessive pharmacological effects on the nervous system and ethanol is thus rarely used now.

Xylitol is a further alternative sugar which has gained some popularity, particularly in Germany. A mixture of glucose/fructose/xylitol in a ratio of 2:1:1 has been suggested to be the most effective solution in the post-injury period. Xylitol infusion has been associated with various metabolic abnormalities, and there would seem little benefit in its use.

From the practical point of view, it would seem most appropriate to use just the one carbohydrate source, glucose. Hyperglycaemia is rarely a problem, particularly if some of the energy requirements are met by fat emulsions. When glucose is used as the sole energy substrate, up to 750 g/day in adults or 25 g/kg per day in infants has been shown to be well tolerated, particularly if the intake is built up slowly over a few days. There would therefore appear to be little justification to use any carbohydrate other than glucose in intravenous nutrition.

III. Fat

The main advantage of fat emulsions is that large amounts of energy can be given in a small volume of isotonic fluid. This is due to the high calorific value of triglycerides, together with the fact that the fat emulsion particles are in suspension, and do not themselves contribute to the osmolarity of the solution. Isotonicity is achieved by addition of a small amount of carbohydrate; for example glycerol is added in the fat emulsion Intralipid [R] (soya oil). Because of the isotonicity of the solution, thrombophlebitis is infrequent, and Intralipid can be satisfactorily infused into a peripheral vein, sometimes in combination with other more hypertonic nutrients.[3, 11]

A further advantage of the use of fat emulsions is that they supply the body with essential fatty acids. These substances are of importance in maintaining normal cell membrane composition and function and as precursors of prostaglandins. Linoleic acid is known to be essential and it is likely that linolenic acid is also essential. Both of these fatty acids are present in substantial amounts in Intralipid [R]. Essential fatty acid deficiency has been observed in patients receiving intravenous nutrition where essential fatty acids have not been provided. Such deficiency states are characterized by scaly skin, hair loss and thrombocytopenia and are readily reversed by infusion of fat emulsions.

Fat emulsions for intravenous nutrition contain a vegetable oil and water and emulsifiers to stabilize the mixture. In Intralipid [R], the triglyceride source is soya bean oil with egg yolk phospholipids as emulsifiers. It has been clearly shown that Intralipid is readily metabolized and can be utilized as an energy source to promote protein synthesis. Clearance of Intralipid from the blood stream occurs with similar kinetics to natural chylomicrons, but such kinetics are not necessarily the same for all synthetic fat emulsions. One interesting feature of fat infusions is that they are made directly into the systemic circulation, in a similar way to natural chylomicrons absorbed after a fatty meal which are transported via the thoracic duct to the subclavian vein. Most individuals clear an infusion of Intralipid within 6 h of the termination of the infusion. If the plasma is still 'milky' after this time, the possibility of some failure of clearance should be investigated. This is an unusual event, but has been said to be associated with sepsis due to Gram-negative organisms.

Fat emulsions have been used to provide up to 85% of the energy intake per day. More commonly, a smaller proportion of daily energy intake is provided by fat, perhaps some 30–50%. Regular infusion of fat emulsions in this way is associated with a reduction in metabolic complications, notably hyperglycaemia and hypophosphataemia, which are commonly associated with high dose glucose infusions. There are many workers who give fat emulsions much less frequently, the bulk of the energy being provided in the form of carbohydrate, one or two 500-ml infusions of fat emulsions per week ensuring an adequate intake of essential fatty acids.

How to obtain Optimal Utilization of Infused Nutrients

1. The amino acid preparation should contain a balanced mixture of the essential amino acids and the non-essential amino acids.
2. An adequate provision of energy should be ensured throughout the period of amino acid infusion, so that gluconeogenesis from the infused amino acids is kept to a minimum.
3. The supply of non-protein energy substrates should be between 125 and 200 kcal/g of amino acid nitrogen infused.
4. High levels of carbohydrate may be particularly effective in promoting nitrogen retention in very catabolic patients, particularly if exogenous insulin is added.
5. Adequate supply of minerals and vitamins are necessary for optimal utilization of the major nutrients.

IV. Minerals

Of the large number of minerals now recognized as being essential for normal nutrition, a classification can be made into those required in relatively large amounts (mmol/day), the major minerals, and those required in micromolar or less amounts per day, the minor minerals. Attempts to estimate, from the oral diets, the amount of these minerals to provide intravenously, are hampered by a lack of basic knowledge of mineral metabolism: in particular, the proportion of each mineral absorbed from the oral diet, the factors which affect absorption, and intestinal and plasma transport systems. These are complex problems, which cannot be related directly to intravenous infusions. As with amino acid infusions, provision of minerals intravenously is empirical, and based upon attempts to maintain apparent biochemical normality and prevention of known clinical deficiency states. Recommendations have been made for the requirements of these various minerals during parenteral nutrition[12-14] (Table 7.1), but such recommendations should only be used as broad guidelines. In situations with abnormal losses of minerals, due to loss of body fluids or to excessive breakdown of tissues, it is impossible to predict mineral requirements. The best estimates can be obtained by careful measurement of losses and monitoring the effect of replacement on blood and urine concentration of the minerals.

Major Minerals

The minerals required in greatest amount are sodium, potassium, phosphorus, magnesium and calcium. The requirement for each of these, with the possible exception of calcium, is variable from patient to patient, from day to day in the same patient, and depends upon changes in fluid and electrolyte status, urine output, fistula or other fluid loss, and relative states of anabolism or catabolism. The major mineral requirements are usually met by the mineral content of the amino acid solution (*Table* 7.3), together with specific additives of individual minerals. Additions can be made to the infused nutrients, provided compatibility requirements are met. The concentrated nature of each additive means that only a relatively small extra volume of fluid is added.

Table 7.3. **Major mineral requirements and additives**

Mineral	Daily requirement, mmol	Concn in amino acid solutions, mmol/l	Additives
Sodium	50–200	0–73	NaCl: 5 mmol/ml
Potassium	50–200	0–60	KCl: 2 mmol/ml
Phosphorus	10–50	0–30	Na phosphate/K phosphate: 1 mmol P/ml
			K phosphate/ } 0·4 mmol P/ml
			K acetate } 2 mmol K/ml
Magnesium	3–25	0–5	50% MgSO$_4$: 2 mmol Mg/ml
Calcium	7–14	0–2·5	Ca chloride: 0·9 mmol Ca/ml

Minor Minerals (Trace Elements)

The list of trace elements known to be essential for nutrition in man is extensive, but these elements can be divided into three main groups:
1. Those in which depletion or deficiency states are relatively common in intravenous nutrition, e.g. zinc, copper or iron. Clinical deficiency syndromes as well as biochemical tests of mineral depletion are clearly documented for these minerals.
2. Those in which depletion or deficiency states are rare. There have been isolated reports of chromium and selenium deficiency in patients receiving long-term intravenous feeding.
3. A large group of minerals in which it is questionable whether a clear depletion or deficiency syndrome exists. However, based on work in other animal species and a knowledge of the metal co-factors for various enzymes, minerals such as manganese and molybdenum are almost certainly essential.

Which trace elements should be given and at what point in therapy they are necessary is a matter of debate. It is now generally accepted that zinc and copper should be provided to most patients; there is also a clear requirement for iron, although the possible role of iron in promoting certain bacterial infections makes it important not to saturate transferrin, the iron-transporting protein. This is particularly relevant because transferrin concentrations are often reduced in concentration in patients who have undergone a period of inadequate protein–energy intake. Many patients have had a period of inadequate intake of trace minerals prior to commencing intravenous feeding. Since it is uncertain how long intravenous feeding will continue, it is therefore logical to attempt to meet the daily requirements of these minerals from the commencement of intravenous feeding; in other words it is better practice to prevent deficiencies from occurring than to treat them after they have developed.

If this basic philosophy is accepted and, to some extent, this area becomes a matter of philosophy rather than hard scientific fact, it seems reasonable to provide as many of the minor minerals as possible. Provision of these minerals must, however, be subject to constraints of practicality and cost.

Provision of minor minerals

1. AS CONTAMINANTS IN INFUSION SOLUTIONS. It is now well recognized that variable amounts of many trace elements are present in solutions of intravenous nutrients, particularly amino acid solutions. The highest concentrations have been found in protein hydrolysates, but, with the increasing use of crystalline amino acid preparations, this source of trace elements has been reduced. Nevertheless, as shown in *Table* 7.4, the amount of various metals, particularly of zinc or chromium, present even in crystalline amino acid solutions, may form a significant proportion of the daily requirement.

The source of trace elements in these solutions is uncertain, although much is likely to have arisen from the rubber bung used in the bottles,

Table 7.4. **Trace elements present as contaminants in infusion solutions**

Solution	Zn µmol/l	Cu µmol/l	Cr µmol/l	Fe µmol/l
Aminosol [R]	46·5	1·9	1·9–3·3	16·0
Vamin [R] glucose	10·0	0·9	0·1–0·3	1·1
Synthamin [R]	2·2	0·3	0·12	3·5
Intralipid (soya oil) 10%	3·2	1·3	0·02	0·02
Daily requirements µmol	20–200	5–50	0·2–0·4	15–50

together with small amounts introduced during manufacture of the solution, or from the raw materials used.

2. AS PLASMA. It has been suggested that intermittent infusion of a unit of plasma may provide an adequate intake of various trace metals. Although this may be the case for some metals in which the plasma concentration is relatively high and the daily requirements relatively low, this practice cannot be recommended. For example, the daily requirement of zinc is usually 50–100 μmol, whereas the plasma concentration of zinc is only about 15 μmol/l. Hence, at least 3 l of plasma per day would be required to deliver the appropriate amount of zinc. On the other hand, infusion of plasma will ensure that the mineral is provided in a biologically active form.

3. AS INDIVIDUAL SUPPLEMENTS. In a recent review[12] of trace metal requirements in intravenous feeding, an expert panel of the American Medical Association indicated that the safest and most flexible way to provide such supplements was by provision of individual trace elements. They recommended the usage of individual supplements of zinc, copper, chromium and manganese. Although the rationale for the use of such a system is clear in terms of tailoring the provision of each trace element to each patient's requirement, such a system would be labour intensive.

4. AS TRACE ELEMENT COCKTAILS. Mixtures of various elements have been proposed, the most comprehensive being Addamel[R] (Kabi Vitrum) which contains calcium, magnesium, iron, zinc, copper, manganese, fluoride and iodide. There is little doubt, however, that the use of such cocktails restricts flexibility, since patients with an increased requirement of only one trace element will receive excessive amounts of the other elements if the total intake of the mixture is increased. For this reason, a practical approach to the provision of trace elements would be use of a mixture of elements to meet the requirements of most patients, and to supplement this where necessary with additional quantities of single trace element solutions to meet individual patient's needs.

V. Vitamins

In comparison to the other components of the diet, the provision of vitamins in intravenous nutrition has received scant attention. Only rarely have patients been observed to have a clinical deficiency state during intravenous feeding, although biochemical evidence of depletion has been widely reported. Vitamin abnormalities are common at the commencement of intravenous feeding. In particular, folic acid, ascorbic acid and vitamin

A and E levels are frequently reduced. Folate deficiency may develop, especially in patients receiving ethanol as an energy source, or when receiving large amounts of methionine from the amino acid infusion. B vitamin requirements are closely related to the level of provision of energy substrates. Recommended levels of intake of vitamins for patients with basal requirements and the levels of supply of vitamins from some widely used vitamin supplements are shown in *Table* 7.5[14, 15] Vitamin requirements may vary considerably with the disease process; in the very sick patient, levels of intake five to ten times those suggested may be necessary. It is clear that most of the available vitamin preparations are poorly balanced with respect to the requirements for intravenous feeding purposes. However, in the majority of patients, the combination of Solivito[R] and Vitlipid[R] as shown in *Table* 7.5 provides an adequate intake of most vitamins for correction of pre-existing deficits.

Table 7.5. **Vitamin requirements and supply in TPN**

Vitamin	Basal requirement[a]	Parentrovite[b] (1 pair amps)	Multibionta[c] (MVI)[e]	Solivito[d]	Vitlipid[d]
Thiamin, mg	1·4	250	50	1·2	
Riboflavin, mg	2·1	4	10	1·8	
Nicotinamide, mg	14	160	100	10	
Pyridoxine, mg	2·1	50	15	2	
Folic acid, mg	0·21			0·2	
Cyanocobalamin, µg	2·1			2	
Pantothenic acid, mg	14		25	10	
Biotin, mg	0·35				
Ascorbic acid, mg	35	500	500	300	
Retinol, mg	0·7		3		0·75
Cholecalciferol, mg	2·8		(25)		3
Phytylmenaquinone, mg	0·14				0·15
Tocopherol, i.u.	35		5		30–35[f]

[a] From Shenkin and Wretlind.[14]   [b] Bencard, Middlesex.   [c] BDH, Bilton.   [d] Kabi Vitrum, Stockholm, Sweden.
[e] USV Lab, New York.   [f] From 500 ml Intralipid (soya oil).

The method of infusion of the vitamins should be carefully considered. It is now appreciated that considerable degradation of some vitamins may occur with exposure to light. In particular, riboflavin and ascorbic acid may be rapidly reduced in concentration unless the solution containing the water-soluble vitamins is shielded from daylight. Alternatively, the injection of water-soluble vitamins into a bottle of fat emulsion may be effective as the opacity of the fat emulsion lends some protection from the action of light. One further possible advantage of infusing the water-soluble vitamins with fat emulsion is the separation of vitamins from trace elements, thus preventing any possible chemical interaction. For example, copper and, to a lesser extent, iron may cause oxidation of ascorbic acid to dehydroascorbic acid and hence inactivate vitamin C. The precise value of inclusion of both water- and fat-soluble vitamins in the fat emulsion has, however, still to be fully established.

METHODS OF INFUSION

Parenteral nutrition is performed either through a central venous catheter with the tip in the superior vena cava or right atrium or by infusion through a cannula in a peripheral vein. In the majority of cases, the infusions are given into a central vein and continuously over the 24-hour period. Occasionally, and particularly in ambulant patients, it may be possible to complete the infusion in 12 or 16 hours. In such cases, the central venous catheter is filled with a dilute heparin solution when not in use. In neonates and infants infusions have usually been made continuously during 24 h/day.

Central venous access can be achieved in a number of ways. Dudrick and coworkers[2] have popularized the use of direct insertion into the subclavian vein, using an infraclavicular approach. Access to the subclavian vein can also be made by the supraclavicular approach or by a cut-down onto the cephalic vein in the deltopectoral groove. Although internal jugular vein catheterization is commonly used in intensive care units, this tends to be less practical from a feeding point of view because of restrictions of the patient's movements and the difficulty in applying dressings. As a general rule, catheters which are being used for intravenous feeding should not also be used for measurement of central venous pressure, because of the risk of infection.

For long-term feeding, a Silastic catheter is tunnelled subcutaneously from the site of venous insertion. A Dacron cuff may be attached to the catheter so that, after insertion, the cuff lies a short distance from the skin exit site and provides a mechanical barrier to the spread of organisms from the skin surface. It is apparent that tunnelling of the catheter prolongs its life as well as facilitating changes of the catheter dressings. The precise role of subcutaneous tunnelling in short-term parenteral nutrition has yet to be established.

Central venous catheters to be used for intravenous nutrition should always be inserted with aseptic techniques, preferably in an operating theatre.

Usage of the 3-l infusion bag has proved to be a major practical advance in nutrient provision. This system permits the mixing of all the aqueous components of the regimen, amino acids, carbohydrates, electrolytes, trace elements and possibly also of water-soluble vitamins. This mixture, which may amount to between 2 and 3 l/day, is a homogeneous solution with a uniform composition and tonicity, and is stable and suitable for continuous infusion. An important benefit is the ease of administration from the nursing point of view, since only one bag need be changed per day. Irregularities in infusion rate should be minimized because such a bag necessitates the use of an accurate infusion system, such as a constant infusion pump. Moreover, this system should also be considerably safer than use of separate bottles, since the additives should have been made by an experienced pharmacist under aseptic conditions. When a fat emulsion is to be given, it is infused from a separate giving set with a V-junction connection. The fat emulsion is infused over 6–8 hours. Once the infusion of fat emulsion is complete, the line is closed off for the remainder of the 24 hour period. One limitation to the general applicability of this system is the requirement for laminar flow facilities within the hospital pharmacy for preparation of infusions. There is an increasing acceptance that this is a worthwhile service in hospitals in which intravenous nutrition is used.

Solassol and Joyeux, from the Centre Anticancereux in Montpellier, France, have pioneered the mixing of fat emulsions with water-soluble nutrients in one container, producing a 'complete nutritive mixture'. They have achieved satisfactory clinical results for many years. However, it is feared that the fat emulsion might separate under these conditions with production of large fat particles which could lead to fat embolism. If it can be established that the fat emulsion remains stable when mixed in this way, this complete mixture would further simplify the administration of parenteral nutrition.

Peripheral vein feeding, using separate bottles of water-soluble nutrients and fat emulsion, or the 3-l bag with separate fat emulsion, has been proved to be effective. It has been of particular value in feeding neonates, where scalp vein feeding can be achieved for prolonged periods. In adults, parenteral feeding for 3 months or more has been possible by this route alone. With peripheral vein feeding, the fat emulsion should be infused continuously throughout the day. The use of a fine Teflon cannula, inserted into as large a peripheral vein as possible, allows adequate blood flow to dilute the hypertonic infusion solution. Frequent cannula changes (as often as every 24 hours) are necessary to avoid thrombophlebitis. Nevertheless it may be difficult to achieve a satisfactory and constant flow rate via peripheral veins.

A central venous catheter, inserted under sterile conditions and managed with appropriate nursing techniques during the changes of dressing and giving set, may last for many weeks or even months. This greater degree of convenience and reliability as far as administration is concerned has led to the central venous catheter technique being the method of choice in most hospitals. It is important to remember, however, that almost all the serious complications associated with the administration of intravenous feeding occur with central venous catheters. It is recommended that insertion and maintenance of central venous catheters should be the responsibility of a small group of interested individuals in each hospital.

COMPILATION OF A PARENTERAL NUTRITION REGIMEN

I. Precise Calculation of Requirements

1. Based upon clinical examination, and fluid balance charts, estimate the volume of fluid to be infused.
2. Based upon urine nitrogen measurements, or theoretical estimate based upon clinical condition and tables, estimate total nitrogen to be infused.
3. Choose an appropriate amino acid source and estimate the volume necessary to meet nitrogen requirements.
4. Estimate the approximate energy requirements based upon 200 kcal/g N.
5. Choose the ratio of carbohydrate to fat which are to be infused, and estimate the total volumes of fat emulsion (10% or 20%) and 50% dextrose.
6. Based upon the relevant biochemistry, estimate the amount of sodium, potassium, magnesium, phosphorus and other trace elements which are to be infused. Calculate the amount of these present in the amino acid solution, and hence calculate the amount of appropriate additives necessary.
7. Add appropriate vitamins, both water- and fat-soluble. Ensure all vitamin requirements have been met.
8. Calculate the total volume and adjust to the desired volume either by addition of water, or by alteration of the concentrations of the amino acid, carbohydrate or fat emulsion.

II. Use of a Standard Regimen

The above approach may be considered to be too difficult in attempting to tailor precisely the nutritional input to the requirements of the patient. A more practical approach for the majority of patients may be to use a fairly standard regimen. For example, we have found that the following procedure is usually satisfactory: for the first 48 hours a 2-l regimen provides 9 g N and 2000 kcal (1000 as glucose and 1000 as fat emulsion). Thereafter a 3-l regimen is used, providing 14 g N and 3000 kcal (2000 as carbohydrate and 1000 as fat). One hundred and fifty mmol sodium, 80 mmol potassium, 7·5 mmol magnesium, 15 mmol phosphate, 100 μmol zinc plus water- and fat-soluble vitamins are given.

With this approach, it is particularly important to monitor the adequacy of the regimen by regular serum and urine analysis. Whether the intravenous regimen is obtained from precise calculation or from a standard procedure, three important rules remain.
1. Discuss the prescription with the pharmacist who is to prepare the solutions.
2. Re-assess the prescription regularly, on the basis of changes in the patient's condition, and changes in the biochemistry.

3. Ensure good communications are maintained between all the personnel involved in the provision of the intravenous nutrition, clinicians, nursing staff, biochemists, pharmacist and dietitians.

Special Types of Parenteral Nutrition

I. Glucose and Insulin Therapy

In the very catabolic patient, it has been clearly shown that infusion of 50% glucose at a rate of 50 ml/h together with adequate insulin (5–25 U/h) and potassium (about 5–10 mmol/h) can lead to a dramatic reduction in urinary nitrogen excretion, from 20 g or more per day to less than 10 g per day.[16] It has been concluded that this effect is due to the increased uptake of glucose into skeletal muscle cells and increased oxidation of glucose by these cells, thus decreasing the stimulus for catabolism of muscle protein. Moreover, insulin stimulates protein synthesis in skeletal muscle. In the absence of glucose infusions, much of the energy required by skeletal muscle would be obtained from oxidation of branched chain amino acids, generated by muscle protein catabolism. The other amino acids released would be transported to the liver for gluconeogenesis and protein synthesis.

This therapy has been shown to have considerable benefits in the short term, both in improving function of certain tissues, especially cardiac function, and also in 'correcting' certain biochemical abnormalities, e.g. 'sick-cell' syndrome, as well as the excess nitrogen excretion. However, concern has been expressed that such an improvement in nitrogen balance may not be beneficial in the long term, if the flow of amino acids from muscle to liver is suppressed. This flow is essential for synthesis of liver proteins such as albumin, clotting factors, and other serum proteins. In other words, visceral protein synthesis may be more important than prevention of skeletal muscle catabolism. It is, therefore, not advisable to continue glucose plus insulin therapy alone for more than 3–4 days, after which (or even during this period) amino acids should be included in the regimen to ensure an adequate supply to the liver.

II. Peripheral Vein Amino Acid Infusion

Blackburn and co-workers[17] have suggested that infusion of amino acids by peripheral vein will lead to an improved nitrogen balance in the postoperative period when compared with standard crystalloid infusions, such as 5% dextrose.

They proposed that this was due to the relatively low insulin response to amino acid infusions, and hence fatty acids would be mobilized readily from adipose tissue. Such fatty acids would therefore be available as an energy substrate for utilization of the amino acids in protein synthesis.

Attractive as this hypothesis is, it has not, however, been proved experimentally. There is little doubt, nevertheless, that peripheral amino acids do improve nitrogen balance in this period, although the mechanism of action appears to be related directly to the amino acids themselves.

Whether such therapy is beneficial to the patient remains to be proved; if clearly demonstrated this would necessitate a major change in postoperative intravenous fluid therapy. At present, such infusions represent a possible 'holding' measure to allow time to assess if the patient requires total parenteral nutrition by the central venous route. It is important to remember that these infusions are hypocaloric, and hence catabolism of stored energy substrates is inevitable. Such infusions should not, therefore, be used in depleted patients.

COMPLICATIONS OF INTRAVENOUS NUTRITION

I. Complications associated with the Catheter

The major complication associated with peripheral vein feeding is the development of superficial thrombophlebitis. This is uncommon when infusions are short and fat emulsions are used.

A wide variety of complications have been reported in association with the insertion of the central venous catheter. These include pneumothorax, subcutaneous haematomas, haemothorax, intrapleural infusion, damage to the carotid or subclavian artery, the thoracic duct and the brachial plexus. Because of the large diameter of the central vein, and the high flow rate of blood through it, complete thrombosis of the subclavian vein or superior vena cava is uncommon. There is, however, increasing evidence that lesser degrees of thrombosis do occur particularly when non-Silastic catheters are used.

The most serious complication of intravenous nutrition is infection of the central venous catheter. This complication may be life-threatening, and must be acted upon promptly. The initial problem is in recognizing the source of the infection; most of the patients involved have a variety of possible sources of infection, particularly if they have had abdominal surgery. Initial action should include blood culture (from peripheral vein and draw back through the catheter), and culture of sputum, urine and wound swabs. If the central venous line is under suspicion, it may be appropriate to discontinue the infusion temporarily and a heparin lock used to seal the central venous catheter. Bacteriology results should be available within 48 hours. If no clear site of infection is identified and if the temperature remains elevated, or if the pyrexia settles within this period only to recommence when the infusion is restarted, then a presumptive catheter sepsis is present, and the catheter should be removed. Meticulous attention to detail during insertion and maintenance of the catheter is essential if the infection rate is to be kept to a minimum.

II. Metabolic Complications

A number of metabolic complications have been observed in patients receiving intravenous nutrition.

1. Hyperglycaemia

Normal adults can usually metabolize glucose at an infusion rate of at least $0.5\,g/kg$ per h. However, in the post-traumatic period or in sepsis, the impaired glucose tolerance may lead to hyperglycaemia and glycosuria. One of the most serious complications of the use of hypertonic glucose infusions is, therefore, hyperosmolar, non-ketotic hyperglycaemic coma. Patients should never be allowed to develop this serious condition, and should be appropriately monitored with 6-hourly testing of urine for glucose.

2. Hypoglycaemia

Insulin secretion from the pancreas increases in response to glucose infusion. If the intravenous glucose is stopped suddenly, there is an immediate fall in blood sugar but serum insulin may remain high leading to rebound hypoglycaemia. This is potentially a dangerous complication, but it can be readily prevented by a policy of gradual reduction in the glucose infusion rate and by giving isotonic glucose for several hours after cessation of hypertonic glucose.

3. Metabolic Acidosis

Acid–base abnormalities are rarely due to parenteral nutrition alone. Amino acid solutions contain a considerable amount of amino acid hydrochlorides, which release hydrochloric acid on their metabolism. Certain amino acid solutions now contain a proportion of acetate and phosphate to reduce the danger of metabolic acidosis.

4. Hyperammonaemia

This was particularly associated with the use of protein hydrolysates. More recently, it has been associated with the use of preparations containing large amounts of glycine. Because hyperammonaemia may be secondary to a relative arginine deficiency, which decreases the efficiency of the urea cycle, arginine supplements to the amino acid solutions may be helpful, especially in patients who are considered to be at risk, such as those with hepatic disease.

5. Essential Fatty Acid Deficiency

This syndrome has been described earlier, and is associated with the use of fat-free intravenous nutrition. Regular infusion of fat emulsion will prevent the characteristic skin rash and haematological changes.

6. Hypophosphataemia

This is a common problem in individuals receiving high dose glucose, fructose or sorbitol infusions. Paraesthesiae, weakness and respiratory failure have been associated with a low serum phosphate. Hypophosphataemia can be prevented by inclusion of 10–20 mmol of phosphate per day in the infusion.

7. Hypomagnesaemia

A low serum magnesium is a common accompaniment to intravenous feeding, especially in individuals with large losses of intestinal fluid. If appropriate serum and urine measurements are made to monitor magnesium status, adequate supplementation can be provided.

8. Other Mineral Deficiencies

A number of other mineral deficiencies have been observed during intravenous feeding, including zinc, copper, chromium and selenium. These deficiencies can all be prevented by provision of the appropriate mineral.

9. Vitamins

Hypovitaminosis states have been reported for many vitamins. Most of these could have been prevented by appropriate vitamin supplementation from the commencement of intravenous feeding.

10. Hepatic Abnormalities

Abnormal liver function tests developing during intravenous feeding pose a particular problem. The question to be answered is whether this is due to the feeding itself, or to some other factor, e.g. abdominal sepsis. Elevation of liver enzymes, either alkaline phosphatase and γ-glutamyltrans-peptidase, implying a cholestatic element, or of transaminases suggesting hepatocellular damage, have been frequently observed. A causal link with intravenous feeding has been clearly implicated in those patients in whom the cessation of intravenous feeding has been associated with a marked improvement in biochemical liver function tests. The cause of this abnorm-ality remains uncertain. Some studies have suggested an association with the use of particular amino acid preparations, both in relation to the amino acid profile and to the presence of metabisulphite as stabilizer. On the other hand, high dose glucose infusions have led, in some cases, to the development of a fatty liver, which is improved by infusion of fat emulsion. One therapeutic suggestion is to stimulate flow of bile by introducing a small amount of oral feeding, if possible, whilst continuing the intravenous feeding. The main guideline for action in this situation is to observe liver function once or twice per week, and if a progressive deterioration is observed, it may become necessary to stop intravenous feeding.

ENTERAL NUTRITION

Recent advances in this field have involved the manufacture of fine bore nasogastric tubes, the development of homogeneous chemically defined diets, and the possibility of using both the new type of tube and diet to provide a constant drip feed rather than bolus feeding. Collectively, these advances have led to a much greater acceptance of tube feeding by the patient, because of the much reduced incidence of side effects. It is now clear that many individuals who previously required intravenous nutrition can achieve an adequate intake by the enteral route.

Tubes for Nasogastric or Nasojejunal Feeding

With the aid of a guide wire, fine bore flexible tubes (6–8 Fr or less) can readily be passed into the stomach for nasogastric feeding. If nasojejunal feeding is indicated, long fine bore tubes with weighted ends are available, which, when placed in the stomach, will often pass spontaneously into the jejunum. If this procedure fails (at least 50% of cases), the nasojejunal tube can be positioned under X-ray screening by use of a guide wire.

Prior to commencement of feeding, it is first necessary to check the position of the tube. Aspiration of fluid and testing with litmus paper, as with standard bore tubes, is often not possible due to the fine bore. Rapid installation of 10 ml air down the tube and auscultation over the epigas-trium is the best way to ensure that nasogastric tubes lie in the stomach. Should this fail, X-ray of the upper abdomen will confirm whether the tube lies beneath the diaphragm. X-ray is, of course, always necessary to check the position of nasojejunal tubes.

It should be remembered that gastric or jejunal feeding tubes can also be placed directly at operation in patients who are expected to require postoperative nutritional support. Once in place, the tubes are taped without tension to the nose or cheek. Daily flushing with 10 ml of water helps to maintain potency. The lack of discomfort associated with their use can allow such tubes to be left in place for many days.

Preparations for Tube Feeding

The successful use of the fine bore tubes requires a non-particulate feed. Thus homogenized ward diets and certain commercial tube feeds prepared from powdered materials may have a somewhat 'lumpy' consistency which will not flow evenly through the tube. A plethora of premixed proprietary feeds, specifically designed for this type of administration, are now available. The basic composition of some of these feeds is summarized in *Table* 7.6.

The major differences between these various feeds are:

1. The type of protein source used. Most feeds use whole proteins of high biological value. However, the elemental diets such as Vivonex[R] or Flexical[R] consist of individual amino acids, or a mixture of amino acids and small peptides.

2. The amount of carbohydrate and fat as an energy source varies considerably. In some preparations there is very little fat present, whereas up to 40% of the energy may be provided by triglycerides.

3. The type of carbohydrate present is variable. The presence of lactose has caused some concern in certain patients, because of possible lactase deficiency states associated either with an inherent lactose intolerance, or due to depletion of brush-border enzymes resulting from chronic malnutrition. The overall osmolality of the feed is also important. This is dependent to a large extent upon the amount of polymerized carbohydrate present, in comparison with the amount of monosaccharides and disaccharides.

4. The energy to nitrogen ratio varies from about 150 kcal/g N to 300 kcal/g N. Preparations which are considered to be short of energy substrates can be supplemented with an additional carbohydrate source such as 'Caloreen[R]', a glucose pentamer.

5. The amounts of minerals and vitamins vary from preparation to preparation. Many do not appear to contain adequate amounts of the minor minerals.

The choice of tube feed will depend on prior experience and confidence in a particular preparation, the nutritional content and finally the cost.

Table 7.6. Tube feeds—amount per 2000 kcal

	RDA[a]	Clinifeed[b] 400	Ensure[c]	Flexical[d]	Isocal[d]	Nutrauxil[e]	Triosorbon[f]	Vivonex[g]	Vivonex HN[g]	Complan[h]/Caloreen[b]
N source	—	Milk/corn protein	Caseinate/soya proteins	Amino acid/peptides	Caseinate/soya proteins	Milk/soya proteins	Caseinate/whey proteins	Amino acids	Amino acids	Milk protein
Carbohydrate	—	Sucrose/lactose dextrins	Sucrose/corn syrup	Sucrose/dextrins	Corn syrup	Partially hydrolysed starch	Oligosaccharides	Glucose	Glucose	Lactose/dextrins
Fat source	—	Soya oil	Corn oil	Soya oil/MCT	Soya oil/MCT	Sunflower oil	MCT	Safflower oil	Safflower oil	Milk fats
No. of pkts/cans for 2000 kcal	—	5 cans	~8	5 cans	5 cans	4 bottles	5 pkts	6 2/3 pkts	6 2/3 pkts	
Carbohydrate, g	—	275	282	305	250	276	224	452	420	352
Fat, g	15–30	67	72	68	85	68	81	2·9	1·7	45
Protein, g	54–84	75	72	45	65	76	81	42	86	56
N, g	8·6–13·4	12	11·5	7	10	12·2	13	6·7	13·3	9·0
Osmolality, mmol/kg	—	450 (undiluted)	450	723	290	350	238	500	840	
Sodium mmol	—	53	63	30	44	66	85	74	67	43
Potassium mmol	—	62	64	64	65	64	85	60	36	61
Calcium, mmol	20	25	26	30	31	25	25	22	13	51

Phosphate, mmol	27	37	33	32	33	39	38	29	17	52
Magnesium, mmol	13	10	17	16	17	11	15	16	10	—
Iron, µmol	200	134	340	322	320	180	286	400	240	350
Zinc, µmol	200	230	480	306	310	64[i]	44[i]	424	260	—
Copper, µmol	40	15	34	32	38	4[i]	7[i]	68	40	22
Thiamin, mg	1·4	2·3	3·2	3·8	4·0	2·2	1·6	1·3	0·8	3·4
Riboflavin, mg	1·6	3·0	3·6	4·3	4·3	3·0	1·9	1·3	0·8	3·1
Pyridoxin, mg	2·0	3·5	4·0	5·0	5·2	2·4	2·2	2·2	1·3	1·1
Niacin, mg	18	17	41	50	53	18	22	15	8·9	21·6
Folic acid, µg	400	754	408	400	400	1000	200	107	67	154
Vitamin B_{12}, µg	3·0	25	12·2	15	15	6·0	3·2	5·5	3·3	6·2
Ascorbic acid, mg	60	136	312	300	320	100	65	78	40	28
Vitamin A, µg	1000	1250	1557	1500	1546	1200	1610	1670	1000	980
Vitamin D, µg	10	13	10	10	10	6	10	11	6·7	3·9
Vitamin E, mg	10	55	62	33	78	30	16	31	20	14·9
Vitamin K, µg	70–140	—	2000	250	250	2200	1050	74	44	3·1

[a] Compiled from *Recommended Dietary Allowances*[19], and *Recommended Daily Amounts* of Food Energy and Nutrients, for Group of People in the United Kingdom[20]

[b] Roussel, Middlesex, England.
[c] Abbot Laboratories, Kent, England.
[d] Mead Johnson, Slough, England.
[e] Kabi Vitrum, London.
[f] BDH, Bilton, Hampshire.
[g] Eaton Labs, London.
[h] Glaxo–Farley Ltd, Middlesex.
[i] Analysed in our laboratories.

Continuous Administration

Constant provision of a tube feed across the 24-hour period is fundamental to the successful use of enteral feeding. Probably the greatest single cause of diarrhoea in patients previously fed by tube was the intermittent syringing of large volumes of hypertonic nutrients into stomach and small intestine. With fine bore tubes and homogeneous feeds, the nutrient can be dripped slowly, either under the influence of gravity, or using a simple constant infusion pump, across the 24-hour period. Indeed it is very difficult to deliver a feed too rapidly when using the fine bore tubes. Constant infusion gives the stomach and small intestine every opportunity to adapt to the rate of infusion and will minimize the problem of sudden shifts of fluid into the small intestine to cope with an osmotic load.

Nevertheless, a carefully structured programme for building up the volume and concentration of the feed is necessary if diarrhoea is to be prevented. For nasogastric feeding, the full strength feed can usually be used from the outset, and the volume increased to the total desired over 3–4 days. Where nasojejunal feeding is being instituted, the feed will usually be introduced at quarter to half strength and approximately 25–50 ml/h and progressively built up, first in the volume and then in concentration, until the full amount is being given.

If diarrhoea still occurs, it can usually be prevented by use of codeine phosphate, 30 mg into the tube, after each bowel movement. If diarrhoea becomes established it may become necessary to reduce both the strength and the volume of the feed before progressively increasing them once again.

Apart from the reduction in side effects, constant administration has other advantages. A marked saving in nursing time is achieved in comparison with bolus feeding; some studies have suggested as much as 1 hour of nursing time per patient per day. Furthermore, accurate ward charts of intake can be kept, allowing a more rational assessment of the patient's response to a particular nutritional regimen.

Monitoring the Provision of Tube Feeding

A similar programme of assessment and monitoring of nutritional status should be provided as outlined below for the use of intravenous feeding. However, most of the tests need not be performed as regularly as those suggested for intravenous feeding. Once the patient is fully established on tube feeding, it seems probable that a nutritional assessment need be carried out only once each fortnight or so to assess overall progress, unless some complication, such as diarrhoea or fistula losses, has developed.

As with intravenous feeding, if the biochemical monitoring indicates that provision of particular nutrients is inadequate, then appropriate supplements should be made into the tube feed, either of additional energy sources, if nitrogen balance is to be improved, or of particular mineral or vitamin supplements. For example, we have found that additional magnesium supplements are frequently necessary for patients with intestinal fistulas who are fed by nasojejunal tube beyond the site of the fistula.

NUTRITIONAL ASSESSMENT AND MONITORING OF NUTRITIONAL SUPPORT

The decision to institute a form of nutritional support is generally taken on clinical grounds. These will not be considered in detail here, but will usually include the recent dietary intake, the patient's general condition and the likelihood of resumption of a normal oral diet. A form of nutritional assessment at the beginning of a period of nutritional support is of importance for a number of reasons. First, this assessment should confirm whether a state of nutritional depletion does exist, and the magnitude of the problem. This also provides a baseline for subsequent measurements. Secondly, the assessment will allow an estimate of the relative amounts of the various nutrients required during nutritional support. Finally, and probably most useful, repeated assessments permit an objective evaluation of the success of therapy, and will indicate the requirement for changing the various components of the nutritional regimen.

Assessment of Protein Energy Nutrition

Energy status is usually considered at the same time as protein status, since protein metabolism interacts so closely with overall energy balance, as described earlier. Body weight is probably the best single measurement in assessment of overall nutritional status. A normal body weight, in comparison with published ranges, indicates that the individual's reserves of energy are probably satisfactory. However, normal values are notoriously variable, and an individual's ideal weight when in perfect health may well be much higher or lower than the value quoted in tables. Moreover, changes in total body weight do not indicate which tissue or body compartment has been affected; changes in fluid balance, in the amount of depot fat or the amount of skeletal muscle may all lead to marked alterations in body weight. Measurement of the triceps skinfold thickness (TST) as an estimate of body fat stores may be useful. Although measurement of skinfold thickness at four separate sites (biceps, triceps, suprailiac and subscapular) leads to a better correlation with whole body fat, these measurements are rarely possible in ill patients, and the TST alone is usually acceptable. This measurement is especially useful when evaluating changes in response to therapy. The mid-arm muscle circumference (mid-arm circumference $- \pi \times$ TST) provides an estimate of whole body skeletal muscle mass. Both the TST and the mid-arm muscle circumference can be compared with standards and values of less than 90% can be considered to indicate mild protein-energy depletion, whereas values of less than 60% of standard indicate very severe depletion. The problem with this approach is the difficulty in obtaining appropriate standards; most of those available are not necessarily representative of the hospital population to which they are being applied.

The severity of protein-energy depletion may also be assessed by delayed hypersensitivity skin tests to recall antigens, such as tuberculin PPD, candida, streptokinase/streptodornase or mumps. These tests provide an in vivo assessment of immunocompetence. The absence of a cell-mediated immune response (anergy) has been said by many workers to be associated with an increased risk of infection and mortality. Anergy has been found to correlate with a reduction in body cell mass. Nutritional repletion in such patients may be followed by return in skin reactivity. It must be stressed, however, that these suggestions have not been confirmed in all studies; several studies have failed to demonstrate the relationship between anergy and morbidity or mortality. Furthermore, conversion of an anergic skin test response to positive is not always associated with an improvement in nutritional status. Such tests, therefore, are not good nutritional markers.

Energy requirements may range from 30 kcal/kg to more than 60 kcal/kg. The most rational method in assessing adequacy of energy intake is to measure energy utilization, usually by indirect calorimetry. However, the collection of expired O_2 and CO_2 is technically difficult, and the gas analysers necessary are not widely available. This method is therefore unlikely to become of widespread use. It has also been suggested that if basal energy expenditure (BEE) is estimated using Harris–Benedict nomograms (which relate height, weight and age to BEE), $1.75 \times$ BEE will provide an adequate energy intake for most patients being fed intravenously. Although this method probably correlates satisfactorily for many patients, the BEE does not allow for sepsis or severity of illness which can have a variable effect on resting energy expenditure. When anabolism is desired, provision of intravenous energy substrates to a level of 50% above this calculated or measured value may be required.

These estimates of energy requirements are only approximate, and probably the best test of adequacy of energy intake is based upon nitrogen (N) balance. An estimate of nitrogen excretion is the corner stone of a nutritional support regimen. Twenty-four hour urine nitrogen can vary from less than 10 g/day to more than 30 g/day depending upon the degree of net protein catabolism. Total urine nitrogen can be readily measured; where this analysis is not available, urea measurements provide a convenient alternative. Provided there is no urinary infection or excessive excretion of amino acids, the urine urea nitrogen usually (but not invariably) comprises about 80% of the total urine nitrogen. An estimate of other losses of nitrogen in faeces, skin, etc. of about 2 g/day (or more if there are fistula or exudate losses) should be added to this. In accurate nitrogen balance studies, an allowance should also be made for changes in blood urea, since urea is distributed throughout body water, a rise in plasma urea of 1 mmol/l being equivalent to retention of about 1 g nitrogen. Having estimated the total amount of nitrogen losses, the adequacy of the nitrogen intake can then be observed. In general, if the object is to achieve a positive nitrogen balance, approximately 3–4 g more nitrogen per day should be provided than the observed daily nitrogen losses.

Based upon the amount of nitrogen which must be provided to achieve the desired nitrogen balance, a more accurate estimate can be made of the amount of dietary energy substrates which should be supplied. As mentioned earlier most studies would suggest that up to 200 kcal/g N should be provided to ensure optimal utilization of amino acid nitrogen, although in individuals in whom large amounts of nitrogen may be required (>20 g/day), a smaller amount of energy, perhaps 125–150 kcal/g N may be adequate. This is an area which is subject to continuous reassessment of the patient's requirements. If the appropriate nitrogen balance cannot be achieved at one particular energy intake, then the nitrogen intake alone, the energy intake alone, or both, may be increased. No firm rules can be given on how to handle this situation.

A number of serum proteins have been proposed to be of some value in assessing protein status, particularly in terms of synthesis of liver proteins. Although the synthetic and catabolic rates of many of these proteins depend upon amino acid nutrition, much of the change in serum level of proteins in ill patients is due to an alteration in the distribution of the protein between intravascular and extravascular fluid. Moreover, since serum albumin has a relatively long half-life, it is of little value as a nutritional marker, especially in the acute situation. A low serum albumin is, nevertheless, a poor prognostic sign.

Shorter half-life proteins, such as transferrin, pre-albumin and retinol binding protein, have been proved useful in diagnosis and treatment of chronic protein–calorie malnutrition. The levels of these proteins fall during acute illness and following injury, and at this time there is little correlation between serum level and nitrogen balance. The change in plasma level in such patients may therefore be a non-specific response, possibly of reduced synthetic rate, which is unrelated to nutrition. Having fallen to low plasma levels, these proteins may still be of value in monitoring the anabolic phase following recovery. Measurement of these serum proteins may be of greater value in assessing progress of relatively stable patients in whom the early effects of the metabolic response to trauma have subsided.

There are, of course, many other measurements which have been suggested to be of value, including plasma measurements of various enzymes, and plasma amino acid profiles, as well as urine measurements of creatinine, creatine and 3-methylhistidine. Although many of these are of considerable interest, none of them really provide much in the way of clinically relevant information which would be used to modify the nutritional intake.

Assessment of Mineral Status

Although subject to the major criticism that serum levels do not represent body stores, the serum level of most minerals is the most commonly used estimate of mineral status. In cases of severe depletion or toxicity of a particular mineral, the diagnosis can usually be confirmed by plasma measurement. Plasma levels alone are, however, of limited value. For example, trauma or infection causes a non-specific fall in the level of serum iron and zinc. Urine analysis may often provide a more sensitive index than serum in reflecting inadequate intake; urine concentrations of magnesium or phosphorus may be low when serum levels are normal. Moreover, measurement of the urine levels allows an estimate of retention of the mineral during repletion. There is little doubt that the best test of mineral status is observation of the response to a supplement of the mineral in question. The extent to which mineral status can be monitored will, of course, vary depending upon the resources of the biochemistry laboratory.

Assessment of Vitamin Status

A variety of tests are available to permit a comprehensive assessment of vitamin status. It is, however, unlikely that many of these need be routinely used. Probably the most relevant are measurements of serum and red cell folate, because of the high incidence of folate deficiency during intravenous feeding. The other tests of B, C and fat-soluble vitamins need only be performed when there is a high level of suspicion of a particular abnormality. From a research point of view, however, it would be of considerable value to determine the optimal levels of provision of vitamins in different illnesses, and for this reason it would be helpful to have more quantitative information of the vitamin status of patients at different levels of vitamin intake.

Protocol for Nutritional Assessment and Monitoring

Based upon the above comments, a protocol for initial assessment of patients who may require nutritional support, and for monitoring such patients can be suggested (*Table* 7.7).

Table 7.7. **Protocol for assessment and monitoring of nutritional status**

Clinical	*Laboratory*	
	Blood	Urine
Height	Urea and electrolyte (A)	Creatinine (B)
Weight (B)	Glucose (E)	Glucose (A)
Weight, % of ideal (B)	Ketones (E)	Nitrogen (urea, total) (B)
Triceps skinfold thickness (C)	Albumin, transferrin, etc. (B)	Ketones (E)
Mid-arm muscle circumference (C)	Liver function tests (B)	3-Methylhistidine (E)
Cell-mediated immunity—		Creatine (E)
skin tests (D)	Ca, P, Mg, Zn, (B)	Ca, P, Mg, Zn (B)
	Vitamin A, C, folic acid (C)	
	Haemoglobin (C)	
	Lymphocyte count (C)	

Key to frequency of measurements:
A—for initial assessment, daily when commencing nutritional support, twice weekly when stable.
B—for initial assessment, then twice weekly.
C—for initial assessment, then weekly.
D—for initial assessment, then every 2–4 weeks.
E—as required or when special indications.

CONCLUSIONS

It is now possible to meet the nutritional requirements of most patients by the intravenous route. Recent developments in enteral nutrition have permitted an adequate nasogastric or nasojejunal intake in many patients who would previously have required intravenous feeding. An appropriate nutritional intake is an important part of therapy in aiding recovery from disease and injury.

REFERENCES

1. Cuthbertson D. P. (1980) Historical background to parenteral nutrition. *Acta Chir. Scand.* [*Suppl.*] **498**, 1–11.
2. Dudrick S. J., Wilmore D. W., Vars H. M. et al. (1969) Can intravenous feeding as the sole means of nutrition support growth in the child and restore weight loss in an adult? An affirmative answer. *Ann. Surg.* **169**, 974–984.
3. Hallberg D., Schuberth O. and Wretlind A. (1966) Experimental and clinical studies with fat emulsion for intravenous nutrition. *Nutr. Dieta* **8**, 245–281.
4. Cuthbertson D. P. (1930) The disturbance of metabolism produced by bony and non-bony injury, with notes on certain abnormal conditions of bone. *Biochem. J.* **24**, 1244–1263.
5. Kinney J. M., Duke J. H., Long C. L. et al. (1970) Carbohydrate and nitrogen metabolism after injury. *J. Clin. Pathol.* **23**, Suppl 4, 65–72.
6. Kinney J. M. (1980) Energy flow—a vital theme in injury and infection. *Acta Chir. Scand.* [*Suppl.*] **498**, 20–25.

7. Long J. M., Wilmore D. W., Mason A. D. et al. (1974) Fat carbohydrate interaction. Effects on nitrogen sparing in total intravenous feeding. *Surg. Forum* **25**, 61–63.
8. Jeejeebhoy K. N., Anderson G. H., Nakhooda A. F. et al. (1976) Metabolic studies in total parenteral nutrition with lipid in man. *J. Clin. Invest.* **57**, 125–136.
9. Askanazi J., Carpentier Y. A., Elwyn D. H. et al. (1980) Influence of total parenteral nutrition on full utilisation in injury and sepsis. *Ann. Surg.* **191**, 40–46.
10. Munro H. N. (1972) Amino acid requirements and metabolism and their relevance to parenteral nutrition. In: Wilkinson A. W., ed., *Parenteral Nutrition*, pp. 34–67. London, Churchill Livingstone.
11. Coran A. G. (1974) Total intravenous feeding of infants and children without the use of a central venous catheter. *Ann. Surg.* **179**, 445–449.
12. American Medical Association (1979) Guidelines for essential trace element preparations for parenteral use. *JAMA* **241**, 2051–2054.
13. Jacobson S. and Wester P. O. (1977) Balance studies of twenty trace elements during total parenteral nutrition in man. *Br. J. Nutr.* **37**, 107–126.
14. Shenkin A. and Wretlind A. (1978) Parenteral nutrition. *World Rev. Nutr. and Diet.* **28**, 1–111.
15. American Medical Association (1975) *Guidelines for Multivitamin Preparations for Parenteral Use.* Chicago, AMA Department of Food and Nutrition.
16. Hinton P., Allison S. P., Littlejohn S. et al. (1971) Insulin and glucose to reduce catabolic response to injury. *Lancet* **1**, 767–769.
17. Blackburn G. L., Flatt J. P. and Hensle T. W. (1976) Peripheral amino acid infusions. In: Fischer J., ed., *Total Parenteral Nutrition*, pp. 363–394. Boston, Little Brown.
18. Woolfson A. M. J. (1979) Metabolic considerations in nutritional support. *Res. Clin. Forums* **1**, 35–47.
19. *Recommended Dietary Allowances*, 9th ed (1980) Washington D.C., Academy of Sciences.
20. *Recommended Daily Amounts of Food Energy and Nutrients for Groups of People in the United Kingdom,* (1979) London, H.M.S.O.

SELECTED REFERENCES FOR FURTHER READING

1. Karran S. J. and Alberti K. G. M. M. (1980) *Practical Nutritional Support.* Tunbridge Wells, Pitman Medical.
2. Richards J. R. and Kinney J. M. (1977) *Nutritional Aspects of Care in the Critically Ill.* Edinburgh, Churchill-Livingstone.
3. Wretlind A. (1972) Complete intravenous nutrition. Theoretical and experimental background. *Nutr. Metab. [Suppl.]* 14, 1–57.

Chapter 8

The Sick-cell Concept and Hyponatraemia

Cecil T. G. Flear and C. M. Singh

The normal functioning of tissues in our bodies derives from the activities of their component cells. Individually, healthy cells as well as healthy tissues respond to neuro-endocrine and other specific stimulation.

Sick cells will not function as healthy cells. They may have abnormalities in aspects of their *specific* functioning. Here we think of inborn errors of metabolism due to enzyme deficiencies, of muscular dystrophy, of malabsorption, of impaired calcification of bone matrix, etc. Cells may also be deficient in respect to the basic activities. Cell membranes may be abnormally leaky, and cells develop altered responsiveness to specific stimulation. Non-specific changes in permeability may mimic some of the ionic accompaniments of specific stimulation, thereby non-specifically initiating increased hormone secretion, etc. Cellular abnormalities at this level can have several consequences to which we shall allude later; but at the outset we would stress that one such consequence is to cause the plasma concentration of sodium to fall. This will form the main topic of this chapter.

Plasma sodium concentrations are low in patients who are critically ill for whatever reason—the result of injuries and surgery, acute infections, abrupt myocardial infarction, long sustained and progressive organ or systems disease (e.g. congestive heart failure, liver failure, malabsorption syndromes, etc.), or neoplasia. They are low, too, in long-sustained chronic disease in which patients are not actually critically ill and may be transiently reduced during febrile episodes in otherwise healthy people. Plasma sodium concentrations are reduced in malnourished infants admitted to hospital, but, since most infants actually admitted to hospital have superadded infections, infection rather than malnutrition may cause the lowering of sodium concentrations. Almost all hyponatraemic patients are either wasted or wasting (to judge by increased excretion of urea and 3-

165

methylhistidine and by the often raised or rising plasma urea concentration, etc.) and most are also excreting unusually high quantities of potassium. Critically ill patients also have an altered pattern of hormone release: increase of the catabolic hormones cortisol, catecholamines, glucagon, together with a relative or absolute reduction of insulin. This fact led to the concept of the 'response to trauma, etc.' which is envisaged as a response package of homeostatic worth 'forged' in our evolutionary past. Increased secretion of antidiuretic hormone in patients has been suggested in most of these situations. This increase has, however, been regarded as inappropriate and the term 'syndrome of inappropriate antidiuretic hormone secretion' introduced.

Although such patients are often excreting little or no sodium in their urine, they are not salt depleted and giving salt neither helps clinically nor raises in a sustained manner the plasma sodium concentration. Clinical improvement or remission is accompanied by a rise in plasma sodium; recovery is accompanied by return of plasma concentration to normal. Prolonged illness protracts hyponatraemia; superadded complications cause further fall in plasma sodium concentration.

We believe that hyponatraemia is a non-specific manifestation of widespread cellular disturbance throughout the body and in 1973 introduced the term 'sick cells' in this connection.[1] Neither author likes the expression 'sick-cell syndrome'. The consequences of sick liver cells will not be those caused by sickness of heart, nor indeed of brain cells. Nevertheless, we consider that it is helpful to recognize that sick cells will not function as effectively as well cells and, providing a large enough mass of body cells is similarly affected, this will have consequences. Clearly there can be no one unique syndrome. The consequences even of disturbances at the rather basic level already discussed will differ depending on how many cells are disturbed. There will be little general effect from disturbances in membrane permeability of 1% of the body cell mass, but much effect when the permeability of 90% of the body cells is changed. The consequences are also likely to be dynamic. At any one time the proportion of cells that are disturbed is likely to vary as some recover and as others deteriorate or become disturbed. We believe that the concept has many useful implications for treatment, that with it many otherwise paradoxical facts become clear, and that it prompts the asking of many questions in such a way that possible answers can be tested in practice.

FACTORS INVOLVED IN MAINTENANCE OF BODY FLUID AND CELLULAR OSMOLALITY

Substrates (including oxygen), intermediates and end products of metabolism (including CO_2) and salts are all dissolved in our body water. Reserves of glycogen and neutral fat are not effectively in solution. Most solutes are unevenly distributed throughout body fluids. Sodium ions are largely confined to extracellular fluids; potassium ions are largely found within cells. Most substrates and intermediates are present at a higher concentration in cell fluids than in the fluid bathing them. Despite this unevenness in concentrations of individual solutes throughout body fluids, uniform *total solute* concentration (and hence osmolality) exists throughout the water in all tissues except the kidney. A high osmolality is achieved within the kidney medulla (some 1800 mosmol/kg water) by a structurally contrived deployment of active sodium transport. Elsewhere throughout the body, fluids in healthy people have an osmolality of about 300 mosmol per kg water.

Uniformity of osmolality throughout body fluids is created by three factors.

1. Active extrusion of sodium ions from cells as fast as they leak into them from the sodium-rich extracellular fluids (ECF) bathing them, which creates the conditions necessary for osmotic equilibrium between cellular and extracellular fluids. Sodium pump activity creates a double-Donnan equilibrium across the cell outer membrane (organic anions constrained within cells; the cation Na^+ effectively constrained in extracellular fluids). Without sodium pumping, there would be a single-Donnan equilibrium (organic anions constrained within cells). A double-Donnan equilibrium is compatible with uniform osmolality of fluids on either side of the cell membrane: a single-Donnan equilibrium is not.[2]

2. The speed with which water diffuses through body fluids and across cell membranes. Because of this and the shortness of distances between cells and capillaries, osmotic gradients arising within a tissue during metabolism and tissue functioning are rapidly dissipated by the appropriate net shifts of water.

3. An efficient circulation which combines iterative perfusion of tissues with central mixing of regional blood. This accomplishes both the appropriate net shifts of water and solutes between tissues and the blood perfusing them, and the effective 'stirring' of extracellular fluids throughout the body.

In tissues like heart and kidney, with a dense, well-perfused capillary network having short intercapillary distances, net redistribution of water is complete within a few milliseconds. In less well-perfused tissues like *resting* skeletal muscle, mesentery and cool skin, it still only takes seconds. Diffusion of solutes, such as glucose and creatinine, is complete in heart tissue within seconds.

Extracellular fluids constitute a common *source-sink* for the millions of cells throughout the body, each of which is an open system in exchange of materials with this source-sink. In health, we can regard body fluids as comprising two well-stirred fluid compartments exchanging water and solutes with one another and with the external environment across specialized cells lining the interface within the lungs, gut and kidney tubules (*Fig.* 8.1).

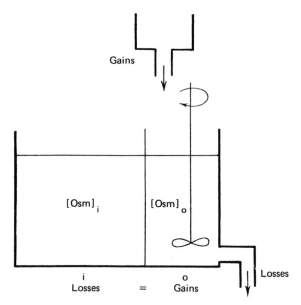

Fig. 8.1. Body water shown as comprised of two well-stirred fluid compartments in osmotic equilibrium, but separated by a membrane; i = cell water and o = extracellular water. The paddle represents the action of the heart and circulation. Matching gains (via lungs and gut) and losses (again via lungs, gut, kidneys and skin are also depicted. $[Osm]_i = [Osm]_o \simeq 300$ mosmol/kg water.

In health, Na^+ with accompanying anions (which are also largely monovalent, i.e. Cl^-, HCO_3^-) comprise some 90% of total solute content of extracellular fluids (interstitial fluid or ISF and plasma). This fact is frequently used to predict plasma osmolality in patients (*see* the appendix). Such predictions have some general validity for healthy people, but are unreliable in most patients. Osmolality should be measured. Comparison of measured and predicted osmolalities in patients is valuable in diagnosing the pathogenesis of hyponatraemia. Plasma sodium levels are quoted in mmol/l plasma, although sodium ions are dissolved in the plasma water.

Generalizing, the sodium concentration in plasma water is higher than that in extravascular water. The effective constraint of more plasma proteins within the blood than is present in ECF creates a Donnan equilibrium across capillary membranes.* This promotes asymmetry in the sodium concentration in fluid on either side of the capillary membrane.

The actual plasma sodium level in a given person varies very little from day to day, reflecting the precision with which osmolality is regulated.

---

*The perceptive reader will recall that earlier it was stated that a single-Donnan equilibrium is incompatible with osmotic equilibrium and yet osmotic equilibrium is usually said to exist across capillary membranes. It would seem likely that, effectively, the presence within extravascular fluids, of molecules of hyaluronic acid, which are also negatively charged, must convert a single to a double-Donnan equilibrium.[3]

Constancy in health, of osmolality of body fluids from day to day and so of its sodium levels throughout the ECF depends on:
1. Balance in the body's gains and losses of water.
2. Disposal from the body of inorganic salts of sodium and potassium gained from food and drink which are in excess of needs and disposal of solutes produced by metabolism. The latter include the end-products CO_2, urea and creatinine.
3. Each of the millions of cells throughout the body maintaining a constant total solute content.

Balance in the Body's Gains and Losses of Sodium and Potassium

Balance in Sodium Exchanges

This balance derives from matching sodium losses to intake less obligatory losses in sweat and faeces. It is achieved by modulated secretion of an, as yet, unidentified circulating natriuretic factor and of the antinatriuretic hormone, aldosterone. Together they regulate sodium excretion by adjusting reabsorption from the collecting ducts. The review by de Wardener[4] gives an excellent discussion of these matters. Expansion or contraction of the extracellular fluid (ECF), or subcompartments thereof, is the trigger for changes in release of antinatriuretic and natriuretic hormones. The controlled release of renin plays a contributory role in modulating aldosterone secretion. Normal activity of sodium pumps in tissue throughout the body is a prerequisite for normal sodium homeostasis. It ensures that net sodium gains by the body are retained within the ECF so that volume or pressure changes within the ECF are sensitive indices of altered body sodium content.

Balance in Potassium Exchanges

Each of the cells throughout our bodies balances its own transmembrane potassium exchanges. In adults, balance in our external exchanges is, therefore, largely a matter of getting rid of unavoidable potassium gained from the food we eat.

In balancing their potassium exchanges, cells maintain constancy of their internal potassium concentration and also of potassium levels throughout the ECF. It was established in the 1930s that net potassium gains distribute evenly throughout all of the body water to bring about an equal rise in both levels of potassium in cellular and extracellular fluids ($[K]_i$ and $[K]_o$, respectively). The rise in $[K]_o$ directly and indirectly initiates prompt increase in potassium excretion: directly by increasing potassium secretion by cells of the collecting ducts; indirectly by increasing secretion of aldosterone which promotes similar effects.

Constancy in Total Solute Content of Cells

The relative impermeability of the outer cell membrane to intermediates and substrates, etc. creates the need to control or regulate the total molar quantity of such non-diffusible solutes within the cell and their net anionic charge. This control is a central feature of metabolic self-regulation by the cell. Without it, osmolality of cell and body fluids would fluctuate as more or less solute was accumulated or produced metabolically. Aspects of this control are embodied in the regulation of glycogen synthesis and breakdown, nucleotide interconversion, storage of fat droplets within cells, protein anabolism and catabolism and in the regulation of cell pH. The pH of cell fluid determines the valence of many of the non-diffusible anions within cells.

The cell content of such constrained anions largely determines cell potassium content. Sodium pump activity plays a contributory role in this by determining cell sodium content. Sodium and potassium jointly serve as counterions to non-diffusible anions within cells.

The Role of Antidiuretic Hormone in the Maintenance of Cellular Osmolality

The thrust of the first section is that the modulated release of antidiuretic hormone into the circulation simply serves to damp down the fluctuations in osmolality that variability in dietary gains of water and solutes would otherwise provoke. However, it neither 'sets' the osmolality nor would it be sufficient alone to stabilize it. For the latter, it is also necessary for cells throughout the body to regulate individually their total content of solutes. This capacity, and the resulting sustained level of osmolality, are twin outcomes of normal cell membrane integrity and metabolic capacity and self-regulation. This viewpoint envisages that a 'desired' level of osmolality is not imposed on the body fluids by *'an osmostat'*, which inbuilt homeostatic mechanisms then conserve and regulate; osmolality and its regulation both derive from the balance and self-regulation of metabolism in health and from the membrane characteristics of healthy cells. It follows from this that osmolality *reflects* the normality of these basic attributes of cell function and membrane integrity and that so, too, does the level of sodium throughout the extracellular fluids, for the major determinant of the sodium level is the osmolality established within cells. Plasma osmolality and the plasma level of sodium will, therefore, both afford indices of cellular well-being. Different animal species maintain their individual and characteristic osmolalities. These can differ markedly: the osmolality of the common British frog is about 200 mosmol/kg water and that of man some 300 mosmol/kg.

This viewpoint would lead one to expect that:

1. Hyponatraemia (a plasma level less than the lower 95% confidence level seen in a reference group of healthy people) would arise in all kinds of disease (*Tables* 8.1–8.3).

2. The duration and extent of hyponatraemia would be more pronounced in severe disease than in lesser illnesses and would parallel the severity of the affliction whatever the disease. These expectations appear also to be confirmed by previous studies (*Tables* 8.2, 8.4–8.6; *Fig.* 8.2).

3. Hyponatraemia would lessen or revert as the clinical condition improves and worsen as the patient's condition deteriorates, whether from progression of the disease or from the supervention of complications. Confirmation of the former expectation is abundantly established as a reality in

Table **8.1. Incidence of hyponatraemia in hospital patients, defined as [Na]$_p$ below the lower 95% confidence limits (CL) of normals investigated by quoted authors**

Observed incidence (frequency), %	Analyses requested	Reference
36	1000	28
39[a]	7695 (Hospital 1)	29
40[a]	1697 (Hospital 2)	
50[b]	1500	30
> 50[c]	324	31
22[a]	600	32
20[a]	11 007	Data from Table 8.2

[a] Lower 95% CL = 135 mmol/l.
[b] Lower 95% CL = 134 mmol/l.
[c] Lower 95% CL = 137 mmol/l (> 50% is an approximation from summarizing information from Payne and Levell,[31] Table 1).

Table **8.2. Incidence (FO) of hyponatraemia ([Na]$_p$ < 135 mmol/l) in patients (consecutive admission) at the Royal Victoria Infirmary, Newcastle upon Tyne**

Department	FO, %	n
Intensive therapy	27	495[a]
Surgical	23	4715
Medical	17	4234
Dermatology		
Inpatient	8	549[a]
Outpatient	0	113
Paediatric[b]	16·7	1014

n Analyses requested by clinicians.
[a] All patients admitted in three separate periods each of 3 months.
[b] Aged 2–14 years.

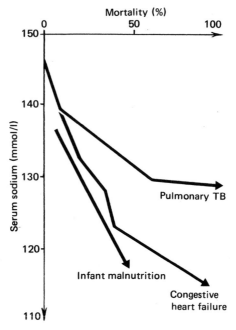

Fig. 8.2. Serum sodium concentration and immediate mortality in illness. Data sources: pulmonary tuberculosis;[36] heart failure;[6, 7] infantile nutrition.[35]

Table **8.3. Incidence (FO) of hyponatraemia ($[Na]_p < 135\,mmol/l$) in infants and children at Royal Victoria Infirmary, Newcastle upon Tyne**

Age	FO, %	n
0–1 months	48	198
1–23 months	33	226
2–5 years	19	450
6–14 years	15	564

n Analyses requested by clinicians.

heart disease and when circulatory improvement follows operative replacement of damaged heart valves, in infantile malnutrition, pulmonary tuberculosis, liver failure, pneumonia, surgery, accidental injuries including burns, sepsis, following recovery from abrupt myocardial infarction and in many other diseases. The latter expectation is equally well established as a clinical reality in a variety of circumstances. Abrupt lowering of plasma sodium has been noted to attend such complications, in congestive heart failure, as chest infection, pulmonary infarct, digitalis toxicity or escape, acute falls in blood pressure from rupture or aneurysm, onset of ventricular fibrillation, etc.,[5–7] to accompany clinical deterioration after abrupt

Table 8.4. Incidence (FO) of hyponatraemia[a] in different diseases

Disease	FO, %	n
Congestive heart disease	62	397[b]
Infantile malnutrition	{ 62	219[c]
	46	304[d]
Liver failure	41	112[e]
Bronchopneumonia	56	45[f]
Myocardial infarction	46	190[g]
Pulmonary tuberculosis	29	169[h]

[a] Hyponatraemia is here defined as a $[Na]_p$ below the lower 95% confidence limits of normals investigated by the authors listed.
[b] *See* Flear.[6, 7]
[c] *See* Chirinos and Ramos-Galvan.[34]
[d] *See* Garrow et al.[35] where hyponatraemia denotes $[Na]_p < 134$ mmol/l. Garrow et al. found lowest $[Na]_p$ in 36 normal infants to be 136 mmol/l; 46% is, therefore, an underestimate.
[e] *See* Sherlock et al.[33] where hyponatraemia denotes $[Na]_p < 130$ mmol/l (normal range not specified by them).
[f] Singh, unpublished observations.
[g] *See* Flear and Hilton.[8]
[h] *See* Westwater et al.[36]

Table 8.5. Incidence (FO) of hyponatraemia ($[Na]_p < 135$ mmol/l) by disease severity

Disease	FO, %	n
Congestive heart failure[a]		
Severe[b]	83	150
Moderate[b]	61	91
Mild[b]	42	156
Consecutive admission to coronary care unit[c]		
Fatal	67	29
Non-fatal	42	161
Ischaemia, no infarct	3	30
Other causes	13	15

[a] *See* Flear.[6, 7]
[b] Pragmatic classification:
Mild: immediate improvement following admission to hospital; no congestive heart failure after 3 weeks.
Moderate: no improvement for 2 weeks after admission; no congestive heart failure after a further few weeks.
Severe: no reduction in oedema for at least 6 weeks, with persisting signs of congestive heart failure or death.
[c] *See* Flear and Hilton.[8]

myocardial infarction[8] and to accompany complications, such as wound or peritoneal infection, rupture of anastomoses after abdominal operations, or infections following open fractures. Indeed, it is our practice to re-evaluate patients for complications if the plasma sodium level falls or remains low for an unduly long period.

Table 8.6. Incidence of a fatal outcome, related to the lowest plasma sodium level attained during admission: 397 patients admitted in congestive heart failure[7]

Lowest $[Na]_p$, mmol/l	Mortality, %
>135	7
135–132	16
132–126	28
125–121	35
≤120	90

SICK CELLS AND HYPONATRAEMIA

In 1973, Flear and Singh[1] pointed out that if the plasma sodium concentration is an outcome of cell metabolism and the integrity of the outer membrane, it will fall when a sufficient mass of cells (a) develop leaky outer membranes or (b) for metabolic reasons become unable to sustain within them the usual molar quantity of non-diffusible solutes, most of which are anions or have a net excess of negative charges in them.

Leaky Outer Membranes

Escape of normally non-diffusible solutes through leaky membranes may arise more or less abruptly. When cells lose solutes in this way, the osmolality of their fluids falls and an osmotic transient arises across the outer membrane. Water shifts into the ECF from cells to negate the transient, and the sodium concentration within the ECF is reduced. Body fluid osmolality does not change, since the body has neither gained nor lost solutes. Increased membrane permeability also causes increased sodium influx which may induce imbalance in transmembrane sodium exchanges and cell sodium gain (*Fig.* 8.3A).

It is, however, the escape of solutes previously constrained inside cells that causes the extracellular (including plasma) concentration of sodium to fall, even when the cells conterminously gain sodium. Shift of sodium into cells from the ECF does *not* cause sodium concentration throughout extracellular fluids to fall.[1, 9–14] Whether inside or outside cells, sodium remains in aqueous solution. Increased sodium influx may cause net gain of sodium by cells, but it can be shown theoretically[15] and it has been shown by experiments in vitro[2] that, when cells gain sodium, they also gain water and chloride. Thus cells effectively gain isosmotic fluid and, in vivo, would swell at the expense of the ECF which itself would shrink. The sodium concentration throughout the ECF therefore remains unchanged. When a balanced state has been attained with a raised internal sodium content and concentration, K^+ will have been lost from cells, and accompanied by Cl^- which entered with Na^+. Potassium loss quantitively equals sodium gain. The rise in extracellular potassium concentration, so provoked, initiates increase in potassium, chloride and water excretion, and the ECF shrinks. Extracellular fluid shrinkage triggers increase in secretion of aldosterone and antidiuretic hormone, thereby re-expanding the ECF, again without change in sodium or chloride concentrations.

If the body gains solutes during these happenings, the fall in plasma sodium concentration will be accompanied by a rise in its osmolality (*Fig. 8.3A*).

Metabolic generation of solutes, for example during imbalance between anabolism and catabolism of protein or caused by substrate mobilization

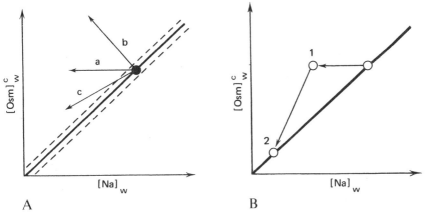

A   B

Fig. 8.3. (A) Functional relationships between plasma sodium levels (sodium in mmol/kg plasma water—$[Na]_w$) and osmolality corrected for plasma urea and glucose ($[Osm]_w^c$, mosmol/kg water) displayed diagrammatically, and flanked by limits within which normally occurring variability falls from day to day (dotted lines). Consequences of leak of some normally non-diffusible solute from cells are shown: (a) alone, with neither gain of solutes by or loss from body fluids; (b) accompanied by conterminous metabolic generation of solutes; (c) with conterminous water gain (oral or i.v.—here 5%, w/v, dextrose is included) or/and solute loss (by solute diuresis). All sequences have been observed during: (i) experimental induction of circulatory collapse in dogs by blood loss, infusion of a killed suspension of *E. coli* and by catecholamine infusion; (ii) dog kidney perfusion in vitro; (iii) clinical circumstances, which include the week following uncomplicated elective surgery, during onset of complication arising after surgery or injury, during developing myocardial infarction, in congestive heart failure, in liver failure, renal uraemia and in bronchopneumonia.[1,13] (B) Consequences of leak of solutes from cells (1) followed by secondary excretion in urine at osmolality in excess of plasma osmolality (2). In this combined sequence hyponatraemia initially (at 1) results from isosmotic water re-distribution and subsequently converts to dilutional hyponatraemia (at 2). At 1, observed $[Osm]_w^c$ is greater than predicted $[Osm]_w^c$ (which is predicted from $[Na]_w$). At 2, observed $[Osm]_w^c$ = predicted $[Osm]_w^c$; *see Fig.* 8.4. The heavy oblique line depicts the functional relationship (concentration/dilution) between $[Osm]_w^c$ and $[Na]_w$. Simple calculations show that $[Na]_w$ could rise and $[Osm]_w^c$ fall, if normally non-diffusible anions and potassium both leak out of cells and are subsequently excreted in urine.

from fuel, such as glycogenolysis and gluconeogenesis, raises osmolality within cells. If these solutes leak from cells so attaining the same concentration outside as inside, generation of solutes will not provoke net shifts of water or lower the concentration of sodium throughout the extracellular fluid. Net hepatic 'release' of glucose into the circulation increases osmolality and lowers sodium concentration. Glucose does not penetrate evenly into all of the remaining cells in the body. Increased ureagenesis, on the other hand, also promotes osmolality increase, but not a fall in extracellular sodium concentration. Urea attains uniform concentration throughout the whole of the body water.

Hyponatraemia provoked by isosmotic redistribution of water and without osmolality reduction (*Fig.* 8.3A) persists as long as the solutes which escape from cells remain within the ECF. Their filtration through glomeruli and into nephrons *causes* their loss from the ECF, unless metabolic replacement and further cellular leak keep pace with excretion. Their excretion from the body can cause the plasma sodium concentration to remain low, to fall still further and even to rise depending on related happenings (*Fig.* 8.3B). *Fig.* 8.4 presents data which suggest that the sequence displayed in *Fig.* 8.3B arises even during experimental situations set up as models of the syndrome of inappropriate antidiuretic hormone secretion (SIADH). Their filtration into nephrons also promotes an osmotic diuresis, which has two other consequences of some relevance:

1. It promotes increased sodium loss.
2. During hydropenia, with maximal antidiuretic hormone, urine osmolality falls to a level a little *above* that of plasma; during a provoked water diuresis, urine osmolality rises to only a little *below* plasma osmolality.

Clearly consequences of abnormal increase in cell membrane permeability are very dynamic. Spillage of normally non-diffusible solutes from cells is unlike emptying a can of beans, since living cells will metabolically replace solutes which leak from them. Much of the escape from skeletal muscle cells will be across leaky sarcoplasmic reticulum (SR) membranes. The surface area of SR membrane in a fibre is some 90 times greater than that of the sarcolemma. Solutes leaking from cells into the SR tubules, must diffuse from these tubules and into interstitial fluid via the SR–transverse (T) tubular junctions and the T-tubule openings on the sarcolemma. Escape of solutes will be slow and will be held up at both of these 'bottle-necks'. This will not, however, significantly delay the general fall in sodium concentration throughout the ECF. Solute gain by SR tubules provokes osmotic transients between the fluid within them and the fluid in both cellular and interstitial fluid (ISF) which provokes net water shifts from both cells and the ISF. This water gain will lower the sodium concentration in SR fluid. Much evidence supports the belief that, normally, sodium is present within SR fluid at the same concentration as in the remainder of the body's extracellular fluids. Lowering of the SR sodium concentration prompts secondary gain of sodium from ISF creating further

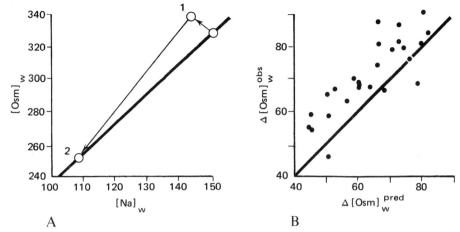

Fig. 8.4. (A) Mean values for plasma sodium and osmolality (mmol/kg and mosmol/kg plasma water) in untreated rats (●) and rats given one unit of vasopressin in oil twice daily for 1 and 2 days (1 and 2 on graph). Data of Dila and Pappius:[58] values for $[Na]_w$ calculated assuming fractional plasma water of 0.93. The oblique line projected from values in untreated rats has the average slope determined by dilution in vitro on plasma separated from dogs and healthy people; *see* Flear and Singh.[1] (B) Correspondence between observed fall in plasma osmolality (mosmol/kg water) and that calculated from the observed fall in plasma sodium in dogs given vasopressin for some 4–18 days. Plasma sodium on day of lowest osmolality was compared with that first measured on the second or third day after the start of vasopressin administration (earliest levels available). Data from Lowance et al.[59] Fall in osmolality was calculated as $1.824 ([Na]_p/0.93)$, where 0.93 is the assumed fractional plasma water content and 1.824 is an empirically determined, functional relationship between change in plasma sodium (mmol/kg water) and osmolality in man and dogs; *see* Flear and Singh.[1] Observed fall in osmolality was greater than that expected. This was compatible with a preliminary fall in plasma sodium during the first 2–3 days of vasopressin administration unaccompanied by fall in osmolality.

osmotic transients, and so on. Conterminously, there will be a slow escape from SR tubules of solutes gained from cells.

These various happenings create a very dynamic situation, which is further compounded by changing proportions of healthy and non-specifically 'sick' cells. Not surprisingly, sequential observation in ill patients may reveal a 'scribble-type' pattern in the relationship between $[Osm]_w^c$ and $[Na]_w$ (where $[Osm]_w^c$ is the osmolality corrected for plasma urea and glucose and $[Na]_w$ is the sodium concentration per kg plasma water (*Fig.* 8.5)).

Cell Inability to Sustain Normal Osmolality

The inorganic cations, K^+ and Na^+, in solution in cell fluids are together responsible for some 60% of the cell's osmolality. Substrates and intermediates, the dipeptides carnosine and anserine, and the 'energy-rich'

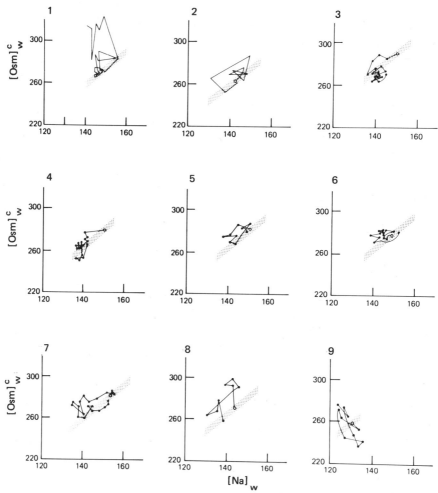

Fig. 8.5. Consecutive measurements of $[Na]_w$ and $[Osm]_w^c$ in patients with various illnesses, to illustrate the increased variability displayed by patients when compared with the variability shown in healthy people. The shaded bands define the expected daily variability in values measured in healthy people. They span twice the average of the observed s.d. on either side of the initial observations and are projected from the observation along the mean slope of dilution-concentration. Data presented from the following patients: (1) and (2) patients with bronchopneumonia following influenza; (3) and (4) patients with chest pains, etc. and shown to developing a myocardial infarction; (5–8) data from patients who had undergone major elective surgery; (9) data from a patient in congestive failure. Initial observations in all patients indicated by open circles and/or i.

compounds ATP and creatine phosphate are constrained within cells and are largely responsible for the remainder. Most of these solutes are anions or have an excess of negative charges. Virtually all of the Na^+ and K^+ ions within cells are in solution and serve as counterions to these multivalent organic anions. In contrast, almost all of the divalent cations (Ca^{2+} and

Mg^{2+}) are bound to proteins which comprise the structural 'scaffolding' of cells. Very little of either of the divalent cations is in solution and their combined contribution to osmolality is entirely negligible. For example, in resting cells the ionized level of Ca^{2+} is only about 10^{-7} M. In health, together with regulation of the cell pH, the maintained constancy of the molar quantity of non-diffusible solutes constrained within cells (A) also brings about constancy in net cationic equivalence (zA where z is the average valence of these solutes). In many diseases, cells fail to sustain the usual molar quantity of these solutes and/or to sustain their normal valence.

Failure to sustain normal amounts of A and zA reduces osmolality of cell fluids. Where zA falls, cells also lose potassium (this possibility was considered by Maffly and Edelman[16]); reduced amounts of A without fall in zA will not cause potassium depletion (see Table 8.7.). Reduction in phosphate esters (all negatively charged) or in anionic intermediates, such as pyruvate, phosphoenolpyruvate, oxoglutarate, oxaloacetate, etc., would reduce both z and zA. These changes are seen in undernutrition (pigs[17] and babies[18]) and congestive heart failure.[19] A fall in the ratio of creatine phosphate to creatine or in cell pH would reduce zA alone. These are all happenings that would provoke potassium depletion, the extent of which would parallel the lowering of osmolality and, therefore, of hyponatraemia. Such an association has been reported in congestive heart failure.[1, 20] They would also bring about a parallel between plasma sodium lowering and a reduction in the combined concentration of sodium and potassium in total tissue water in muscle biopsies. This is also found in congestive heart failure (Flear, unpublished observations). No parallel was found in patients with adult steatorrhea, ulcerative colitis and regional ileitis[1] (Flear and Singh, unpublished observations). Edelman suggested that hyponatraemia might be caused by potassium depletion in congestive heart failure.[21] Reduction in A without reduction in zA will lower osmolality causing hyponatraemia, without also causing potassium depletion. Our body and muscle composition findings in patients with alimentary tract disease are, therefore, explicable. Reduction in cell amino acids or in the dipeptides carnosine and anserine would lower A. The former occurrence would leave zA constant, the latter would raise zA.

Leaf has drawn attention to one obstacle to the notion that hyponatraemia can be caused by a primary fall in cell fluid osmolality.[9, 22] This is that the net shift of water from a sufficient mass of cells would expand the ECF, which would inhibit antidiuretic hormone release and allow the kidney to reduce the ECF expansion. Why, therefore, is the water which is transferred from cells to the ECF not promptly excreted with correction of the serum sodium and osmolality? Leaf and Cotran[22] suggest that perhaps this is because the osmoreceptor cells share the intracellular deficit. Alternatively, it should be noted that, whilst an abrupt fall in osmolality of cell fluids will certainly create a substantial osmotic transient across outer

Table 8.7. Mechanisms of hyponatraemia

Causing dilution of body fluids[a]	Not causing dilution of body fluids

1. Increase in body water without a matching increase in body solute
2. Decrease in body solute without a matching loss of water
  i. From ECF
    Na^+ and anions
  ii. From cells
    a. K^+ accompanied by normally non-diffusible anions or caused by reduced valence of organic anions
    b. Non-diffusible solutes accompanied by potassium (solutes uncharged or, if charged, conterminous increase in valence of residual anions)
  iii. From both—initiated by tissue wasting
	3. *False hyponatraemia* caused by reduction in fractional water content of plasma—hyperlipidaemia; raised plasma protein content[b]
	4. *False hyponatraemia* caused by decrease in net cationic equivalence of plasma proteins[c]
	5. Isosmotic redistribution of water caused by ECF gain of sodium-free solute
	  i. Exogenous—i.v. dextrose, hyperosmotic or isosmotic
	    —i.v. amino acids, frequently hyperosmotic
	  ii. Endogenous—hepatic glucose release (in diabetes mellitus—increased glycogenolysis; after trauma—increased gluconeogenesis)
	    —escape of normally non-diffusible solutes from cells *throughout* the body with leaky outer membranes

[a] Dilution is often confounded by pre-existing or conterminous uraemia or hyperglycaemia. To avoid this, dilution is here defined as decrease in $[Osm]_w^c$, where

$$[Osm]_w^c = [Osm]_w - [G]_w - [U]_w$$

$[Osm]_w$ = measured plasma osmolality (mosmol/kg plasma water)

$[G]_w$ = mmol glucose/kg plasma water

$[U]_w$ = mmol urea/kg plasma water

[b] Here, neither $[Na]_w$ nor $[Na]_o$ throughout ECF *are reduced*; sodium activity determined in plasma by sodium-selective electrodes is *not reduced*.

[c] Here $[Na]_w$ and activity measured by sodium-selective electrodes *are reduced*; $[Na]_o$ throughout ECF *is not reduced*.

cell membranes, an *insidious* fall in osmolality will not. At no time will a substantial gradient arise and there will be no substantial ECF swelling. If the reduction in osmolality results from a faster leak of A and/or zA from cells, than from their metabolic replacement, then their presence in ECF will cause osmoreceptor cells to shrink and, therefore, promote *increased* antidiuretic hormone release. If osmoreceptor cells are not affected similarly to the 'sick cells' throughout the body, the normally non-diffusible solutes leaking from these affected cells will not be able to penetrate osmoreceptor cells. The 'effective osmolality' of plasma and the ECF bathing osmoreceptor cells will, therefore, be raised. In other words, this ECF will no longer be *isotonic* for osmoreceptor cells. It will cause these cells to shrink and initiate *increased* antidiuretic hormone release into the circulation.[14]

RECOGNITION AND MANAGEMENT OF HYPONATRAEMIA FROM 'SICK CELLS'

This diagnosis is largely made by clinical exclusion of the more obvious clinical features and signs of other causes of hyponatraemia (H_2O excess or salt depletion), or by the results of physiological and biochemical tests made to exclude other causes (*see Table 8.7*), for example reduction of a low fractional water content of plasma (presence of abnormal plasma proteins or a very lipaemic plasma) or hyperglycaemia in a diabetic patient. After this it remains to discriminate between 'sick cells' and the syndrome of inappropriate antidiuretic hormone secretion (*Table 8.8*). This is

Table **8.8. Discrimination between cells and syndrome of inappropriate antidiuretic hormone secretion as causes of hyponatraemia; comparison of effects and pathogenesis with explanatory notes**

	'Sick cells'		
Factors measured	*Abrupt and widespread increase in cell membrane permeability*	*Primary lowering of cell osmolality*	*Syndrome of inappropriate antidiuretic hormone secretion*
Onset	Abrupt	Usually slow and insidious	Abrupt or slow
Body weight	No change or fall	Fall[a]	Rise, when onset abrupt[b]
Plasma concn			
K	Often raised or rising	High, normal or low	Fall
Urea, creatinine	Often raised or rising	Normal or high	Fall
Plasma protein	Often reduced	Often reduced	Fall

Table **8.8.** (*cont.*)

Factors measured	'Sick cells'		
	Abrupt and widespread increase in cell membrane permeability	*Primary lowering of cell osmolality*	*Syndrome of inappropriate antidiuretic hormone secretion*
Day-to-day variability			
$[K]_p$	Increased	Normal or increased	Normal
$[Na]_p$	Increased	Normal or increased	Normal or reduced
Product			
$[K]_p.[Cl]_p$	Increased[c]	Normal	Normal
MCHC, Hb	Normal	Normal	Reduced
Total body water	Determined by conterminous events	Determined by conterminous events	Raised[w]
$(Na_e + K_e^f)$/body water	Normal	Normal or reduced[d]	Reduced[e]
$[Na^+ K]_t^g$	Normal	Normal or reduced[d]	Reduced
K_e and/or TBK[h]	Determined by events[i]	Normal or reduced[d]	Reduced[j]
Na excretion			
During onset or persistence of hyponatraemia	Often low or very low[k]	= Intake	Typically raised[l]
During recovery or improvement	Usually > intake and $[Na]_p$ rising		= Intake
Plasma osmolality (corrected for urea and glucose $[Osm]_w^c$)	Raised, normal or reduced[m]	Low[n]	Low[n]
Relationship between $[Osm]_w^c$ and $[Na]_w$	Consecutive measurement often display 'scribble' pattern (*see Fig. 8.7*)	Cluster tightly about normal functional relationship	Cluster tightly about normal functional relationship
Urine osmolality	Depends on intake, on catabolic generation of solutes, on pre-renal oliguria or solute diuresis	*See* previous column: during TPN[p] or GKI[q] depends on metabolic storage of dietary substrates and whether spilled in urine	Uncorrected plasma osmolality $([Osm]_w)^o$

Table 8.8 (cont.)

Factors measured	'Sick cells'		
	Abrupt and wide-spread increase in cell membrane permeability	Primary lowering of cell osmolality	Syndrome of inappropriate antidiuretic hormone secretion
Renal response to water load	Impaired by presence of solute diuresis	Usually excreted and urine diluted[r]	Waterload *not* excreted; urine not diluted[s]
Plasma arginine vasopressin[t]	Raised[u]	May be raised	Sometimes raised Sometimes normal[v]

[a] Due to tissue wasting.
[b] Confounding factors include oedema accumulation and tissue wastage.
[c] See *Fig.* 8.6.
[d] Not reduced if reduction in cell osmolality caused by failure to sustain A; reduced if zA and K are reduced.
[e] Not reduced in patients investigated by Burke.[44]
[f] Na_e = total exchangeable body Na; K_e = total exchangeable body K.
[g] $[Na + K]_t$ = the combined tissue contents of Na and K, expressed as a concentration (mM/l total tissue water). $[Na + K]_i > [Na + K]_t > [Na + K]_o$, where i and o indicate the concentrations of ICF and ECF, respectively.[42] Reduction in $[Na + K]_i$ will reduce $[Na + K]_o$, but so too will an increase in the relative contribution of ECF to total tissue water. Maximal decrease in $[Na + K]_t$ occurs when caused by decrease in z without fall in A.
[h] TBK = total body K.
[i] For example K depletion or tissue wasting.
[j] Reduced in one patient in Schwartz et al.,[39] and in patients investigated by Baraclough[43] and Burke.[44]
[k] Low when there is peripheral circulatory failure (septic shock, blood loss shock, cardiogenic shock), burn injuries, etc. Excretion increased when osmotic diuresis present.
[l] Schwartz et al.,[39] *but* prolonged administration of pitressin to man[45] eventually leads to a state of Na balance (excretion = intake)
[m] Nevertheless greater osmolality predicted from $[Na]_p$ (predicted $[Osm]_w^c = 2 [Na]_p$; see *Table* 8.9 and *Fig.* 8.5B). Others have also noted this gap between observed and predicted $[Osm]_w^c$.[46-50] Because of dynamic nature of underlying cell happenings (proportion of cell mass with leaky membranes; some improving, some worsening, etc.) and of renal sequelae (osmotic diuresis, etc.), measured $[Osm]_w^c$ does not always exceed predicted $[Osm]_w^c$ (see Leaky outer membranes, *Fig.* 8.5 and *Fig.* 8.7).
[n] Observed $[Osm]_w^c$ not significantly different from predicted.
[o] See *Table* 8.9; *but* can be reduced to only just above plasma osmolality—by conterminous solute diuresis.
[p] TPN = total parenteral nutrition.
[q] GKI = glucose, K and insulin.
[r] Several factors may however impair or prevent this—including inversion of diurnal rhythms of excretion, poor delivery of pre-urine to the diluting segment of nephrons.
[s] But *see* Zerbe et al.[27]
[t] Arginine vasopressin = antidiuretic hormone.
[u] In response to haemodynamic influences.[51-53]
[v] See Zerbe et al.[27] and Gupta.[54]
[w] Body water *reduced* in hyponatraemic patients with bronchial carcinoma investigated by Burke.[44]

particularly difficult for patients with chronic illness. In these patients, osmolality is low, as predicted from plasma sodium concentration. Acutely ill patients can more often be noted to have a significant osmotic gap (measured $[Osm]_w^c$ − predicted $[Osm]_w^c$) although this is not a constant finding in what is a very dynamic and changing situation (*Fig.* 8.5). For practical purposes, failure to discriminate probably does not matter all that much. Therapy is said, by proponents of both diagnoses, to be a matter of treatment of the underlying condition.

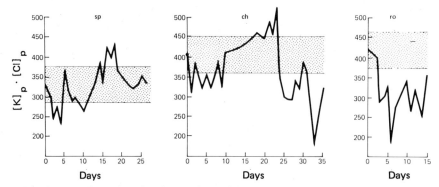

Fig. 8.6. Consecutive values for the product of the plasma concentration of potassium and chloride $\{[K]_p \cdot [Cl]_p \, (mmol/l)^2\}$ from each of three patients with bronchopneumonia following influenza. In each patient, the stippled band projected from the initial observation projects an area which spans ± 2 s.d. about the initial product (where s.d. is the average standard deviation determined for the value of this product in healthy people, calculated from concentrations of $[K]_p$ and $[Cl]_p$ measured daily for a period of some 11–14 days).

There are, however, other important differences of emphasis for treatment (*Table* 8.9). *The syndrome of inappropriate antidiuretic hormone secretion* places considerable emphasis on the need to *restrict* fluid intake and, at times, to give loop diuretics intravenously to achieve rapid rise in plasma sodium.[23] In our opinion, unless there is clear indication that the lowering of plasma sodium concentration, in a given patient, has been both abrupt and caused by equally rapid water retention, it is unnecessary, unhelpful and even unkind to restrict water intake.

In contrast, the *sick-cell* concept suggests and explains several very useful therapeutic practices (*Table* 8.9). Intravenous administration of glucose,

Table 8.9. Treatments proposed for sick-cell hyponatraemia and the syndrome of inappropriate antidiuretic hormone secretion (SIADH)

Treatment	Sick cell	SIADH
Blood transfusion[a]	Yes	—
Total parenteral nutrition of hyperalimentation[b]	Yes	—
Glucose, potassium, insulin	Yes	—
Elevation of $[Na]_p$ and plasma osmolality	No	Yes[c]
Treatment of underlying disease and its complications	Yes	Yes

[a] To replace losses. Flear and Clarke[55] and, more recently, Flear et al.[12,13] showed that prompt replacement in major long bone fractures lessens or prevents metabolic and endocrine changes. Hinton et al.[56] showed that blood transfusion corrected hyponatraemia arising after burn injuries. Flear[57] showed that blood transfusion lessened both pyrexia and weight loss after thoracic surgery.
[b] *See* Flear et al.[13]
[c] By restricting fluids or intravenous frusemide.

potassium and insulin has found very wide use (cases 5, 13–15 in *Table* 8.10[24, 25]). So too has the use of high caloric intakes to sustain the increased resting metabolic expenditure (RME) seen after injury or surgery (particularly when compounded by post-operative complication, sepsis or infection), in the critically ill, in congestive heart failure, cancer and during acute infections. We suggest that this increase in our cost of living (RME) is promoted by inflated sodium pump activity in skeletal muscle cells.[12, 13, 26]

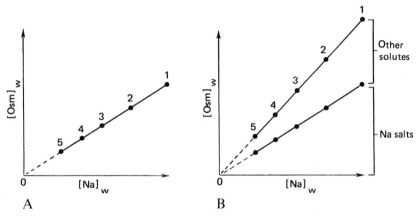

Fig. 8.7. Theoretical depiction (qualitative) of the functional relationship between osmolality ($[Osm]_w$) and the concentration of sodium ($[Na]_w$) in (A) aqueous solution of NaCl and (B) plasma.

Increased pump activity arises from the need to balance faster sodium influx, which is caused by the non-specific increase in membrane permeability in these sick-cell situations. In direct extension of these considerations, the sick-cell concept prompts reflection that to return a reduced plasma sodium level to normal would provoke further inflationary increase in the cost of living and might even provoke imbalance in transmembrane sodium exchanges causing cell gain of sodium. An increased intracellular sodium concentration would impair tissue function and metabolism. As an example, such imbalance in heart fibres would reduce myocardial contractility. We consider that impairment of anabolic recovery would be prominent amongst the consequences that a diminished transmembrane sodium gradient would have, if widespread. Its reduction would lessen the potential energy store, in cell membranes, available for transduction into amino acid accumulation and protein anabolism.

For these and other reasons, we believe that hyponatraemia, although abnormal, is more appropriate to the circumstances that provoke it than a normal level would be. We believe that attempts should not be made to increase plasma sodium levels directly, but rather to improve the basic metabolic activities in those cells that are sick.

Table 8.10. Illustrative cases

Cases	$[Na]_p$, mmol/l	Comments
1. Chronic alcoholic female: after acute binges i. Collapsed but just rousable; answers yes to all questions ii. Collapsed at home surrounded by empty beer bottles—rousable, alcohol not detectable in plasma	i. 100 ii. 92	Measured osmolalities were those expected for $[Na]_p$ levels i. 202 mosmol/kg Gradual and uneventful (no fits) return to her 'usual' hyponatraemic level of around 133 mmol/l with only moderate fluid restriction (osmolality range 266–276 mosmol/kg)
2. Healthy male of 100-kg weight, 16 pints *drunk in 20 min*; subject not drunk, speech and mental processes clear, good co-ordination	143 before beer 127 after beer	Osmolality before = 286 mosmol/kg H_2O; $[Na]_w$ = 153 mmol/kg H_2O; 262 and 133, respectively, after beer. Osmolality of beer = 772 mosmol/kg; $[Na]$ = 1·5 mmol/l; equal dilution $[Na]_p$ and osmolality; expected dilution from gain of 9 l H_2O (16 pints) $[Na]_w$ = 61/70 of 153 = 133; $[Osm]_w$ = 61/70 of 285 = 248; assumed initial body H_2O = 61 kg Conclusion—much practice and a healthy liver enabled subject to metabolize almost all alcohol[37]
3. Whipple's disease, severely ill; maintained throughout on constant nasogastric milk drip	118	6 hours previously $[Na]_p$ = 142; 6 h later $[Na]_p$ = 130; no treatment given for hyponatraemia. $[Na]_p$ fell again to 118 in a further 21 hours and rose to 130 in another 27h; no fits; no disturbance of consciousness; $[K]_p$ varied greatly[1]
4. Liver failure	104	96 h previously $[Na]_p$ = 138 and 135; no treatment given for hyponatraemia and no change in consciousness or apparent clinical state; no fits; $[K]_p$ varied greatly[1]
5. Fulminant hepatic failure	123	Clinical recovery with insulin glucose treatment; $[Na]_p$ rose to 130[38]

6. Sudden onset confusion and weakness 12 hours before admission; history (from relatives) of cough, sputum, breathlessness for 12 years; intermittant oedema for 4 weeks; digitalis 9 years; 5 g chlorothiazide in 5 days before admission; confused and drowsy	105	ECG pattern suggestive of K depletion; RBC K low, low muscle K; treatment with substantial K supplements—excellent recovery; [Na]$_p$ rise to 130; no fits; increase in muscle and RBC K
7. Cardiac failure with increasing oedema and resistant to thiazide diuretics	114	Clinical improvement with loss of all oedema and rise of [Na]$_p$ to 142 on low salt diet (less than 10 mmol/day); no disturbance of consciousness, no fits
8. Cardiac failure with oedema, admitted for drainage of recurrent pleural effusion	110	[Na]$_p$ 3 days after blood loss shock treated with some success by blood (13 pints), but accompanied by profuse sweating and relapse of circulatory state; only intake water. Oral sodium salts stabilized circulation and returned [Na]$_p$ to 130—level obtaining before episode; further salt without effect on [Na]$_p$ but increased oedema[60]
9. Admitted in coma; blood glucose 55 mmol/l; normal anion gap	117	Coma presumed due to net shift H$_2$O from brain cells in response to abrupt rise glucose; hypertonic saline would escalate situation
10. Newborn male, 3·64 kg; urinary retention; uraemia	133 (Day 0)	[K]$_p$ = 82 day 0, 1·61 hypo-osmotic infusions day 0–5 inclusive—caused considerable oedema, progressive fall [Na]$_p$ and fits
	80 (Day 5)	Osmolality = 218 mosmol/kg; on day 6, 100 mg chlorothiazide 100 ml triple strength NaCl i.v.; day 7 drip stopped; steady rise in [Na]$_p$ to 130 mmol/l; fall in [K]$_p$, rise in urea
11. Oedematous, anuric newborn; L-sided abdominal mass; small non-functioning polycystic R kidney, (hydronephrosis and calyceal diverticulum in L kidney Pelviureteroplasty	125	Post-operative convulsions relieved by i.v. Ca (plasma Ca very low), i.v. saline and triple saline promoted further oedema without sustained rise in [Na]$_p$ (125–114 mmol/l); measured [Osm]$_w^c$ close to predicted from [Na]$_p$. Plasma K very high at times (8·2 mmol/l); always greater than 5·2 mmol/l; plasma urea range 17–23 mmol/l

Table 8.10. (cont.)

Cases	$[Na]_p$, mmol/l	Comments
12. Female, 46 years old; rheumatic heart disease; mitral stenosis and incompetence; tricuspid stenosis; auricular fibrillation; digitalis and diuretics with initial improvement; became progressively more oedematous (wt gain 3·25 lb), weak, apathetic with enlarged liver	Admission = 135	$[Na]_p$ fell steadily to 113 mmol/l; despite gross oedema dyspnoea and maximal neck vein distension, 2·5 pints NaCl (1·8 g/dl) given i.v.: transient rise in $[Na]_p$ to 122 mmol/l falling to 117 mmol/l; $[K]_p$ *rose* to 7·2, and $[urea]_p$ to 22 mmol/l; 3 lb wt gain in 24 hours following i.v. NaCl; over next 6 days further 7·25 lb wt gain, onset of peripheral circulatory collapse and death
13. Female, 35 years old with severe wound infection (β-haemolytic strept.) following tubal ligation; admitted in septicaemic shock with high fever; BP 80/60 mm Hg, pulse 140/min; given 2 l glucose saline i.v.; deteriorated	134 (Admission) 118 (After 4 hours) 132 (After 24 hours)	$[K]_p$ 4·5 mmol/l at 0 hours $[K]_p$ now 5·6; condition worse; BP unstable and falling, antibiotics given, suture removed for drainage; plasma expanded with dextraven and 1 l blood. Given 3 l GKI[a]; by 16 hours condition improved: BP > 120/80, pulse 110/min $[K]_p = 3·2$ mmol/l, continued improvement—discharged in 14 days

	Plasma Na	
14. Female, 65 years old; TB with superadded Klebsiella bronchopneumonia: rising fever for 8 days; given massive infusion saline Ringer and glucose–saline—became stuporose and hypoxic BP range 100/60 and 80/40 mmHg; pulse 120–130/min	128 (Admission)	$[K]_p = 3 \cdot 2$ mmol/l; over 8 days given 3200 mmol Na and 80 mmol **K**; became markedly oedematous; day 8–9, 24 hours urine loss, Na = 40 mmol, K = 60 mmol
	108 (Day 8)	Given frusemide and GKI[a] (*no Na* included), oxygen, anti-TB drugs and antibiotics; condition improved over next 4 days; plasma urea concentration fell from 11 to 2·6 mmol/l; discharged after 1 month
15. Well 24-year-old male with gunshot injury; admitted in shock 36 hours later; **BP**—90/50 mmHg; peritonitis on admission operated on for bowel resection after 4 l blood and 1·5 l l dextraven; 5 l Ringers saline also given	124 (Admission) Fell to 115	$[K]_p = 4 \cdot 8$ mmol/l
		$[K]_p$, then = 4·6; very sick, Hb 9 g/dl; wound infected with *E. coli*, *Klebsiella* and *Pseudomonas*; treatment, wound lavage (saline), i.v. GKI[a] (77 mmol Na/day; 80–120 mmol K); some 500 ml blood per day
	132 (10 days later)	$[K]_p = 4 \cdot 2$ mmol/l, cumulative balances = over 10 days Na = + 120 mmol, **K** = 1200 mmol

[a] GKI—glucose, potassium and insulin; outline regime.

Is the Syndrome of Inappropriate Antidiuretic Hormone Secretion a Consequence or a Cause of Sick Cells?

We have suggested that leak of A and zA from a sufficiently large mass of cells throughout the body may *specifically* induce increased antidiuretic hormone release. These solutes would be unable to penetrate normal osmoreceptor cells, so that ECF would have a raised *effective* osmolality and initiate osmoreceptor cell shrinkage. This would trigger antidiuretic hormone release. When osmoreceptor cells are themselves sick, increased antidiuretic hormone release may result from the *non-specific* increase in their membrane permeability and the resulting change in sodium and calcium fluxes. These will be akin to those initiated by *specific* stimulation of osmoreceptors.[11,14] Consequently, patients with sick-cell hyponatraemia are likely to have raised circulating levels of antidiuretic hormone, not promoted by either increase in osmolality or baroreceptor stimulation. Increased antidiuretic hormone release arising *non-specifically* may or may not be turned off, or down, by reduction in plasma effective osmolality, depending on whether osmoreceptor cells remain responsive to further stimulation. In these ways the differing patterns of antidiuretic hormone levels and their response to hyperosmotic saline and to water described by Zerbe et al.[27] can be explained.

Table 8.11. Criteria for diagnosis of the syndrome of inappropriate antidiuretic hormone secretion[39-41]

1. Hyponatraemia with low osmolality	
2. Urine osmolality > Plasma (or serum)[a]	'. . . need not be
3. Urinary sodium > Sodium intake	met in a case'[b]

[a] '. . . higher than that appropriate for the corresponding tonicity of serum'.[41]
[b] Bartter.[41]

We further suggest that a sustained increase in circulating antidiuretic hormone levels may provoke directly non-specific increase in cell membrane permeability, i.e. in widespread sick cells.

In conclusion, we believe that several considerations favour the sick cell concept as the 'prime mover' in non-specific hyponatraemia. It favours plausible mechanisms which explain the onset of hyponatraemia and its reversal during clinical recovery, and explains why the plasma sodium level is such a sensitive index of cellular and tissue well-being. It prompts a number of therapeutic suggestions and is supported by their success. The concept satisfactorily accounts for the variety noted in circulating antidiuretic hormone levels and in their response to hyperosmotic and hypo-osmotic fluid infusions. At the same time it also explains the several related metabolic and other endocrine accompaniments to hyponatraemia, the impairment of tissue functioning that attends disease, and anabolic recovery. Finally, this concept alone satisfactorily accounts for a rise in circulating antidiuretic hormone levels in such a variety of disease situations and for their return to normal with clinical recovery.

Acknowledgements

Researches referred to or presented in this chapter were supported by The Royal Society (equipment grant) and the Wellcome Trust. Some researches were made whilst one of us (C.M.S.) was a visiting Fellow in the Department of Surgery, Royal Victoria Infirmary, Newcastle upon Tyne.

REFERENCES

1. Flear C. T. G. and Singh C. M. (1973) Hyponatraemia and sick cells. *Br. J. Anaesth.* **45**, 976–994.
2. Leaf A. (1956) On the mechanism of fluid exchange of tissues in vitro. *Biochem. J.* **62**, 241–248.
3. Laurent T. G. and Ogston A. G. (1963) The interaction between polysaccharides and other macromolecules. The osmotic pressure of mixtures of serum albumin and hyaluronic acid. *Biochem. J.* **89**, 249–253.
4. de Wardener H. E. (1978) The control of sodium excretion. *Am. J. Physiol.* **253**, F163–F173.
5. Weston R. E., Grossman J., Borun E. R. et al. (1958) The pathogenesis and treatment of hyponatraemia in congestive heart failure. *Am. J. Med.* **25**, 558–572.
6. Flear C. T. G. (1960) Studies in congestive heart failure: therapeutic and theoretical problems. Birmingham University, MD Thesis.
7. Flear C. T. G. (1960) Water and electrolyte metabolism in congestive heart failure. *Postgrad. Med. J.* **36**, 104–119.
8. Flear C. T. G. and Hilton P. (1979) Hyponatraemia and severity and outcome of myocardial infarction. *Br. Med. J.* **1**, 1242–1246.
9. Leaf A. (1962) The clinical and physiologic significance of the serum sodium concentration. *N. Engl. J. Med.* **267**, 24–30 and 77–83.
10. Leaf A. (1974) Hyponatraemia. *Lancet* **1**, 1119–1120.
11. Flear C. T. G. (1974) Hyponatraemia. *Lancet* **2**, 164–166.
12. Flear C. T. G., Bhattachrya S. S. and Nandra G. S. (1977) Cellular exchanges and happenings after injury and in the critically ill. In: Richards J. R. and Kinney J. M., ed., *Nutritional Aspects of Care in the Critically Ill*, pp. 195–224. Edinburgh, Churchill Livingstone.
13. Flear C. T. G., Bhattacharya S. S. and Singh C. M. (1980) Solute and water exchanges between cells and extracellular fluids in health and disturbances after trauma. *J. Parent. Ent. Nutr.* **4**, 98–119.
14. Flear C. T. G., Gill G. V. and Burn J. (1981) Hyponatraemia: mechanism and management. *Lancet* **2**, 26–31.
15. Flear C. T. G. (1970) Electrolyte and body water changes after trauma. *J. Clin. Pathol.* [*Suppl.*] **23**(1), 16–31.
16. Maffly R. H. and Edelman I. S. (1961) Role of sodium, potassium and water in hypo-osmotic states of heart failure. *Prog. Cardiovasc. Dis.* **4**, 88–104.
17. Widdowson E. M., Dickerson J. W. T. and McCance R. A. (1960) Severe undernutrition in growing and adult animals: 4, the impact of severe undernutrition on the chemical composition of the soft tissues. *Br. J. Nutr.* **14**, 457–471.

18. Metcoff J., Frenk S., Yoshida T. et al. (1966) Cell composition and metabolism in Kwashiorkor. *Medicine* **45**, 365–390.
19. Mangun G. H., Reicle H. S. and Myers V. C. (1965) Further studies in human cardiac and voluntary muscle. *Arch. Intern. Med.* **67**, 320–332.
20. Flear C. T. G. (1966) Disturbance of volume and composition of body fluids in congestive heart failure. In: Bajusz E., ed., *Electrolytes and Cardiovascular Diseases*, Vol. 2, pp. 357–385. Basel, S. Karger.
21. Edelman T. S. (1956) The pathogenesis of hyponatraemia: physiologic and therapeutic implications. *Metabolism* **5**, 500–507.
22. Leaf A. and Cotran R. S. (1976) *Renal Pathophysiology*. New York, Oxford Press.
23. Hantman D., Rossler B., Zohlman R. et al. (1973) Rapid correction of hyponatraemia in the syndrome of inappropriate secretion of antidiuretic hormone. *Ann. Intern. Med.* **78**, 870–875.
24. Hinton P., Allison S. P. and Littlejohn S. (1973) Electrolyte changes after burn injury and effect of treatment. *Lancet* **2**, 218–221.
25. Woolfson A. M. J., Heatley R. V. and Allison S. P. (1979) Insulin to inhibit protein catabolism after injury. *N. Engl. J. Med.* **300**, 14–17.
26. Flear C. T. G. (1973) Changes in extracellular fluid after trauma. *Proc. R. Soc. Med.* **66**, 481–484.
27. Zerbe R., Stropes L. and Robertson G. (1980) Vasopressin function in the syndrome of inappropriate antidiuresis. *Annu. Rev. Med.* **31**, 315–327.
28. Bradham G. B. and Gadsden R. H. (1962) Electrolyte patterns for 1000 hospital patients. *Surg. Gynecol. Obstet.* **114**, 535–538.
29. Lindberg D. A. B., Van Peenen H. J. and Couch R. D. (1965) Patterns in clinical chemistry, low serum sodium and chloride in hospitalised patients. *Am. J. Clin. Pathol.* **44**, 315–321.
30. Owen J. A. and Campbell D. G. (1968) A comparison of plasma electrolyte and urea values in healthy persons and in hospital patients. *Clin. Chim. Acta* **22**, 611–618.
31. Payne R. B. and Levell M. J. (1968) Redefinition of the normal range for serum sodium. *Clin. Chem.* **14**, 172–178.
32. O'Halloran M. W. O., Studley-Ruxton J. and Welby M. L. (1970) A comparison of conventionally derived normal ranges with those obtained from patients results. *Clin. Chim. Acta* **27**, 35–46.
33. Sherlock S., Senewiratnie B., Scott A. et al. (1966) Complications of diuretic therapy in hepatic cirrhosis. *Lancet* **1**, 1049.
34. Chirinos P. G. and Ramos-Galvan R. (1964) *Bol. Med. Hosp. Infant. Mex.* **21**, 89.
35. Garrow J. S., Smith R. and Ward E. E. (1968) *Electrolyte Metabolism in Severe Infantile Malnutrition*. Oxford, Pergamon Press.
36. Westwater J. O., Stiven D. and Garry R. C. (1939) A note on the serum sodium level in patients suffering from tuberculosis. *Clin. Sci.* **4**, 73–77.
37. Flear C. T. G., Gill G. V. and Burn J. (1981) Beer drinking and hyponatraemia. *Lancet* **2**, 477.
38. Burn J. H. and Williams W. D. C. (1978) The effects of insulin glucose administration in fulminant hepatic failure. *Intensive Care Med.* **4**, 133–136.
39. Schwartz W. B., Bennett W., Curelop S. et al. (1957) A syndrome of renal sodium loss and hyponatraemia probably resulting from inappropriate secretion of antidiuretic hormone. *Am. J. Med.* **23**, 529–542.
40. Bartter F. C. and Schwartz W. B. (1967) The syndrome of inappropriate secretion of antidiuretic hormone. *Am. J. Med.* **42**, 790–806.
41. Bartter. F. C. (1970) The syndrome of inappropriate secretion of antidiuretic hormone. *J. R. Coll. Physicians Lond.* **4**, 264–272.
42. Flear C. T. G. (1969) Alterations in water and electrolyte distribution in congestive heart failure and their significance. *Ann. N.Y. Acad. Sci.* **155**, Art. 1, 421–444.
43. Baraclough M. A. (1971) Inappropriate secretion of antidiuretic hormone and potassium depletion. *Proc. R. Soc. Med.* **64**, 1069–1070.

44. Burke B. J. (1979) An investigation into the nature of hyponatraemia in patients with carcinoma of the bronchus. Bristol University, MD Dissertation.
45. Jaenike J. R. and Waterhouse C. (1961) The renal response to sustained administration of vasopressin and water in man. *J. Clin. Endocrinol. Metab.* **21**, 231–242.
46. Rubin A. L., Braveman W. S., Dexter R. L. et al. (1956) The relationship between plasma osmolality and concentration in disease states. *Circ. Res.* **4**, 129.
47. Olmstead E. G. and Roth D. A. (1958) The use of serum freezing point depression in evaluating salt and water balance in pre-operative and postoperative states. *Surg. Gynecol. Obstet.* **106**, 41–48.
48. Boyd D. R. and Mansberger A. R. (1968) Serum water and osmolal changes in haemorrhagic shock: an experimental and clinical study. *Am. Surg.* **34**, 744–749.
49. Boyd D. R., Fock F. A., Condon R. E. et al. (1970) Predictive value of serum osmolality in shock following major trauma. *Surg. Forum* **21**, 32–33.
50. Tindall S. F. and Clark R. G. (1976) Hyponatraemia in surgical practice. *Br. J. Surg.* **63**, 150.
51. Kirsch K. and Gauer O. H. (1980) Identification of receptor groups. Concept of two interacting volume control systems. *J. Parent. Ent. Nutr.* **4**, 71–76.
52. Schrier R. W. and Bichet D. G. (1981) Osmotic and non-osmotic control of vasopressin release and the pathogenesis of impaired water excretion in adrenal, thyroid and edematous disorders. *J. Lab. Clin. Med.* **98**, 1–15.
53. Robertson G. L., Athar S. and Shelton R. L. (1977) Osmotic control of vasopressin function. In: Andreoli T. E., Grantham J. J. and Rector F. C., ed., *Disturbances in Body Fluid Osmolality*, pp. 125–148. Bethesda, American Physiological Society.
54. Gupta K. K. (1971) Syndrome of inappropriate secretion of antidiuretic hormone. *Lancet* **1**, 866.
55. Flear C. T. G. and Clarke R. (1955) Influence of blood loss and blood transfusion upon changes in metabolism of water, electrolytes and nitrogen following civilian trauma. *Clin. Sci.* **14**, 575–599.
56. Hinton P., Allison S. P. and Farrow S. (1972) Blood volume changes and transfusion requirements of burned patients after the shock phase of injury. *Lancet* **1**, 913–915.
57. Flear C. T. G. (1956) Influence of transfusion adequacy on clinical progress in thoracic surgery. *Br. J. Clin. Pract.* **10**, 787–790.
58. Dila C. J. and Pappins H. M. (1972) Cerebral water and electrolytes: an experimental model on inappropriate secretion of antidiuretic hormone. *Arch. Neurol.* **26**, 85–90.
59. Lowance D. C., Garfinkel H. B., Mattern W. D. et al. (1972) The effect of chronic hypotonic volume expansion on the renal regulation of acid–base equilibrium. *J. Clin. Invest.* **51**, 2928–2940.
60. Flear C. T. G. and Hill M. (1957) Massive haemorrhage in chronic congestive heart failure followed by sodium depletion. *Lancet* **1**, 966–968.
61. Singh C. M. (1972) Cellular factors causing disturbances of water and electrolyte metabolism in clinical situations. University of Newcastle upon Tyne, PhD Thesis.
62. Edelman I. S., Leibman J., O'Meara M. P. et al. (1958) Interrelations between serum sodium concentration, serum osmolality and total exchangeable sodium, total exchangeable potassium and total body water. *J. Clin. Invest.* **37**, 1236–1256.

APPENDIX

Plasma Osmolality: Measurement and Prediction, and Their Comparison
Measurement by Freezing Point Depression

Several important points should be stressed.[61]
1. Blood should be centrifuged, and its plasma separated immediately after

withdrawal from a patient. If this is not done, the osmolality eventually measured will exceed that present in vivo. This is because blood cells continue to metabolize in vitro, generating additional solutes. We find that osmolality rises steadily after blood withdrawal. After 2 hours, osmolality increases by some 5 mosmol per kg water.

2. If measurement *cannot* be made immediately, store plasma in a refrigerator at some 4 °C. Never deep freeze plasma. We find that osmolality measured on thawed plasma that has been frozen and stored differs unpredictably from that measured on unfrozen fresh plasma immediately after its collection.

3. Plasma can be stored in a refrigerator for up to a week without significant changes occurring in its osmolality. It is not certain that this is true for plasma from patients with bacteraemia.

4. Only one measurement should be made on any given sample of plasma. Subsequent measurements on thawed plasma differ unpredictably from the original measurement, even after stirring (and by as much as 8 mosmol/kg from each other).

Prediction of Plasma Osmolality

Typically, plasma from a healthy person has the composition shown below.

Solute	mosmol/kg H_2O
Na^+ + anions	262·8
K^+ + anions	10
Ca^{2+} + anions	4
Mg^{2+} + anions	2
Urea	3
Glucose	5
Creatinine	1
Dissolved CO_2	1
Plasma protein	1·4
Total	290·2

In this example, sodium and its anions comprise 91% of the total osmolality. This is generally true in patients also[62]. Plasma osmolality can therefore be predicted approximately from the concentration of sodium.

$$[Osm]_w^{pred} = n\phi^1 [Na]_w \qquad (1)$$

where $[Na]_w$ is the concentration of Na in mmol/kg plasma water.

If ϕ^1 is presumed to have a value of 0·93 (the osmotic coefficient of a dilute aqueous solution of NaCl), equation (1) would be further simplified to

$$[Osm]_w^{pred} = 2[Na]_p$$

since

$$[Na]_w = [Na]_p/[H_2O]_w$$

and $[H_2O]_w$, the fractional water content of plasma (kg/l plasma), averages 0·93.

Chapter 9

Infection and Septic Shock

Iain McA. Ledingham, J. A. Bradley, Christine McCartney and Penelope J. Redding

Infection is one of the most taxing problems in the practice of intensive care, particularly in units with a large proportion of acute general surgical, burns or trauma referrals.[3,47,53,67,71] Transplant recipients[8,19] and patients undergoing treatment for leukaemia[68] and other malignant diseases[17] are also at risk, and sepsis is not unknown in units with predominantly elective admissions, e.g. following open heart surgery.[18,50] The potential consequences of infection in such patients range from death within a short period (usually as a result of septic shock) to an extended stay in hospital often with severe single or multiple organ failure.

COMMON SYNDROMES AND BASIC MANAGEMENT

In the context of intensive care, patients suffering from infection may be subdivided into two main categories. Patients in the first category become infected outside the intensive therapy unit (ITU) and are admitted primarily because of the severity or rapidly progressive nature of the infective process. Characteristic clinical features are present and a specific pathogenic organism or combination of organisms can often be isolated. Examples of this type of infection are tetanus, gas gangrene, necrotizing fasciitis, and some fulminating forms of cellulitis and pneumonia. Patients in the second category become infected whilst receiving treatment in the ITU for any of the usual assortment of life-threatening cardiovascular, respiratory or neurological conditions for which intenstive care is normally sought. This type of infection is commonly non-specific in character, and convincing demonstration of pathogenic organisms is often difficult.

Inevitably, the two categories of infection have a number of features in common. Complications, e.g. septicaemia and organ failure (especially

196

respiratory and renal), readily occur in both groups, and the ultimate metabolic and cellular consequences may be indistinguishable.

Specific Infections

Of the various more or less specific syndromes in the first category of infection, only tetanus is automatically associated with treatment in an ITU.[33] The major risk of respiratory failure secondary to the severe muscle spasm associated with tetanus has, for a long time, constituted a clear indication for the use of relaxant drugs and mechanical ventilation. Recognition of the role of intensive therapy in the management of other infections in this category has been slower to emerge, partly because these conditions are not associated with early respiratory failure and partly because of the fear of cross-infection. Nevertheless, the fact that ITUs have more to offer than ventilatory care is gradually being appreciated and the benefits to be gained from a combination of intensive care and aggressive surgery are becoming obvious.

Mortality in this group of infections was very high in the past, but earlier clinical recognition, together with rapid institution of intensive care, antibiotic therapy and, where relevant, surgery, has transformed the outcome.[24,33,39] Morbidity remains a problem and the legacy of severe infection, compounded by delayed or inadequate treatment, may be measured in months or, in some cases, years of suffering. Extensive tissue loss and the need for reconstructive plastic surgery are not uncommon.

Non-specific Infections

The types of infection described in the previous section attract considerable attention, but they are much less numerous than the non-specific variety presenting within the ITU. The latter are harder to describe in precise terms although no-one who has experience of intensive therapy would have any difficulty recognizing the sequence of events. The young man with multiple trauma, for example, or the elderly obese lady after colonic surgery seem to be making good immediate progress. A measure of haemodynamic instability or respiratory insufficiency warrants careful observation and management, but only when the expected full recovery is not achieved does anxiety arise.

The early warning signs may present in different ways: inability to wean from mechanical ventilation, rising blood urea and falling urine output, persistent ileus, increasing insulin requirement, etc. These features are usually associated with a moderate fever and a variable degree of leucocytosis; bacteriological analysis shows a change from normal commensal organisms to colonization with an assortment of bacteria, predominantly Gram-negative. Characteristically, the duration of stay in the ITU by this stage is in excess of 1 week.

Management of these patients is complex and often frustrating. The main objective is to maintain haemodynamic and respiratory stability whilst leaving no stone unturned in the search for a source of infection. Not infrequently, the search proves fruitless or at best unconvincing, in which case the only course of action is to continue with antibiotics and endeavour to maintain optimum host defence. In most instances this is easier said than done since the underlying pathophysiological mechanisms are unclear and medication may exacerbate existing vicious cycles, e.g. by adversely affecting hepatorenal function. Ultimately, many of these patients die from multiple organ failure—in part the consequence of increasingly successful techniques of acute resuscitation. Sometimes a superadded infection with *Nocardia* species, yeasts such as *Candida albicans* and true fungi, such as *Aspergillus* species, viruses such as cytomegalovirus, and protozoa such as *Pneumocystis carinii* may be incriminated, but most often no organism is isolated other than those previously considered to be relatively innocuous colonizers.

In the past, such patients were kept alive for many weeks or months. Nowadays, with increasing use of clinical and laboratory prognostic indices[11, 26, 63] and greater awareness of the present limitations of intensive therapy, it is the policy of most units to discontinue active support at a considerably earlier stage in the event of failure of appropriate treatment. The patient is thus spared a lingering death.

MEASUREMENTS AND MONITORING

Bacteriological and Immunological Techniques

1. Isolation of pathogenic organisms.
2. Identification of defective host defence.
3. Environmental assessment.

The submission of suitable bacteriological specimens for culture and analysis is the first step towards effective treatment. Pus, tissue and fluid samples must be sent promptly to the laboratory for immediate Gram-staining and plating on culture media. Isolation of anaerobic bacteria is improved if fluid samples are sent in a capped syringe or, with larger volumes, in a universal container; bacteriological swabs are an unacceptable compromise except when tissue or fluid are unavailable. The initial Gram-stain is of value in detecting the presence of Gram-positive and/or Gram-negative organisms. This may enable 'best guess' antibiotics to be started and is especially useful in the case of clostridial, staphylococcal and streptococcal infections. Rarely can bacteria be specifically identified. It is now possible, using gas–liquid chromatography, to distinguish very rapidly (less than 1 hour) between anaerobic and aerobic infection on specimens of pus; anaerobic bacteria are recognized by the production of specific fatty acids.[62]

Careful examination of serial blood cultures is an important diagnostic and prognostic manoeuvre. Blood samples must be taken atraumatically using a sterile technique after adequate skin preparation. The correct volume of blood is transferred to aerobic (meat extract broth) and anaerobic (thioglycollate broth) bottles using separate needles and these bottles then sent directly to the bacteriology department for incubation at 37 °C. Samples are normally taken from the blood culture bottles at 18–24 h, 48 h and 1 week for Gram-staining and subculturing. The presence of bacteraemia may be detected as early as 18–24 h by Gram-staining, but it may take 48–72 h for full identification of the organisms and determination of antibiotic sensitivities. If the patient is receiving antibiotics it may take longer to isolate the organisms. It is essential to take blood cultures even though the patient is receiving antibiotics for the following reasons:
1. Certain antibiotics (penicillins and sulphonamides) may be inactivated.
2. The antibiotic concentration may be below therapeutic levels or inappropriate.
3. Bacteria which fail to be isolated on subculture may be demonstrated in the Gram-stain.
4. A variety of organisms may be isolated from a septic source, but only rarely is more than one organism isolated on blood culture, and antibiotic therapy may need to be modified accordingly.

It is recommended that three sets of blood cultures be taken within 24 h in order to increase the chance of isolating an organism.[6,82,89] However, the time interval between collections is determined by circumstances and the urgency to initiate antibiotic therapy, though a minimum of two specimens should always be possible in the acute situation. When a blood culture is reported positive, samples should be repeated once or twice daily until consecutive samples are sterile over a 48 hour period.

Experience from this centre indicates that, at best, half the patients with septic shock have detectable organisms in the blood stream.[38] It is possible that newer methods will improve the rate of isolation. One such method is based on the fact that as bacteria multiply they convert complex nutrients to end-products whose chemical composition is reflected in the electrical properties of the media. The resulting increase in the number of ions produces an increase in conductivity or decrease in impedence, which can easily be measured. This technique is not only more rapid than conventional methods, but is also more sensitive in detecting bacteraemia.[31] A similar claim is made for an even more recent method[80] which involves the removal of antibiotics and other bacterial inhibitors from blood cultures using a mixed-resin system. The absolute number of organisms in the blood is not routinely measured in clinical practice, but there is some evidence that this quantitative measurement may have prognositic significance.

The observation that blood cultures from patients in septic shock are often negative has contributed to the current interest in detection of endotoxin in the blood. Endotoxin is a lipopolysaccharide component of the cell wall of Gram-negative bacteria and its toxic properties are believed to reside in the phospholipid part of the molecule: the so-called lipid A. It is possible to estimate the level of circulating endotoxin by employing the limulus lysate gelation test.[73]

The precise role of the Limulus test in clinical practice has yet to be defined, but it is clear that misleading results may arise if the technique is

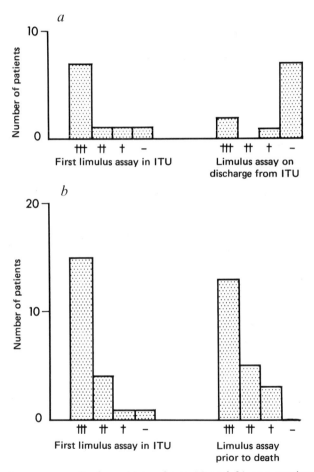

Fig. 9.1. Limulus assay results from 10 survivors (a) and 21 non-survivors (b); + + +, strong positive gel; + +, positive gel; +, weak positive gel. The majority of non-survivors had persistent endotoxaemia until death. In the 10 survivors, the disappearance of detectable endotoxaemia was associated with clinical improvement which often preceded a negative Limulus amoebocyte lysate (LAL) assay by as much as three days.

not performed under strictly controlled laboratory conditions with pains-taking attention to detail. Perhaps one of the most useful applications of the test will be in monitoring the course of patients with residual sepsis following surgery; preliminary clinical investigations in this centre have suggested that the continued presence of endotoxin is associated with a poor prognosis (*Fig.* 9.1).

A modification of the Limulus test using a chromogenic substrate has recently been reported.[54, 27] This assay uses a spectrophotometrically determined end-point which is considerably more satisfactory than the conventional gelation assay end-point.

Host Defence

Measurements

Clearly, the pathogenicity of invading organisms contributes to the severity of clinical infection, but recent studies in critically ill patients point increasingly to the importance of reduced host defence in the aetiology of refractory sepsis. The finding of a markedly impaired immune response in ITU patients suggests that they may be as vulnerable as other im-munosuppressed patients, e.g. transplant recipients.

The body's defence mechanisms may be divided into local mechanisms, e.g. gastric acid, cilia and lysozyme, and the general defence mechanisms to which this discussion refers. It is convenient for descriptive purposes to divide the general host defence mechanisms into three categories: phago-cytic function, cell-mediated immunity and humoral immunity. Some of the clinical and laboratory tests currently used to assess these three aspects of host defence are listed in *Table* 9.1 and certain of these are outlined in the

Table **9.1. Assessment of host defences**

Phagocytic function	Neutrophil and monocyte count
	Neutrophil—Adherence
	Local mobilization
	(Rebuck window)
	Chemotaxis
	Phagocytosis
	Bacterial killing
Cell-mediated immunity	Allograft rejection
	New antigens
	Recall skin antigens
	Lymphocyte count, T cell count
	T cell mitogens
	Mixed lymphocyte reaction
Humoral immunity	Immunoglobin levels
	Antibody response to antigen
	B cell count
	B cell mitogens

following discussion. It should be remembered that these tests are usually more informative when used serially rather than as a single measurement.

The complement system is an integral component of the host response to infection, but since complement activation has other important sequelae, this system will be discussed separately.

Phagocytic Function

Differential peripheral blood leucocyte counts are a routine laboratory investigation in any patient suspected of having infection. Leucopenia is a feature of the early stages of septic shock and is usually followed by a marked leucocytosis; absence of the latter is of sinister significance (*Fig. 9.2a*). Even when there is a normal or increased number of circulating neutrophils, these cells may have impaired function leading to increased susceptibility to infection. Indeed, altered neutrophil function appears to be an important component in the development of bacteraemia in patients with burns, after trauma or in surgical patients with a high risk of infection.[2]

Several in-vitro tests of neutrophil function are available, including measurements of neutrophil adherence, chemotaxis, phagocytosis and bactericidal activity. None of these tests used in isolation will reflect effectively overall neutrophil function, and it should be remembered that in vivo the defects in phagocyte function may be added to by changes in migration of cells round the body and passage into and out of the circulation. Recent evidence suggests that altered neutrophil function, as shown by reduced chemotaxis, may be of value in predicting sepsis and mortality in ill surgical patients.[12] Although neutrophil chemotaxis can be assessed by several different methods, a variant of the Boyden chamber technique is one of the most popular.[85] A similar technique may also be used to measure monocyte and lymphocyte chemotaxis. It should be remembered that the total response in vivo is the sum of the *number* of cells and their *activity*.

Cell-mediated Immunity

Simple skin testing with recall antigens, i.e. proteins to which the patient is already sensitized, is a safe and easily performed method in vivo of measuring cell-mediated immunity. In order to test cell-mediated immunity effectively, a variety of commonly encountered antigens should be used. This increases the chances of any individual patient having previously met one or more of these antigens and therefore increases the implications of an absent response. Increasing evidence suggests that the response to recall skin antigens is of prognostic value in critically ill patients admitted to the

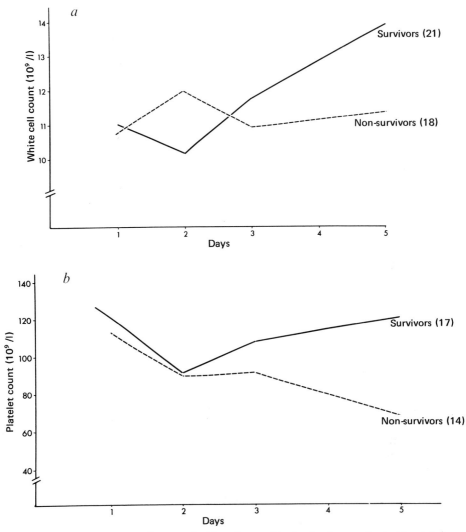

Fig. 9.2. (a) Mean white cell counts in 39 patients with shock who survived at least 5 days. The white cell count rose in survivors between day 2 and day 5 ($P = 0.06$) and also between day 3 and day 5 ($P = 0.039$). (b) Mean platelet count in 31 patients with shock who survived at least 5 days. Ultimate survivors had higher counts at day 5 ($P = 0.037$). The fall in platelet count between day 1 and day 5 in non-survivors was also significant ($P = 0.035$).

ITU, and that initial and persisting anergy is associated with a poor outcome.[15,52] In such patients it has been found that anergy is a generalized phenomenon, rather than a specific lack of reaction to individual antigens.

In this centre, we routinely skin test patients admitted to the ITU with four commercially available recall antigens: (1) purified protein derivative

(PPD), (2) 1% *Candida albicans*, (3) streptokinase 10 units plus strepto-dornase 2·5 units (Varidase) and (4) mumps antigen. The antigens used, however, should be chosen to suit the population being tested and, for example, in some geographical areas PPD may be inappropriate as a recall antigen, whilst *Trichophyton rubrum* may be a useful recall antigen. Each of these antigens (0·1 ml) is injected intradermally several centimetres apart on the volar aspect of the forearm. The response to each antigen is then measured as the diameter of induration at 24 and 48 h. The result of this test may conveniently be quantified using a simple scoring system.

Induration, mm	Score
5	0
5–9	1
10–19	2
19	3

Total score range for four antigens 0–12

Alternatively, a positive response can be taken as one with 5 mm or more of induration and patients can be arbitrarily divided either into non-reactors to any of the antigens and reactors to one or more antigens, or, into anergic, relatively anergic and normal.

Repeat skin testing may be performed on seriously ill patients at weekly intervals and this may be of additional value in giving an objective measure of the response of these patients to their treatment whilst in the ITU. When used in this way, however, the effects of recent previous skin testing may amplify the response to antigens on repeat testing and this must be borne in mind when interpreting the results.

One defect in using recall antigens is the fact that immunological memory is being tested. An in-vivo estimation of cell-mediated immunity to a *new* antigen may be made by measuring the response to the chemical hapten 2,4-dinitro-1-chlorobenzene. When applied to the skin this chemical becomes conjugated with a carrier protein and acts as a new antigen. Its advantage is that, after a sensitizing dose, nearly 95% of normal subjects will show a response when tested 14 days later with a challenge dose of 2,4-dinitro-1-chlorobenzene. However, this delay between sensitization and testing reduces the practical value of the test in the critically ill patient.

Several tests are available to measure the in-vitro function of isolated peripheral blood lymphocytes. Studies of the proportion of T and B cells in immunosuppressed states have, in general, not shown clear trends. The blastogenic response to stimulation by polyclonal or specific mitogens (e.g. phytohaemagglutinin) or by antigens (e.g. *Candida albicans*) can be measured by the uptake of ^{14}C or tritiated thymidine into stimulated lymphocytes. T cell mitogens (e.g. concanavalin A) predominantly measure cell-mediated immunity whilst B cell mitogens (e.g. pokeweed mitogen) will predominantly measure humoral immunity. However, studies using these tests in critically ill patients have produced conflicting results.[49, 52]

Humoral Immunity

Humoral immunity is less easily measured than phagocytic function or cell-mediated immunity. The serum levels of the various immunoglobulins (IgG, IgA, IgM, IgE) may readily be measured in the laboratory by radial diffusion or radio-immunoassay. Although these may sometimes be useful as a screening investigation, they are altered by many factors and non-specific disease processes and hence are of limited value in the majority of patients in the ITU. In burns patients, there is a transient decrease in all the immunoglobulins, although this is not clearly related to outcome.

A clearer assessment of humoral immunity could be made by measuring the antibody response after administration of an antigen already met (e.g. tetanus toxoid) or a new antigen, such as keyhole limpet haemocyanin which produces a primary humoral (and also a cell-mediated) response. There is, surprisingly as yet, little information available about the effects of injury, burns or infection on this type of specific antibody response.

Environmental Screening

In addition to isolation of pathogenic organisms and identification of host defence defects assessment of the environment of the critically ill patient may be important. A number of elements which are an essential part of patient care may at the same time increase the risk of infection. Mechanical ventilation systems, for example, are a ready vehicle for the introduction of sepsis via endotracheal and tracheostomy tubes. Likewise, nasogastric tubes encourage aspiration of infected material into the lungs, and bladder catheters may cause urinary tract sepsis. Intravascular catheters are particularly liable to initiate or sustain blood-borne infection.

In most ITUs, patients are subjected to detailed bacteriological scrutiny at least twice a week and, in addition, all tubes, drains and catheters are sent for culture after use. In the event of an outbreak of infection, more detailed studies are made of other possible sources including ventilator circuits, sinks, feeding solutions and ITU personnel. In this centre for a number of years the practice of wearing gowns or uniforms covered with plastic aprons (*Fig.* 9.3) has been obligatory for all staff; even senior surgeons are not exempt from this ritual! No patient is handled without preliminary hand-washing in a solution of hibitane/glycerine/alcohol and gloves are worn as an additional precaution during such procedures as tracheal suction, etc. Isolation rooms appear to be of value in reducing the risk of cross-infection but adequate barrier-nursing can only be achieved if a transfer airlock is incorporated.

Much can be learned from routine study of the bacteriological pattern in the ITU, particularly when an unexpected change in pattern is revealed. Three such episodes occurred in this centre during a period of 2 years and

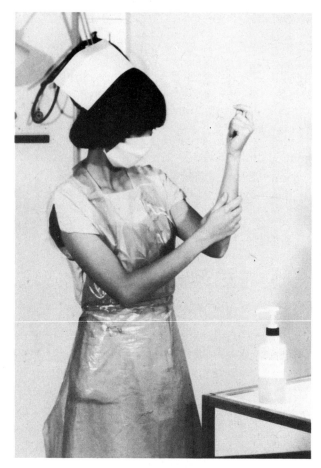

Fig. 9.3. ITU nurse wearing disposable plastic apron and applying antiseptic hand lotion prior to patient contact.

the resultant bacteriological detective work served to emphasize the importance of constant vigilance and meticulous attention to detail in all aspects of management of the critically ill patient. The closest possible collaboration should exist between the ITU staff and their microbiological advisors, perferably as partners in the clinical team.

Episodes of Infection

Pathogenic or potentially pathogenic bacteria are often isolated from the respiratory tract of patients who are intubated and ventilated. These organisms can persist without causing infection but pulmonary sepsis and even bacteraemia are not uncommon. The possible routes by which the organisms reach the trachea include the following: airborne, via equipment, via the hands of staff and via food. Three illustrative examples from this centre are outlined.

Example 1

During twice-weekly monitoring of the ITU it became clear that *Pseudomonas fluorescens* was being consistently isolated from the tracheal aspirates of those patients who had been ventilated for 4 days or more. *Ps. fluorescens* was isolated from the humidifier water of all the ventilators in use, from the inspiratory tubing and from the pre-filter expiratory tubing. Further investigation revealed that the humidifier water was contaminated before use although this was not true of the humidifiers or the tubing. At this time it was noted that the temperature of the humidifiers during use was between 38 and 41 °C. After a thorough environmental screen of the unit, the 8-1 plastic containers, in which the distilled water was delivered from the pharmacy, were discovered to be acting as a reservoir. The water direct from the distillation plant was sterile, but the plastic containers were neither sterilized nor dried out before refilling. Fortunately, only one of the seven patients involved in this episode required specific antibiotic treatment. The others responded to supportive management only and were gradually weaned from mechanical ventilation.

As a result of this experience, each patient is now allocated his own container of sterile water and the humidifier water temperature is regularly checked to lie between 48 and 51 °C. The humidifier water is sampled twice weekly. The disposable tubing is changed on a daily basis and the humidifiers sent for autoclaving thrice weekly. Since this procedure came into practice there have been only a few unrelated isolates of *Ps. fluorescens.*

Example 2

On another occasion *Klebsiella pneumoniae* was consistently isolated from the tracheal aspirates of those patients receiving nasogastric feeding. At that time, food was supplied from the hospital diet kitchen and some feeds were homogenized in the ITU. The organism was isolated from the unit liquidizer, some of the feeds and the nasogastric giving sets. *Klebsiella pneumoniae*, together with other coliforms, was traced to the work surfaces, refrigerator and some utensils in the hospital diet kitchen. Spread from the gastric aspirate via the mouth, nasopharynx and tracheostomy wounds to the trachea was established, confirming the observation of others[5] that the stomach can act as a source of potentially pathogenic bacteria.

Only one patient of this series required specific antibiotic treatment.

Subsequently, the nasogastric sets have been changed daily and the homogenized feeds have been replaced by sterile cans of commercial enteral preparations. *Klebsiella pneumoniae* is now only rarely isolated.

Example 3

Acinetobacter calcoaceticus var. *anitratus* has emerged recently as a colonizing organism in this ITU. The organism was introduced from a urological ward and although originally sensitive to tobramycin and amikacin it gradually became resistant to all antibiotics except colistin.

Environmental screening of the unit confirmed the presence of *A. calcoaceticus* on the hands of staff and in the sink traps. Once established as part of the residential flora, this organism is extremely difficult to eradicate; in the case of the authors' unit reappearing after closure of the unit for thorough washing, redecorating and replacement of sink traps. The possibility of carriage on the hands of staff remains the most likely explanation of this continuing problem.[20] Unfortunately, shortage of staff may not allow scrupulous hand-washing between patients and one nurse per patient plus another pair of hands for lifting is rarely available. Naturally the problem extends beyond the ITU to the rest of the hospital as patients are discharged to various wards which then act as reservoirs for further cross-infection. Orthopaedic and urological wards are at particular risk.

Other Laboratory Findings

No distinctive pattern of biochemical disturbances is observed in septic patients. Blood gas analysis often reveals a combination of hypoxaemia, hypocapnia and metabolic acidosis. Many patients have a raised blood urea and almost all are hypocalcaemic and hypoalbuminaemic. The prognostic significance of reduced protein levels in the critically ill septic patient and the relationship of these levels to the response to recall skin antigens is a matter of current controversy.

Anaemia of varying magnitude is a common feature of sepsis. The significance of leucopenia and leucocytosis has already been mentioned. Undoubtedly, the most consistent haematological observation in severe Gram-negative sepsis is thrombocytopenia with platelet counts falling below 50 000/μl;[7,48,58] thrombocytopenia is not a striking feature of Gram-positive sepsis. Persistent thrombocytopenia appears to be indicative of continuing infection and carries a poor prognosis (*Fig.* 9.2b). Abnormalities of prothrombin and partial thromboplastin times occur in some patients with sepsis but have not been found to be particularly helpful in diagnosis. Generalized bleeding supervenes in less than 10% of patients with Gram-negative septic shock;[48] its appearance usually marks a downward turn in the patient's clinical course. The diagnosis of disseminated intravascular coagulation is made when bleeding is associated with progressive thrombocytopenia, an abnormal coagulation profile and raised fibrinogen degradation products.

Haemodynamic and Respiratory Monitoring

Frequent careful monitoring of the cardiovascular and respiratory systems is essential in the management of any infected patient in the ITU. The aim of monitoring is not necessarily to maintain all the measured variables within the normal range but to determine what combination of values produces optimal perfusion and oxygenation.

Routine bedside monitoring of these patients includes repeated or continuous measurement of pulse rate and rhythm (from the electrocardiogram), arterial blood pressure and central venous pressure (via intravascular catheters), central and peripheral temperatures, respiratory rate and depth, blood gases and urine output. While most of these routine measurements can be made in a general surgical ward, it is customary nowadays to transfer patients requiring this level of monitoring to an ITU. Nevertheless, close collaboration between surgical staff and their ITU colleagues is mandatory since, in many cases, the acute phase of resuscitation is followed by surgical intervention, the optimal timing of which requires careful, co-ordinated judgement.

A number of more sophisticated monitoring techniques have recently become available, which have helped to increase the efficacy of acute resuscitation of patients suffering from septic shock. Catheterization of the pulmonary artery by means of a Swan–Ganz catheter[74] allows measurement of pulmonary artery pressure and cardiac output; pulmonary angiography may also be performed. In the often complex haemodynamic circumstances of septic shock the Swan–Ganz catheter may be of value as a guide for fluid management, in the simultaneous evaluation of right and left ventricular function, as an aid in the management of acute interstitial pulmonary oedema and in the diagnosis of pulmonary embolism.[55]

The measurement of plasma oncotic (or osmotic) pressure may be of additional value as a guide for fluid management and in helping to differentiate between the various causes of pulmonary oedema. Colloid oncotic pressure is frequently below normal in patients suffering from septic shock, and pulmonary oedema is an obvious risk particularly if pulmonary wedge pressure is simultaneously elevated.[16]

Mixed venous oxygen tension or saturation is a reliable measure of the overall adequacy of tissue perfusion and oxygenation.[32] Ideally, a true mixed venous sample should be obtained through a pulmonary artery catheter but samples withdrawn from the right atrium are usually an acceptable alternative. In the presence of major sepsis, interpretation of changes in this parameter is more difficult since a number of factors may be changing simultaneously. Mixed venous oxygen saturation is often well above the normal value of 70%, coincident with an elevated cardiac output and 'normal' oxygen consumption; low values (<50%) are uncommon except as a preterminal event.

Oxygen consumption is an important measurement in the critically ill septic patient as a guide to resuscitative and nutritional requirements. It may also be a valuable prognostic indicator, although in the septic patient this possibility remains unconfirmed. Part of the difficulty is that, since oxygen consumption is not a routine measurement, baseline values prior to the onset of infection or shock are rarely available. For this reason, alternative measurements, such as that of blood lactate, have been preferred. A number of studies have shown a good correlation between arterial lactate levels and prognosis in various forms of shock.[9, 60, 83] Few of these studies, however, contained significant numbers of septic patients and this may be important in view of the observations of Perret[61] who found that lactate values were significantly lower in septic shock than in other forms of shock, and that there appeared to be no correlation with the outcome. Furthermore, arterial hypoxaemia, liver disease and intravenous feeding may all increase blood lactate. If these factors can be excluded, lactate values in excess of 9 mmol/l are indicative of a poor prognosis.

New Developments

It is scarcely surprising that the problem of serious infection has stimulated abundant research. The following section cites only a few of the clinical measurements emerging from recent investigations which are likely to be of some practical value in the future.

A number of vasoactive substances of probable aetiological importance in the cardiovascular and respiratory disturbances of shock can now be accurately and readily measured in patients. Catecholamines, angiotensin II, histamine and 5-hydroxytryptamine have been extensively investigated; more recently plasma kinins and, in particular, prostaglandins, have raised a variety of attractive therapeutic possibilities.

The plasma complement system is an integral part of the body's antimicrobial defence system. The system consists of several enzymes capable of sequential activation in at least two different ways. The 'classic' pathway involves antibodies attached to cell walls or to soluble antigens in circulating immune complexes. The 'alternative' pathway can be activated without involving antibodies by a number of substances, one of which is endotoxin. A terminal sequence of reactions, common to both pathways, initiates a number of reactions throughout the body including the release of vasoactive substances, enhanced phagocytosis and cytolysis. Measurement of complement activity in the septic patient may indicate a recovery pattern (*Fig.* 9.4), herald a further shock episode, or forecast a complication such as the adult respiratory distress syndrome (ARDS). In the latter regard, a new test of the tendency for granulocytes to aggregate within the blood stream, reflecting C5a activation, appears to be of particular value.[28] When

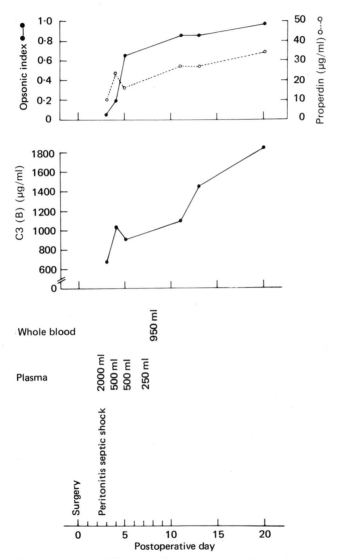

Fig. 9.4. Serial measurements of C3 properdin (O----O), and opsonic index (●——●) in a 31-year-old woman with severe bacterial peritonitis secondary to a ruptured appendix. Fresh frozen plasma in large amounts resulted in restoration of normal values and a marked improvement in her clinical condition. After Alexander, 1980.[1]

this test was performed in a recent prospective study of 32 patients, all six who demonstrated a positive result developed ARDS; none of the remainder developed progressive lung dysfunction.[22]

An assortment of new techniques is now available to measure hypoperfusion. Transcutaneous Po_2 and Pco_2 electrodes reflect arterial blood gas values reasonably accurately until cardiac output falls to an extent which causes peripheral vasoconstriction.[78] At this point the electrode values closely correspond to flow changes (*Fig.* 9.5). Similarly, direct monitoring of tissue pH, via an electrode placed on the surface of a muscle, may be used to quantitate the severity of ischaemia in shocked patients.[34]

In view of the increased capillary permeability associated with sepsis, methods have been devised to quantify the degree of 'leak' into vital organs, such as the lung. It is possible to relate the protein content of

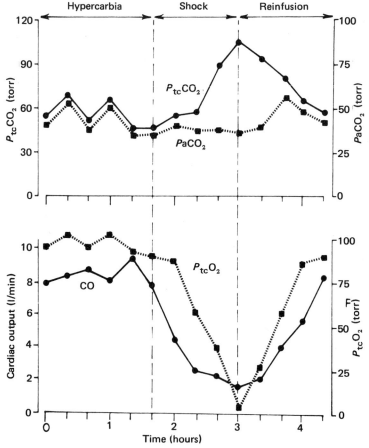

Fig. 9.5. Transcutaneous Pco_2 ($P_{tc}co_2$), $Paco_2$, transcutaneous Po_2 ($P_{tc}o_2$) and cardiac output (CO) during hypercarbia, shock and reinfusion in the dog. With the onset of hypovolaemia CO and $P_{tc}o_2$ fell and the $P_{tc}co_2$ rose abruptly.

bronchopulmonary aspirates to that of plasma or to measure 'clearance' of radiolabelled albumin from blood to broncho-alveolar secretions and thus distinguish between cardiogenic and non-cardiogenic pulmonary oedema.[4]

Hepatic dysfunction in sepsis and septic shock is becoming increasingly recognized as an important determinant of outcome, and liver function tests are therefore of value in assessing clinical progress.[57,65] Attention has recently centred on the role of the Kupffer cell in major infection and measurement of serum opsonic α_2 surface-binding glycoprotein may serve as an index of the functional state of the reticuloendothelial system.[70]

PATHOPHYSIOLOGICAL MECHANISMS

The factors initiating the onset of infection clearly vary. In the case of 'specific infection', a well-recognized pathogenic organism contaminates damaged or diseased tissue and the subsequent illness pursues a more or less predictable course. In 'non-specific infection', diminished host defence seems to play a more important role and the clinical course is less certain. Septic shock may ensue at any stage during the development of either type of infection.

Specific Infections

No attempt will be made to discuss the mechanisms underlying all the conditions included in this category but two, necrotizing fasciitis and Legionnaires' disease, are discussed further. These have been chosen because they are perhaps less well known than the others and because they are undoubtedly susceptible to expert management in an ITU.

Necrotizing Fasciitis

Necrotizing fasciitis is a relentlessly destructive bacterial infection characterized by extensive necrosis of the subcutaneous tissues of the abdominal wall and, less frequently, the extremities. The condition is fortunately uncommon but is potentially fatal and demands early recognition in order that treatment may be effective.[39,75,76]

Pathogenic organisms undoubtedly play a major role in initiating and spreading the necrotizing process. The type of bacteria now encountered, however, seem to differ from those in earlier reports. In Meleney's classic report[45] bacterial culture showed that the haemolytic streptococcus 'was the only organism invariably present'. In Wilson's series of 22 patients,[86] haemolytic organisms were found in pure culture in 58% and in combination with non-haemolytic bacteria in an additional 26% of the patients.

The majority of organisms (88%) were pathogenic staphylococci. Rea and Wyrick[64] reported 44 patients with necrotizing fasciitis seen during 15 years at Parkland Memorial Hospital in Dallas. In this group, haemolytic streptococci and pathogenic staphylococci together accounted for 89% of the wound infections with enteric Gram-negative organisms responsible for the remaining 11%. Wilson and Haltalin[87] described 11 children with necrotizing fasciitis. Haemolytic streptococci were found in 50% of cases. The other organisms were staphylococci and *Pseudomonas aeruginosa*. In the report by Ledingham and Tehrani,[39] the predominant organisms in initial wound culture, obtained through fresh incisions in the affected areas, were coliforms in combination, most frequently, with enterococci and streptococci: in only one case was the streptococcus of the β-haemolytic variety. Other organisms included *Bacteroides* species, *Clostridium welchii*, *Proteus* species, *Staphylococcus* species, *Ps. aeruginosa* and diphtheroids. Since colonizing bacteria rapidly invade the affected area, bacteriological cultures, both aerobic and anaerobic, must be taken from several sites at an early stage in the course of the disease. Irrespective of the species of organism involved, the initial bacterial growth takes place in the subcutaneous tissues, i.e. the subcutaneous fat, superficial fascia and the superficial layer of the deep fascia, most commonly of the abdominal wall and lower extemities. The initiating injury responsible for introduction of the infection may follow minor trauma or surgical incision. At times, no obvious cause is found.

After the initial bacterial insult, the infection spreads rapidly along the fascial plane causing massive necrosis. The presence of ischaemic tissue further facilitates spread of the necrotizing process. The skin remains intact initially, but later develops patchy necrosis and becomes gangrenous as a result of thrombotic occlusion of both venules and arterioles supplying the skin. The factors responsible for this alarming spread are unknown. An anaphylactic reaction similar to the Schwartzmann or Arthus phenomenon was suggested by Meleney.[46] McCafferty and Lyons[51] postulated activation by streptokinase or staphylokinase of a serum proteolytic enzyme, present in the inflammatory exudate, causing progressive collagen necrosis. Other organisms, such as *Pseudomonas* species, are known to produce collagenase with a primary effect on subcutaneous tissues and fascia.

Another important factor in any major infection of this sort is reduction in host defence. Primarily, local reduction in tissue resistance is achieved by the action of bacterial toxins added to the effect of kinases. This action is further enhanced by the general reduction in host defence mechanisms occurring in the postoperative period, or by pre-existing systemic diseases such as diabetes, arteriosclerosis, agamma- or hypogammaglobulinaemia, rheumatoid arthritis, malnutrition and gastrointestinal haemorrhage (*Fig.* 9.6). Infection, local ischaemia and reduced host defence combine to form a vicious cycle which is responsible for the initiation and spread of the process.

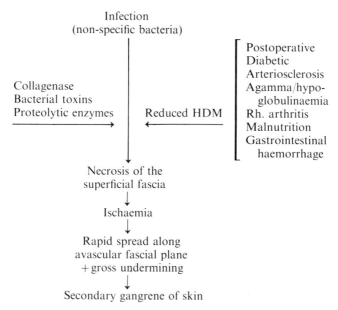

Fig. 9.6. Factors involved in the pathogenesis of necrotizing fasciitis. HDM = host defence mechanisms.

Legionnaires' Disease

This recently described form of atypical pneumonia is attributable to the pathogenic organism *Legionella pneumophila*.[37,66] The bacterium gains access to the body through the gastrointestinal tract via drinking water or through the lungs by inhalation. The disease usually presents as a pneumonic illness although other systems of the body may be affected including the gastrointestinal, hepatic, renal and central nervous system; some patients have developed disseminated intravascular coagulation.

Pathological findings are frequently limited to the lungs and although initially only one lung appears to be involved, bilateral infiltrates occur in over 50% of cases. Microscopically, most changes are confined to the alveoli and bronchioles which are filled with polymorphonuclear leucocytes, macrophages, cellular debris and fibrin. Vessels are normal in appearances. Organisms may be demonstrated within lung tissue using a special silver staining technique.

Non-specific Infection

The replacement of normal commensal flora by the predominant bacteria in the environment is inevitable in patients spending more than a few days in an ITU. Previous exposure to broad-spectrum antibiotics contributes, at least in part, to this process of colonization. The type of colonizing organism depends on whether the process has involved endogenous spread or exogenous contamination. In patients admitted following general surgery or trauma, the most frequently isolated organisms are Gram-negative in type (*Table* 9.2) and often several species are present simultaneously. A similar pattern occurs in patients suffering from malignant disease. In burns, however, a recent study showed that *Staphylococcus aureus* was the most commonly recovered organism, colonizing 85% of the wounds[53] β-Haemolytic streptococcus was recovered from only 5–10% of the patients. *Pseudomonas aeruginosa* showed a decrease in colonization rate from 50% in 1970 to 21% in 1976. In all patients whose illness is protracted and who have received various courses of broad-spectrum antibiotics, the risk of superadded infection with fungi and other unusual microbes is high.

Table 9.2. **Trauma and infection and types of organism**

Organism type	Incidence, %
Predominance of Gram-negative	70
Pseudomonas	24
Candida	16
Klebsiella	10
Enterobacter	8
Escherichia coli	6
Coag. neg. *Staphylococcus*	6

After Miller et al., 1973.[47]

One of the most difficult decisions that has to be made in interpreting bacteriological results in this type of infection is whether or not the organisms isolated are invasive and, therefore, the cause of significant clinical infection. Two or more positive blood cultures leave little room for doubt but tissue isolates alone often present a quandary, and the clinical features of infection may be masked in a severely ill patient who may also be receiving immunosuppressive agents. The distinction between colonization and infection is particularly troublesome in the respiratory system although some helpful pointers may be present (*Table* 9.3).

Host Defence

Over the past few years, the importance of reduced host defence has become increasingly obvious as techniques for demonstrating defects of this system have been developed.

When considering the pathophysiology of altered host defence mechanisms in patients in the ITU, it is convenient to consider three categories of patient. First, a small number of patients may coincidentally have one of

Table 9.3. **Factors that may help to differentiate between colonization and infection in the respiratory tract**

I. *Bacteriological*		
1. Gram-stain	Colonization	Infection
Epithelial cells	+ +	
White cells	± (+ + with endotracheal tube)	+ + +
Organisms	± mixed	+ + one species
2. Comparison of upper and lower respiratory tract flora	Same in both; or organisms present only in upper respiratory tract specimen	Different species in the two specimens
3. Type of growth obtained	Light or moderate pure growth or a mixed growth (even if heavy)	Heavy pure growth
4. Change in flora over a period of days		+
5. Species isolated	Usually: *Pseudomonas* spp. *C. albicans* *Staph. aureus*	Usually: *Strep. pneumoniae* *H. influenzae* 'Coliforms' *Klebsiella* spp.
II. *Clinical* Including: Mechanical ventilation Antibiotic regimen General symptoms of infection Local symptoms of infection		

After Shield et al., 1979.[71]

the many types of uncommon primary immunodeficiency diseases which usually become apparent in early life, e.g. one of the different types of agammaglobulinaemia. Secondly, a number of patients may have a disease or be receiving treatment which is known to produce secondary immunosuppression. Examples of the miscellaneous 'high risk' group include cancer patients on chemotherapy, renal transplant patients receiving immunosuppressive drugs including steroids, and patients with lympho-proliferative diseases, such as Hodgkin's disease. Radiotherapy and splenectomy can also reduce immunocompetence.

The third and largest category of patients met with in the ITU are those where the acquired deficiency is secondary to factors such as age, injury, anaesthesia, operation, shock, haemorrhage, sepsis or malnutrition. The severity of the immunological defect in this last and heterogeneous group may be variable and knowledge of the defects occurring in host defences is not yet clear.

The remainder of the discussion is concerned mainly with this latter group. A common finding in the majority of these patients is a lowered response to recall skin antigens. In this centre, initial skin testing in critically ill surgical patients admitted to the ITU has shown that of 82 patients, 59 were non-reactors to skin testing (anergic). Such testing had prognostic significance (*Fig.* 9.7) since, in those patients who were initially

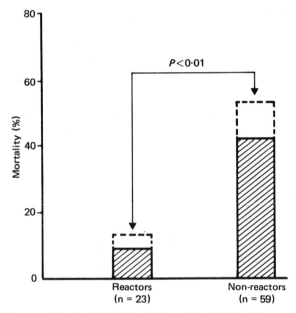

Fig. 9.7. Mortality according to initial skin testing. Mortality in 59 non-reactors was 40% and in 23 reactors was 9% ($P<0.01$).

non-reactors, the mortality was 40% compared to 9% in the 23 patients who initially reacted to skin testing ($P<0.01$). Furthermore, 30 of the patients who were initially non-reactors and remained in the ITU for more than one week were skin tested at weekly intervals. Ten of these patients subsequently converted to reactors and the mortality in this group was 20%, compared with a mortality of 80% in the 20 patients who remained anergic. These results emphasize the fact that initial and persisting anergy to recall antigens is associated with a poor prognosis.

Since a defect in any component of this response may prevent a normal reaction to the antigen, the mechanism of anergy is difficult to identify. Some studies of patients after burns[49] have reported an altered in-vitro lymphocyte response to mitogens and it may be that, in these patients, anergy is partly due to an acute defect in lymphocyte function. Other studies suggest that there is a decreased inflammatory response as the responsible mechanism.[14] The localization of polymorphs in an inflammatory response requires the generation of chemotactic mediators and a trophic response by the cells. However, there are conflicting reports on whether neutrophil chemotaxis is altered in anergic patients.[12,29]

A possible mechanism for anergy in some patients may be the presence of inhibitory serum factors which may prevent the response to recall antigens. It has been suggested that these inhibitory factors may decrease chemotaxis and prevent the movement of non-specific inflammatory cells, i.e. neutrophils and monocytes, therefore inhibiting the expression of a cell-mediated response.[13]

Septic Shock

The commonly held view that septic shock is easily recognized and readily distinguished from other forms of shock is, in many cases, erroneous. Certainly the young otherwise healthy individual in whom bacteraemia occurs secondary to urological intervention, will manifest fever and hypotension, the cause of which is obvious. The majority of patients who develop septic shock, however, are either older or have some associated systemic disease, may be frankly hypovolaemic and, not infrequently, have latent cardiac disease. The pathophysiological basis of shock in these patients is a complex mixture of factors, only one of which is the presence of infection.

Shock occurs in association with both Gram-positive and Gram-negative infections—less frequently in the former (about one in ten patients) than in the latter (about one in three patients). In the past, it was believed possible to discriminate between Gram-positive and Gram-negative septic shock on clinical grounds, but recent evidence makes it clear that this is untrue. In a study of 59 patients,[84] Wiles and his colleagues were unable to detect a difference in any physiological variable between organism group, or indeed between specific organisms. After initial resuscitation, all patients exhibited a hyperdynamic cardiovascular response with abnormal vascular tone; some degree of myocardial depression was evident in most patients. Mortality was over 70% in both Gram-positive and Gram-negative septi-caemia. The conclusion reached in this study was that while the exact pathogenesis of the septic response remained unclear, it did not seem to be peculiar to a specific micro-organism. This supports the contention that the fate of patients suffering from septic shock is determined by the speed and adequacy of initial resuscitation and, thereafter, by the nature of the underlying disease process.

In the early stages of septic shock (the hyperdynamic phase), cardiac output is often high and the skin warm and dry. Urine output may be elevated and some patients may exhibit an inappropriate polyuria at the expense of effective circulating plasma volume. These effects are related to the presence in the circulation of various pyrogens and to the release by bacterial products of plasma kinins, histamine and prostaglandins of the E series. These agents may later contribute (by direct effects on capillary permeability) to the transudation of fluid from capillaries. The primary respiratory response is hyperventilation, mediated by both central and peripheral mechanisms, and arterial blood gas analysis may reveal only some reduction in P_{CO_2}. Metabolic acidosis in septic shock is more variable than in other forms of shock and, therefore, less reliable as a prognostic indicator.

In the later stages of septic shock (the hypodynamic phase), cardiac output falls and there is marked hypotension, peripheral vasoconstriction and oliguria. These effects are almost certainly caused by the release of catecholamines and angiotensin II. More recently discovered substances such as thromboxane B_2, derived from damaged platelets, may augment this reaction particularly in the pulmonary circulation[59] and contribute to a deterioration in pulmonary gas exchange with a progressive fall in arterial P_{O_2}.

Metabolic disturbances appear earlier in septic than in other forms of shock. Characteristically, the arteriovenous oxygen difference falls and in some patients' oxygen consumption may be very low.[88] There is agreement that the most likely explanation for this observation is impaired cell metabolism. This metabolic defect interferes with capillary and cell membrane function and prevents the cells from utilizing oxygen and energy substrates properly to form ATP. Lipolysis occurs with high circulating levels of free fatty acids and serum triglycerides.[81] In muscle there is a block to the intracellular oxidation of glucose, which, together with an inability to utilize ketone bodies, leads to increased catabolism of branched-chain amino acids. The disturbance in carbohydrate metabolism may be due to inhibition of certain of the reactions within the citric acid cycle which may account for the lower than expected levels of lactate in septic shock. Hypophosphataemia and hypocalcaemia are also common.

Many of the haemodynamic and metabolic effects which have been described may be attributable to circulating endotoxin, the complex lipopolysaccharide coating of Gram-negative bacteria, and in particular the lipid-A moiety. Endotoxin causes aggregation of platelets by direct damage to the cell wall, and of white cells by an indirect action via activated complement. Platelet aggregation leads to the formation of thrombi in the microcirculation at a rate which may swamp fibrinolytic and reticuloendothelial phagocytic mechanisms. White cell aggregation may also cause plugging of the microvasculature with damage of the capillary endothelium resulting from direct contact with toxic oxygen radicals, such as superoxide anion and hydrogen peroxide, released from the leucocytes.[22, 28]

These microcirculatory disturbances may be observed widely throughout the body and may result in focal necrosis in the lung, kidneys and liver, as well as other organs.

In the lung, damage to the capillary endothelium leads to the development of protein-rich pulmonary oedema which, if not arrested early, may progress to the fully developed adult respiratory distress syndrome. In the kidney, endotoxaemia may cause an already reduced glomerular filtration rate to fall further and precipitate acute renal failure. If the source of sepsis can be successfully eradicated recovery is possible.

Jaundice may occur in the presence of extra-hepatic Gram-negative infection. The jaundice is of a cholestatic type, typically reflected in elevation of conjugated serum bilirubin and alkaline phosphatase, with modest increases in serum transaminases. The histological appearances in the liver are those of intercellular and intra-canalicular bile stasis with little or no evidence of parenchymal damage. The observed cholestasis in sepsis may be caused by the inhibitory effect of endotoxin on the active sodium transport mechanism of hepatocytes.[79]

Failure of liver function abnormalities to return to normal within a few days of a septic insult often indicates a persisting source of major infection.[57,65] Attention has once again begun to centre on the role of the hepatic Kupffer cells in the removal of bacteria and their breakdown products, including endotoxin, from the circulation. The activity of these cells is inhibited during an episode of septic shock[70] and the success of treatment may well be determined by the degree of functional recovery which ensues after the phase of resuscitation.

TREATMENT

No single treatment can be expected to cure severe infection in the critically ill patient. Indeed, the only possibility of success lies in the prompt institution of a combination of therapeutic manoeuvres with subsequent careful observation of the patient in order that modification or reinforcement of treatment may be effected without delay. The high mortality associated with invasive infection emphasizes the fact that prevention is infinitely superior to attempted cure. In the following account, mention will be made of (1) general antibiotic policy for severe infections in the ITU, (2) clinical management of the 'specific' and 'non-specific' conditions previously outlined, and finally (3) the principles of resuscitation of the patient suffering from septic shock.

Antibiotic Policy for Severe Infections

There are certain guidelines which should be followed before and during antimicrobial therapy:

I. Confirm as far as possible the presence of clinically significant infection.

II. Use an antibiotic or combination of antibiotics appropriate to the infection; consider dosage, route and penetration.

III. Some antibiotics are more appropriate than others for specific organisms.

IV. Review possible complications of antibiotic therapy.

V. Be alert to causes of treatment failure.

VI. Avoid misuse of antibiotics.

I. Bacteriological and clinical information should always be considered together. Differentiation must be made between normal flora, colonization and infection[71] (*Table* 9.3). For example, *Streptococcus pyogenes* nearly always requires treatment whereas a *Pseudomonas* species rarely does. Immunosuppressed patients are more difficult to assess since they are liable to become infected with so-called 'non-pathogenic' organisms.

II. The choice of antibiotics is straightforward in the case of some specific infections and can be based initially on clinical findings; examples include gas gangrene, lobar pneumonia and scarlet fever. More often a 'best guess' choice of antimicrobials has to be made while the bacteriological diagnosis and sensitivity results are awaited. In severe infections a broad-spectrum regimen, active against all likely pathogens, should be chosen. This can be modified in the light of subsequent laboratory data. Inappropriate antibiotics should be discontinued immediately and a narrow spectrum used thereafter in order to minimize the effect on normal flora. Combinations of antibiotics are justified in four situations: severe infections of unknown aetiology, tuberculosis, when synergy is of value, and when the treatment of more than one organism is required (and cannot be achieved with a single agent).

There is rarely any need to exceed the recommended dose of an antibiotic although a reduction in dose may be required in the presence of impaired renal function. The oral and intramuscular routes are not generally relevant in the critically ill septic patient. Intravenous administration may be by bolus or infusion. In the latter case, chemical incompatibilities should always be considered (e.g. the penicillins and gentamicin), and no drugs should be added to blood, plasma, parenteral feeding solutions, mannitol or sodium bicarbonate. Electrolyte and fluid overload are hazards if antibiotic carrier fluids are not included in the anticipated daily requirements (e.g. sodium carbenicillin). Some antibiotics may be administered efficiently by the rectal route, e.g. metronidazole, thus avoiding the problems of intravenous administration. Local and topical antibiotics are appropriate in the treatment of eye and ear infections which are always a risk in those severely ill patients. Antibiotics capable of penetration must be considered in infections of bone, joint, eye and cerebrospinal fluid.

III. If the causative organism(s) is *unknown* the following combinations of antibiotics are appropriate:

1. Ampicillin/amoxycillin or benzylpenicillin together with gentamicin and metronidazole.

2. Erythromycin (in penicillin-sensitive patients) together with gentamicin and metronidazole.

The foregoing combinations are preferable if there is a likelihood of anaerobic organisms, as in intra-abdominal sepsis.

3. Co-trimoxazole.

4. Mezlocillin together with gentamicin or cephuroxime—this combination covers most organisms including *Staphylococcus aureus*: mezlocillin is inactivated by β-lactamase from Gram-positive or Gram-negative organisms.

If the causative organisms are known to be *Gram-negative* the following choice of antibiotics is available:

1. For *Escherichia coli, Klebsiella* species, *Proteus* species:
   Ampicillin with or without gentamicin
   Co-trimoxazole
   A cephalosporin; not cephaloridine if there is impaired renal function

2. For *Pseudomonas* species: rarely requires treatment but when it does treatment with combined antibiotics should be aggressive.
   Gentamicin together with carbenicillin, ticarcillin or azlocillin

If the causative organisms are known to be *Gram-positive* the following choice is available:

1. For *Staphylococcus aureus*:
   Fusidic acid together with flucloxacillin or penicillin (if organism sensitive), erythromycin, clindamycin, cephalosporin or gentamicin

Fusidic acid should never be used alone because of the rapid emergence of resistance; the intravenous preparation is associated with jaundice.[25]

2. For *Streptococcus pyogenes*:
   Benzylpenicillin; alternatives include erythromycin, clindamycin and cephalosporin

3. For *Clostridium welchii*:
   Benzylpenicillin with or without metronidazole

The various antibiotics recommended for severe respiratory tract infections are listed in *Table* 9.4.

The examples of antibotic usage outlined above are based on experience in this centre. Each hospital has its own commensal organisms and 'antibiotic policy' must be modified according to local requirement.

IV. The complications of antibiotic administration. Three examples relate particularly to ITU practice.

1. *Aminoglycosides*: the risks of nephrotoxicity and ototoxicity (8th nerve) are well documented. Serum assays, both trough (just before) and peak (half an hour after intravenous and one hour after intramuscular dose) must be made to confirm adequacy and safety of dosage. The trough level should not exceed 2 mg/l and the peak should be between 5 and 10 mg/l. In order to maintain an adequate peak level it may be necessary to give a higher dose, e.g. 120 or 160 mg of gentamicin 12-hourly rather than the usual 80 mg 8-hourly. The extra four hours enables excretion of the drug to bring the trough level to below 2 mg/l. A single dose per day may be adequate in patients with renal failure.

Table 9.4. Respiratory tract infections

Clinical diagnosis	Possible causal organisms	Appropriate antimicrobials
Chronic bronchitis	*Haemophilus influenzae* *Streptococcus pneumoniae*	Ampicillin Co-trimoxazole Erythromycin
Lobar pneumonia	*Streptococcus pneumoniae*	Penicillin Erythromycin Clindamycin
Aspiration pneumonia	Mouth organisms, including anaerobes	Penicillin and metronidazole *or* Clindamycin
Post-influenzal pneumonia	Culture essential *Staphylococcus aureus* *Streptococcus pneumoniae*	Staphylococcal: fusidic acid + flucloxacillin or chloramphenicol (modify after culture results) *See above*
Primary atypical pneumonia	*Mycoplasma pneumoniae* *Chlamydia psittaci* *Coxiella burneti*	Erythromycin *or* Tetracycline
Legionnaires' disease	*Legionella pneumophila*	Erythromycin alone or initially with rifampicin
Bronchopneumonia	Primary pathogen may be difficult to find, culture and sensitivities essential *Haemophilus influenzae* *Streptococcus pneumoniae* less common *Staphylococcus aureus* Coliforms *Pseudomonas*	Modify according to culture results Ampicillin Co-trimoxazole Severe—benzylpenicillin and gentamicin } Consult laboratory before treating as they } may not be significant
Lung abscess	*Streptococcus milleri* *Staphylococcus aureus* anaerobes, etc.	Consult laboratory

2. *Penicillin*: hypersensitivity may prompt replacement with a non-penicillin antibiotic.

3. Several antibiotics have now been implicated as a cause of pseudo-membranous colitis[35] including ampicillin, lincomycin, clindamycin, co-trimoxazole and metronidazole. The disease appears to be due to a toxin-producing strain of *Clostridium difficile*. All antibiotics should be stopped and *oral* vancomycin commenced.

V. Treatment failure may be due to a number of causes. The antibiotic may not have been given or not absorbed. The dose may have been inadequate or the antibiotic inappropriate for penetration. The original bacteriological assay may not have been representative or overgrown with another organism. Perhaps the commonest reason for failure is that surgical drainage of persistent localized sepsis is required.

VI. Misuse of antibiotics can lead to the emergence of multiresistant organisms with attendant problems of antimicrobial therapy in the case of bacteraemia, e.g. the previously mentioned *Acinetobacter* species. Patients with aminoglycoside-resistant *Staphylococcus aureus* or coliform infections should always be barrier-nursed to prevent cross-infection. There is always a risk of plasmid transfer of resistance to other organisms.

Clinical Management

Specific Infections

Obviously each of the conditions in this category demands a different treatment regimen. The ITU offers an opportunity for integrated and sustained endeavour, not only during the phase of acute resuscitation, but also during the subsequent phase of recovery when skilled nursing care and optimum nutrition become crucially important. The main points of this approach to treatment will be illustrated with reference to two brief case histories—one concerning necrotizing fasciitis (*Case 1*) and the other Legionnaires' disease (*Case 2*).

Case 1

A 17-year-old girl was crushed by a block of ice in the Swiss Alps. Her injuries included fractures of the superior and inferior pubic rami, diastasis of the sacro-iliac joint and a Le Fort II fracture of the maxilla.

The pelvic fractures were treated conservatively and she remained well until eight days after the accident when her condition deteriorated and she became toxaemic with swelling of her left leg. An initial diagnosis of gas gangrene was made and appropriate therapy, including hyperbaric oxygen and multiple incisions, was instituted. No clostridial organisms were cultured. Her condition continued to deteriorate and she was transferred to Glasgow five days later.

On admission, the clinical picture was suggestive of necrotizing fasciitis and this was confirmed at operation when it was found that the necrosis involved only the subcutaneous layer. The characteristic grey gelatinous appearance of the fascia was obvious and the underlying muscle was quite normal. All the undermined skin and subcutaneous tissue was excised from the left lower abdomen, left thigh and half the left lower leg. Because of the possibility that bowel organisms might have contributed to the condition, possibly from a silent perforation of the sigmoid colon or rectum, and also to prevent faecal soiling of the denuded area, a defunctioning colostomy was performed. The organisms cultured were β-haemolytic streptococci, *Bacteroides* species and Gram-positive diphtheroids.

Not surprisingly, the patient had a stormy postoperative few days. Specific antibiotic therapy was maintained throughout this period, together with abundant intravenous fluids including an adequate supply of calories and nitrogen. Fortunately, no major respiratory or renal complication ensued. The skin excised at the time of the operation was prepared as a free skin graft, stored at 4 °C, and re-applied to the denuded area one week later. Two secondary grafting procedures were required and finally the colostomy was closed.

Confusion in diagnosis between necrotizing fasciitis and clostridial myositis can be avoided if early incision is performed and the underlying tissues carefully examined. The combination of aggressive surgery and intensive therapy has transformed the outcome of necrotizing fasciitis in much the same way that the development of specialized centres has in the case of burns.

Case 2

A previously healthy 49-year-old man presented with a short history of malaise and breathlessness. The initial diagnosis of pneumonia was confirmed by chest X-ray and the possibilty of an atypical organism was considered.Despite treatment with erythromycin and rifampicin, his condition deteriorated and he became confused and exhausted with an arterial Po_2 of 30 mmHg and a Pco_2 of 20 mmHg when breathing 40% O_2.

The patient was transferred to the ITU for mechanical ventilation. Over the next 24 h his condition deteriorated with evidence of cardiovascular instability which responded to treatment with digoxin and peripheral vasodilator agents. An inspired oxygen concentration of 65% and a positive end-expiratory pressure of 10 cm H_2O was required to maintain adequate gas exchange. Biochemical analysis revealed hyponatraemia with a very low serum albumin and grossly abnormal liver enzymes, but renal function was unimpaired.

The patient's condition improved slowly and he was successfully weaned from mechanical ventilation after eight days despite a severe confusional state.

He went on to make a full recovery.

The atypical pneumonias and in particular those due to *Legionella pneumophila* are frequently multisystem disorders in which the pulmonary lesion is complicated by signs of cerebral, cardiac, hepatic, renal and gastrointestinal involvement. This may progress to organ failure and there is no doubt that many of these patients can benefit from intensive supportive therapy, in addition to treatment of the respiratory failure with mechanical ventilation and physiotherapy.

The combination of cerebral and gastrointestinal involvement with vomiting in the presence of depressed consciousness leads to a very real risk of the primary pneumonia being complicated by bronchopulmonary aspiration of gastric contents. Careful observation or intubation with a cuffed endotracheal tube may minimize this risk. Hyponatraemia and hypoalbuminaemia are common complications, making careful management of fluid therapy important, particularly as myocardial and renal involvement may compromise the patient's ability to handle fluids. In severe cases, the development of ileus may make intravenous nutrition necessary and should renal failure develop dialysis will be required.

Unfortunately, there is little evidence that antibiotic therapy has much influence on the course of severe cases with multisystem failure.

Non-specific Infections

Colonization of the immunologically compromised critically ill patient with potentially pathogenic organisms seems inevitable. Prophylactic antibiotics and antiseptic solutions cannot prevent this process and, indeed, merely complicate the problem by increasing the incidence of resistant organisms.[43] Nevertheless, there is evidence that many patients come to terms with the colonizing organisms, provided that the latter are not highly pathogenic, do not gain access to the bloodstream or become otherwise invasive.

The aim of management of the critically ill patient should be to reduce, by every means available, the risk of invasion by colonizing bacteria. The only way to achieve this aim is for each member of staff to maintain a continually positive attitude to the control of infection and constantly guard against the temptation to 'cut corners'. The highest possible standards of aseptic and antiseptic technique are required whenever the skin has to be breached, e.g. during the insertion of intravascular catheters or shunts, or when tubes are placed in previously sterile organs, e.g. the bladder, or body cavities, e.g. the thorax.

When clinically significant infection supervenes, the single most important therapeutic manoeuvre is to establish adequate drainage; further extension of infection may thus be limited. Antibiotics may be of some value if prescribed for brief periods in adequate doses, but are ineffective in the presence of deep-seated or loculated infection, irrespective of site. Drainage under these circumstances offers the only hope of success and this principle holds true for chest infections where postural drainage, physiotherapy and regular tracheal suction are the usual combination of choice, as well as for intra-abdominal sepsis, where surgical drainage is indicated. In a few cases, no overt source of infection can be identified although the patient's clinical condition would seem to suggest the presence of infection. The prognosis for these patients is poor and the commonest mode of death is multiple organ failure.

In the absence of a consistent response to antibiotics in this category of infection and in the knowledge that the host defence mechanisms are often defective, the concept of immunotherapy is becoming increasingly popular. This form of treatment includes the use of immunostimulant agents, parenteral nutrition and vaccination.

Several agents have been proposed as possible immunomodulators. These include bacille Calmette–Guérin (BCG) vaccine, *Corynebacterium parvum*, thymosin and levamisole. In some instances, a degree of immunostimulation, as judged by improvements in in-vitro measurements of immunological function, has been shown, but none of these agents has yet been shown to have a convincing clinical effect in critically ill patients. In a recent double blind study from France,[21] no decrease in mortality occurred in anergic septic patients given the immunostimulant, isoprinosine. In another study from Canada,[44] the administration of levamisole to ill surgical patients produced a slight, but unconvincing, improvement in sepsis and mortality.

An alternative or additional approach lies in the vaccination of critically ill patients against specific organisms where these are known to be a common threat. In burns patients, where *Pseudomonas aeruginosa* infection is common, early trials[30] of the prophylactic administration of a polyvalent pseudomonas vaccine (PEV-01) soon after the burn injury have shown encouraging results. An increase in protective antibody and increased phagocytic activity against *Pseudomonas* species occur and are associated with a reduced mortality from pseudomonas infection. Future trends may lead to the development of other polyvalent vaccines for prophylactic use in other types of critically ill patients at risk of infection.[81]

Septic Shock

Treatment should be directed towards immediate resuscitation followed, when appropriate, by eradication of the source of sepsis. Fluid repletion and correction of hypoxaemia are the two primary considerations in the treatment of all forms of shock and are no less relevant in the case of major sepsis. Various pharmacological agents have come to play an increasingly important complementary role in management.

Fluid Repletion

Hypovolaemia is almost invariably present in septic shock. Fluid intake has often been inadequate and fluid losses due to pyrexia, hyperventilation and gastrointestinal disturbances are often excessive. An absolute volume deficit is compounded by complex fluid shifts between the intravascular, interstitial and intracellular compartments. The principal aim of fluid replacement is rapid restoration of blood volume and return to normal of impaired tissue perfusion. If central venous pressure, core-peripheral temperature gradient and urine output are restored to normal, it is usual to find that the pulse rate, blood pressure and acid–base balance rapidly follow suit.

In the acute treatment of hypovolaemia, the speed and volume of fluid administered are more important than the type of fluid used. The colloid versus crystalloid debate remains unresolved, but clinical evidence suggests that neither approach is convincingly superior to the other.

It is the practice in this centre to use colloids in the first instance—principally plasma protein fraction or gelatin solution rather than dextran.[38] Thereafter crystalloid solutions are administered, the type and amount depending on estimated deficits and measurement of serum electrolytes, plasma proteins, plasma osmolality, colloid oncotic pressure and haematocrit. Transfusion of whole blood or packed cells is often required, though it is recognized that haemodilution may improve oxygen availability and oxygen consumption.

Once haemodynamic stability has been achieved, it is important to take immediate stock of further fluid needs since even small amounts in excess of requirement will tend to provoke pulmonary oedema,[72] whilst mild dehydration may increase the risk of renal failure.[42]

Oxygen and Ventilation

Of equal importance to restoration of impaired tissue perfusion is correction of reduced oxygen content. The association of anaemia and septic shock has already been noted. In addition, not only is there commonly a reduction in arterial oxygen tension but there may be a shift to the left of the oxygen dissociation curve.

Correction of hypoxaemia may be achieved, in the first instance, by an increase in the inspired oxygen concentration but, in the presence of low blood flow, the magnitude of increase in arterial Po_2 will frequently be disappointing. Many centres now advocate the early use of intermittent positive pressure ventilation (IPPV) with the aim of preventing the onset of significant alveolar damage which precedes the fully developed adult respiratory distress syndrome. IPPV has the additional advantage of reducing oxygen consumption directly by eliminating the oxygen cost of breathing and indirectly by allowing adequate safe analgesia and sedation.

Once initial fluid repletion had been completed and cardiac output has increased, the addition of positive end-expiratory pressure to the ventilator circuit may be of considerable value in further improving and maintaining pulmonary gas exchange.

Pharmacological Support

The principal drugs which may be of advantage in the management of a patient with septic shock, include those with an effect on the cardiovascular system, on the coagulation/fibrinolytic system, on metabolism and those with combined effects.

If hypoperfusion persists after volume expansion and correction of hypoxaemia, methods of increasing cardiac output and improving perfusion become an important priority. Many drugs are now available which can help to achieve these aims.

The oldest, yet perhaps still the most controversial, of the inotropic drugs is digoxin. Digitalization is practiced at an early stage in this centre amongst older patients suffering from septic shock.[38] The advantages of this practice appear to outweigh the disadvantages, although the indications for continuing the administration of digoxin should be reviewed on a daily basis. Cardiac glycosides are known to produce vasoconstriction, particularly in the splanchnic circulation,[40] and for this and other reasons, many clinicians are attracted to alternative inotropic drugs such as isoprenaline, dopamine and dobutamine.

Dopamine is now favoured in the treatment of septic shock. Not only does this drug exert an inotropic effect by stimulating cardiac B_1-adrenoceptors but it also has a unique action in dilating the mesenteric and renal blood vessels. Dopamine undeniably produces beneficial haemodynamic and renal effects in the majority of patients with septic shock (*Fig. 9.8*) and is, therefore, of value in 'buying time' to allow surgical intervention. On the other hand, whether the drug reduces mortality or prevents long-term complications is doubtful. Dopamine would appear to be of particular value when the haemodynamic combination of lowered arterial pressure and vasodilation is present, especially if urine volume is also reduced. In the case of high cardiac filling pressures combined with severe peripheral vasoconstriction, other inotropic agents, e.g. dobutamine, may be preferred since dopamine, in this situation, may produce excessive increases in left ventricular work. Vasodilator drugs have recently attracted

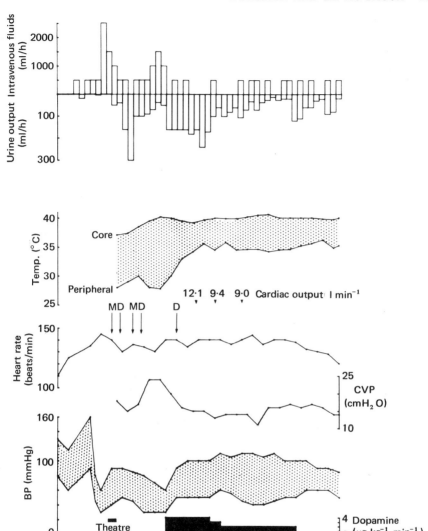

Fig. 9.8. 41-year-old male patient with faecal peritonitis. Two hours prior to laparotomy shock ensued; resuscitation with fluids, oxygen and antibiotics was continued throughout operation. Continuing hypotension, vasoconstriction and, finally, oliguria during the early postoperative phase prompted the use of dopamine with good effect.

considerable attention. Not only may peripheral vasoconstriction be relieved but cardiac function may also improve.[36] No convincing evidence exists as to which of the vasodilator drugs is most efficient; selection should be based on the predominant cardiovascular disturbance. A combination of dopamine with one of the vasodilators may be beneficial in some patients with septic shock.[10]

The possible relationship between disseminated intravascular coagulation and endotoxic shock[23] suggests that heparin should be of therapeutic value. Convincing evidence, however, is lacking and heparin is rarely given routinely in surgical practice. Even in patients with frank generalized bleeding, the first priority should be the controlled administration of platelet concentrates and coagulation factors. If heparin is to be given, the dose should be adjusted to produce a prolongation of activated partial thromboplastin time.

High doses of glucocorticoids, principally methylprednisolone, have been advocated in the treatment of septic shock,[41] although uncertainty about their value remains. A single dose of 30 mg/kg of methylprednisolone sodium succinate, repeated four hours later if necessary, is recommended. The only clinical control study which has been published indicates a beneficial action of steroids.[69] Others have been unable to demonstrate a decrease in mortality with the use of steroids[77] and further clinical trials are necessary. Perhaps selective use of glucocorticoids, for example in patients with excessive C5a activation,[22] will prove more rewarding.

Antimicrobial Agents

The correct choice of antibiotic is clearly important, although the evidence that mortality following Gram-negative septicaemia has been reduced by antibiotics is not convincing. In a recent extensive review[89] it was concluded that in both aerobic and anaerobic Gram-negative infections, resuscitation and surgical drainage 'may be more important to a successful outcome than optimal antibiotic selection'. If antibiotics are to be of value in septic shock they must be used early and in appropriate dosage.

In most instances, the immediate choice of antibiotic is determined by knowledge of the source of infection, the likely organisms involved, and their probable sensitivities. At the present time, the practice in this centre is to use a combination of gentamicin, metronidazole and ampicillin for severe infection suspected to be due to faecal organisms. Ampicillin is used because of its effectiveness against enterococci—which are resistant to gentamicin and metronidazole.

Surgical Intervention

A substantial proportion of patients suffering from septic shock will require some form of surgical intervention during the course of their illness. The importance of this component of treatment in relation to final outcome cannot be over-emphasized although, in the individual case, it is often difficult to know precisely what course of action to take. Evaluation of the acutely ill patient with septic shock, constitutes one of the greatest challenges to the diagnostic skills and clinical acumen of the surgeon. Indications for surgery (and its timing), identification of the septic source, and surgical procedure all demand a high degree of surgical skill and experience. The best results are undoubtedly achieved when those decisions are reached in collaboration with ITU, anaesthetic and bacteriological colleagues.

Although ultrasound scanning and radioisotope imaging,[56] amongst several new diagnostic procedures, may help in the detection and localization of intra-abdominal sepsis, the surgeon must often make his judgement on the basis of clinical experience and in the knowledge that the most probable explanation for failure to respond to adequate resuscitation is continuing sepsis. Under these circumstances adequate exposure and careful exploration of the abdomen offer the only real chance of success.

New Developments

A number of new concepts relating to treatment of the severely infected patient are currently under investigation. Two of the more promising of these are the administration of fresh frozen plasma in patients with a persistent depression of C3 and of cryoprecipitate[70] in patients with low circulating serum opsonic α_2 surface-binding glycoprotein.

REFERENCES

1. Alexander J. W. (1980) The role of host defense mechanisms in surgical infections. *Surg. Clin. North Am.* **60**, 107–116.
2. Alexander J. W., Stinnett J. D., Ogle K. et al. (1979) A comparison of immunologic profiles and their influence on bacteraemia in surgical patients with a high risk of infection. *Surgery* **86**, 94–104.
3. Allgower M., Durig M. and Wolff G. (1980) Infection and trauma. *Surg. Clin. North Am.* **60**, 133–144.
4. Anderson R. R., Holliday R. L., Driedger A. A. et al. (1979) Documentation of pulmonary capillary permeability in the adult respiratory distress syndrome (ARDS) accompanying human sepsis. *Am. Rev. Resp. Dis.* **119**, 869–877.
5. Atherton S. T. and White D. J. (1978) Stomach as a source of bacteria colonising respiratory tract during artificial ventilation. *Lancet* **2**, 968–969.
6. Bartlett R. C., Ellner P. D. and Washington J. A. (1974) Blood cultures. In: Sherris J. C. ed., *Cumulative Techniques and Procedures in Clinical Microbiology (Cumitech)*, Vol. 1, pp. 1–6. Washington, American Society for Microbiology.
7. Beller F. K. and Douglas G. W. (1973) Thrombocytopenia indicating Gram-negative infection and endotoxemia. *Obstet. Gynecol.* **41**, 521–524.
8. Briggs J. D. (1980) Renal transplantation. In: Chapman A., ed., *Clinics in Critical Care Medicine*, Vol. 1, *Acute Renal Failure*, pp. 149–171. Edinburgh, Churchill Livingstone.
9. Broader G. and Weil M. H. (1964) Excess lactate: an index of reversibility of shock in human patients. *Science* **143**, 1457–1459.
10. Cerra F. B., Hassett J. and Siegel J. H. (1978) Vasodilator therapy in clinical sepsis with low output syndrome. *J. Surg. Res.* **25**, 180–183.

11. Chang P. C., Weil M. H., Portigal L. D. et al. (1977) Prognostic indices and predictors for patients in circulatory shock. In: Ledingham I. McA., ed., *Recent Advances in Intensive Therapy*, pp. 19–31. Edinburgh, Churchill Livingstone.

12. Christou N. V. and Meakins J. L. (1979) Neutrophil function in anergic surgical patients. *Ann. Surg.* **190**, 557–564.

13. Christou N. V. and Meakins J. L. (1979) Neutrophil function in surgical patients: two inhibitors of granulocyte chemotaxis associated with sepsis. *J. Surg. Res.* **26**, 355–364.

14. Christou N. V. and Meakins J. L. (1979) Delayed hypersensitivity in surgical patients: a mechanism for anergy. *Surgery* **86**, 78–85.

15. Christou N. V., Meakins J. L. and MacLean D. (1981) The predictive role of delayed hypersensitivity on preoperative patients. *Surg. Gynecol. Obstet.* **152**, 297–300.

16. Da Luz P. L., Shubin H., Weil M. H. et al. (1975) Pulmonary edema related to changes in colloid osmotic and pulmonary artery wedge pressure in patients after acute myocardial infection. *Circulation* **51**, 350–357.

17. Dionigi R., Dominioni L. and Campani M. (1980) Infections in cancer patients. *Surg. Clin. North Am.* **60**, 145–159.

18. Engelman R. M., Chase R. M., Boyd A. D. et al. (1973) Lethal post operative infections following cardiac surgery. *Circulation* **48**, 31–36.

19. Evans D. B. (1981) Invasive fungal infections in transplant patients. *Hospital Update* **7**, 701–708.

20. French G. L., Casewell N. W., Roncoroni A. J. et al. (1980) A hospital outbreak of antibiotic-resistant *Acinetobacter anitratus*: epidemiology and control. *J. Hosp. Infect.* **I**, 125–131.

21. George G., Matamis D., Sabatier C. et al. (1980) Randomised assay of an immunostimulant (Isoprinosine) in anergic patients. *Intens. Care Med.* **6**, 52.

22. Hammerschmidt D. E., Weaver L. J., Hudson L. D. et al. (1980) Association of complement activation and elevated plasma-C5a with adult respiratory distress syndrome. *Lancet* **1**, 947–949.

23. Hardaway R. M. (1966) *Syndromes of Disseminated Intravascular Coagulation.* Springfield, Illinois, Thomas.

24. Heimbach R. D., Boerema I., Brummelkamp W. H. et al. In: Davis J. C. and Hunt T. K., ed., *Current Therapy of Gas Gangrene, in Hyperbaric Oxygen Therapy*, pp. 153–176. Bethesda, Undersea Medical Society.

25. Humble W., Eykyn Susannah and Phillips I. (1980) Staphylococcal bacteraemia, fusidic acid and jaundice. *Br. Med. J.* **1**, 1495–1498.

26. Imrie C. W., Benjamin I. S., Ferguson J. C. et al. (1978) A single centre double blind trial of trasylol therapy in primary acute pancreatitis. *Br. J. Surg.* **65**, 337–341.

27. Iwanaga S., Morita T., Harada T. et al. (1978) Chromogenic substrates for horseshoe crab clotting enzyme—its application for the assay of bacterial endotoxins. *Haemostatis* **7**, 183–188.

28. Jacob H. S., Craddock P. R., Hammerschmidt D. E. et al. (1980) Complement-induced granulocyte aggregation: an unexpected mechanism of disease. *N. Engl. J. Med.* **302**, 789–794.

29. Johnson W. C., Ulrich F., Medguid M. M. et al. (1979) Role of delayed hypersensitivity in predicting post-operative morbidity and mortality. *Am. J. Surg.* **137**, 536–542.

30. Jones R. J., Rue E. A. and Gupta J. L. (1979) Controlled trials of a polyvalent pseudomonas vaccine in burns. *Lancet* **2**, 977–982.

31. Kagan R. L., Schuette W. H., Zierdt C. M. et al. (1977) Rapid automated diagnosis of bacteremia by impedence detection. *J. Clin. Microbiol.* **5**, 51–57.

32. Kasnitz P., Druger G., Yorra F. et al. (1976) Mixed venous oxygen tension and hyperlactatemia. Survival in severe cardiopulmonary disease. *J. Am. Med. Assoc.* **236**, 570–574.

33. Kerr J. A. (1979) Current topics in tetanus. *Intens. Care Med.* **5**, 105–110.

34. Kung T., LeBlanc O. and Moss G. (1976) Percutaneous microsensing of muscle pH during shock and resuscitation. *J. Surg. Res.* **21**, 285–289.

35. Larson E. H. (1979) Pseudomembranous colitis is an infection. *J. Infect.* **1**, 221–226.

36. Leading Article (1978) Vasodilators in heart failure. *Lancet* **1**, 972–973.

37. Leading Article (1979) Legionnaires' disease. *Br. Med. J.* **2**, 81.

38. Ledingham I. McA. and McArdle C. S. (1978) Prospective study in the treatment of septic shock. *Lancet* **1**, 1194–1197.

39. Ledingham I. McA. and Tehrani M. A. (1975) Diagnosis, clinical course and treatment of acute dermal gangrene. *Br. J. Surg.* **62**, 364–372.

40. Lefer A. M., Glen T. M., Lopez-Rasi A. M. et al. (1971) Mechanism of the lack of a beneficial response to inotropic drugs in hemorrhagic shock. *Clin. Pharmacol. Ther.* **12**, 506–516.

41. Lillehei R. C., Motsay G. J. and Dietzman R. H. (1972) The use of corticosteroids in the treatment of shock. *Int. J. Clin. Pharmacol. Ther. Toxicol.* **5**, 423–433.

42. Lucas C. E., Rector F. E., Werner M. et al. (1973) Altered renal homeostasis with acute sepsis. Clinical significance. *Arch. Surg.* **106**, 444–449.

43. Meakins J. L., Wicklund B., Forse R. A. et al. (1980) The surgical intensive care unit: current concepts in infection. *Surg. Clin. North Am.* **60**, 117–132.

44. Meakins J. L., Christou N. V., Shizgal H. M. et al. (1979) Therapeutic approaches to anergy in surgical patients. *Ann. Surg.* **190**, 286–296.

45. Meleney F. L. (1924) Hemolytic streptococcus gangrene. *Arch. Surg.* **9**, 317.

46. Meleney F. L. (1933) Differential diagnosis between certain types of infectious gangrene of the skin. *Surg. Gynecol. Obstet.* **56**, 847.

47. Miller R. M., Polakavetz S. H., Hornick R. B. et al. (1973) Analysis of infections acquired by the severely injured patient. *Surg. Gynecol. Obstet.* **137**, 7–10.

48. Milligan G. F., MacDonald J. A. E., Mellon A. et al. (1974) Pulmonary and hematological disturbances in septic shock. *Surg. Gynecol. Obstet.* **138**, 43–49.

49. Munster A. W., Winchurch R. A., Birmingham W. J. et al. (1980) Longitudinal assay of lymphocyte responsiveness in patients with major burns. *Surgery* **192**, 772–775.

50. Myerowitz P. D., Caswell Karen, Lindsay W. G. et al. (1977) Antibiotic prophylaxis for open heart surgery. *J. Thorac. Cardiovasc. Surg.* **73**, 625–629.

51. McCafferty E. L. and Lyons C. (1948) Suppurative fasciitis as the essential feature of haemolytic streptococcus gangrene with notes of fasciotomy and early wound closure as treatment of choice. *Surgery* **24**, 438–442.

52. MacLean L. D., Meakins J. L., Taguchi K. et al. (1975) Host resistance in sepsis and trauma. *Ann. Surg.* **182**, 207–217.

53. MacMillan B. G. (1981) The control of burn wound sepsis. *Intens. Care Med.* **7**, 63–69.

54. Nakamura A., Morita S., Iwanaga M. et al. (1977) A sensitive substrate for the clotting enzyme in horseshoe crab hemocytes. *J. Biochem. (Tokyo)* **81**, 1567–1569.

55. Nichols W. W., Nichols M. A. and Barbour H. (1978) Hemodynamic monitoring with thermodilution flow-directed catheters. *J. Cardiovasc. Pulmon. Technol.* **6**, 13–20.

56. Norton L., Eule J. and Burdick D. (1978) Accuracy of techniques to detect intra-peritoneal abscess. *Surgery* **84**, 370–378.

57. Norton L., Moore G. and Eiseman B. (1975) Liver failure in the postoperative patient: the role of sepsis and immunologic deficiency. *Surgery* **78**, 6–13.

58. Oppenheimer L., Hryniuk W. M. and Bishop A. J. (1976) Thrombocytopenia in severe bacterial infections. *J. Surg. Res.* **20**, 211–214.

59. Parratt J. R., Coker Susan J., Hughes Bernadette et al. (1981) In: McConn Rita, ed., *The Possible Role of Prostaglandins and Thromboxanes in the Pulmonary Consequences of Experimental Endotoxin Shock and Clinical Sepsis*. New York, Raven Press. (In Press.)

60. Peretz D. E., Scott H. M., Duff J. et al. (1965) The significance of lactacidemia in the shock syndrome. *Ann. N.Y. Acad. Sci.* **119**, 1133–1141.

61. Perret C. and Enrico J. F. (1978) In: Bossart A. and Perret C., ed., *Lactate in Acute Circulatory Failure in Lactate in Acute Conditions*, pp. 69–82. Basel, S. Karger.
62. Phillips K. D., Tearle P. U. and Willis A. T. (1976) Rapid diagnosis of anaerobic infection by gas liquid chromatography of clinical material. *J. Clin. Pathol.* **29**, 428–432.
63. Ranson J. H. C., Rifkind K. M. and Turner J. W. (1976) Prognostic signs and non-operative lavage in acute pancreatitis. *Surg. Gynecol. Obstet.* **143**, 209–215.
64. Rea W. J. and Wyrick W. J. (1970) Necrotizing fasciitis. *Ann. Surg.* **172**, 957–964.
65. Royle G. T. and Kettlewell M. G. W. (1980) Liver function tests in surgical infection and malnutrition. *Ann. Surg.* **192**, 192–194.
66. Sanford J. P. (1979) Legionnaires' disease—the first thousand days. *N. Engl. J. Med.* **300**, 654–656.
67. Schimpff S. C., Miller R. M., Polakavetz S. H. et al. (1974) Infection in the severely traumatized patient. *Ann. Surg.* **179**, 352–357.
68. Schimpff S. C., Young V. and Greene W. (1972) Origin of infection in acute nonlymphocytic leukemia—significance of hospital acquisition of potential pathogens. *Ann. Inter. Med.* **77**, 707–714.
69. Schumer W. (1976) Steroids in the treatment of clinical septic shock. *Ann. Surg.* **184**, 333–341.
70. Scovill W. A., Saba T. M., Blumenstock F. A. et al. (1978) Opsonic α_2 surface binding glycoprotein therapy during sepsis. *Ann. Surg.* **188**, 521–529.
71. Shield M. J., Hammill H. J. and Neale D. A. (1979) Systematic bacteriological monitoring of intensive care unit patients: the results of a twelve month study. *Intens. Care Med.* **5**, 171–181.
72. Shoemaker W. C. (1976) Comparison of the relative effectiveness of whole blood transfusions and various types of fluid therapy in resuscitation. *Crit. Care Med.* **4**, 71–78.
73. Siegel S. E. and Nachum R. (1977) Use of the limulus lysate assay (LAL) for the detection and quantitation of endotoxin. In: Bernheimer A. W., ed., *Prospective in Toxicology*, pp. 61–86. New York, Wiley Medical.
74. Swan H. J. C., Ganz W., Forrester J. et al. (1970) Cardiac catheterisation with a flow-directed balloon-tipped catheter. *N. Engl. J. Med.* **283**, 447–451.
75. Tehrani M. A. and Ledingham I. McA. (1977) Necrotizing fasciitis. *Postgrad. Med. J.* **53**, 237–242.
76. Tehrani M. A., Webster M. H. C., Robinson D. W. et al. (1976) Necrotising fasciitis treated by radical excision of the overlying skin. *Br. J. Plast. Surg.* **29**, 74–77.
77. Thompson W. L. (1977) Dopamine in the management of shock. *Proc. R. Soc. Med.* **70**, 25–33.
78. Trumper K. K., Mentelos R. A. and Shoemaker W. C. (1980) Effect of hypercarbia and shock on transcutaneous carbon dioxide at different electrode temperatures. *Crit. Care Med.* **8**, 608–612.
79. Utili R., Abernethy C. O. and Zimmerman M. J. (1977) Studies on the effects of *E. coli* endotoxin and canalicular bile formation in the isolated perfused rat liver. *J. Lab. Clin. Med.* **89**, 471–482.
80. Wallis C., Melnick J. L., Wende D. et al. (1980) Rapid isolation of bacteria from septicemic patients by use of an antimicrobial agent removal device. *J. Clin. Microbiol.* **11**, 462–464.
81. Wardle N. (1979) Shock: bacteraemic and endotoxic shock. *Br. J. Hosp. Med.* **1**, 223–231.
82. Washington J. A. (1975) Blood culture: principles and techniques. *Mayo Clin. Proc.* **50**, 91–98.
83. Weil M. H. and Afifi A. A. (1970) Experimental and clinical studies on lactate and pyruvate as indicators of the severity of acute circulatory failure. *Circulation* **41**, 989–1001.

84. Wiles J. B., Cerra F. B., Siegel J. H. et al. (1980) The systemic septic response: does the organism matter? *Crit. Care Med.* **8**, 55–60.

85. Wilkinson P. C. (1977) Neutrophil leucocyte function tests. In: Thompson R. A., ed., *Techniques in Clinical Immunology*, pp. 201–218. Oxford, Blackwell Scientific Publications.

86. Wilson B. (1952) Necrotizing fasciitis. *Am. Surg.* **18**, 416.

87. Wilson H. D. and Haltalin K. (1973) Acute necrotizing fasciitis in childhood. *Am. J. Dis. Child.* **125**, 591–595.

88. Wilson R. F. and Gibson B. S. (1978) The use of arterial-central venous oxygen differences to calculate cardiac output and oxygen consumption in critically ill surgical patients. *Surgery* **84**, 362–369.

89. Young L. S., Martin W. J., Meyer R. D. et al. (1977) Gram-negative rod bacteremia: microbiologic, immunologic and therapeutic considerations. *Ann. Int. Med.* **86**, 456–471.

Chapter 10

Blood Transfusion and Haematology

D. Hopkins

Blood is a complex mixture of diffuse tissues some of which share common stem cells and each of which lies partly within and partly without the cardiovascular system. The intravascular component of each tissue consists of many individual units of short life span and of varying ages. The intravascular size of each tissue can vary within wide limits, the more so when the rate of change is slow and the individual is otherwise fit. An excess of one tissue may compensate in part for a deficiency in another, while pathological overproduction of one may deny space or precursor cells to another. All can be grafted, although stem cell graft is often impractical and is not within the remit of an intensive care unit.

Blood is both a transport and control system and a part of the store of defence mechanisms. It contains part of a complex leak plugging system because the pressure and flow rates, which are essential for efficient function, depend largely upon the blood volume being maintained.

COMMON SYNDROMES AND BASIC MANAGEMENT

The circulating level of each fraction of blood is the result of a balance between production and destruction. Functional failure results from any unacceptable imbalance which causes a low blood level of the fraction, be it the result of excessive loss or of deficient or pathological production. Syndromes include acute and chronic blood volume loss, red cell and plasma fraction shortfall, coagulation deficiencies. In each case the management objectives are to identify the fraction and the approximate severity of the shortfall, to stop further loss, and to make good the functional deficiency.

Until the mid 1960s, the replacement substance of choice following

238

blood volume and red cell loss was 'whole blood' consisting of 400–420 ml of blood collected into a glass bottle which contained 120 ml of acid citrate dextrose anticoagulant solution. The shelf life was 21 days at 4 °C. Sometimes red cell concentrates were prepared to correct anaemia, and the plasma so obtained together with that from time-expired blood was freeze-dried. Such dried plasma was used in the management of acute plasma loss, particularly in burnt patients, and as an initial volume expander.

Three developments have had a profound effect on basic management:

For many years there had been increasing concern about the frequency with which serum hepatitis was transmitted by pooled freeze-dried plasma. It was found that plasma protein fraction, alias plasma protein solution (PPS), which was mainly albumin, could be heated to 60 °C for 10 hours without significant protein aggregation, which treatment was believed to eliminate hepatitis risk. Unfortunately a given volume of plasma yields considerably less PPS then freeze-dried plasma; at least 450 ml of plasma is required to produce 250 ml of PPS.[1]

Secondly, a steadily increasing requirement for Factor VIII products, platelets, and other coagulation factors led to plasma separation from increasing quantities of blood before it was transfused.

Thirdly, it was shown that injured hypovolaemic adults could be rendered normotensive quickly and safely by immediate infusion of large volumes of crystalloid solution.[2-5]

The coincidence of increased plasma requirement and a swing to initial crystalloid resuscitation led to increased separation of fresh donor blood into plasma for processing, and red cell concentrates. Thus red cell concentrates became much more readily available, whole blood less so, and production logistics made it impractical to replace all the plasma removed from the red cells with plasma protein solution. Subsequent developments which have increased demands for plasma and PPS still further include cell separators used for plasma exchange, and increasingly successful treatment of patients with massive protein loss.

The debate about the extent to which colloid and crystalloid solutions should be used for blood volume replacement continues.

Crystalloid protagonists emphasize experimental work in which a very high proportion of the blood volume has been replaced by electrolyte solution and work indicating that, after haemorrhagic shock, there is increased pulmonary vascular permeability to plasma proteins anyway.[6-8] It is argued that electrolyte solutions are just as effective as colloid in restoring circulation and do not promote pulmonary oedema.[8] Other reports indicated that colloid resuscitation might be associated with an increased risk of pulmonary oedema and an elevated pulmonary capillary wedge pressure,[9,10] while albumin therapy could be associated with impaired coagulation and an increased blood transfusion requirement,[11] although admittedly patients in the last study received in the order of 600 g of albumin over 4 or 5 days (one 400-ml bottle of PPS contains 16–20 g of protein).

Vietnam war experiences during the late 1960s and the early 1970s showed that it was entirely practical to resuscitate hypovolaemic battle and accident casualties with electrolyte solution.[2-5] However, conditions were not typical of civilian hospital practice. Most patients studied were previously healthy young male adults injured by blast or gunfire and who reached hospital very quickly indeed. Intravenous crystalloid was given en route if need be.[2,3] It was found that many litres of solution could be given through two to four large-bore intravenous cannulae with only a transient fall in total serum protein levels and a weight gain of 3–4 g over a few days.[2]

While crystalloid solutions and whole blood were readily available, colloid solutions were not, and tended to be limited to 25% albumin.[4] Whole blood was given after a quick and partial cross-match. Case records might state only the major blood substitute and the total quantity of all substitutes transfused, and seriously burnt patients were rapidly evacuated out of the country.[4]

It was apparent that while blood volume and pressure could be maintained by crystalloid infusion if enough were given and, indeed, haemodilution sponsored better tissue perfusion by decreasing blood viscosity,[12] the position of middle-aged and elderly patients who are more typical of civilian hospitals differed. After crystalloid resuscitation, the total body albumin mass redistributes partially to restore plasma albumin levels and, once the patient's oncotic gradient is more or less restored, copious diuresis follows. Such 'drying out' of a patient without restoring some colloid can produce hypovolaemia and even frank shock.[7,13]

Prospective and retrospective trials studied the advantages and disadvantages of crystalloid against colloid.[3,9,10,12,14-16] Results, like conditions, varied. Against the puzzle of why albumin therapy appeared to associate with an increased risk of pulmonary distress and pulmonary oedema[10] and appreciation that in any case there is only a small difference in albumin concentration between plasma and pulmonary interstitium,[16] crystalloid alone was shown to have hazards[13] and some elderly patients did not tolerate even transient hypoalbuminaemia.[13]

Other background factors are that human albumin resources are limited, yet may be overused on an emotional basis and in an unscientific way.[10] A recent paper[17] reports albumin for infusion as making up 10% of a hospital's total drug bill with 91% given to surgical patients for which the decision to give albumin was judged correct in only 29% of cases.

Red cell deficiency on its own can be the result of production failure, or of plasma expansion after haemorrhage. A healthy adult can tolerate an acute loss of over half his red cell mass if his blood volume is maintained, and a greater loss if this is spread over several weeks or months. But an individual who is already red-cell deficient has lost much of his reserve, and will decompensate the sooner if there is further haemorrhage. One of the aims of intensive care management is, therefore, to keep the patient's reserve intact.

Plasma deficiency on its own arises from plasma loss, for example after burns or severe and prolonged infection or certain renal and hepatic malfunctions. There are two further subtle iatrogenic forms: a patient whose blood loss has been replaced fully and entirely by red cell concentrates, and a patient whose fluid intake has been unwittingly curtailed. An example of the latter is the elderly lady who lies still in bed for several days after her femoral neck has been pinned, drinks little, and whose case notes accumulate reports of a steadily rising haemoglobin level.

White cell deficiency results from production failure; haematological disorders including leukaemias where there may be overproduction of non-functioning pathological cells, drug suppression, and severe infection which has depressed marrow function. Management is both symptomatic and preventive and includes all attempts to prevent further infection. Occasionally some white cell replacement may be possible.

Coagulation deficiency can arise from many different causes and may indicate multiple factor deficiency.

Some individuals have a congenital deficiency of one or more coagulation factors. Haemophiliacs have low or absent Factor VIII levels, patients with Christmas disease have low Factor IX levels, and there are several other rarer syndromes. If a congenital deficiency is sufficiently severe to cause a functional coagulation defect, the intensive care patient requires specialized haematological supervision, preferably from the appropriate unit with adequate system replacement. Factor VIII is replaced as cryoprecipitate or as Factor VIII concentrate, Factor IX by fresh frozen plasma or Factor IX concentrate. The dose varies greatly from one patient to another and the best guide will be given by the unit at which the individual patient is known.

Several factors, prothrombin, VII, IX, X, are produced in the liver and production requires vitamin K. Production is blocked by coumarin-type drugs and may be severely retarded in hepatic insufficiency.

A patient who has impaired liver function, or who is taking coumarin drugs, may acquire a coagulation defect involving both the intrinsic and extrinsic coagulation systems. The defect must be identified and monitored while replacement therapy is given.

Intravascular fibrin formation from fibrinogen and lysis of the fibrin so formed, is the basis of the group of syndromes termed disseminated intravascular coagulation (DIC), defibrination syndrome or consumption coagulopathy. Fibrinogen levels fall, sometimes to zero, and there may be steady or uncontrolled haemorrhage. This is well known as a complication of childbirth but is also caused by haemolytic transfusion reactions resulting from incompatible blood transfusion, Gram-negative septicaemia, and some snake bites. It can also occur during or after cardiopulmonary bypass and in some other surgical conditions and in association with neoplasia. Untreated, the mortality is high. The difficult management objective is to restore equilibrium without making matters worse.

Platelet deficiency can arise from a wash-out effect of blood transfusion, in certain haematological disorders, and when drugs or irradiation depress bone marrow function. In the absence of injury, spontaneous haemorrhage is not expected until the platelet level is well below 20 000 per mm^3 and is usually preceded by the appearance of petechiae. Post-surgical patients require considerably higher platelet levels for initial wound healing. Management is by platelet transfusion.

MEASUREMENTS AND MONITORING

The *total blood volume* cannot be measured quickly or easily. The first estimate was by Bischoff[18] with condemned criminals. More modern and less Draconian methods require separate assessment of red cell and plasma masses using isotopes measured over several hours, with calculations to compensate for differential plasma and red cell pooling. In the average adult, blood makes up 7–8% of the total body weight, around 75 ml/kg in males, 67 ml/kg in females. An approximate, but practical, guide is one transfusion unit (approximately half a litre) for each 7 kg (or 1 stone) of body weight.

The *haematocrit* (or red cell : total blood volume ratio) and haemoglobin level are measured quickly and easily in the laboratory from a citrated venous blood sample or from an immediately diluted capillary blood sample. The venous haematocrit varies above and below 43% in normal adults while the whole body haematocrit can be up to 10% lower. The subject and its variation can be studied in any standard haematological textbook.

Haemoglobin is an oxygen-carrying substance contained within red cells which normally have a 120-day life following on a 6–7 day manufacturing time from stem cells in the marrow. Its level is measured as g haemoglobin in 1 dl (100 ml) of blood. Haemoglobin levels vary widely from one individual to another and there is no such thing as a single normal level. Useful approximate ranges for healthy adults at sea level are 13·5–17 g/dl for males, 12–15·5 g/dl for females. The precise value for any individual depends upon such variables as posture, time of day, the degree of venous stasis before collection, and such laboratory factors as dilution accuracy and calibration. Differences in successive haemoglobin estimations of less than 1 g/dl should be regarded with caution.

Otherwise healthy individuals can tolerate substantial red cell loss if this takes place over weeks or months. Patients with megaloblastic anaemia may be ambulatory with haemoglobin levels under 2 g/dl. On the other hand, an individual who is polycythaemic because of chronic respiratory damage may be seriously embarrassed if his haemoglobin level falls to 'normal adult' levels.

Within these limits, haemoglobin levels should be measured initially and, thereafter, as frequently as every 1–2 days if substantial rapid change is taking place.

Plasma consists of water, various plasma proteins, crystalloids, and a variety of substances in low concentration for which plasma is the transport medium.

Plasma proteins are classified as albumins, globulins, fibrinogen and others together totalling 60–80 g/l of which normally 35–55 g is albumin, 15–30 g globulins and 3 g fibrinogen. The common laboratory measurement is total plasma protein, with albumin and globulin levels. For many purposes the concentration of each main class of globulin, IgC, IgM, IgA, is measured. Fibrinogen levels are measured separately if deficiency or fibrinolysis is suspected as part of a coagulation defect.

The differential between intracapillary and tissue pressure is in the order of 25–40 mmHg and the conventional 'Starling' concept is that plasma proteins prevent excess fluid loss across this differential by increasing the capillary osmotic pressure. However, albumin and, to a lesser extent, globulins circulate out of the vascular system through lymphatics and back into the vascular system at a rate estimated in normal subjects[19] as 5% of the plasma albumin mass per hour, 1–3% of the various globulin fractions per hour. The rate of transcapillary protein escape depends upon local capillary leakiness. Hypoproteinaemia is not necessarily associated with oedema, especially in individuals who have congenitally very low levels of one protein fraction.[14] Since plasma proteins are but part of a protein pool which redistributes after blood loss, frequent measurements are only necessary if there is continuing severe protein loss and replacement therapy which requires close monitoring.

Platelets are measured as the number in 1 mm^3 of blood counted in a laboratory electronic counter. Venous blood for platelet counts is collected into an appropriate anticoagulant, usually EDTA. Normal platelet levels are in the range 250 000–400 000 per mm^3 but, as indicated later in the absence of surgery, bleeding is not expected until platelet levels are well under 20 000 per mm^3. Platelet levels should be measured whenever a significant platelet deficiency is suspected.

Coagulation factor measurement and monitoring is a specialized haematology laboratory process and each individual hospital laboratory will indicate which tests it is programmed to carry out on what basis together with blood sample details.

If bleeding is suspected to be due to a coagulation factor defect four tests usually are readily available and produce useful results within a reasonable time: platelet count, prothrombin time, partial thromboplastin time and tests for evidence of disseminated intravascular coagulation. The second and third measure test and control reaction times under preset laboratory conditions; a prolonged prothrombin time suggesting an extrinsic pathway deficiency, and a prolonged partial thromboplastin time suggesting an intrinsic pathway defect. Where Factor VIII or IX deficiency is proven, factor assays may be required to monitor therapy, particularly when an individual patient's response to therapy is not well known. Tests for disseminated intravascular coagulation are carried out whenever the condition is suspected; the tests detect circulating products of fibrinolysis and measure plasma fibrinogen levels which in this condition can fall near to zero.

There are several dozen independent human red cell *blood group* systems each indicating differences at a molecular level in the red cell envelope. The practical importance of any blood group system to an individual patient depends upon whether or not his plasma contains an antibody to one or more components of that system, and whether or not the plasma of a transfused unit of blood contains such an antibody. If there are no antibodies either way, that blood group system can be ignored so far as immediate therapy is concerned although long-term effects must be considered.

The ABO blood group system is the most important both because almost all patients and donations of blood have naturally occurring ABO blood group antibodies, and because ABO-incompatible therapy can be lethal. The very complex rhesus blood group system is next in importance because a high proportion of individuals who lack certain rhesus antigens, particularly Rh(D), form antibody readily on antigen exposure.

For most remaining blood group systems, antigens are less immunogenic and naturally-occurring antibodies rare. Therefore, to allow red cell replacement to remain a practical proposition, each of the many other blood group systems is disregarded unless the patient or potential blood donor has a blood group antibody within one of the systems. In addition, for most purposes the rhesus system is simplified into Rh(D)-negative and Rh(D)-positive for patients, 'rhesus negative' (CDE-negative) and 'rhesus positive' (everything else) for donations of blood. This gives the eight transfusion blood groups in descending frequency $0+$, $A+$, $B+$, $0-$, $A-$, $AB+$, $B-$ and $AB-$. One practical point which should be remembered is that, because of the particular way in which the rhesus blood group system is simplified and the slightly different criteria for patients and for donations of blood, approximately 2% of a Caucasian population are 'rhesus negative' as patients, but 'rhesus positive' if they are blood donors.

For blood group determination, an accurately identified blood sample is sent to the hospital's transfusion laboratory. The exact form and size of the sample will vary from one hospital to another and, in particular, upon whether manual or automated techniques are used. The laboratory will determine the ABO and rhesus (D) status of the sample and will screen for non-ABO blood group antibodies, using a selected mixture of type O blood.

If red cell or whole blood replacement is required, the transfusion laboratory cross-matches units of donor blood against the patient's serum using a variety of techniques. If the donor units appear to be compatible they are tagged with the patient's identification and reserved for a period, usually 1 or 2 days. It must be remembered that blood transfusion is inherently dangerous, and that human blood and blood products are limited human resources which, if squandered on one patient, are not available for another.

Elapsed time is important. A full blood group determination with antibody-screen requires at least $1\frac{1}{2}$–2 hours from the time the patient's blood sample reached the laboratory bench. Donor blood cannot be selected for cross-match until the patient's blood group is known, and blood may have to come from many miles away. A complete cross-match requires a further $1\frac{1}{2}$–2 hours by current routine techniques. In practice, a considerable further time can elapse while the hospital messenger system transits the patient's blood sample, and a very busy routine laboratory which has to operate a batch system may require longer.

To circumvent part of the elapsed time, any patient who may require transfusion at a later stage must be blood grouped and screened for antibodies on admission. A patient who has a difficult antibody or a rare blood group can be identified, and the laboratory will hold each patient's serum for up to a week cutting out transit time when blood is required.

In a clinical emergency times can be shortened and tests overlapped. This increases the risk of an incompatible transfusion and is only justified if the risk of waiting is even greater.

Protein, white cell and platelet antibodies exist and are rare causes of transfusion reactions. The laboratory techniques for identification are specialized and are not routine screening procedures.

PATHOPHYSIOLOGICAL MECHANISMS

Blood loss involves both red cells and plasma. Initially whole blood or red cell loss is compensated by a shift of fluid and albumin into the intra-vascular space and, if the loss is acute, by peripheral vasoconstriction and an increased circulatory rate. Substantial or continuing loss evokes increased plasma protein, platelet and red cell production; the latter can increase five- to ten-fold if need be and, after severe haemorrhage, immature red cells may appear in the peripheral blood.

The extent to which physiological compensation for red cell loss or blood loss is possible varies enormously from one individual to another. Each day, many thousands of adults each lose 10–13% of their blood volume within 3–5 minutes without ill effect. They are called blood donors. Chronic red cell loss in which blood volume is maintained can be surprisingly well tolerated: one 70-year-old man who had lost an estimated

10–15 l of blood over 3–6 months from a chronic gastric ulcer and whose haemoglobin level was found to be less than 4 g/dl, had as his only symptom some tiredness after walking his dog half a mile instead of his customary 3 miles.

Each individual has his limit beyond which further physiological compensation fails. The limit of tolerated acute haemorrhage can be reached very rapidly if there is a pre-existing defect, such as severe anaemia or myocardial damage.

In contrast to red cell and blood volume loss where the immediate compensatory mechanism includes plasma volume expansion to restore the total blood volume, plasma loss is less well tolerated and the compensation limit is reached sooner.

Platelet deficiency can arise from the wash-out effect of fluid or blood replacement after haemorrhage, especially if surgery or injury leaves a raw area which increases platelet utilization. There is a compensatory increase in platelet production, but this requires several days to be effective. There are many haematological conditions which result in increased platelet consumption, defective platelet production, or decreased platelet production in any of which supportive platelet transfusion may be required.

Blood coagulation is a multistage process the end step of which is fibrin formation from fibrinogen in dynamic equilibrium with fibrinolysis. Adequate platelet function is required to form an effective contractile fibrin network and to plug capillary leaks.

Fibrinogen conversion to fibrin requires thrombin, ionized calcium and other factors. Thrombin can be formed from prothrombin in two ways, by an intrinsic or intravascular cascade process which requires Factors VIII, IX and others, and by a shorter extrinsic or extravascular cascade process triggered when thromboplastins released by injured tissue react with plasma Factor VII. The latter stages of both processes require Factors V and X. A severe deficiency of any factor, whether congenital or acquired, can disrupt either or both of the extrinsic and intrinsic coagulation processes.

Any infection or severe injury will normally evoke increased white cell production, mainly neutrophils. Overwhelming infection or marrow failure from any other cause can result in severe neutrophil deficiency. White cell replacement is at present not generally practical and, in this sense, unless the patient has an underlying haematological disorder white cell monitoring of an acutely ill patient is often only academic.

THERAPY INCLUDING SYSTEM REPLACEMENT

Treatment of whole blood or plasma loss has as basic objectives to stop further loss, to restore and maintain adequate organ perfusion, and to maintain sufficient oxygen transport ability in the circulating fluid.

Venous blood samples should be taken immediately for haemoglobin estimation, blood grouping and antibody screen. The haemoglobin result indicates whether or not there was pre-existing anaemia, and provides a baseline. The grouping sample allow immediate blood grouping and antibody screen against a possible future transfusion requirement, and invaluable advance warning if the patient has a 'difficult antibody' or is of a rare blood type. Further, if within a few hours or days transfusion becomes necessary, the laboratory will already have a sample of the patient's serum with which to cross-match and which is free from volume expanders which may cause cross-matching difficulties.

Blood group information from case notes of an earlier admission or in the patient's pocket has to be read with a little caution. Blood group information can be inserted in the wrong case notes or typed incorrectly on a summary sheet, a patient may form an antibody even during a single admission and, as indicated above, a person's blood group may differ with the situation.

There has been much recent debate over which substance to use for initial blood volume restoration: electrolyte solution or colloid. The range of substances which is available is wide but each has disadvantages as well as advantages. In alphabetical order:

Crystalloid. These comprise electrolyte solutions, such as intravenous saline and intravenous Ringer lactate. No preparatory tests are required other than to check that the solution is clear and has not passed its expiry date.

Dextrans are long chain glucose molecules with molecular weights in the 20 000–200 000 plus range. Clinical dextran preparations make acceptable plasma substitutes in many circumstances.[20] There are disadvantages: dextrans with molecular weights below 70 000 pass rapidly into the extravascular space and are excreted, while as the molecular weight rises there is increasing sludging in vivo and rouleaux formation in vitro. Rouleaux formation causes great difficulty when cross-matching blood. Common clinical preparations are 'Macrodex' (average molecular weight 70 000, although the range is considerable) as a 6% solution in either saline or glucose, and 'Rheomacrodex' (average molecular weight 40 000), a 10% solution in either saline or glucose. The immediate colloid effect of dextran depends upon the molecular concentration and the 10% solution is hyperosmolar, but this effect of low-molecular-weight dextrans is very short lived.[20]

Dried plasma is supplied in capped glass bottles, each containing the freeze-dried residue from 400 ml of pooled human plasma. Dried, its shelf life is 4 years at room temperature. It is reconstituted by adding the 400 ml of pyrogen-free, sterile distilled water which is supplied in another bottle with a shelf life of 1–2 years. The reconstituted material contains 5·5–6% of protein, and must be used immediately. Although dried plasma is prepared from a pool of plasma of mixed ABO groups it may still contain anti-A and anti-B and large quantities may cause some haemolysis of the recipient's red cells, particularly if the recipient is group AB. In some areas, dried plasma may not be widely available.

Fresh frozen plasma is plasma removed from one or two donations of blood within a few hours of collection and supplied in 50 ml, 200 ml or 400 ml packs. Fresh frozen plasma is issued mainly to supply coagulation factors but can be used to supplement other volume expanders. Thawing is more rapid in a water bath at 37 °C; this temperature must not be exceeded and the bag should be dried, particularly around the covers of the entry ports, before use.

Plasma protein fraction or plasma protein solution (PPS) is manufactured from bulk human plasma. The manufacturing process is balanced between a high yield of an impure product and a very low yield of a pure product, and a typical balance may yield only 40–50% of the starting volume of plasma as PPS. It is supplied in 250 or 400 ml volumes as a 4·3–5% solution of material of which 92–97% is albumin, the remainder mainly globulin. Particularly if the starting material was plasma from time-expired blood, there may be traces of haemoglobin. The shelf life is 4 years at room temperature, sodium content 130–150 mmol/l, potassium content usually less than 2 mmol/l. Some batches contain serotonins which should be inactivated on passage through the lungs.

Red cell concentrate is a donation of blood from which between 150 and 250 ml of the plasma/anticoagulant mixture has been withdrawn. Units from which less than 150 ml of plasma has been withdrawn may be given a name such as 'partly deplasmatized blood'.

Whole blood, despite its name, is diluted blood; 400–450 ml of venous blood is removed from a donor into a prepared plastic pack containing 63–70 ml of acid citrate dextrose (ACD) or citrate phosphate dextrose (CPD) anticoagulant solution and stored at 4 ± 2 °C. The exact quantity of anticoagulant varies a little with the manufacturer of the collecting pack, but a typical quantity is 1·65 g of sodium citrate, 0·206 g of citric acid, 0·158 g of sodium acid phosphate, together with 1·46 g of dextrose as an aid to red cell survival. With correct storage the shelf life of CPD blood is 28 days. All tested units have had the red cells and serum ABO grouped, the red cells Rh(D) typed with additional Rh(C) and (E) typing of D-negative units, have been screened for other blood group antibodies using a mixture of cells containing all common and some rare red cell antigens, and have shown negative tests for syphilis and hepatitis-B antigen.

Full testing of donor blood requires most of the day after collection, and it is unwise to assume that blood from a registered donor can be transfused safely before tests have been completed. Such an assumption is akin to overtaking in a car on a blind corner.

Other substances prepared from whole blood include:

Frozen red cells. Red cells from a donation of blood that has been frozen in liquid nitrogen will keep for several years. Frozen blood must be thawed, washed and resuspended before transfusion. This process takes several hours, and so frozen cells are not generally a first choice. It may, however, be the quickest or only available means of obtaining blood for a patient who requires blood of a rare type.

Cryoprecipitate is prepared by freezing fresh plasma and subsequently thawing at just above its freezing point. Cryoprecipitate contains most of the Factor VIII of the plasma and appreciable quantities of fibrinogen. It is supplied in approximately 25 ml units from single donations of blood.

Factor concentrates, Factor VIII concentrate, Factor IX concentrate (which also contains Factors II and X) and Factor II-VII-IX-X concentrate are supplied for specific treatment of coagulation factor deficiency. The material is freeze dried, stored at 4 °C, and resuspended with sterile, pyrogen-free water before intravenous injection.

Various *immunoglobulins* are supplied for specific therapy, almost always by intramuscular injection except in dire emergency.

Platelet concentrates are prepared as platelets from single units of blood contained in 25–50 ml of plasma. The maximum shelf life of the product is 72 hours when stored at 20 °C with continuous agitation, which can cause logistic problems. Platelets should be obtained from donations of blood which are ABO-compatible with the patient, either from donors of the same ABO group or from group O donors. One unit of platelets is expected to raise the platelet level of a thrombocytopoenic patient by 10 000 per mm^3 and, for an adult, several units will be required. Normally five or six units are pooled into a single administration bag. Recent surgery or raw areas of tissue are among the indications for a higher initial dose.

A pragmatic approach to the initial therapy of blood volume deficiency is to restore blood volume as rapidly as is practical with a mixture of crystalloid solution, colloid, red cell concentrates and whole blood. Initial therapy is aimed at restoring and maintaining peripheral tissue perfusion and a central venous pressure of at least 6 cm water. A useful guide is a urine output of more than 30 ml/h.

The choice of replacement will depend upon the patient, the severity and rate of volume loss, and what is available within which time span. A basic plan for the average adult is to infuse up to 1 l of electrolyte solution immediately the initial blood samples have been taken. If blood pressure and pulse rate are not restored to acceptable values, further electrolyte solution and plasma protein solution or plasma or dextran solution is given. A guide limit is 1 l of dextran solution (a 40 000 molecular weight dextran will be hyperosmolar). Plasma protein solution or other albumin preparations are given in the absence of other special factors only if there is hypotension *and* at least 1 l of electrolyte solution has been infused first.[17] Electrolyte solutions are practical for a blood loss of up to 4 l in an average adult, but at the expense of increased interstitial pressure and weight gain;[21] for blood loss in this range, if crystalloid is given without colloid, volumes of approximately three times the blood loss are required. Elderly patients may take less kindly to these volumes.

When cross-matched red cell concentrate and/or whole blood is available this should be given to maintain the haemoglobin level in the 10–14 g/dl range and to constitute an increasing part of volume replacement therapy. The decision when to transfuse blood and the quantity to transfuse is based on the individual patient and on the initial haemoglobin level. If further blood loss is not expected a final haemoglobin level of 10–11 g/dl may be adequate. Routine blood transfusion given only because a patient's haemoglobin level is in the 11·5–12·5 g/dl range implies the question, 'Who will transfuse the donor?'.[22] But if there is a chance that the patient may bleed again, for example from a peptic ulcer or oesophageal varices, and particularly if the patient is old, it is wise to aim for a final haemoglobin level of 12–14 g/dl by the time normovolaemia has been attained. This high haemoglobin level is, in itself, unnecessary but allows greater tolerance of immediate crystalloid or colloid resuscitation should this be required days later. A patient whose haemoglobin level is already low is less tolerant of further haemorrhage.

After initial crystalloid and colloid resuscitation, the first two units of blood can be given as red cell concentrate. Thereafter, cell concentrate and whole blood might be given in a 2:1 ratio with, if need be, an additional 200 ml of colloid or 200–400 ml of dextran for each one or two units of red cell concentrate. If the initial haemoglobin level was low, or if large volumes of fluid have already been given, red cells can be given on their own to raise or restore the circulating haemoglobin level and assist oxygenation.

When initial blood loss is rapid and massive, or the patient presents a cross-match problem or is of a rare blood group, logistics must be considered. In practice, to take a blood sample from the patient, transport it to the hospital transfusion laboratory, carry out a shortened blood grouping and rapid emergency cross-match, and transport the blood back to the patient, can easily take an hour, a relatively small proportion of which is taken up by the cross-match. If the laboratory has a recent sample of the patient's serum on a 'group and retain serum' policy the time is considerably shortened. Further time is saved if blood is dispatched to the patient pending telephone confirmation of the cross-match result. On the other hand, if the patient and the laboratory are some miles apart, or if the patient requires blood of a rare type, many hours may elapse.

If such delay is unacceptable, and the patient is not known to have a blood group antibody, the risk of transfusing uncross-matched or scarcely cross-matched blood must be balanced against the risk of waiting. Very few patients' plasma will react with group O red cells and, if an unknown patient has a red cell antibody, it is most likely to be against one or more of the rhesus antigens D, C and E, none of which are carried by 'rhesus negative' (CDE-negative) donor blood. Therefore, if immediate transfusion of uncross-matched blood is essential, group O rhesus negative blood is the least bad choice, preferably as red cell concentrate. Plasma from such blood will contain anti-A and anti-B which, if given in quantity and particularly if it contains alpha or beta haemolysins, may react with some of a group A or B or AB recipient's red cells.

A small minority of patients have other blood group antibodies which will produce a severe, possibly fatal, reaction with random O-negative cells. Antibodies may form within a few weeks of transfusion or during or after pregnancy and even a recent 'no antibodies' report in case notes is not a guarantee that this is still the position.

If blood loss is so massive and continuing that not only is there no time for any form of cross-match but the hospital's stock of O-negative blood is inadequate, there must be immediate consultation with the laboratory. A compromise may have to be made of transfusion with ABO-homologous blood without cross-match in the hope that, if the patient does have an antibody, this will be 'washed out' by what in effect will be an exchange transfusion.

Red-cell deficit on its own with an unacceptably low haemoglobin level may be best treated by specific therapy, such as oral or parenteral iron, vitamin B_{12} or folic acid. If blood transfusion is given, this must be as red cell concentrate and, as a general guide, one unit will raise the haemoglobin level of a 70-kg patient by approximately 1 g/dl. The infusion rate must be slow. Very anaemic and elderly patients, in particular, are intolerant of circulatory overload and as little as 200 ml of blood given rapidly to such a patient can cause fatal pulmonary oedema.[20] If such a patient must be transfused it is advisable to give, at most, only a single unit of red cell concentrate in any one day, along with a diuretic, and using the central venous pressure as an indicator of impending cardiac decomposition.

Heavy and continuing plasma loss requires continuing colloid infusion, the greater part as plasma protein solution or plasma. The aim should be to maintain plasma albumin levels at 20–30 g/l after the first 24 hours.[14] In burnt patients there is a massive protein and water shift into tissues during the first 24 hours when capillary permeability is at its maximum.[14, 19]

One undesirable risk of infusion is local thrombophlebitis. The risk increases the longer the same delivery system is used at the same site, yet too frequent changes are not desirable. One suggestion[23] is to change the administration set routinely after 48 hours, but more frequently 24 hours or less, if blood or blood products are given.

Whole blood and red cells must be transfused through an efficient filter, which should be changed at the intervals recommended by the manufacturer or earlier if it becomes blocked to the extent that the required flow rate cannot be maintained. Platelets must be given through a platelet infusion set and not through a blood filter which will mop up the platelets. Certain fluid combinations should be avoided; blood and dextrose should not be given through the same set for fear of sludging during change-over, and units of blood of differing ABO groups must not be given through the same administration set or filter because of incompatibility between the plasma of one unit and the red cells of the other. Drugs or other additives should never be added to blood or blood products.

Each unit of whole blood contains approximately 6·5 mmol of citrate as sodium citrate and citric acid. A unit of red cell concentrate contains approximately 2·5 mmol, a 200-ml unit of fresh frozen plasma 4 mmol, a 400-ml unit of freeze-dried or fresh frozen plasma 8 mmol. Normally such infused citrate is metabolized. A recent study[24] of patients who received from five to over ten units of blood, and who lacked any history of liver disease, found that while the chelating effect of citrate did depress plasma-ionized calcium levels, this depression was transient and levels returned rapidly to normal as citrate was redistributed and metabolized. It was concluded there is no need to administer intravenous calcium empirically or calculated from the volume of transfused blood so long as the circulating volume is maintained.

A transfusion reaction may occur during or shortly after transfusion. Any reaction must be notified to the transfusion laboratory for investigation and all of the evidence retained: for this reason used containers must not be discarded or washed out. Whenever a reaction is suspected, transfusion of the current unit of blood or other fluid must be stopped, the unit labelled and refrigerated together with an immediate post-reaction blood sample preferably at least 10 ml in volume. The safest policy is to discontinue all further transfusion until the cause of the reaction has been established, but this is not always possible.

Many urticarial and mild febrile reactions are due to antibodies against donor white cells, globulins or platelets. If such a reaction is a problem, future transfusions can be of washed red cell concentrates or of frozen blood suitably thawed and resuspended.

More serious reactions may be due to donor red cell incompatibility. The most common cause is a clerical error which can arise in identifying the patient or his blood sample, transposing samples, filing information incorrectly, transcribing errors or withdrawing the wrong unit of blood from the holding refrigerator. Alternatively, an antibody in the patient's plasma may not have been detected by in vitro tests. The most serious reactions of all are due to gross red cell incompatibility or to infected blood, blood product or crystalloid solution. Intravascular haemolysis, circulatory collapse and disseminated intravascular coagulation may occur in any combination.

The immediate treatment of intravascular haemolysis is to promote diuresis in an effort to prevent or minimize renal tubular necrosis. A standard regime is 100 ml of 20%mannitol given intravenously along with 40 mg of frusemide, while ensuring adequate circulatory haemodynamics and hydration. A urine flow in excess of 100 ml/h is the objective.

A patient with 'generalized oozing' following massive replacement of blood loss, particularly after surgery, is most likely to have dilutional platelet deficiency possibly with other factor deficiencies in addition. If a platelet count shows a platelet level in the 20 000–50 000 range, platelet adminstration is indicated. The platelet deficiency may not be sufficiently severe to be the prime cause of continuing bleeding, but it will fall further after further blood transfusion. If more than ten units of blood have been given a lowered platelet count is almost certain. A standard initial five or six units of platelets, pooled if possible, are given through a platelet administration set. More may be required later. If there is a large area of traumatized tissue an initial 10–12 units of platelets may be desirable.

Where multiple deficiencies are suspected and rapid treatment of a changing situation is desired, the available rapid laboratory tests may do little more than indicate the general area in which the deficiency lies. Here block therapy may be a practical solution. For the average adult who is continuing to bleed from suspected factor deficiency, restore the platelet count first, then give two to three units of fresh frozen plasma (400–600 ml) together with four donor units of cryoprecipitate. This regime will usually bring a dilutional factor deficiency under control. One must always be alert to the possibility that continuing postoperative blood loss may be due to an untied blood vessel and not to capillary bleeding with a coagulation defect.

Congenital factor deficiencies require specialized and individual replacement therapy. A haemophiliac patient, for example, will be known to his haemophilia centre which will have information of the usual quantity of Factor VIII which he requires and whether or not he has an inhibitor. Such information makes management more precise with less frequently required factor assays.

Where rapid reversal of a coumarin anticoagulant is essential, or when haemorrhage from a coagulation deficiency follows hepatic malfunction, prothrombin complex which contains Factors II, VII, IX and X can be used. The concentrate is supplied freeze-dried in a vial containing 200–250 units in approximately 0·5 g of protein and is reconstituted with 10 ml of distilled water. A basic intravenous dose where there is Factor VII deficiency is 10 units (0·5 ml) per kg of body weight, but this should be controlled and adjusted by coagulation tests. Prothrombin complex should not be used in place of the more plentiful Factor IX concentrate to treat a pure Factor IX deficiency. Some prothrombin complex preparations carry a very significant risk of transmitting hepatitis-B,[25] but this risk should be minimal if all donor units of blood used in its preparation were tested for hepatitis-B antigen by a sensitive and reliable method.

Disseminated intravascular coagulation or DIC should be suspected in situations where there is continuing blood loss from multiple sites, a predisposing factor, no platelet deficiency and no response to fresh frozen plasma. The diagnosis should be considered if a blood sample fails to clot, or if the clot becomes fluid again. Diagnosis is indicated by laboratory detection of intravascular products of fibrinolysis, and is supported by a low fibrinogen level. Once the haematological diagnosis has been made, the cause must be removed if possible; indeed by the time DIC has been diagnosed the precipitating events may have ceased. When the sequence of events has stopped, fresh frozen plasma (400–600 ml) and four to six units of cryoprecipitate should provide adequate haemostasis. Platelets may be required, if a dilution effect has been added.

If DIC continues, fibrinogen is usually withheld on the grounds that it simply provides more fuel for the process without assisting haemostasis. The alternatives are to interrupt coagulation with intravenous heparin, or to inhibit primary fibrinolysis if this is the main factor using ε-aminocaproic acid or other available products. A loading dose of 10 000 units of heparin, in an adult, is followed by supplements with assessment by the haematology laboratory by serial sampling. Heparin overdose itself will result in bleeding, but this is rapidly reversed by intravenous protamine sulphate given slowly. Primary fibrinolysis is inhibited by intravenous ε-aminocaproic acid under laboratory control; an appropriate loading dose is 5 g followed by 1 g per hour. Results can be dramatic.

DEVELOPMENTS

A small minority of patients have circulating antibodies against platelets of certain tissue groups. Here, platelets of the appropriate tissue type are to be preferred but if donors of suitable known tissue types are not available the only recourse is to increase the quantity of platelets which is given.

The current recommendation is for each unit of platelets to be prepared in 50 ml of plasma. Patients who have severe thrombocytopoenia from cytotoxic drugs may require twelve units of platelets at a time. If these were contained in 600 ml of plasma patients could experience circulatory embarrassment, so platelet concentrates may still be supplied in approximately 25 ml of plasma.

White cell replacement therapy has a very useful potential for patients with neutropenia from suppressed bone marrow function, especially if there is concurrent infection. It is not practical to obtain suitable white cells from multiple donations of blood, but white cells can be obtained from a single pre-selected donor using a cell separator. Similarly, it is possible to obtain sufficient platelets for one administration from a single matched donor.

Recently oxygen-carrying blood volume expanders have been studied as possible blood substitutes. Haemoglobin solution has been considered. It is essential that the solution is free from red cell stroma.[26] Such a solution is a better oxygen carrier than plasma or PPS, but free haemoglobin has a higher oxygen affinity than haemoglobin in red cells while renal excretion is both rapid and causes water loss.

Fluorocarbons have been studied.[26] Compared to haemoglobin in circulating red cells these have a low oxygen content at ambient pressure, and there are unresolved doubts about the safety of tissue accummulation.

Many specific immunoglobulins are now available. Normally these are given by intramuscular injection but, in an extreme situation, these have been given intravenously after dilution in saline to a 5% protein concentration. There may be a severe vasomotor reaction, especially if there are protein aggregates in the material, and close medical supervision is essential.

REFERENCES

1. Counts R. B., Haisch C., Simon T. L. et al. (1979) Hemostasis in massively transfused patients. *Ann. Surg.* **190**, 91–99.
2. Cloutier C. T., Lowery B. D. and Carey M. D. (1979) The effect of hemodilutional resuscitation on serum protein levels in humans in hemorrhagic shock. *J. Trauma* **9**, 514–521.
3. Mendelson J. A. (1974) The selection of plasma volume expanders for mass-casualty planning. *J. Trauma* **14**, 987–989.
4. Mendelson J. A. (1975) The use of whole blood and blood volume expanders in US military medical facilities in Vietnam 1966–1971. *J. Trauma* **15**, 1.
5. Procter H. J., Ballantine T. V. N. and Broussard N. D. (1970) An analysis of pulmonary function following non-thoracic trauma, with recommendations for therapy. *Ann. Surg.* **172**, 180–189.
6. Northrup W. F. and Humphrey E. W. (1978) The effect of hemorrhagic shock on pulmonary vascular permeability to plasma proteins. *Surgery* **83**, 264–273.
7. Cervera A. L. and Moss G. (1978) Crystalloid requirements and distribution when resuscitating with RBCs and non-colloid solutions during hemorrhage. *Circ. Shock* **5**, 357–364.
8. Moss G. S. (1972) An argument in favor of electrolyte solution for early resuscitation. *Surg. Clin. North Am.* **52**, 3–17.
9. Virgilio R. W., Rice C. L., Smith D. E. et al. (1979) Crystalloid vs colloid resuscitation—is one better? *Surgery* **85**, 129–139.
10. Weaver D. W., Ledgerwood A. M., Lucas C. E. et al. (1978) Pulmonary effects of albumin resuscitation for severe hypovolemic shock. *Arch. Surg.* **113**, 387–392.
11. Johnson S. D., Lucas C. E., Gerrick S. J. et al. (1979) Altered coagulation after albumin supplements for treatment of oligemic shock. *Arch. Surg.* **114**, 379–383.
12. Rush B. F., Richardson D., Bosomworth P. et al. (1969) Limitations of blood replacement with electrolyte solutions. *Arch. Surg.* **98**, 49–52.
13. Cervera A. L. and Moss G. (1975) Progressive hypovolemia leading to shock after continuous hemorrhage and 3:1 crystalloid replacement. *Am. J. Surg.* **129**, 670–674.
14. Tullis J. L. (1977) Albumin. 1. Background and use. 2. Guidelines for clinical use. *J. Am. Med. Assoc.* **237**, 355–360; 460–463.

15. Skillman J. J., Restall D. S. and Salzman E. W. (1975) Randomized trial of albumin vs electrolyte solutions during abdominal aortic operations. *Surgery* **78**, 291–303.
16. Lowe R. J., Moss G. S., Jilek J. et al. (1977) Crystalloid vs colloid in the etiology or pulmonary failure after trauma: a randomized trial in man. *Surgery* **81**, 676–683.
17. Alexander R. M., Ambre J. J., Liskow B. I. et al. (1979) Therapeutic use of albumin. *J. Am. Med. Assoc.* **241**, 2527–2529.
18. Rowntree L. G. (1929) *The Volume of Blood and Plasma in Health and Disease.* Philadelphia, W. B. Saunders.
19. Rossing N. (1978) Intra- and extravascular distribution of albumin and immuno-globulin in man. *Lymphology* **11**, 138–142.
20. Mollison P. L. (1972) *Blood Transfusion in Clinical Medicine.* Oxford, Blackwell.
21. Editorial (1979) *Lancet* **1**, 1385–1386.
22. Bowley C. C. Personal communication.
23. Band J. D. and Maki D. G. (1979) Safety of changing delivery systems at longer than 24-hour intervals. *Ann. Intern. Med.* **91**, 173–178.
24. Kahn R. C., Jascoff D., Carlon G. C. et al. (1979) Massive blood replacement: correlation of ionized calcium, citrate, and hydrogen ion concentration. *Anesth. Analg.* **58**, 274–278.
25. Rossiter S. J., Miller C., Raney A. A. et al. (1979) Hepatitis risk in cardiac surgery patients receiving factor IX concentrates. *J. Thorac. Cardiovasc. Surg.* **78**, 203–207.
26. De Venuto F., Friedman H. I., Neville J. R. et al. (1979) Appraisal of hemaglobin solution as a blood substitute. *Surg. Gynecol. Obstet.* **149**, 417–436.

Chapter 11

Radiology

B. Moule

The radiological investigations of intensive care patients can be divided into two groups:
1. Examinations carried out in the intensive care unit (ICU). These will mainly be portable X-ray examinations of the chest and abdomen but may now also include examinations performed with portable ultrasonic machines.
2. Examinations, which because of their complexity have to be carried out in various parts of the X-ray department where the appropriate non-portable equipment is installed. These examinations include arteriography, computerized axial tomography (CT scanning), most ultrasonic procedures, myelography, venography, contrast examination of the alimentary tract where fluoroscopy is needed, isotope scanning, percutaneous transhepatic cholangiography or venography, splenic venography, etc. In fact almost all present-day radiological procedures can be used to investigate intensive care patients provided appropriate care is taken and the patients are carefully monitored in the usual ways. Recently, an exciting development has occurred in radiological practice which has significance in the management of some intensive care patients. This is the so-called 'interventional' radiology whereby the radiologist extends his diagnostic techniques to perform therapeutic manoeuvres. Examples are therapeutic embolization of arterial vessels to stop arterial bleeding, and percutaneous transhepatic biliary drainage to relieve obstructive jaundice. These techniques will be described in more detail later.

As far as selecting the appropriate radiological procedure is concerned it cannot be stressed too strongly that good co-operation and regular communication between the radiological and ICU staff is of paramount importance. Regular meetings between the people involved will help to solve difficult diagnostic problems, and the radiologist may be able to bring to the attention of the intensive care staff variations of radiographic technique or new radiological procedures which can prove rewarding.

Many patients in the ICU may have had radiological examinations prior to their admission to the unit. Trauma patients, for example, have frequently had films taken of chest, abdomen, skull and parts of the skeletal system in the casualty X-ray department. Patients transferred to the unit from other departments in the hospital will have already had radiological investigations appropriate to their condition. All radiographs of such patients should be readily available to the radiologist and intensive care staff and subsequent changes in the radiological appearances can then be noted when compared with these earlier radiographs.

I. Radiological Examinations Performed Within the Intensive Care Unit

1. *Chest*

Radiographs of the chest taken with portable X-ray equipment in the ICU can provide much useful and important information. As with other radiological examinations it is necessary to insist on good technique in the taking of these films, e.g. the patient should not be rotated significantly from the AP plane, the film should be properly exposed so that all important structures and inserts such as the endotracheal tube and central venous pressure (CVP) line can be seen, there should be no movement blurring and the film should be taken at inspiration. Variations of the technique may be required, such as expiration, lateral and decubitus films, and an oblique or rotated view sometimes shows the position of the endotracheal tube quite clearly, and may reveal rib fractures. Therefore, although a straight AP chest film is the radiographer's aim, any films that have been taken should be looked at carefully before being rejected.

The films should provide the following information:

a. The position of the endotracheal or tracheostomy tube and other inserts and of electrodes. The tip of the endotracheal tube should, in the neutral position of the head and neck, be about 5–7 cm from the carina.[1] This allows for a tube movement downwards of 2 cm in full flexion of the head and neck, and an upward movement of 2 cm in extension.

Ideally, the endotracheal tube will be between one-half to two-thirds of the width of the trachea and the inflated cuff should fill the tracheal lumen but not bulge the lateral walls. Faulty positioning can result in the tube entering a main stem bronchus, usually the right, with resultant over-inflation of that lung and poor ventilation of the opposite lung. *Fig.* 11.1, which is an oblique view from an emergency arch aortogram series, shows the endotracheal tube in good position.

The tip of the CVP line should be in the superior vena cava to reflect right atrial pressure and blood volume changes. Complications of

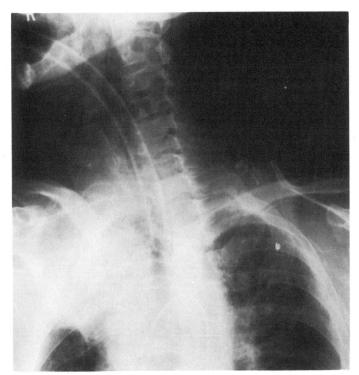

Fig. 11.1. Tip of endotracheal tube in correct position above the carina.

insertion of the CVP line include catheter fragmentation and this should be looked for.

If a catheter, such as a No. 5 balloon-tipped Swan–Ganz catheter, has been inserted to measure pulmonary capillary wedge (PCW) pressure, its position should be checked on the radiographs. The tip should be in the right or left pulmonary artery, 5 or 6 cm from the bifurcation of the main pulmonary artery. Balloon inflation will cause the catheter to drift into the 'wedge' position, and deflation allows the catheter to return to its original position.

A transvenous cardiac pacemaker, if inserted, can be localized by AP and lateral views. Ideally, the tip should be in the apex of the right ventricle, and on the lateral view it should lie anteriorly 3 or 4 mm beneath the epicardial fat stripe.[2] Complications, such as detachment of the pacemaker wires from the pulse unit, can be easily recognized but fractures of the electrode wires are more difficult to see on radiographs because the insulating sheath may hold the broken wires together. Fluoroscopic examination may then be helpful.

It should be noted whether pleural drainage tubes are in a good position. In bedridden patients, lying supine, pleural air collects beneath the sternum whilst pleural fluid collects posteriorly. The position of the drainage tube should be modified accordingly, and a horizontal beam lateral radiograph will show the position of the tube relative to air or fluid.

b. The condition of the lung fields. Areas of opacity or shadowing in the lungs should be noted and an attempt made to determine the cause, e.g. whether there is pleural fluid, pulmonary oedema or consolidation–collapse. Adams[3] has pointed out difficulties in determining the exact cause of pulmonary shadowing in intensive care patients, due to some of the technical difficulties associated with the portable film (vertical X-ray beam) examination.

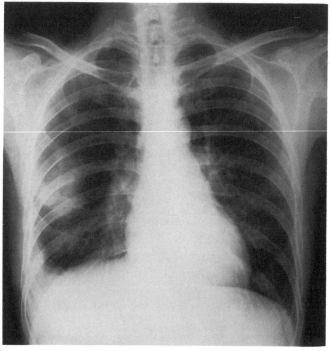

Fig. 11.2. Pulmonary infarcts in right lung.

A confident diagnosis of the cause of pulmonary shadows may be made if relevant clinical information is available. In *Fig.* 11.2, for example, the pulmonary shadows were considered to be due to pulmonary infarcts since venography had already shown deep vein thromboses in leg and pelvic veins (*see Fig.* 11.22a), or the pulmonary shadowing may have a characteristic appearance as in *Fig.* 11.3 and 11.4a, which show collapse of the right upper lobe. Note also the low position of the endotracheal tube in *Fig.* 11.4a curving towards the right. *Fig.* 11.4b shows improvement in the right upper lobe collapse after bronchoscopy and aspiration of mucous plugs and, on this film, the endotracheal tube

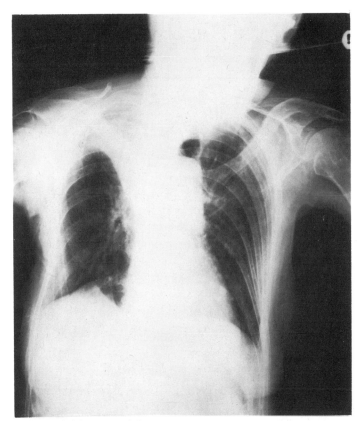

Fig. 11.3. Collapse of right upper lobe.

is in better position. However, there is 'elevation' of the right dome of the diaphragm where a subpulmonary pleural effusion developed (*Fig.* 11.4c). Lateral views of the chest can be helpful in locating an area of shadowing and deciding its nature as illustrated in *Fig.* 11.5a, b and c. *Fig.* 11.5a shows shadowing in the lower parts of both lungs. The appearances in the left lower zone suggest collapse in the left lower lobe with patchy shadowing probably due to inflammatory change in the lingula, whilst the right lower zone shadowing is probably due to consolidation. A lateral view was not obtained at this time, but several days later, the PA film (*Fig.* 11.5b) shows clearing of the left lower zone shadows, but persistence of the right lower zone shadow which is seen on the lateral view (*Fig.* 11.5c) to be in the lower posterior part of the right lower lobe. This was, in fact, a lung abscess. The area behind the heart should always be looked at carefully since a triangular opacity there suggests an area of collapse in the left lower lobe (*Fig.* 11.6). It is of course difficult to distinguish pulmonary infarcts from other causes of pulmonary shadows, unless the clinical information points to it, or there

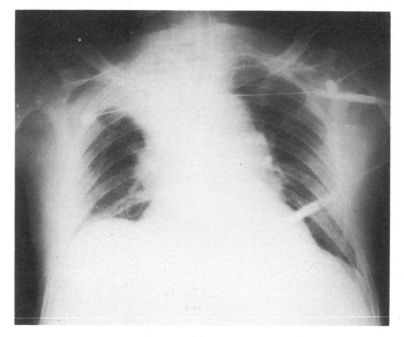

(a)

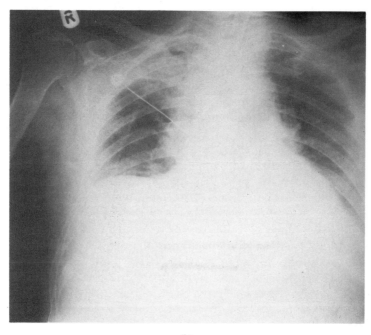

(b)

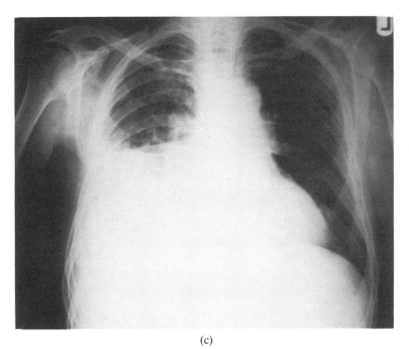

(c)

Fig. 11.4. (a) Consolidation–collapse of right upper lobe. (b) Improved after aspiration through bronchoscope. (c) Right subpulmonary effusion.

are other appropriate radiological signs, such as elevation of the dome of the diaphragm or pleural reaction on the same side as the pulmonary infarcts.

Pulmonary oedema occurs in intensive care patients in the same way as in other patients and can be due to cardiac failure as in *Fig.* 11.7, over-transfusion of intravenous fluids, etc. In addition, the condition referred to as 'shock lung' or adult respiratory distress syndrome occurs in intensive care patients due to septicaemia, severe trauma, fat embolism and a host of other causes,[4, 5] and after an initial radiograph which may seem 'normal', diffuse parenchymal infiltrates develop, serial radiographs may show perihilar haze, then interstitial oedema progressing to confluent pulmonary oedema within twenty-four hours. There may then be little change for several days. Treatment by positive end-expiratory pressure (PEEP) may dramatically improve the condition by increasing the aeration of the lungs, and the radiograph may return to 'normal' after several days, though some patients seem to proceed to interstitial pulmonary fibrosis. Underlying chest disease, such as chronic obstructive airways disease or congestive cardiac failure, may alter the radiological appearances to those of the underlying disease. PEEP can produce an apparent improvement in the radiological appearances of the

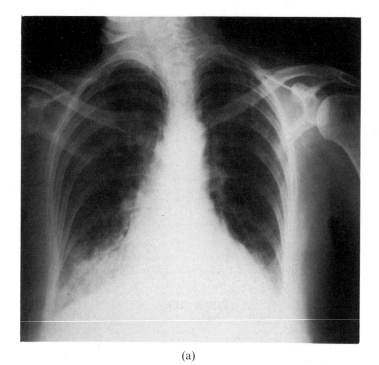

(a)

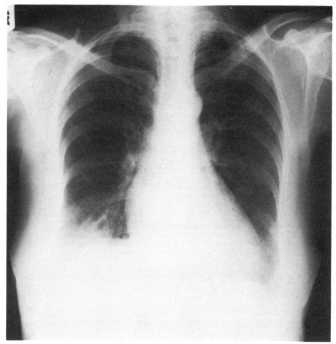

(b)

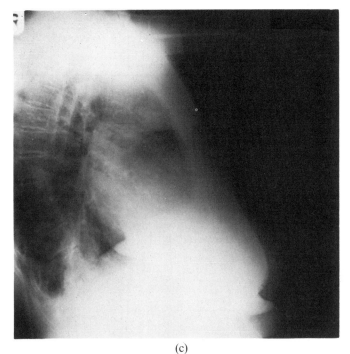

(c)

Fig. 11.5. (a) Consolidation in right and left lower zones. (c) Pulmonary abscess in right lower lobe. (b) Left lung now appears clear.

chest making infiltrates and atelectases less prominent due to the greater lung expansion, and the radiologist should always know whether or not the patient is receiving this treatment. In trying to decide whether pulmonary oedema is due to cardiac failure or a non-cardiac cause measurements of the pulmonary capillary wedge pressure as well as the central venous pressure is helpful.

In addition to the AP supine chest film, the influence of gravity on pulmonary oedema can be used to distinguish it from other pulmonary infiltrates. Thus, after the initial film, if the patient can be placed in the lateral decubitus position for about two hours, with the affected lung up, a later film will show a tendency for pulmonary oedema to shift to the dependent lung whilst other pulmonary infiltrates remain unchanged in position.[6]

Pleural effusions frequently occur in intensive care patients and, if an erect chest radiograph has been obtained, the usual radiographic appearances will be seen, such as the meniscus sign. However, if the patient has been lying supine for some time before the erect film is taken, the meniscus sign may not have developed completely. *Fig.* 11.8 shows some pleural fluid at both lung bases probably with a meniscus sign developing at the right base, but most of the pleural fluid appearing as

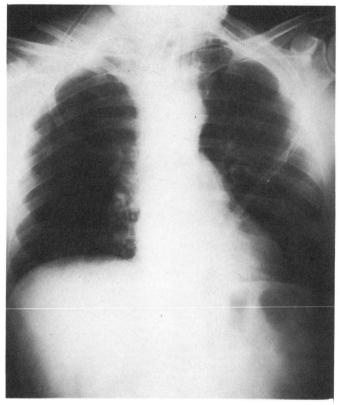

Fig. 11.6. Triangular opacity behind the heart in left lower zone, due to partial atelectasis of left lower lobe.

hazy opacity in the lower zones with obliteration of the costophrenic angles. If the film is taken with the patient supine and using a vertical X-ray beam, then only the hazy lung shadowing and obliteration of the costophrenic angles may be seen. In *Fig.* 11.8 there is also pulmonary oedema and enlargement of the heart. *Fig.* 11.9a shows pleural fluid obliterating the costophrenic angles and causing hazy shadowing in both lower zones whilst passing into the interlobar fissures in the right lung. Subpulmonary effusion can be suspected on the supine film by the difference in height of the domes of the diaphragm and the hazy opacity at the right base in *Fig.* 11.9b; but an erect film (*Fig.* 11.9c) will increase the height difference of the diaphragmatic domes and make the diagnosis of subpulmonary effusion easier.

Since pleural fluid accumulates posteriorly in patients who are lying supine, lateral decubitus chest radiographs are very helpful in distinguishing pleural fluid from pleural thickening or pulmonary infiltrates.

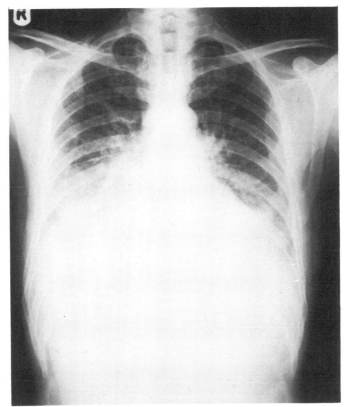

Fig. 11.7. Bilateral pulmonary oedema due to cardiac failure.

c. The presence or absence of abnormal air collections. Extra-alveolar escape of air is seen in from 5 to 15% of patients on intermittent positive-pressure ventilation. Furthermore, up to two-thirds of pneumothoraces in respirator patients are of tension type and urgent drainage of these will be required. Air leaks occur most often in patients with chronic obstructive airways disease, interstitial pulmonary fibrosis or cavitary lung disease.

It must be remembered that, in the supine patient, pleural air will collect beneath the sternum and, if the patient cannot be placed to obtain sitting or erect chest films, horizontal beam lateral radiographs combined with the AP view will be useful. Also radiographs exposed in both inspiratory and expiratory phase may reveal a pneumothorax which may be missed on the inspiration film alone. A lateral decubitus film with affected side uppermost is also worth taking.

Pneumomediastinum may precede pneumothorax and a pneumoperi-cardium may be seen as in *Fig.* 11.10, which also shows a tracheostomy and wide superior mediastinum.

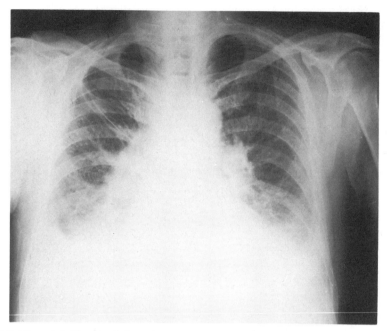

Fig. 11.8. Pleural fluid at both lung bases, with pulmonary oedema.

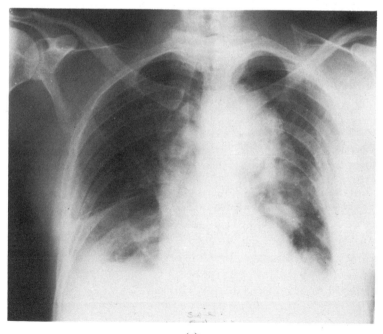

(a)

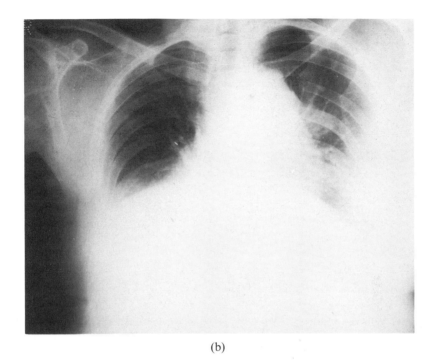

(b)

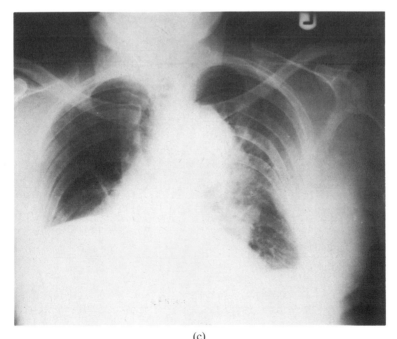

(c)

Fig. 11.9. (a) Pleural fluid in the lower zones. (b and c) Right subpulmonary effusion. (*see* text.)

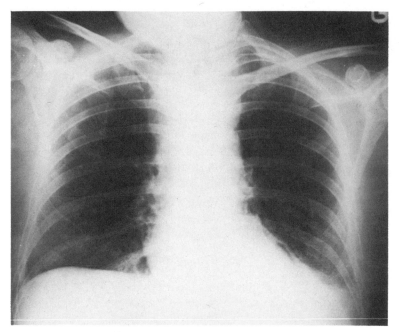

Fig. 11.10. Pneumomediastinum with pneumopericardium.

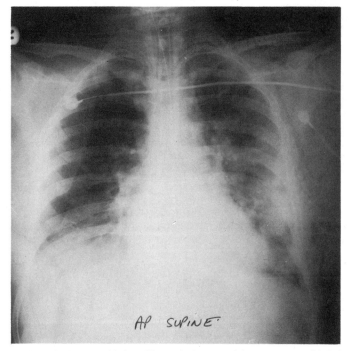

Fig. 11.11. Air in soft tissues of left axilla and chest, and haematoma of left lung.

Air may be seen in the soft tissues ('surgical' emphysema) as a complication of trauma or after tracheostomy. *Fig.* 11.11 shows surgical emphysema in the left axilla and soft tissues of the lateral wall of the left side of the chest, with pleural reaction at the right base and haematoma of the left lung.

d. The condition of the bony thoracic cage. A correctly exposed AP supine film may reveal rib fractures, but these are more likely to be seen if oblique views are obtained and, sometimes, may be shown on a more penetrated AP film when they are not clearly seen on a film which shows the lung fields well but the ribs, particularly their posterior parts, not too clearly. *Fig.* 11.12 shows multiple fractures of the right ribs, surgical emphysema in the right axilla and neck, right-sided pleural fluid or haematoma, segmental consolidation–collapse in the right lung, a drainage tube in the right side of the chest, enlarged heart and elevated domes of diaphragm.

A well-penetrated AP film may also reveal fractures of the dorsal spine.

e. The width of the mediastinum. This is important since a wide mediastinum can imply a tear or dissection of the aorta. Serial films may

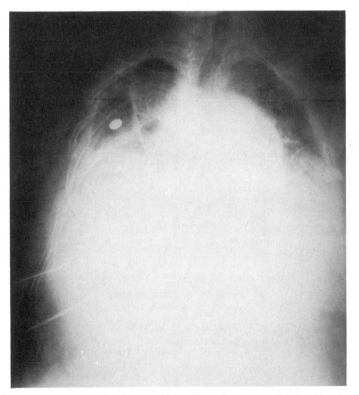

Fig. 11.12. Severe trauma to the chest, with multiple fractures of right ribs, (*see* text).

reveal that the widening of the mediastinum is increasing. Damage to the great vessels arising from the aortic arch or to the arch itself will result in widening of the superior mediastinum. If the site of the tear is near the attachment of the ligamentum arteriosum, there may, in addition to the superior mediastinal widening, be displacement of the trachea to the right and a haemothorax (particularly on the left side). Fractures of the first and second ribs may be seen, which are uncommon except in severe chest trauma.

Fig. 11.13 shows widening of the mediastinal shadow below the aortic knuckle with a double shadow due to spontaneous aortic dissection below the left subclavian artery.

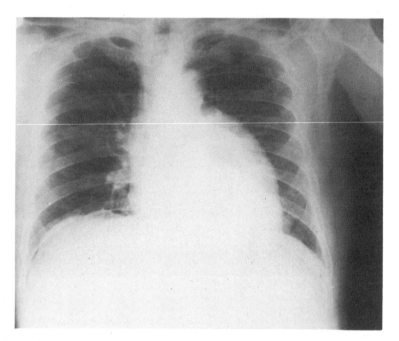

Fig. 11.13. Dissection of aorta below the aortic knuckle.

f. The size of the heart and the shape of the heart and thoracic aorta. Transverse cardiac enlargement can be exaggerated by portable supine radiographs as obtained in most intensive care patients. Likewise the shape of the aorta can be difficult to assess. However, if a standard PA chest film of good quality has been taken, the size of the heart in the transverse diameter can be assessed and a reasonable opinion formed of the shape of the heart and thoracic aorta. Abnormalities such as mitral value disease may be apparent. *Fig.* 11.14a shows an aneurysm of the ascending thoracic aorta, and the lateral view (*Fig.* 11.14b) shows the

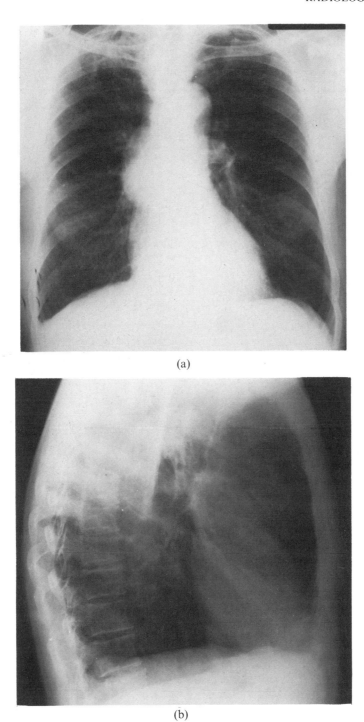

(a)

(b)

Fig. 11.14. Aneurysm of ascending thoracic aorta.

curved shadow of the aneurysm lying anterior in the lower superior mediastinum (*see* Aortogram in *Fig.* 11.21; p. 283).

g. The position and shape of the domes of the diaphragm. An AP supine film of the chest taken in expiration will show the diaphragmatic domes to be high in position. However, a significant difference in height between the two domes, particularly if the film has been exposed in inspiration, suggests the presence of an abnormality. (*Fig.* 11.15 shows elevated right dome, right pleural effusion and drainage tube.)

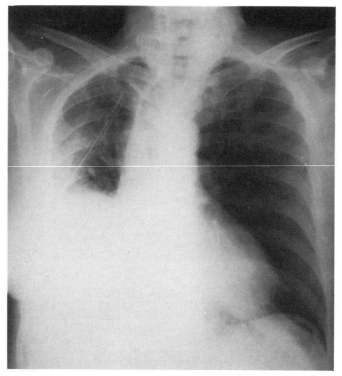

Fig. 11.15. Marked elevation of right dome of diaphragm with some right-sided pleural effusion.

Pulmonary infarction or collapse can cause elevation of the dome on the same side as also may traumatic rupture of the dome, particularly if the liver projects through a damaged right dome. Subphrenic abscess can also cause elevation of the dome on the same side with irregularity in its outline due to pleural reaction. Fluoroscopy provides information about the mobility of the diaphragm but may not be a suitable examination for the intensive care patient, though chest films exposed at expiration and inspiration are a limited alternative. Phrenic nerve damage will elevate and immobilize the diaphragmatic dome on that side.

2. *Abdomen*

Abdominal radiographs taken in the ICU can indicate whether there is intra-abdominal pathology and locate support apparatus. Thus the correct position of nasogastric, small bowel, gastrostomy and rectal tubes can be determined. If a Sengstaken–Blakemore tube has been inserted to stop bleeding from lower oesophageal varices, both the position of the tube and any complication of its insertion, such as oesophageal rupture or pneumonitis, can be seen.

Various types of abdominal pathology can be diagnosed by correctly exposed portable radiographs, particularly if a combination of supine, erect or lateral decubitus, and horizontal beam lateral films can be obtained, including the following.

a. Abnormal gas collections. Pneumoperitoneum due, for example, to intra-abdominal perforation will be shown by erect or lateral decubitus films where the air rises to the highest point in the abdominal cavity, unless it is loculated. It may be suspected on the supine film if both sides of the wall of a gas-filled viscus are outlined. Gas should also be looked for retroperitoneally and in the liver where the bile ducts may fill with gas. In some very seriously ill patients gas may be seen in the portal circulation. Gas may be seen in intra-abdominal abscesses or in the wall of the bowel, gall bladder and urinary bladder where disease is present. Pneumatosis cystoides intestinalis may be recognized on plain abdomen films. In the absence of intra-abdominal perforation, pneumoperitoneum and pneumoretroperitoneum related to ventilator therapy are invariably accompanied by pncumomcdiastinum.

b. Abnormal gas patterns. The following can be recognized on plain abdominal films.

   i. Acute dilatation of the stomach.

   ii. Intestinal obstruction. There is dilatation of bowel down to the level of obstruction, and erect or lateral decubitus films show fluid levels.

   iii. Adynamic ileus. There is proportionate dilatation of small and large bowel, including rectum, with a relatively small amount of intraluminal fluid and therefore less obvious fluid levels.

   iv. Colonic distension due to ileus or obstruction. Severe, acute ulcerative colitis may produce a markedly dilated colon.

   v. Bowel infarction. This may show as gas distension of bowel, gas in the bowel wall and, in severe cases, gas in the portal venous circulation. The radiological signs, however, are often non-specific.

c. Abnormal calcifications. These include gall stones, concretions in the appendix, urinary calculi, pancreatic calcification, calcified aortic aneurysm and others.

Other examinations which can be undertaken in the ICU include:

Urinary tract. Excretion urography (IVP) can be performed without prior preparation of the patient. An intravenous injection of the usual volume of water-soluble contrast medium can be given as in other IVP examinations. Films can be taken at the usual intervals of time with the vertical beam AP supine view of abdomen being used. A more limited examination could involve films being taken of abdomen and pelvis at, e.g. 1, 10, 20 and 30 min after injection. Information such as whether both kidneys are excreting the contrast is useful, and damage to the kidneys, ureters or bladder may be suspected from the available films. Compression of the abdomen is usually not feasible.

Fluoroscopy. Portable fluoroscopic machines can be used in the ICU to assist in the placement of a cardiac pacemaker by the transvenous method. Other fluoroscopic examinations such as locating broken catheters or contrast examinations of the upper gastro-intestinal tract are possible by use of a portable machine. However, it is recommended that, whenever possible, fluoroscopy should be performed within the X-ray department. This is partly due to the problems of radiation protection involved in the use of a portable fluoroscopy machine within the ICU, and partly to the fact that a better more informative examination can be achieved on the fluoroscopy table in the X-ray department.

II. Radiological Examinations Performed Outside the Intensive Care Unit

Many of these investigative techniques have been mentioned in the introductory paragraphs, and this chapter is not intended to provide a catologue of every available type of radiological investigation, but to indicate examples of situations where more complex radiology can be helpful in resolving clinical problems in intensive care patients.

1. *Angiography*

For several reasons, angiographic investigations are best carried out in the angiography room of the radiology department. First, the film changer will be able to provide rapid sequence radiographs, e.g. six films per second, and some lesions may only be seen on one of these rapidly taken films (*Fig. 11.16*). Also fluoroscopy will be available to provide accurate localization of the catheter and, therefore, enable selective catheterization to be performed. This, in turn, gives the radiologist the option to extend the diagnostic procedure to therapeutic intervention as in the case of therapeutic arterial embolization to stop arterial bleeding.

The indications for angiography are similar to those in other patients, e.g. trauma to an artery, acute arterial embolization, haemorrhage and sometimes to show tumour circulation. It is, however, likely that there will be a preponderance of trauma cases. The angiogram will almost always be performed by the Seldinger method of arterial catheterization via a femoral, axillary or brachial artery. Translumbar aortography could be used to demonstrate a block of the lower abdominal aorta or occlusions of the arteries of the lower limbs.

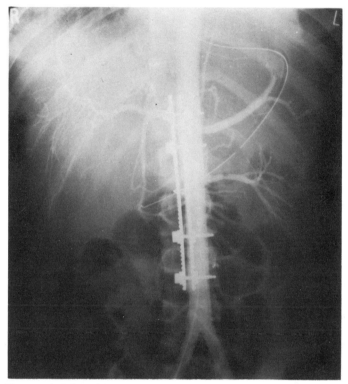

Fig. 11.16. Traumatic left renal artery stenosis with no filling of right renal artery due to avulsion. (*see* text).

Local anaesthesia will be used with premedication if necessary, though an intensive care patient may be unconscious. General anaesthesia is often used for the translumbar technique, though the placing of a seriously ill patient in the prone position for this type of aortogram may give rise to problems.

The following cases provide examples of the usefullness of angiography in intensive care patients.

Case 1. (*Fig.* 11.16) A 15-year-old male was transferred from a peripheral hospital having sustained a traumatic vertebral dislocation at the dorso-lumbar junction. There was no sensory or motor deficiency in the lower limbs. He was anuric and an IVP performed in the other hospital had shown no excretion of contrast by the kidneys. His blood pressure was high (205/100) and damage to the renal arteries was suspected. After reduction of the spinal dislocation and fixation by metallic plating, an abdominal aortogram was performed and showed a stenotic lesion of the left renal artery (due to a traumatic tear) and no filling of the right renal artery due to an avulsion of its origin from the aorta. The lesion of the left renal artery was clearly seen on only one of the rapid sequence films. The left renal artery was repaired by a graft, and the right kidney was removed.

Case 2. (*Fig.* 11.17) A teenage male patient who had been injured in a road traffic accident. Plain AP chest films suggested widening of the superior mediastinum. Arch aortography shows a tear of the innominate artery producing an irregular traumatic aneurysm.

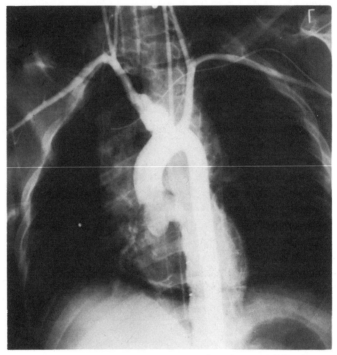

Fig. 11.17. Traumatic aneurysm and tear of innominate artery following a road traffic accident.

Case 3. (*Fig.* 11.18a, b) A male patient aged 53 years presenting with sudden, very severe and increasing chest pain. Plain AP film of the chest showed a wide superior mediastinum and descending thoracic aorta with transversely enlarged heart. Arch aortography shows a dissecting aneurysm of the thoracic aorta beginning near the left subclavian artery and the dissection extended as far as the upper abdominal aorta where re-entry occurred.

Case 4. (*Fig.* 11.19a, b, c) A 69-year-old man with severe increasing chest pain, whose plain chest radiograph has already been described in *Fig.* 11.13. Arch aortography demonstrates an aneurysm of the thoracic aorta, just distal to the left subclavian artery with aortic dissection extending as far as the upper abdominal aorta. This patient was catheterized by the right axillary artery as both femoral pulses were poor.

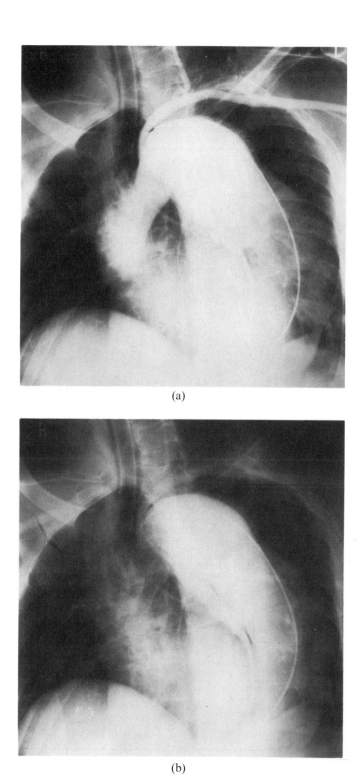

(a)

(b)

Fig. 11.18. Dissection of distal arch and descending thoracic aorta.

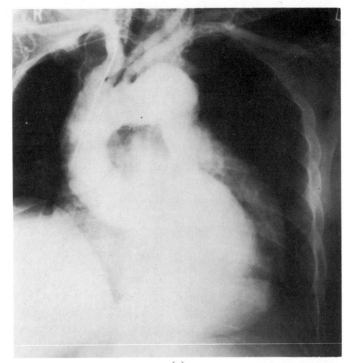

(a)

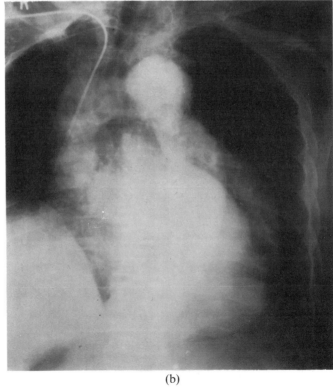

(b)

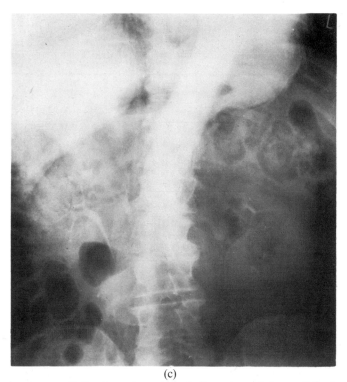

(c)

Fig. 11.19. Aneurysm of distal aortic arch and dissection of descending thoracic aorta extending to upper abdominal aorta.

Case 5. (*Fig.* 11.20a, b) A 62-year-old female with severe chest pain, with a wide aortic arch shadow and also a wide descending thoracic aorta. Seldinger aortography via the right femoral artery was able to show only the thoracic aorta distal to the innominate artery (*Fig.* 11.20a) as neither guide wire nor catheter could be manipulated into the ascending aorta due, presumably, to excessive aortic tortuosity. A catheter was therefore passed into the ascending aorta via the right axillary artery (*Fig.* 11.20b) and shows a more complete picture of the thoracic aorta. There is a large aneurysm of the aortic arch with tortuosity and kinking of the descending thoracic aorta and a shadow beyond but parallel to the dye-filled descending thoracic aorta suggesting aortic dissection.

Case 6. (*Fig.* 11.21) A 60-year-old male patient with clinical and plain radiographic features (*Fig.* 11.14a, b), suggestive of an enlarging aneurysm of the ascending aorta. This was confirmed by arch aortography as shown in *Fig.* 11.21.

Aortography or selective arteriography relevant to the anatomical region where a lesion is suspected can be performed on intensive care patients under strict monitoring. Computed tomography of the head has reduced the need for carotid angiography in neurological intensive care patients, but there is still a place for this and vertebral angiography, e.g. in locating arterial aneurysms in subarachnoid haemorrhage.

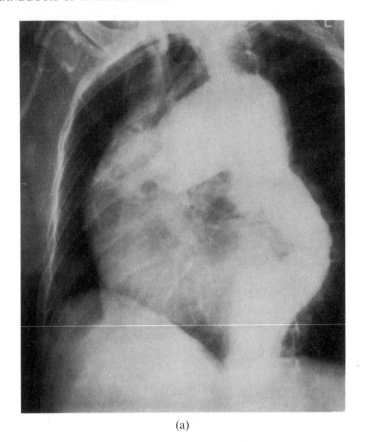

(a)

2. Leg Venography and Pulmonary Angiography

The patient whose chest radiograph was shown in *Fig.* 11.2 was suspected of having pulmonary infarcts due to deep vein thrombosis in the right leg. The presence of deep vein thrombosis in the right calf and thigh was confirmed by leg venography (*Fig.* 11.22a) and this also shows thrombus in the right iliac vein. (*Fig.* 11.22b also shows fractures of the upper right femur fixed by pin-plate.) Leg venography is simple to perform, provided a superficial distal vein can be located and, although it could be carried out within the ICU, it is better to transfer the patient to the radiology department where the examination is likely to provide a more accurate result due to the serial film changing methods and fluoroscopy available in the department. Per-osseous venography can be used if the superficial distal veins are impossible to locate due to severe swelling of the limb. This, however, may require general anaesthesia or adequate analgesia.

Pulmonary angiography is performed in cases of suspected pulmonary embolism, but is usually preceded by a radionuclide lung scan which will

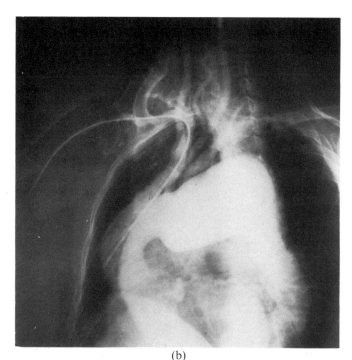

(b)

Fig. 11.20. Aneurysm of thoracic aorta close to left subclavian artery with dissection of descending thoracic aorta.

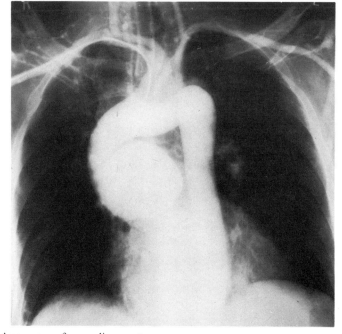

Fig. 11.21. Aneurysm of ascending aorta.

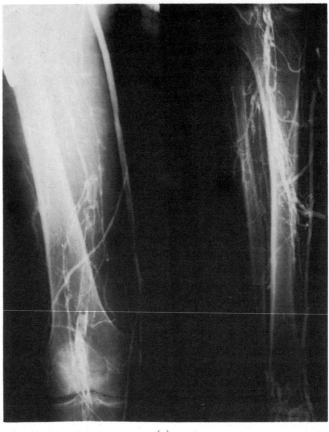

(a)

show decreased perfusion in affected parts of the lungs in most cases of pulmonary embolism.

Although a perfusion lung scan can be performed in the ICU if appropriate equipment is available, it is usually performed within the department of nuclear medicine and the pulmonary angiogram is carried out in the appropriate room in the radiology or pulmonary function department where additional measuring and monitoring devices are available.

3. *Fluoroscopy*

As already indicated, most examinations requiring fluoroscopy should be performed in the radiology department. These will include barium or Gastrografin studies of the alimentary tract, myelography, angiography, splenic or transhepatic venography, percutaneous transhepatic cholangio-

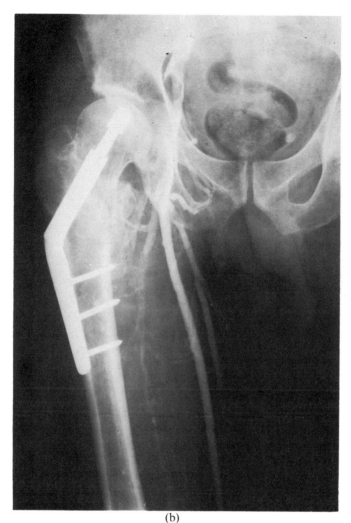

(b)

Fig. 11.22. Deep vein thromboses in right lower limb and right iliofemoral veins.

graphy (PTC) and interventional techniques. Patients with obstructive jaundice may be critically ill due to hepatorenal failure, and may require treatment in the ICU. Prompt diagnosis of the cause of the obstructive jaundice can be made by ultrasonographic examination of the liver and pancreas followed by PTC or, in some situations, endoscopic retrograde choledochopancreatography (ERCP). PTC is simpler and quicker to perform than ERCP and provides extremely accurate results. A 'skinny' Chiba-type needle is used under local anaesthesia, and patient discomfort is minimal.

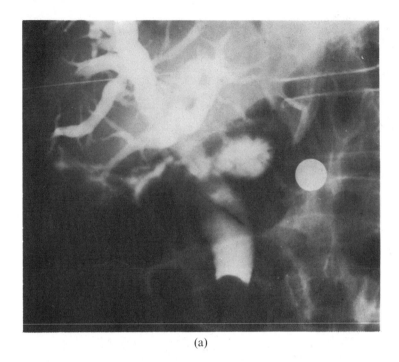

(a)

The following are illustrative cases.

Case 1. A 67-year-old severely jaundiced male patient in hepatorenal failure was examined by PTC and *Fig.* 11.23a, b show obstruction of the lower end of the common bile duct by an impacted gall stone, occlusion of the cystic duct by a gall stone resulting in non-filling of the gall bladder, and dilated intrahepatic and extrahepatic bile ducts.

Case 2. A 40-year-old man with a history of previous obstructive jaundice due to carcinoma of head of pancreas, treated by cholecystojejunostomy drainage several months before his present admission, now presented with recurrence of the jaundice and external bile leakage to the anterior abdominal wall. *Fig.* 11.24 shows the PTC findings, namely some dilatation of the intrahepatic bile ducts, occlusion of the upper common hepatic duct (by tumour) and a fistulous track extending downwards to the anterior abdominal wall from the common hepatic duct. An experienced operator can outline dilated bile ducts by PTC in 100% of cases, and will be successful in outlining about 80% or more non-dilated duct systems.

Case 3. A 57-year-old female patient with severe jaundice and in hepatorenal failure. Ultrasonography and biochemistry had not provided conclusive evidence as to whether the jaundice was obstructive or non-obstructive. PTC (*Fig.* 11.25) shows some of the intrahepatic ducts to be slightly dilated whilst others were not dilated. Contrast passed freely through the extrahepatic ducts into gall bladder (containing gall stones) and duodenum, also outlining the pancreatic duct. However the common hepatic duct and adjoining right hepatic duct are stretched and displaced and the left intrahepatic duct system was not outlined. It was, therefore, considered that an intrahepatic mass such as metastases or hepatoma

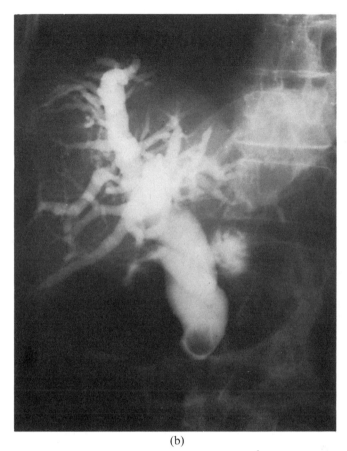

(b)

Fig. 11.23. Lower common bile duct obstruction by a large gall stone.

was present and liver biopsy confirmed the hepatoma. The patient died several days later but post-mortem examination was refused.

III. Interventional Radiology

There are several clinical situations where a radiologist can extend his diagnostic techniques to treat a life-threatening condition.

1. *Active Gastro-intestinal Bleeding*

The source of bleeding can be located by angiography and the bleeding can be stopped by infusing vasopressin into the appropriate artery through the catheter which has been placed in the vessel under fluoroscopic control.[7]

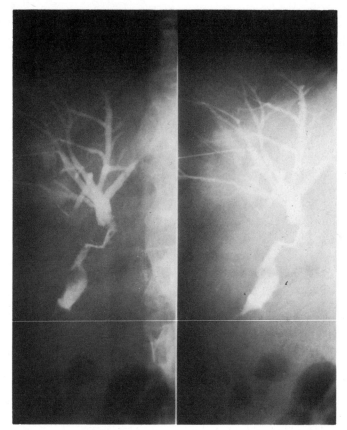

Fig. 11.24. Occlusion of common hepatic bile duct with fistula extending downwards.

Alternatively, the bleeding may be stopped by injecting embolic material, such as sterile absorbable gelatin sponge, through the arterial catheter.[7,8] Angiography is performed both before and after the treatment to decide whether the bleeding has stopped.

It is important to remember the condition of angiodysplasia of the caecum and right colon as a cause of lower gastro-intestinal bleeding which can sometimes be massive. *Fig.* 11.26a and b, which are films of an abdominal aortogram series, and *Fig.* 11.27a and b, a selective superior mesenteric angiogram, show angiodysplasia of the caecum and adjoining ascending colon in an elderly female patient who presented with massive bleeding per rectum. A barium enema showed diverticular disease of sigmoid and descending colon, and some of these diverticula contain barium residues on the angiogram films. It was thought that angiodysplasia should be excluded, and the angiogram was therefore performed.

After vasopressin infusion into the superior mesenteric artery, the bleeding stopped.

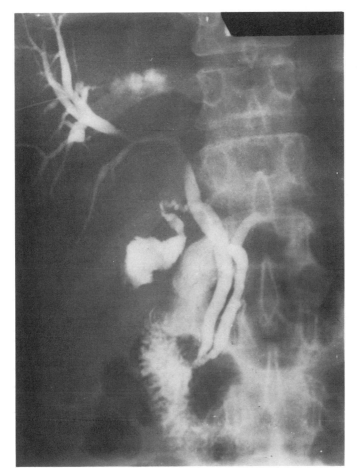

Fig. 11.25. Hepatoma compressing and displacing common hepatic duct.

2. *Active Bleeding from Oesophageal Varices*

Active bleeding from oesophageal varices in cases of portal hypertension can be stopped at least temporarily, by embolization techniques after locating the venous communications by percutaneous transhepatic portal venography,[9] and catheterizing the appropriate veins under fluoroscopic control. Embolic material is then injected through the catheter to occlude the venous communications.

3. *Obstructive Jaundice*

Obstructive jaundice can be relieved by percutaneous transhepatic catheterization. This can be done either to allow a critically ill patient, who may

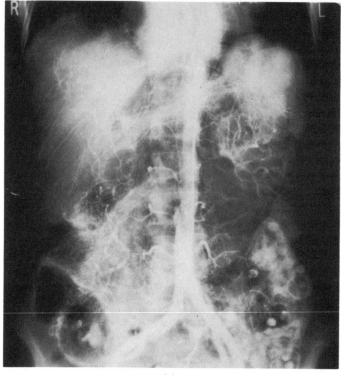

(a)

be in hepatorenal failure, to become fit enought for operation, or as an alternative to surgery where the cause of the obstruction is considered to be inoperable.[10] Drainage can be established through a catheter by the transhepatic method, and the bile allowed to drain externally into a collecting bag or, if the guide wire can be passed through the obstruction into the duodenum, internal drainage after insertion of an endoprosthesis can be achieved and can continue for a long period of time.

Fig. 11.28 shows an impacted gall stone in the lower end of the common bile duct causing severe obstructive jaundice. The patient was in hepatorenal failure, and considered unfit for immediate surgery. External bile drainage was achieved by percutaneous transhepatic catheterization and continued until the patient was fit for operation. In *Fig.* 11.28 the lower end of the drainage catheter is just above the impacted gall stone.

4. *Percutaneous Nephrostomy*

Percutaneous nephrostomy can be established to relieve obstruction of the kidneys and at the same time antegrade pyelography can be performed to

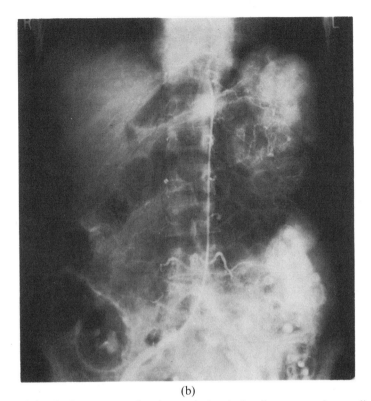

(b)

Fig. 11.26. Abdominal aortogram showing angiodysplasia of caecum and ascending colon.

provide information about the kidney and ureter as far as the level of obstruction. In placing the nephrostomy tube guidance by fluoroscopy, ultrasound and computed tomography have been used.[11]

ULTRASONOGRAPHY

This is a non-invasive technique, completely safe and though requiring a degree of patient co-operation to achieve the best results in many cases, ultrasonic examinations can be very useful in assessing many of the conditions that can arise in intensive care unit patients.

Ultrasonic techniques can be divided into the following types:

I. 'A' mode examinations distinguish fluid from solid tissue and can be useful in determining whether there is a mid-line shift in cases of intracranial pathology. However, the interpretation of mid-line shift can be misleading and the availability of CT scanning will reduce the need for 'A' mode examinations of the brain.

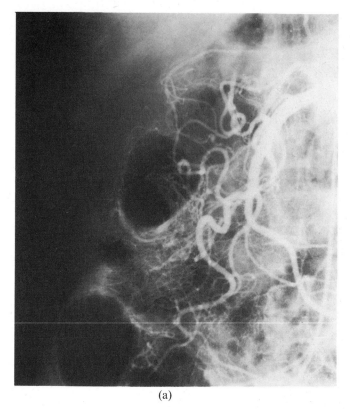

(a)

II. 'M' mode records the motion of structures such as the heart and pericardium and is useful in deciding whether there is a pericardial effusion. It has been said that as little as 16 ml of pericardial fluid can be detected by this method, and ultrasonography can be used to direct a needle tap of the effusion.

III. 'B' mode produces a two-dimensional anatomical picture and, with grey scale, differences in echo transmission patterns within soft tissue structures such as liver and pancreas can be recognized. Fluid-containing structures can be differentiated from solid tissue and the 'B' scan can be combined with the 'A' mode, e.g. in showing the pulsatility of the abdominal aorta.

'A' and 'M' mode equipment is portable and though most 'B' mode equipment is in the ultrasonic department, portable equipment with real-time is available.

The following are some examples of the ways in which ultrasonography can provide information in the intensive care unit patient.

1. Pericardial effusions can be outlined and occasionally ultrasonography is useful in locating pleural effusions and loculated empyemas. Likewise, loculated ascites can be detected. Ultrasound-guided needle tap can be performed.

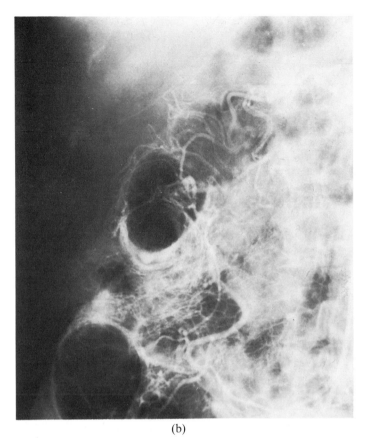

(b)

Fig. 11.27. (a) and (b) Selective superior mesenteric angiogram of the case shown in *Fig.* 11.26.

2. Examinations of the biliary system may reveal the intrahepatic ducts to be dilated in cases of obstructive jaundice. The cause of obstruction, e.g. a mass in the head of pancreas, may be observed. Gall stones may be seen in the gall bladder and external bile ducts. Metastases or other masses may be seen in the liver. The portal vein can be located.

3. Information about the pancreas can be achieved by ultrasonography and as shown in *Fig.* 11.29a and b the presence of a pancreatic pseudocyst can be demonstrated.

4. The size of the lumen of the abdominal aorta can be measured and aortic aneurysm detected, as may dissection of the abdominal aorta or leakage from it.[12, 13]

5. Doppler ultrasound can suggest patency or otherwise of tibial arteries.

6. Kidney scans may show cysts or other space-occupying lesions and demonstrate hydronephrosis. Ultrasound-guided biopsy can be achieved and also guided percutaneous nephrostomy drainage in obstructive urinary tract disease.

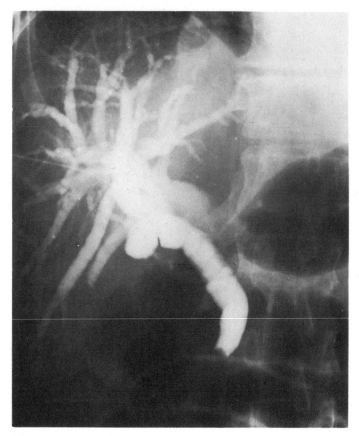

Fig. 11.28. External bile drainage via catheter. Impacted gall stone in lower common bile duct.

Although departmental examinations may be required to provide optimum information, much of the information detailed above could be achieved by bedside examinations using the appropriate portable ultrasonic equipment.

RADIONUCLIDE IMAGING

Many radionuclide imaging procedures can be performed at the bedside in the ICU using portable equipment, though the availability of such equipment depends, of course, on adequate financial resources. Other procedures can be undertaken in the department of nuclear medicine if the patient is suitably monitored (*see below*).

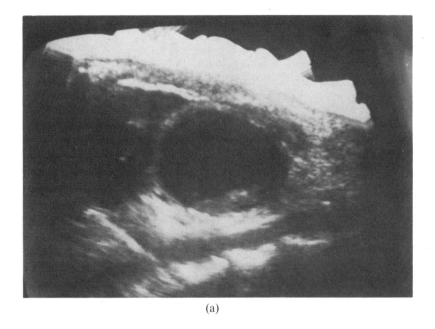

(a)

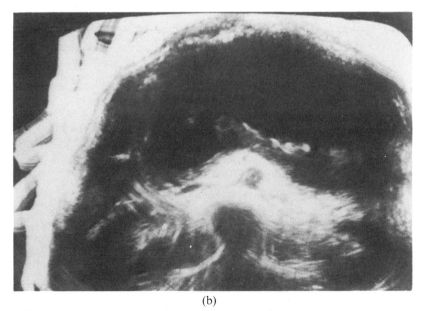

(b)

Fig. 11.29. (a) Longitudinal ultrasound scan showing pancreatic pseudocyst containing debris. (b) Transverse scan of same case.

Cardiovascular System

Two types of study are useful in ICU patients.
1. The adequacy of myocardial perfusion and the presence of myocardial infarction can be estimated either by a thallium 201 scan which shows maximal radionuclide accumulation in normal areas of myocardium and reduced accumulation in infarcted areas, or by a technetium 99m pyrophosphate scan which produces the opposite effect, i.e. maximal accumulation in infarcted zones.

Dual thallium 201 and technetium 99m pyrophosphate imaging improves diagnostic accuracy.[14]
2. Cardiac performance can be assessed either by obtaining a radionuclide angiocardiogram after intravenous injection of technetium 99m sulphur colloid, pertechnetate or human serum albumin or by gated cardiac blood-pool imaging, e.g. using technetium 99m labelled to either human serum albumin or autologous red blood cells.

These methods may prove useful in screening patients for admission to a coronary care unit when the diagnosis of myocardial infarction has been in doubt, for evaluating perioperative myocardial infarction in surgical ICU patients (e.g. after coronary artery bypass surgery), assessing the response of ICU patients to therapy, and evaluating patients with acute myocardial infarction, suspected left ventricular aneurysm and some types of cardiomyopathy.

Lungs

Pulmonary perfusion scanning shows decreased perfusion in areas affected by pulmonary embolism. Thus, 75–90% of patients with a normal chest radiograph, but perfusion scans showing lobar or segmental defects, will show pulmonary emboli on pulmonary arteriography.[15]

The perfusion scans are less convincing in patients with chronic obstructive airways disease (COAD) and pulmonary angiography may be required in more of these patients.

Perfusion scans can be performed at the bedside and serial scans can be used to assess the effectiveness of treatment.

Arteries and Veins

Gross anatomical assessment of the larger arterial vessels may reveal patency or blockage of these vessels, e.g. occlusion of an aortic bifurcation graft.[16]

Occlusion of pelvic or leg veins, or inferior vena cava by blood clots or obstruction of the superior vena cava may be revealed by radionuclide venography.

Kidneys

Renal function and anatomical abnormalities can be shown by radio-nuclides and renal ischaemia due to arterial injury may be suspected. Various types of renal pathology, including tumours, can be detected. Renal transplant patients can be serially examined for evidence of rejection and vascular patency.

Abdomen

Gallium 67 citrate scanning is very useful in localizing intra-abdominal abscesses, since the gallium becomes incorporated in granulocytes and accumulates in areas of active inflammation and in some tumours.

Radionuclide scans can demonstrate the size and position of the liver and spleen and show various abnormalities, such as abscesses, neoplasms and cysts, and are useful in the management of patients with abdominal trauma. Lacerations of the liver may be suspected on the scans. HIDA scanning is useful in deciding whether jaundice is obstructive or non-obstructive, and in the investigation of suspected acute cholecystitis.

Brain

Although radionuclide scans of the brain may reveal many abnormalities, CT scanning of the brain has more applicability to the ICU patient.

Skeleton

Although skeletal imaging can be excellent, there is limited applicability to the ICU situation.

The non-invasive nature of radionuclide investigations make them worth considering in the investigation of the critically ill patient.

COMPUTED TOMOGRAPHY (CT SCANNING)

This technique has proved of immense value in the investigation of brain disorders, outlining and localizing space-occupying lesions within the skull, such as haematomas, neoplasms, etc. Therefore the head scanner has a definite use in the investigation of critically ill patients who are suspected of having intracranial pathology. If a CT head scanner is available, it will reduce the need for other forms of investigation of these patients, e.g. radionuclide imaging of the brain, cerebral angiography and 'A' mode ultrasonography. In this situation a CT brain scan should be one of the earliest investigations to be performed.

As far as the use of CT body scanning is concerned in the investigation of ICU patients the position is far less clear-cut. There are several reasons for this. First, CT body scanners are, at the moment, much less widely available than head scanners in the UK. Secondly, the early generation of body scanners requires relatively long scanning time of approximately twenty seconds. Suspending respiration for such a long time may be difficult in the critically ill patient. Thirdly, the patient has to be transported to the department of CT scanning for the examination to be carried out, though of course, this also applies to angiographic examinations.

The newer generations of body scanners need only a short scanning time of a few seconds, so it seems likely that CT body scanning will have more applicability to intensive care investigations when these scanners are in operation. The body scan could then provide useful information in a wide variety of disorders such as intra-abdominal trauma to liver, spleen and kidneys, retroperitoneal haematomas, pancreatitis, tumours within the abdomen and chest and elsewhere, etc. As mentioned previously, CT can be used to guide a biopsy or drainage needle.

Nuclear Magnetic Resonance (NMR) can produce very good images of the head and body and is likely to be most useful in the investigation of certain types of ICU patients, particularly those with suspected intracranial space-occupying lesions such as haematomas and tumours. It is to be hoped that NMR units will eventually become widely available.

REFERENCES

1. Goodman L. R. and Putman C. E. (1978) *Intensive Care Radiology*, p. 32. St Louis, Mosby.
2. Ormond R. S., Rubenfire M., Anbe D. T. et al. (1971) Radiographic demonstration of myocardial penetration by permanent endocardial pacemakers. *Radiology* **98**, 35.
3. Adams F. G. (1979) A simplified approach to the reporting of intensive therapy unit chest radiographs. *Clin. Radiol.* **30**, 219–226.
4. Adams F. G. and Ledingham I. McA. (1977) The pulmonary manifestations of septic shock. *Clin. Radiol.* **28**, 315–322.
5. Beyer A. (1979) Shock lung. *Br. J. Hosp. Med.* **21**, 248–258.
6. Leeming B. W. A. (1973) Gravitational oedema of the lung observed during assisted respiration. *Chest* **64**, 719.
7. Walker W. J., Goldin A. R., Shaff M. I. et al. (1980) Per catheter control of haemorrhage from the superior and inferior mesenteric arteries. *Clin. Radiol.* **31**, 71–80.
8. Allison D. J. (1980) Gastrointestinal bleeding. Radiological diagnosis. *Br. J. Hosp. Med.* **23**, 358–365.
9. Lunderquist A. and Vang J. (1974) Transhepatic catheterization and obliteration of the coronary vein in patients with portal hypertension and esophageal varices. *N. Engl. J. Med.* **291**, 646–649.
10. Dooley J. S., Dick R., Olney J. et al. (1979) Non-surgical treatment of biliary obstruction. *Lancet* **2**, 1040–1044.
11. Meek D. and Austin C. (1980) Percutaneous nephrostomy and antegrade pyelography guided by computed tomography. *Xtract* **8**, 8–10.

12. McGregor J. C., Pollock J. G. and Anton H. C. (1975) The value of ultrasonography in the diagnosis of abdominal aortic aneurysm. *Scott. Med. J.* **20**, 133.
13. Bresnihan E. R. and Keates P. G. (1980) Ultrasound and dissection of the abdominal aorta. *Clin. Radiol.* **31**, 105–108.
14. Berger H. J., Gottschald A. and Zaret B. L. (1978) Dual radionuclide study of acute myocardial infarction; comparison of thallium-201 and technetium-99m stannous pyrophosphate imaging in man. *Ann. Intern. Med.* **88**, 145.
15. Jackson D. C., Tyson J. W., Johnsrude I. S. et al. (1975) Pulmonary embolic disease; the roles of angiography in lung scanning and diagnosis. *J. Can. Assoc. Radiol.* **26**, 139.
16. Wiener S. N. and Weiss P. H. (1975) Radionuclide imaging in the care of the critically ill patient. *Surg. Clin. North Am.* **55**, 729–753.

Chapter 12

Burns

W. H. Reid

In Great Britain each year approximately 60 000 people sustain burns, and, of these, approximately 20 000 are admitted to hospital. Figures for the United States are difficult to ascertain accurately, but it is thought that 2 000 000 people are burned in that country each year, of whom about 300 000 are admitted to hospital.

Approximately 20% of burns are sustained by children. Most burns are preventable and are due to carelessness on the part of the patients themselves, or, in those not able to look after themselves, carelessness on the part of the people who should be looking after them. Legislative prevention in most countries has been relatively ineffective, as it has been in Great Britain, in reducing the number of burns. Although many advances have taken place with flame-proofing of clothing fabrics and other safety requirements, the number of burns seen each year is not diminishing and, in fact, locally, in spite of a decrease in population in the catchment area of the unit, the number of burns is increasing. Throughout most series reported in the world, there has been a marked increase in numbers of patients with more extensive burns over the past 10 years or so.

MORTALITY

The seriousness of a burn, with its potential mortality, is often under-estimated by lay people and even, regrettably, by medical and nursing staff. A 20% full thickness skin loss burn produces an injury as severe as having both legs crushed by a train. The curve of mortality probability shown in *Fig.* 12.1 is based on the table of Bull[1]. There are many similar tables which give estimates of the probability of death in different parts of the world and all have close correlation. One rule of thumb assessment states that if the extent of the burn, expressed as a percentage of the body surface area, plus the patient's age is 75, that patient has a very poor prognosis. An important fact to be realized is that, if a healthy patient of between 20 and 24 years of age sustains a burn of approximately 60% of the body surface, that person

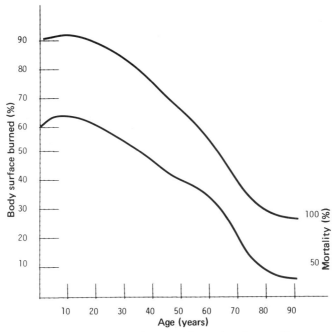

Fig. 12.1. The relationship between surface area burned and mortality.

has only a 50:50 chance of surviving. Because of the differences in the course of pathophysiological changes following a burn compared with other types of injury, a problem is that almost no matter how severe the burning injury, the patient is frequently conscious and able to reply to questions for some time after his admission to hospital. This is in contrast with the patient who has sustained severe multiple injuries, as in road traffic accidents or falls from buildings, where the patient is often unconscious. It is very difficult for the staff attending a seriously burned patient, and even more difficult for that patient's relatives, to accept that such burned patients have a very high risk of dying in the later stages. Thirty-five years ago most of the deaths occurred in the first 2 days or so, but this now rarely happens in the absence of other complicating factors, and the deaths now occur in the second or third week, or even later. The improvement in mortality is less than at first it seems, because of the delay of up to several weeks before the patient's death.

PATHOPHYSIOLOGY

Vascular Injury

After a burn injury, the capillary permeability is increased, especially in the area of a burn.[2] However, in extensive burns the permeability is increased not only in the area of a burn, but throughout the body, resulting in fluid being lost to the circulation. There is a very close relationship between the amount of fluid lost and the area of the body surface burn, which was first emphasized about 50 years ago. The vaso-active substance which is released in the burn has, as yet, not been isolated and allows molecules of less than 125 000 to freely leave the vascular bed and flow into the interstitial space. The fluid lost has the same electrolyte concentration as plasma and approximately 80% of the protein content. This increased capillary permeability is greatest in the few hours following a burn and slowly, after a period of 36–48 hours following the injury, returns to normal. The fluid collecting in the interstitial spaces causes the oedema of burns, which can cause secondary complications, such as compromising the upper airway and the circulation in the limbs. Oedema is little noticed: in a 5ft 8in, 70 kg patient, 8 l of oedema causes 0·5 inch increase in thoracic diameter and 2 inches on the leg. The cardiac output is also reduced immediately after a burn and this is thought to be due to a myocardial depressant factor in the serum[3]. The cardiac output returns to normal usually about 2 days after the injury and may, indeed, be supra-normal for several weeks. Blood glucose increases and carbohydrate metabolism goes from the aerobic towards the anaerobic pathway and acid metabolic products accumulate. The catecholamine and corticosteroid levels increase, but there is no evidence that the administration of steroids or ACTH is helpful. Unless there is good evidence of pre-existing steroid deficiency, these drugs should not be administered. There is a considerable loss of nitrogen as catabolism increases. Sodium is initially retained, sodium and chloride levels in the serum are increased, whereas potassium is lost. When diuresis occurs, usually between the second and third day post-burn, the levels return to normal, but in the first week the paradox of a low serum sodium in the presence of a normal or high total body sodium may be present, and is thought to be due to the intracellular shift of sodium and secondary aldosteronism.

Red Cell Destruction

The destruction of red cells is proportional to the extent and to the depth of the burn.[4] The cells are haemolysed by heat in the capillaries of the burn, and those which are not actually haemolysed are sufficiently damaged that they become sequestrated in the reticulo-endothelial system, and also significant numbers of red blood cells are trapped in the thrombosed vessels of the burn, which is more apparent in deeper burns than superficial ones. Red cell losses of at least 30% have been recorded in extensive deep burns. The phenomenon of 'sludging', as a result of haemoconcentration, leads to a decrease in perfusion of the peripheral tissue and diminution in the number of functioning red cells. Because of the red cell destruction, the appearance of haemoglobinuria is frequent in deep burns, but this is not of serious import unless it persists. Although significant numbers of red cells are destroyed, there is no evidence that the transfusion of whole blood is worthwhile in the first 24–48 hours post-burn, although later in the treatment of an extensive burn multiple transfusions are frequently necessary.

Blood Coagulation

Abnormalities of blood coagulation frequently appear in extensive burns, abnormal macroglobulins are often present and also fibrinolysins. Fibrinogen is increased.

The Injury to the Skin

Normally, skin controls evaporation of water from the body and prevents bacterial invasion. In an extensive burn, the water loss from the surface is greatly increased and, in a given area, the water loss is directly proportional to the depth of the burn. Because of this increase in water loss, there is an obligatory increase in the catabolic expenditure by the body and this, in the second and third weeks onwards in an extensive burn, can impose a critical demand on the patient's ability to provide the necessary calories from carbohydrate, protein and fat. When skin is burned, particularly in its full thickness, not only is the barrier to bacterial invasion destroyed, but in the deeper burns an ideal culture medium for bacteria is formed. A most useful illustration of the complicating factors in a large burn is shown in *Fig.* 12.2, based on the work of Hinton and quoted by Douglas Jackson.[5]

FIRST AID

The most effective way of taking the discomfort out of a burned area at the time of the burn is to apply cold water.[6] This has only comparatively recently been adopted in the first aid textbooks, but has probably been known as long as man has had the ability to make fire. On the basis of the traditional Icelandic method of treating burns, Ofeigsson[7] recommended the treatment of burns by cold water. He carried out extensive experiments on rats. These experiments showed that the application of cold greatly

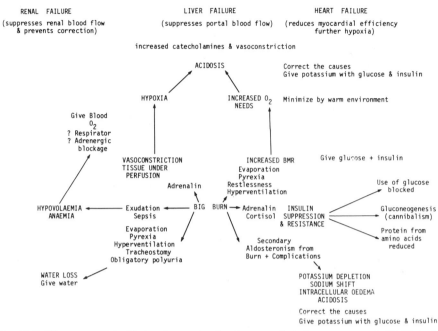

Fig. 12.2. The sequential effects of an extensive burn, and their management. BMR is the basal metabolic rate.

improved the prognosis of the burned animals.[7] Similar experiments were carried out by several other workers, usually on rats; unfortunately, the experimental error caused by the cyclical changes in the hair growth on a rat's skin has invalidated these results, and, from work done on human volunteers, there is no evidence to suggest that the application of cold has more effect than reducing the pain and has no continuing effect on the pathophysiological course of a burn.

INITIAL ASSESSMENT

In the initial assessment of a patient with a burn, the area of the body surface involved is more important than the depth, although, for a given area, the deeper the burn the more severe will be its effect on the patient. There is a close relationship between the area of a burn and the amount of fluid lost to the circulation. For practical purposes, the 'Rule of Nines' (*Fig.* 12.3) gives adequate clinical assessment of the area, but it is to be remembered that, in a child, the proportion of the body surface area of the head and neck to the total surface area is much greater than in an adult (*Fig.* 12.4) and this is significant because of the large number of children who receive scalds involving the head and neck and upper chest, and whose area of burn may be greatly underestimated, to the detriment of the patient.

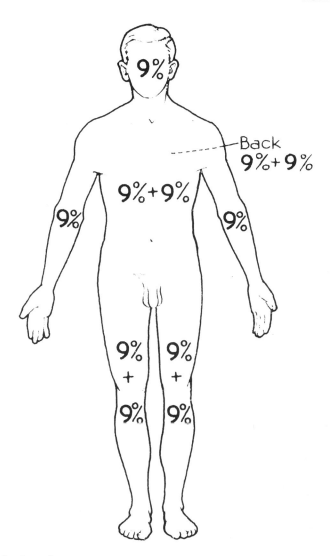

Fig. 12.3. Distribution of
'Rule of Nines' for assessment
of burn areas.

CRITICAL AREAS

In an adult the critical amount in area of the body surface burned is
15–20%, and in a child 10%. Patients with burns involving these amounts
will require, whether or not they are shocked when first seen, intravenous
resuscitation. A useful rule to remember, which is particularly helpful when
the burns are scattered, is that the area of one surface of the patient's hand
is approximately 1% of the body surface area, and a total calculation
of the area involved can be made by using this estimate.

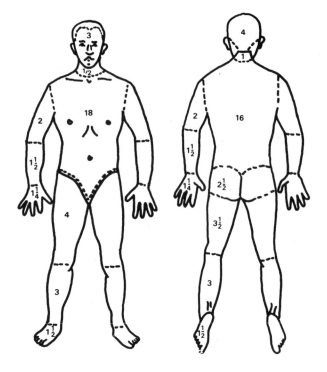

BODY PROPORTIONS MODIFIED FOR AGE

Age	1	2	3	4	5	6	7	8	9	10	11	12	Adult
Head & Neck	20	19	18	17	16	15	14	13	12	11	10	9	9%
Trunk	37	37	37	37	37	37	37	37	37	36	36	36	34%
Upper Limbs	16	16	16	16	16	16	16	16	16	17	17	17	19%
Lower Limbs	27	28	29	30	31	32	33	34	35	36	37	38	38%

N.B.   Figures on body represent
percentages

Fig. 12.4. Surface area related to age.

DEPTH OF BURN

Often burns are described as first, second and third degree. The difficulty in using such terminology is that, although they may mean almost the same thing to different observers in different parts of the world, they do not always do so and it is better to rely on a more anatomically descriptive terminology. An important factor in any burned patient is whether the full thickness of the skin has been destroyed or only the partial thickness of the skin. If the full thickness has been destroyed skin grafting is inevitable, whereas partial thickness burns will heal themselves in varying periods of time according to their depth, increasing in length towards full thickness destruction. An important point is that the deeper partial thickness burns, so-called 'deep dermal burns', take a considerable time to heal and lead to the post-burn hypertrophic scarring which is one of the major problems in plastic surgery.

METHODS OF ASSESSING THE DEPTH OF A BURN

Blanching of the burned area on pressure, with capillary return following release of the pressure, may be regarded as partial thickness skin loss, but there is evidence that the presence of early post-burn dermal circulation does not absolutely indicate partial thickness skin loss; nor does the absence of capillary return indicate full thickness skin loss.

The injection of intravenous dyes began in Glasgow in 1944. Gibson and Brown used Kiton fast green. More recently, disulphine blue has been used. When these dyes are administered intravenously, all the tissues in the patient become stained greenish-blue, apart from non-viable areas. Unfortunately, the dye takes at least 48 hours to disappear and, because of this, cannot be regarded as useful for routine purposes.

The fluorescence of the skin under ultra-violet light, after administering tetracyclines to the patient, has been used. Partial thickness skin loss burns give a golden-yellow fluorescence and full thickness burns do not fluoresce. Fluorescein itself has been used, and the fluroescence observed using a Wood's lamp has been used after the dye was administered intravenously, to estimate the depth of damage.

Thermography has also been used. This technique traces infra-red rays from the skin on to polaroid film, and varying patterns are revealed in shades of grey, and the differentiation between partial thickness skin loss and full thickness skin loss is obtained. This method has, until recently, been very expensive and impractical to use, as the patient had to be taken to the thermograph. However, with recent sophistication and miniaturization of such instruments, this is a more reasonable method of objectively assessing the depth of a burn. However, it is still very expensive.

Another method of assessing the depth, using similar physical principles of heat emitted from the skin, is the use of the radiometer, which also gives reasonable results.

Ultrasonic techniques have also been used to good effect.

Dupuytren[8] recognized, however, the difference in sensation between burns of different degrees and, for practical purposes at present, this method combined with the appearance of the burned tissue is probably the most clinically applicable method of diagnosing the depth of burns. A sterile hypodermic needle is used and the patient's sensitivity to the needle prick gives a guide to the depth of the burn. Partial thickness burns are not anaesthetic and may be hyperaesthetic, whereas in full thickness burns the needle is not appreciated as being sharp. Some burns are mottled white and red in appearance, are moist and are analgesic, but heal: therefore, the sensation to needle prick sign is more significant when present than when absent.

These clinical methods of assessing the depth have the fault of sub-jectivity, with the sensation test being subjective on the part of the patient and the appearance being subjective on the part of the observer. An ideal cheap method of obtaining an objective assessment of the depth of burns is still being sought. This is important if very early surgery is proposed, otherwise time, with the passage of a few days, will distinguish the depth of burn.

TREATMENT

After the initial assessment of the area of the burn and the depth has been made, all the patients with burned areas over the above-mentioned critical levels require resuscitative therapy and intensive care nursing facilities. Most extensive burns are painful, although the amount of pain of which the patient complains is often remarkably little. This is especially so when adequate resuscitation is begun quickly after the burning accident. However, sedation is usually required and an important point is that this sedation should be administered using the intravenous route, which will have to be established in any case, and the patient's response titrated against the amount of drug administered. Analgesics, such as morphine and pethidine, given by the routine subcutaneous or intramuscular routes, may not be adequately absorbed into the circulation and, therefore, they will not have the proper therapeutic effect. The danger is that further drugs may be given by a similar route of administration in order to try and obtain an analgesic effect. When the shock is controlled these deposits of analgesic can be absorbed into the circulation in an amount sufficient to constitute a further danger to the patient, e.g. respiratory depression.

An intravenous cannula should be inserted in a peripheal vein, prefer-ably through unburned skin and, if possible, in the upper rather than the lower limb. A central venous line is not required for routine purposes, certainly in the early stages of treatment of a burn. An important point is to place in the vein as large a diameter of cannula as is possible. The reason for this is related to Poiseuille's law relating to the flow of fluids in a tube. If the diameter of the tube is doubled, the flow in the tube is increased by 16 times for the same head of pressure; but to double the flow in a given bore of tube, four times the pressure is required. It is easy to reduce the flow of fluid in an intravenous drip, but it is frequently very difficult to have the drip flow as rapidly as desired. If possible, cut-downs should be avoided, because of the high risk of these wounds becoming infected, with con-sequent thrombophlebitis which may lead to systemic sepsis. Because of the risk of sepsis in a burned patient, ideally all sites of intravenous cannulae should be changed every 3 days.

Because of the importance of having accurate measurement of the urinary output, an indwelling Foley catheter is placed in the bladder connected to a closed drainage system. The urethral meatus should be cleaned daily and an antibacterial agent applied. A closed system of drainage is to be preferred to an open system as the incidence of bacteriuria is eight times less in the closed system.

Fluid Requirements

Many different regimes have been devised for intravenous resuscitation of seriously burned patients and, although in the past these have been adhered to with almost religious fervour by their advocates, it has been realized increasingly that their effectiveness in dealing with burn shock is almost equivalent. The common factor has not, as yet, been clearly isolated, but the possibility of the sodium ion being the critical one has recently been emphasized. No formula must be rigorously adhered to, as it only provides the clinician with a guide as to the amount of the fluid required by a patient, and it must not be followed slavishly. Moore[9] described the estimated requirement as a budget, which he says is 'a general scheme or forecast plan that must be changed as conditions vary and according to the needs and circumstances. It is a starting plan, it is a blue-print or a roadmap—it is not a precise chemical formula or expression that should be pursued with compulsive desire to avoid change'[9].

The Evans Formula

This formula[10] was the first widely used and was introduced in 1952. The size of the patient and the extent of the ·burn were related to the fluid requirement. In this formula equal parts of electrolyte and colloid solutions were given.

The Brooke Formula

From the Evans formula, the Brooke Army Medical Center developed the Brooke formula. The essential difference was that the colloid in this formula is withheld until the second 24 hours of the burn, only electrolytes being administered during the first 24 hours.

In both the Evans and the Brooke formulae, the fluid requirements are calculated as a maximum of 50% of total body surface. A burn area greater than 50% is calculated at 50% for the amount of fluid to be administered, because of the danger in estimates of over 50% causing pulmonary oedema.

The Parkland Formula

This formula was introduced by Baxter[11] in Dallas and was based on clinical and laboratory studies. This formula calls for 4 ml of Ringer lactate solution per kg for each percent of the burned area, without either colloid or electrolyte-free water during the first 24 hours. The total area of burn is used in calculating the requirement. During the second 24 hours no electrolyte solution is given, and glucose in electrolyte-free water and colloids in varying quantities are administered. The colloids are given either as protein or plasma expander. The more extensive the area of burn, the greater the amount of plasma expander required. The ratio of plasma expander to glucose is at least 1 of plasma expander to 3 of 5% glucose and water.

The above formulae have their origins in the United States and in that country it has always been very difficult to obtain human plasma. Much has been written in the American literature about the waste and ineffectiveness of plasma or protein solutions used in the first 24 hours, particularly the first 8 hours post-burn in the resuscitation of burned patients, but plasma has not been able to be used in the United States in a similar fashion to Great Britain, and its potential drawbacks have been over-emphasized.

$$\text{Give}\left(\frac{\text{wt in kg}}{2} \times \text{percentage area burned}\right)\text{ml of plasma in each of the}$$

following 6 periods over 36 hours from the TIME OF BURNING:

0–4 hours, 4–8 hours, 8–12 hours
12–18 hours, 18–24 hours,
24–36 hours.

Fig. 12.5. Muir and Barclay formula for the calculation of fluid requirements after a burn.[12]

The Muir and Barclay formula

There are several formulae used in Great Britain, but the most widely used is the Muir and Barclay formula[12] (*Fig.* 12.5). An important practical point which, surprisingly, requires emphasis is that the zero time in any formula refers, not to the time of the patient having a drip set up in hospital, but to the actual time of the burning incident. Therefore, because of delays in transportation, a patient may be several hours behind in the intravenous requirements and the calculated amount for the first 4 hours must be administered to the patient as quickly as possible to catch up the deficit.

Choice of Fluids

Plasma

The use of reconstituted freeze-dried human plasma has been said to be wasteful by American workers and, of course, there is the risk of hepatitis borne by the plasma. However, this risk is extremely small and is becoming even less with the use of small donor-pooled plasma. In one major burns unit there has been one proven case in over 1200 patients receiving plasma. Purified plasma substitute contains 92% albumin, 130 mmol sodium, 130 mmol chloride and 2 mmol potassium. In Great Britain recently, because of the development of plasma fractionating equipment, the Blood Transfusion Service has encouraged the use of this material instead of freeze-dried plasma. This solution is hepatitis free, but to obtain an equivalent resuscitation it has been found that between 30 and 40% more of this solution has been required to obtain an equivalent resuscitation than using reconstituted freeze-dried plasma.

Dextran Solutions

These polysaccharide solutions have been developed as plasma substitutes for the treatment of hypovolaemic states and are named according to the average molecular weight of the Dextran content. The two most commonly available in this country are Dextran 40, 'Rheomacrodex' or 'Lowmodex' and Dextran 70. Both of these have been widely used in the resuscitation of burns, but their use has mainly been in Scandinavia and North America.

Blood

Blood is required in any extensive burn, particularly where there is a significant full thickness component to the injury, but its use is generally applicable towards the end of the shock period[13] and in the later stages of burn treatment,[14] and it is not used to a significant degree as an initial resuscitative fluid to maintain the circulatory volume.

Saline

Saline has been used, but its use has largely been replaced by balanced salt solutions, e.g. Ringer's lactate, and it is this solution which is given as the basis of the first 24-hour resuscitation in copious amounts using the Parkland formula.

Hypertonic Lactated Saline

Because of the interest in the sodium ion, Monafo[15] used this solution containing 300 mmol sodium and 200 mmol lactate as the principal resuscitative fluid. This solution is not routinely available in most hospitals, certainly not in Great Britain, and cannot be recommended for routine use because of the significant risk of producing hypernatraemia, unless silver nitrate is used as the topical dressing agent for the burned surface. The silver nitrate leeches sodium ion onto the burned surface.

Metabolic Water

Often the necessary water to balance evaporative and insensible losses of water from the burned surface and from the lungs can be administered orally, provided the patient is not vomiting. The amounts given generally begin with 50 ml/h and are slowly increased to the necessary level. The calculated necessary amount of electrolyte-free water is usually between 1·5 and 2·0 ml per kg of body weight per hour, which may need to be increased if there is an excessive evaporative loss. If the toleration of the fluid administered by mouth is poor, it may be administered intravenously, and should be given as 5% dextrose solution in water. The fluid must not contain salt.

MONITORING THE PATIENT

The Haematocrit

This is normally 42–46% of the blood volume in a sample taken from a peripheral vein. When successful resuscitation is being achieved, this level should be about 35% or slightly higher.

Pulse Rate

The pulse rate is a very sensitive indicator of change in the patient's state. The pulse rate changes at a much earlier stage in worsening shock than does the blood pressure, and should be kept at a level, in an adult, of about 90 beats/min or less.

Blood Pressure

It is often difficult to apply a sphygmomanometer on burned tissue. Any degree of oedema gives a false reading and the blood pressure only drops comparatively late in the development of shock. The use of interarterial cannulation to assess the blood pressure cannot be recommended for routine assessment of resuscitation.

Central Venous Pressure

This measurement is not particularly helpful in assessing the patient's minimum requirements. It does, however, tell when a patient has been overloaded, but this overloading should be readily seen by the other regular measurements which are taken. It can be dangerous,[16] and the dangers quoted have been thrombosis, bacterial contamination, septicaemia, pulmonary and air embolism with haemorrhage. It is not an accurate guide in patients who have cardiac disease, pulmonary hypertension, abdominal distension, or in young children and in some other critically ill patients. In some units the use of a Swan–Ganz catheter[17] has been recommended to give an accurate indication of the intravascular volume, particularly in problem patients, but this technique, again, has the potential complications of thrombosis in the right ventricle with infection and endocarditis, and the technique should probably be reserved for patients with known cardiac disease.

Clinical Status (Vital Signs)

If the peripheral areas of unburned skin are warm, pink and dry, this is an indication that the peripheral circulation is satisfactory. However, if such areas become cold, grey and moist, this is an indication that the peripheral circulation is failing and probably that the central circulation is also inadequate. The response of the patient to questions can also provide useful information. In adults, although alcoholic addiction is prevalent in our cases and may be the cause of irrational answers and even confusion, irrationality and clouding of consciousness is an indication that there is hypoxia of the brain. Children's brains are particularly sensitive to hypoxia and this may be expressed as convulsions. These convulsions are not necessarily to be interpreted as a sign of intracranial abnormality, but an indication that the circulation is not being satisfactorily maintained.

Encephalopathy

The neurological syndrome has been reported mainly in children of cerebral irritability, hyperpyrexia with vomiting, twitching, convulsions and, finally, coma, with frequently a rise in the blood pressure. It is thought to be due to water and electrolyte imbalance, with a shift of water into the brain resulting in cerebral oedema, causing hypothalamic changes which result in hyperpyrexia of the 'core' of the body, whilst the 'shell' remains at a subnormal temperature. The treatment of this problem, should it develop, is usually to give a vasodilating drug, such as chlorpromazine, and heating the patient in an attempt to bring the 'shell' temperature to the level of the 'core'. When equilibration in the temperatures has been achieved, slow cooling is allowed.

Urinary Output

The urinary output is a very useful measurement of the adequacy of resuscitation and *Table* 12.1 shows satisfactory amounts.

Table 12.1 'Safe' levels of urine output in children and adults

Age, years	Urine output, ml/h
0–1	8–20
1–4	20–25
4–10	25–30
10+	30–50

Biochemical Monitoring

Blood and urine chemistry should be estimated at least daily, and the levels of sodium, potassium, chloride, bicarbonate, urea and creatinine assessed. Estimation of blood gases is frequently necessary to assess the acid–base balance of the patient and, also, particularly where there has been lung damage. Other estimations may be made as required, e.g. blood glucose levels if glycosuria appears, and protein levels. Liver function tests may be indicated, particularly if there is a history of pre-existing liver damage. The urine chemistry is usually assessed on an aliquot of a 24-hour collection, but may be done on an hourly specimen and the relative osmolar levels of blood and urine calculated.

Body Weight and Blood Volume

These estimations have been used in some centres to give an accurate guide to the progress of a seriously burned patient in the initial stages, but they require comparatively sophisticated equipment and are not recommended for routine use.

TOPICAL TREATMENT AND AVOIDANCE OF INFECTION

Initially, in the early part of this century, tannic acid was recommended to produce a sterile coagulum. However, with the high incidence of liver damage and necrosis, this was discontinued. In recent years there has been a move away from the topical application of antibiotics, because of the grave risk of producing antibiotic-resistant organisms. It is interesting to note that recently the Federal Drugs Administration of America has banned the topical application of gentamicin.

Silver Nitrate

Silver nitrate, 0·5% solution, is used in some centres as a topical application, with great effect.[18] Its advantages are in keeping the bacterial levels in the wound very low and in diminishing the development of bacteraemia and septicaemia. However, its disadvantages are that the treated area must be kept constantly moist with the solution. The solution stains the area dark brown; any surrounding clothes and bedclothes, etc. are also stained with the solution and this has been found unacceptable in some hospitals. It also leeches sodium from the wound and a very close watch must be kept on the patient's sodium balance.

Sulfamylon (Mafenide)

Sulfamylon, topical sulphonamide, is also used, but has the problem in a large proportion of patients of causing considerable discomfort for 20–30 minutes after its application, and has the risk, when extensive areas are covered, of inhibiting carbonic anhydrase, resulting in renal bicarbonate loss, causing metabolic acidosis.[19]

Because of these problems, *silver sulphadiazine*[20] is most commonly used. It is bacteriostatic and keeps the surface bacteria count low. It is particularly effective against Gram-negative organisms, but penetrates the eschar poorly. If there is any significant degree of Gram-positive contamination, it is recommended in a mixed infection to combine this application with chlorhexidine cream, accepting the fact that because of the relative sizes of the cations and anions in silver sulphadiazine and chlorhexidine when used in combination, the efficacy of chlorhexidine is lessened. An important point in the use of any topical application is to observe one of Joseph Lister's principles, which is to ensure that an adequate amount of active application reaches the appropriate surface and the application should be removed regularly, preferably daily or more often, and a fresh application administered.

ANTIBIOTICS

The tendency to use antibiotics topically, as mentioned above, is decreasing and also their use systemically. If possible, systemic use of antibiotics should be limited to a full therapeutic dose of an effective antibiotic determined by surface cultures and blood cultures, under bacteriological laboratory control. The use of broad-spectrum antibiotics should be curtailed, as it has been clearly shown in most burns centres throughout the world that the indiscriminate use of such antibiotics kills off more aggressive organisms, but leaves behind a culture of relatively non-aggressive but resistant organisms. These organisms flourish greatly and can be extremely difficult to eradicate and have often made a significant contribution to the ultimate death of seriously burned patients. In fact, occasionally, with injudicious use of antibiotics, bacteria have been removed to such an extent that an overgrowth of fungi has occurred and, in one reported series, 25% of the deaths in seriously burned patients showed evidence at post-mortem of fungal septicaemia.[21]

Prophylactic Antibiotics

There is little, if any, need for prophylactic antibiotics to be administered nowadays, except perhaps when the patient has been exposed to the risk of having a β-haemolytic streptococcal infection or harbouring this organism in the nasopharynx. If suspicion of this is held, a course of penicillin is adequate to deal with this particular organism. These organisms are, even today, sensitive to penicillin. Penicillin does not mask the development of other infection or the identification of more seriously pathogenic bacteria.

SPECIFIC BURN TOXIN

The presence of a specific toxin derived from burn skin was proposed by Russian and Czech workers who used convalescent serum obtained from patients who had had a significant burn several months before, which had healed.[22, 23] This serum was administered to patients who had recently been burned and who were at risk of developing 'toxaemia'. Fairly good results have been reported by a few groups, but this work has not, in fact, been corroborated clinically by any subsequent immunological studies and it seems that the beneficial effect of convalescent serum, if any, was, in fact, due to its antibacterial antibodies.[24]

IMMUNIZATION

Passive Immunization

Feller,[25] at the University of Michigan, has used a heat-killed phenol-preserved vaccine of *Pseudomonas*. This vaccine was given to healthy volunteers and an immune response obtained. Human hyperimmune plasma was prepared by vaccinating groups of volunteers, collecting the plasma and storing it frozen. This hyperimmune plasma was administered to patients at serious risk of developing a Gram-negative septicaemia, with a four-fold reduction in the number of deaths. Work in obtaining active immunity to *Pseudomonas* organisms was pioneered by Alexander and, more recently, Jones and Roe,[26] in Birmingham, have prepared a vaccine, which in field work in India, when administered to seriously burned patients within the first few days of burning, results in a significant titre of antibodies being obtained, and this has shown very promising early results in diminishing the death rate.

Tetanus Prophylaxis

The American recommendations and the practice in Great Britain differ widely. The Americans routinely give a booster dose of tetanus toxoid if patients have been immunized in the preceding 10 years and, if not, tetanus toxoid is administered, plus separate passive immunization with tetanus-immune globulin. Tetanus in burned patients is not a problem in Great Britain, and in most units administration of tetanus toxoid is not routine.

LOCAL CARE

The burned surfaces themselves should be gently, but thoroughly, cleaned using a detergent solution, such as cetrimide, followed by chlorhexidine in a watery solution. All loose dead tissue should be snipped off and blisters de-roofed. Blister fluid is initially sterile and, if the integrity of blisters could be ensured, that might be left as a protective cover for the regenerating epithelium at their base. However, in by far the greater proportion of patients, the blister becomes infected and the effect of this is often to damage the viable and regenerating epithelial remnants in the base of the blister, and can readily change the partial thickness self-healing burn to one of full thickness skin loss. After cleansing has been carried out, the burn may be left exposed, but in most centres today dressings are applied using an antibacterial agent, such as silver sulphadiazine and/or chlorhexidine, applied to the burned surface, the dressing then being built up with layers of gauze and, finally, crepe bandages are applied.

Facial and perineal burns are frequently treated by the exposure method, but it should not be assumed that this method is one of neglect, and frequently these burns require even more attention than those treated with dressings. The problem is that the crust which develops tends to crack and, whilst the external surface may appear dry and free from infection, frequently infection has penetrated the cracks and underneath the crust is a collection of pus. Burns of the limbs are generally dressed, because it is difficult to prevent the cracking of the burned surface when movements are carried out.

The drying of the burned surface is recommended in some continental centres using compressed air or oxygen, with apparently good effect, and recently hyperbaric oxygen monochambers have been developed,[27] which dry out the burned surface and are also said to render the environment unsuitable for bacterial proliferation. However, these chambers are not in routine use as they are very expensive, and also a considerable proportion of patients who have been submitted to this form of therapy complained of claustrophobia and could not tolerate being in these chambers for more than short periods at a time.

ESCHAROTOMY

In circumferential burns, particularly of the limbs, the viability of the distal portions of the affected limbs may be seriously at risk, because the development of oedema under the burned surface compromises the distal circulation. In these affected limbs, mid-lateral escharotomies are recommended. These escharotomies may be done without anaesthesia, as the burn is inevitably of full thickness skin loss and, therefore, the patient is insensitive to the burned surface being cut with a scalpel. Such properly placed and used escharotomy incisions often surprisingly spring widely apart, showing the amount of tension in the burned skin. Escharotomies are also frequently of help where there are full thickness burns of the chest wall, which compromise the respiratory excursion. Several vertical incisions in the anterior axillary line, with perhaps transverse incisions at the lower costal margin, are beneficial in restoring a worthwhile degree of chest expansion.

PHYSIOTHERAPY

It is most important that all joints, as far as possible, should be put through a full range of movement at least once a day if not more often, and also chest physiotherapy is extremely important. No matter how seriously burned the patient is, ambulation should be encouraged on as early a date following the injury as is feasible, using supportive bandaging on the legs.

RESPIRATORY, RENAL AND NUTRITIONAL PROBLEMS

With the increasing length of survival of seriously burned patients, three particular problems arise. These are respiratory problems following inhalational burns, renal failure and nutritional problems.

Respiratory Problems

Over the past 15 years or so, although the number of burns sustained from open coal fires has dramatically decreased, this has been more than made up by the increasing frequency of burns sustained in house fires. Many furnishing fabrics, when burned, produce highly dangerous substances, which greatly irritate the lung and which interfere with gaseous exchange in the alveoli. A problem is that the effects of such substances may not be immediately apparent on the patient's arrival at hospital and the respiratory problems only become apparent after 24 hours or even longer.[28] When a patient is seen who has been in a house fire, whether or not there is significant burning of the skin, the patient should be admitted for observation, and a routine chest X-ray taken, which initially is often surprisingly normal even after prolonged exposure to smoke. Blood gases, carboxyhaemoglobin and blood cyanide levels should be measured. Reliance on serial blood gas estimations alone has proved to be inadequate for foretelling the patients who will require ventilation, and a technique which will identify early on the patients who require ventilation is being actively sought. When the respiratory distress syndrome develops, with rapid and significant deterioration in the levels of oxygen and carbon dioxide in the blood, ventilation is mandatory but is often therapeutically ineffectual.

Steroids

The question of administering steroids to patients with respiratory problems is frequently raised. This is a decision which should be taken on a full assessment for each individual involved patient. Steroids may prevent progressive respiratory problems, but, if administered, should be given in one or two large doses at the most, e.g. 120–200 mg of methylprednisolone or 1500–3000 mg of hydrocortisone. It is most important not to put the patient on a continued or maintenance dose of steroid, as this greatly enhances the risk of sepsis.

Because of the difficulty in prognosticating the patients at risk, various regimes are being pursued, e.g. fibreoptic bronchoscopy,[29] which is an invasive technique and, even if it is done properly by an expert, cannot be routinely advocated in all patients who have inhaled smoke. Xenon scintigraphy of the lungs has also been carried out with good effect in some parts of the world[30] but it is not a method which is routinely applicable in most hospitals. It has been recommended by some that all patients exposed to smoke should be ventilated, but this non-critical all-or-nothing response to the injury carries a very considerable morbidity and ventilation should be used only in patients who definitely require it.

Tracheostomy

If ventilation is likely to be required for more than a few days, tracheostomy is probably indicated.

Renal Problems

In extensive burns acute renal failure can occur. A regular assessment of hourly urinary volumes gives a reasonable indication of the function of the kidneys, but urinary output, used as the sole criterion of renal function in very extensive burns, can be fallacious and in such patients, regular observations of blood urine chemistry and the relative osmolalities should be carried out.

Haemoglobinuria

When burns are deep, haemoglobinuria may appear, and when much muscle tissue has been destroyed, particularly by electrical burns, myoglobinuria is often present. The pigment in the urine often clears in a few hours and does not return, and its appearance is not, in itself, of serious import unless there is prolonged or repeated haemoglobinuria or myoglobinuria. The persistent appearance over a prolonged time of pigment in the urine is an ominous predictor of renal failure and, as a first step, diuresis is attempted using mannitol, provided that the fluid load given to the patient has been adequate, in a dose of 1 g per kg body weight given as a 20% solution, over 30–40 minutes.

Dialysis

Once renal failure has become established, it has been our experience that dialysis of such patients is ineffective in tiding the patient over until the renal function returns, and uniformly such patients die.

Nutritional Problems

In extensive burns there is usually a severe nutritional deficit related to excessive catabolism, from the third week onwards. It is inappropriate to discuss this fully here, as dealing with these nutritional problems is part of the continuing care of an extensively burned patient, rather than in the intensive early care.

Hot air

It has been shown, particularly by Swedish workers and corroborated in Birmingham, that keeping the patient at 32 °C very greatly diminishes weight loss and seems to cut down the hypermetabolism. Initially this was carried out using sophisticated and expensive air-conditioning systems, but more recently simpler patient-controlled infra-red heaters have been used to good effect.[31]

Hyperalimentation

As it is infrequent for there to be any alimentary tract absorption problem in burns, the route of enteral feeding should be used, often supplementing patients' normal oral intake, with a fine bore nasogastric tube. If possible, the use of intravenous feeding should be avoided, because of the great risks of infective complications from it.

CURLING'S ULCER

Acute ulceration of the stomach or duodenum associated with burns is known as Curling's ulcer.[32] Complications such as bleeding or perforation, carry a high mortality. As a preventive measure, the administration of antacids to keep the pH of the gastric juice at 7, has been strongly recommended.[33] More recently, H_2-receptor antagonists, e.g. cimetidine, have been used in the prevention of gastrointestinal ulceration.

SURGERY IN THE EARLY STAGES

In most centres aggressive surgery of full thickness skin loss is limited to burns of 15%, or at the most 20%, of the body surface area. The problems of blood loss are very great[34, 35], and the demands on the Blood Transfusion Service enormous. Recently, in the United States, partial excision of extensive deep burns has been carried out at intervals of several days, limiting each excision to approximately 15% of the body surface and using allograft material mainly to cover the resultant defect. This and the other method of excision, combined with immunosuppression and allografting,[36] are methods which can only be carried out in the most specialized units, and cannot, as yet, be routinely recommended.

A full discussion of the surgery of burns is beyond the scope of this chapter, but one indication for early surgery which can, indeed, be life-saving, is in the case of deep high-tension electrical burns,[37] where the damage to the deeper tissues under the skin, particularly the muscles, is such that the risk of anaerobic infection is so great that affected parts of the limbs should be amputated in a guillotine fashion as soon as is reasonably feasible after the admission and resuscitation of the patient.

Tangential Excision

This is a concept introduced in Yugoslavia[38] to deal particularly with burns where the damage is at the deep dermal level. The shaving of such burns within the third or fourth post-burn day, and the immediate application of skin grafts, is helpful in reducing the amount of hypertrophic scarring to which such burns are liable if treated in other fashions. This technique is, however, limited generally to smaller burned areas and not to those burns requiring intensive care treatment.

REFERENCES

1. Bull J. P. (1971) Revised analysis of mortality due to burns. *Lancet* **2**, 1133–1134.
2. Baxter C. R. (1974) Fluid volume and electrolyte changes of the early post burn period. *Clin. Plast. Surg.* **1**, 693–709.
3. Merriam T. W. (1962) Myocardial function following thermal injury. *Circ. Res.* **11**, 669–673.
4. Topley E., Jackson D. M., Cason J. S. et al. (1962) Assessment of red cells in the first two days after severe burns. *Ann. Surg.* **155**, 581–590.
5. Jackson D. M. (1970) Burns as a special problem in trauma. *J. Trauma* **10**, 991–996.
6. Earle J. (1799) *Means of Lessening the Effect of Fire on the Human Body*. London, C. Clarke.
7. Ofgeigsson O. J. (1959) Observations and experiments on the immediate cold water treatment for burns and scalds. *Br. J. Plast. Surg.* **12**, 104–119.
8. Dupuytren G. (1832–34) *Leçons Orales de Clinique Chirurgicale Faites a l'Hotel Dieu de Paris*, Vol. 1. Paris, G. Bailliere.
9. Moore F. D. (1970) The body weight burn budget. *Surg. Clin. North Am.* **50**, 1249–1265.
10. Evans E. I., Purnell O. J. Robinett P. W. et al. (1952) Fluid and electrolyte requirements in severe burns. *Ann. Surg.* **135**, 804–815.
11. Baxter C. R. and Shires T. (1968) Physiological response to crystalloid resuscitation of severe burns. *Ann. N.Y. Acad. Sci.* **150**, 875–894.
12. Muir I. F. K. and Barclay T. L. (1974) *Burns and their Treatment*, 2nd ed. London Lloyd Luke.

13. Muir I. F. K. (1961) Red cell destruction in burns. *Br. J. Plast. Surg.* **14**, 273–302.
14. Loebl E. C., Baxter C. R. and Curreri P. W. (1973) The mechanism of erythrocyte destruction in the early post-burn period. *Ann. Surg.* **178**, 681–686.
15. Monafo W. W. (1970) The treatment of burn shock by the intravenous and oral administration of hypertonic lactated saline solution. *J. Trauma* **10**, 575–586.
16. Warden G. D., Wilmore D. W. and Pruitt B. A. (1973) Central venous thrombosis: a hazard of medical progress. *J. Trauma* **13**, 620–626.
17. Swan J. J. C. (1975) Balloon flotation catheters: their use in haemodynamic monitoring in clinical practice. *J. Am. Med. Assoc.* **233**, 865–867.
18. Constable J. D. (1973) Silver nitrate in the treatment of burns. In: Lynch J. B. and Lewis S. R., ed., *Symposium on Treatment of Burns*. pp. 113–116. St Louis, C. V. Mosby Co.
19. Asch M. G., White M. G. and Pruitt B. A. Jr (1970) Acid-base changes associated with topical Sulfamylon therapy: retrospective study of 100 burned patients. *Ann. Surg.* **172**, 946–950.
20. Fox C. L. Jr (1973) Use of silver sulphadiazine in burned patients. In: Lynch J. B. and Lewis S. R., ed., *Symposium on the Treatment of Burns*, pp. 123–128. St Louis, C. V. Mosby Co.
21. MacMillan B. G., Law E. J. and Holder I. A. (1972) Experience with candida infections in the burned patient. *Arch. Surg.* **104**, 509–514.
22. Feodorof N. A. and Skurkovich S. V. (1962) Immunohaemotherapy of burn sickness. In: Arts C. P., ed., *Research in Burns*, 266. Philadelphia, F. A. Davis.
23. Dobrokovsky M., Dolezalova J. and Pavkova L. (1962) Immunological and biochemical changes in burns. In: Arts C. P., ed., *Research in Burns*, 260.
24. Craig R. D. P. (1965) Immunotherapy for severe burns in children. *Plast. Reconstr. Surg.* **35**, 263–270.
25. Feller I. (1966) The use of pseudomonas vaccine of hyperimmune plasma in the treatment of seriously burned patients. In: *Research in Burns*, 470–473.
26. Jones R. J., Roe E. A. and Gupta J. L. (1978) Low mortality in burned patients in a pseudomonas vaccine trial. *Lancet* **21**, 401–403.
27. Hart G. B., O'Reilly R. R., Broussard N. D. et al. (1974) Treatment of burns with hyperbaric oxygen. *Surg. Gynecol. Obstet* **139**, 693–696.
28. Achauer B. M., Allyn P. A., Furnas D. W. et al. (1973) Pulmonary complications of burns: the major threat to the burned patient. *Ann. Surg.* **177**, 311–319.
29. Moylan J. A., Adib K. and Birnbaum M. (1975) Fiberoptic bronchoscopy following a thermal injury. *Surg. Gynecol. Obstet.* **140**, 541–543.
30. Pegg S. P., Hinckley V. M. and Aidashan N. (1978) Adjunct xenon scintigraphy and bronchoscopy in the early diagnosis of respiratory burns. *Burns* **4**, 86–91.
31. Danielsson U., Arturson G. and Wennberg L. (1975) The elimination of hypermetabolism in burned patients. *Burns* **2**, 110–114.
32. Pruitt B. A., Foley F. D. and Moncrief J. A. (1970) Curling's ulcer: clinicopathological study of 323 cases. *Ann. Surg.* **172**, 523–539.
33. McAlhany J. C. Jr, Czaja A. J. and Pruitt B. A. Jr (1976) Antacid control of complications from acute gastro-duodenal disease after burns. *J. Trauma* **16**, 645–649.
34. Jackson D., Topley E., Cason J. S. et al. (1960) Primary excision and grafting of large burns. *Ann. Surg.* **152**, 167–189.
35. Bennett J. E. and Thompson L. W. (1969) The role of aggressive surgical treatment in the severely burned patient. *J. Trauma* **9**, 776–783.
36. Diethelm A. G., Dimick A. R., Shaw J. F. et al. (1974) Treatment of a severely burned child with skin transplantation modified by immuno-suppressive therapy. *Ann. Surg.* **180**, 814–818.
37. Hunt J. L., Mason A. D., Masterson T. S. et al. (1976) Pathophysiology of acute electric injuries. *J. Trauma* **16**, 335–340.
38. Janzekovic Z. (1970) A new concept in the early excision and immediate grafting of burns. *J. Trauma* **10**, 1103–1108.

Chapter 13

The Alimentary System

D. H. Osborne and D. C. Carter

THE ALIMENTARY SYSTEM AND HOMEOSTASIS

The important functions of the alimentary system are the following.

I. *Digestive*

Mechanical and chemical digestion converts ingested protein, fat and carbohydrate into molecules small enough to be absorbed from the gut lumen. Pepsin initiates protein digestion in the stomach, and all food chemicals are broken down in the small bowel by enzymes in pancreatic and small intestinal secretion. Bile acids aid digestion by emulsifying fat.

II. *Absorptive*

Food chemicals, vitamins, electrolytes and water are absorbed from the small bowel, and absorption of water and electrolytes continues in the large bowel. Useful constituents of bile are reabsorbed largely in the distal small bowel, and an enterohepatic circulation allows the total bile acid pool to circulate 6–10 times a day.

III. *Excretory*

The lower gastrointestinal tract controls excretion of undigested food residue and waste products. Excretion of any compound from the body is governed by water solubility and molecular weight. Water-soluble compounds with mol. wt less than 300 can be excreted by the kidney but heavier less soluble compounds are excreted by the liver, usually after conjugation with glycine or glucuronic acid. Cholesterol is excreted in bile in micellar solution with bile acids and phospholipids.

IV. *Endocrine*

The alimentary system probably contains a greater mass of endocrine cells than all of the discrete endocrine organs of the body taken together. The alimentary endocrine cells are scattered throughout the gastrointestinal mucosa or aggregated in the islets of Langerhans. Most of these endocrine cells appear to regulate motility, intermediate metabolism or exocrine secretion, but only gastrin, cholecystokinin, secretin, gastric inhibitory peptide, insulin and glucagon have established physiological roles.

V. *Barrier Function*

The gastrointestinal mucosa is the largest area of interface between man and his environment, and normally bars entry of luminal micro-organisms. Hydrochloric acid is inimical to bacterial growth but does not entirely sterilize gastric contents. Luminal bacterial counts increase in the distal small bowel and large bowel. The organisms present are anaerobes (*Bacteroides*, clostridia and anaerobic streptococci) and to a much lesser extent, aerobic coliforms, *Proteus, Pseudomonas* and streptococci. Anaerobes normally exceed aerobes by some 1000:1. The biliary tract is normally sterile.

CONSEQUENCES OF ALIMENTARY MALFUNCTION

I. *Digestive Malfunction*

Loss of digestive capacity is seldom a problem in intensive care patients. However, such patients are often unable to maintain an adequate oral intake or clinical circumstances may dictate that the alimentary system be rested. These difficulties can usually be overcome by appropriate recourse to nasogastric or nasoenteric tube feeding, elemental diets or parenteral nutrition (*see* Chapter 7).

Inappropriate digestive function, as in the 'autodigestion' of peptic ulceration or acute pancreatitis, may either cause or complicate critical illness.

II. *Absorptive Malfunction*

Failure to absorb adequate amounts of nutrients from the gut may arise;
1. As an inevitable consequence of maldigestion.
2. Due to temporary or permanent loss of absorptive surface area as in intestinal obstruction, fistula formation or massive intestinal resection.
3. When nutritional demand exceeds intake or absorptive capacity, as for example in burned patients with sepsis.

III. *Excretory Malfunction*

Loss of hepatic excretory function is considered elsewhere (Chapter 18).

IV. *Endocrine Malfunction*

Loss of alimentary endocrine function is a rare but significant problem in critically ill patients under the following circumstances:
1. Transient diabetes mellitus may be a feature of acute pancreatitis but is usually mild and easily controlled. Permanent diabetes often accompanies chronic pancreatitis and is invariable after total pancreatectomy. Post-pancreatectomy patients are particularly sensitive to insulin (possibly because of loss of pancreatic glucagon) and management is often complicated by maldigestion and malabsorption due to loss of pancreatic exocrine function.
2. Gastric hypersecretion and peptic ulceration may follow massive small bowel resection. The cause of hypersecretion is uncertain but it may be due to loss of an intestinal inhibitor of gastric secretion.

V. *Loss of Barrier Function*

Stasis favours bacterial overgrowth in any part of the alimentary system, and promotes colonization of the biliary tree by aerobic organisms (*Escherichia coli, Klebsiella aerogenes* and *Streptococcus faecalis*) and, to a lesser extent, by anaerobes. Achlorhydria allows bacterial proliferation within the stomach and gut organisms (*see above*) may be recovered from gastric aspirates. Luminal bacterial overgrowth increases the risk of septic complications following gastrointestinal surgery.

Bacterial toxins are frequently present in portal venous blood but are normally removed by reticuloendothelial cells within the hepatic sinusoids. Hepatic malfunction (as in obstructive jaundice) may cause this 'filter' to fail with resultant systemic toxaemia.

Bacteria escape from the lumen of the gut and biliary system whenever there is loss of mural viability with gangrene and/or perforation. Bacterial peritonitis follows and organisms are absorbed into the blood stream to produce bacteraemia and septicaemia.

COMMON SYNDROMES OF ALIMENTARY MALFUNCTION

The rest of this chapter is devoted to the common syndromes of alimentary malfunction which may cause or complicate critical illness (*see Table* 13.1). Each problem is considered in terms of its pathophysiology, investigation and management, but the details of operative treatment will not be discussed.

Table **13.1 Common syndromes of alimentary malfunction**

Acute upper gastrointestinal bleeding
   Erosive gastritis
   Acute duodenal ulceration
Intestinal obstruction
Acute pancreatitis
Biliary tract disease
   Acute cholecystitis
   Cholangitis
   Acalculous cholecystitis
   Hepatorenal syndrome
Peritonitis
Acute mesenteric vascular ischaemia
Fistulae

ACUTE UPPER GASTROINTESTINAL BLEEDING

This section is concerned primarily with bleeding as a complication of critical illness although the principles of management apply to all cases of gastrointestinal haemorrhage.

Pathophysiology of Upper Gastrointestinal Bleeding

Gastrointestinal bleeding as a complication of critical illness is almost always due to acid-pepsin digestion of gastroduodenal mucosa resulting in erosive gastritis or acute duodenal ulceration.

I. *Pathophysiology of Erosive Gastritis*

Major operative procedures, multiple trauma, respiratory failure and jaundice may all be complicated by erosive gastritis. The risks are particularly great in patients with hypotension, sepsis and renal failure. The patient develops multiple black-based shallow mucosal erosions with coagulative necrosis and interstitial haemorrhage. Intervening areas of mucosa are also inflamed and the process may affect all or any part of the gastric mucosa.

Gastric Lumen

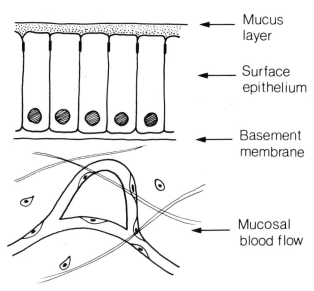

Mucus layer

Surface epithelium

Basement membrane

Mucosal blood flow

Fig. 13.1. Diagrammatic representation of the components of the gastric mucosal barrier.

Under normal circumstances, the gastric mucosa is an effective barrier to back-diffusion of H^+ from the lumen. Factors which maintain this barrier include the covering layer of mucus, the apical cell membrane of surface epithelial cells, normal mucosal acid–base balance and metabolism, and an appropriate mucosal blood flow (*Fig.* 13.1). Failure of any component reduces mucosal resistance to damage by acid-pepsin, allows acid influx from the lumen, and results in inflammation, erosion and bleeding. Gastric hypersecretion is not necessary for erosive gastritis to occur; it is damage to the mucosa which has cardinal importance.

In the context of critical illness, mucosal barrier damage is probably initiated by bile reflux. Bile salts, such as sodium taurocholate, have a detergent action and disrupt apical cell membranes causing cell extrusion. Bile reflux alone does not produce the full spectrum of mucosal damage;

mucosal ischaemia plays a critical role by increasing susceptibility to injury, and acid-pepsin must be on hand to exploit the damaged barrier and exacerbate inflammation.

II. *Pathophysiology of Acute Duodenal Ulceration*

Gastric hypersecretion, rather than mucosal damage, is the primary factor in acute duodenal ulceration during critical illness. Such acute ulcers are associated particularly with severe burn injury (Curling's ulcer) and trauma to the central nervous system (Cushing's ulcer).

Management of Upper Gastrointestinal Bleeding

I. *Resuscitation*

Blood is grouped and cross-matched so that 4–6 units are on hand. A free-flowing line is established to allow *rapid* transfusion; peripheral veins are inadequate for this purpose and a cannula is placed in the subclavian, jugular or basilic veins. If the patient is shocked, plasma or plasma substitute is used until blood is available; otherwise normal saline is infused in the first instance.

A nasogastric tube (16 Fr) is passed to keep the stomach empty, prevent vomiting, and monitor continued or renewed bleeding. Iced saline lavage is said to reduce peptic activity but there is little evidence to support its use and we do not employ it.

Pulse and blood pressure are monitored every 15 minutes, a urinary catheter is inserted to monitor hourly output, temperature is monitored 4-hourly, and haematocrit is checked daily. A separate central venous pressure (CVP) line is an invaluable guide to the rate of fluid replacement in the elderly and those with myocardial insufficiency. Oxygen is given to all shocked patients at 4 l/min through a well-fitting Hudson mask, unless there are anxieties regarding carbon dioxide retention (p. 99). Periodic checks of arterial H^+ concentration, Po_2 and Pco_2 are used to monitor gas exchange and detect derangement in acid–base balance.

Impaired haemostasis is anticipated in patients needing massive transfusion and in those with deranged liver function. Stored blood transfusion quickly results in deficiencies of labile Factors V and VIII, but these defects can be restored by fresh frozen plasma (FFP; one pack for every 3 l of blood transfused). Regular clotting screens to determine thrombin time, prothrombin time, kaolin-cephalin coagulation time and platelet count are of value in patients with massive bleeding. Vitamin K_1 is given routinely to all jaundiced patients when prothrombin time is prolonged (5–50 mg intravenous), but FFP is needed in patients with liver disease who are unresponsive to vitamin K.

II. *Define the Source of Bleeding*

Although the source of bleeding may be suspected clinically, it must always be defined by endoscopy. Resuscitation must be a matter of urgency, the aim being to proceed as quickly as possible to endoscopy so as to place further therapy on a rational basis. Barium meal examination or angiography are reserved for those patients with massive bleeding where endoscopy fails to define the source of bleeding. Endoscopy can be carried out quickly without necessarily moving the patient to another part of the hospital, requires only sedation (in our practice, intravenous diazepam 5–20 mg), and, in competent hands, is safe and accurate.

End-viewing flexible endoscopes allow inspection of the oesophagus and stomach, although it may prove difficult to inspect the gastric fundus and duodenal bulb. The fundus can be viewed from below if the instrument is flexed in the stomach while thorough inspection of the duodenal bulb may mean recourse to an oblique or side-viewing instrument. Massive bleeding may prevent adequate inspection despite lavage with iced water and, on rare occasions, one may have to proceed directly to surgery in the face of life-threatening haemorrhage.

III. *Institute Appropriate Therapy*

1. *Erosive Gastritis*

Histamine H_2-receptor antagonists have been used prophylactically to reduce the incidence of gastrointestinal bleeding in patients with fulminant liver failure,[1] and there is evidence from uncontrolled trials that they prevent further haemorrhage in patients with established gastritis. It has been our practice to prescribe cimetidine (400 mg 6-hourly by intravenous infusion) in all critically ill patients and in those known to be bleeding from erosive gastritis.

All agree that cimetidine reduces the amount of acid-pepsin available to exploit damaged mucosal defences, but there is debate as to whether it has additional 'cytoprotective' properties.[2] It has also been suggested that cimetidine antagonizes histamine-induced vasodilatation at sites of mucosal injury, thereby reducing bleeding.[3]

Antacids also prevent bleeding in critically ill patients[4] and recent reports suggest that they may be more effective than cimetidine. Priebe and colleagues[5] studied 75 intensive care patients randomized to receive cimetidine (300 mg 6-hourly) or intensive antacid therapy (Mylanta II* instilled hourly in amounts needed to keep intragastric pH above 3·5). Upper gastrointestinal bleeding occurred in 7 of 38 cimetidine-treated

---

*Mylanta II is a proprietary preparation containing aluminium, magnesium hydroxide and simethicone.

patients and in none of the 37 antacid-treated patients. In the light of this study, we now supplement cimetidine by 2-hourly instillation of antacid (30 ml Aludrox alternating with 30 ml magnesium trisilicate) until the situation is clarified by further study.

Priebe and colleagues point out that actively secreting mucosa generates bicarbonate (the 'alkaline tide') in amounts equal to the amount of acid secreted into the lumen. They speculate that this alkali may be available to buffer influxing acid during damage to an uninhibited mucosa, whereas lack of available alkali renders a cimetidine-treated mucosa less able to cope with acid back-diffusion.

Maintenance of the gastric microcirculation and avoidance of acidosis are essential. Hypovolaemia reduces gastric mucosal blood flow and causes hypoxia with acidosis, and every effort must be made to restore and maintain circulating blood volume. Intravenous bicarbonate protects against experimentally induced mucosal damage[6] and, in keeping with Priebe's hypothesis, this may relate to enhanced mucosal ability to deal with acid influx.

Other non-operative measures said to prevent further bleeding from erosive gastritis include somatostatin infusion, intragastric instillation of nor-adrenaline and selective arterial infusion of vasopressin. None of these measures are of proven value and we have no experience of them.

Surgery is avoided if at all possible by intensive medical therapy but may be unavoidable if bleeding continues or recurs. There is understandable reluctance to submit ill patients to major surgery and considerable clinical judgement is needed to determine the need for operation (*Table* 13.2). The clinical decision is influenced by the patient's general condition, nature of the underlying critical illness, clotting screen and response to medical treatment.

Table 13.2. Guidelines for operative intervention in patients with massive upper gastro-intestinal haemorrhage

Operation indicated if

Whole blood transfusion exceeds 2500 ml in first 24 hours
Whole blood transfusion exceeds 1500 ml in second 24 hours
Significant rebleeding after 24 hours of intensive medical therapy

Factors favouring early operation

Patient older than 60 years
Patient bleeding from gastric or duodenal ulcer

If surgery is unavoidable, truncal vagotomy and subtotal gastrectomy is probably the best option. Truncal vagotomy and drainage is complicated by re-bleeding in over 25% of cases, whereas total gastrectomy increases operative mortality. Effective prophylaxis and intensive medical therapy have reduced the number of patients requiring surgery for erosive gastritis, but operative mortality rates for those patients who come to surgery range from 50 to 80%.

2. *Acute Duodenal Ulceration*

There is little evidence that cimetidine or antacid therapy prevents further bleeding from established gastric or duodenal ulcers, although both agents may promote ulcer healing. Persisting or recurrent bleeding from acute duodenal ulceration is an indication for surgery (*see Table* 13.2). The choice of operation lies between truncal vagotomy and subtotal gastrectomy, and truncal vagotomy with pyloroplasty after underunning the ulcer with non-absorbable sutures. In general, we advocate truncal vagotomy and pyloroplasty as the safer procedure, accepting that it may carry a slightly greater risk of re-bleeding.

If the patient is deemed unfit for surgery, alternative approaches include:
a. Arteriography with localization and cannulation of the main bleeding vessel which can then be embolized with blood clot or plastic polymer, or infused with vasopressin to cause selective local vasoconstriction.
b. Endoscopic electrocoagulation (monopolar or bipolar).
c. Endoscopic laser photocoagulation.

Success has been reported from uncontrolled trials of all these modalities of therapy. Current interest centres on controlled trials with the neodymium yttrium aluminium garnet (YAG) laser.

INTESTINAL OBSTRUCTION

Simple mechanical obstruction seldom places a patient in need of intensive care unless there is pre-existing cardiovascular, respiratory or renal disease. Strangulation obstruction is a much more serious illness, carries a mortality of around 30%, and frequently places a patient in need of intensive care. Adynamic (paralytic) ileus may complicate the course of a number of illnesses and, not infrequently, poses a problem in diagnosis and management in patients receiving intensive care.

Pathophysiology of Intestinal Obstruction

I. *Simple Mechanical Obstruction*

Fluid and gas accumulate proximal to the site of obstruction and cause bowel distension. The accumulating gas is mainly swallowed air; bacterial fermentation within the bowel makes only a minor contribution. The accumulating liquid is in part swallowed but is mainly gastrointestinal secretion. Some 8–10 l are secreted into the upper gastrointestinal tract each day, but all except 100–200 ml are normally reabsorbed distally. As Shields[7] showed, distension so alters mucosal function that water and electrolytes accumulate in the lumen. Although still within the body, this fluid is effectively lost from the extracellular fluid (ECF) compartment, a fact which should be borne in mind during resuscitation.

ECF loss becomes manifest as dehydration, haemoconcentration, rising blood urea and oliguria. The fluid lost is isotonic with plasma and slightly alkaline, but significant changes in acid–base balance are unusual. Pyloric stenosis is exceptional in that longstanding loss of gastric secretion is associated with significant metabolic alkalosis.

Unrelieved obstruction leads gradually to tachycardia, decreased venous return, hypotension, and finally to hypovolaemic shock. As a rough working guide, 2 l of ECF can be lost before dehydration becomes manifest, loss of 3–4 l is reflected in obvious dehydration, while circulatory collapse in simple mechanical obstruction reflects losses of the order of 5–6 l.

The speed of onset of vomiting and abdominal distension are usually inversely related. Vomiting occurs early with high intestinal obstruction, whereas distension may not be apparent. Conversely, vomiting is a late feature of low intestinal obstruction and distension under these circumstances is marked. Gross abdominal distension impairs venous return from the legs, and diaphragmatic elevation causes respiratory embarrassment.

The number of luminal bacteria increases greatly in obstructed bowel, but, in the absence of strangulation, bacteria and their toxins remain confined to the lumen and are not implicated in the development of shock.

II. *Strangulation Obstruction*

Strangulation can complicate all forms of simple mechanical obstruction. When the bowel and its mesentery are both compressed as, for example, in sigmoid volvulus, venous return is soon occluded and the bowel becomes engorged with blood until ultimately the arterial inflow is also occluded. The amount of blood lost depends on the length of bowel involved; as much as 70% of blood volume can be lost in strangulated sigmoid volvulus. This blood loss is the major cause of hypovolaemia in strangulation obstruction, and overshadows ECF losses from the gut mucosa (*Fig.* 13.2).

The second major feature of strangulation is loss of bowel wall viability. This allows bacteria and their toxins access to the peritoneal cavity and blood stream, resulting in endotoxaemia, bacteraemia and septicaemia.

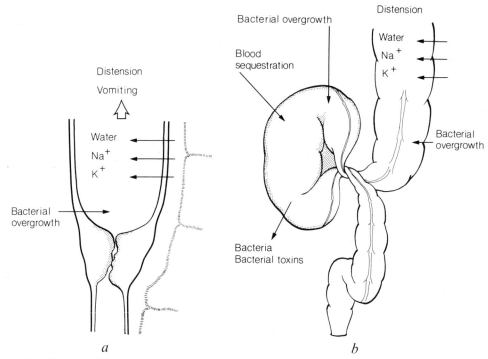

Fig. 13.2. (a) Diagrammatic representation of the consequences of simple mechanical intestinal obstruction. The net flux of water and electrolytes into the lumen is increased and bacterial overgrowth occurs proximal to the obstructing lesion. (b) Diagrammatic representation of the consequences of strangulation obstruction as in sigmoid volvulus. Bacterial overgrowth occurs within the strangulated loop and bacteria and their toxins migrate through the devitalized bowel. Sequestration of blood within the strangulated bowel is a major feature of strangulation and a much more potent cause of hypovolaemia than sequestration of water and electrolytes in the obstructed intestine.

III. *Adynamic Ileus*

The main causes of adynamic ileus are:

1. *Reflex ileus* after retroperitoneal haemorrhage, spinal or pelvic fracture.
2. *Peritonitis* with toxic paralysis of intrinsic nerve plexuses.
3. *Metabolic* causes including uraemia, diabetic coma, and depletion of potassium or magnesium.
4. *Drugs* including atropine, probanthine, hexamethonium and nortryptiline.
5. *Postoperative ileus* due to handling of the bowel, peritoneal contamination, electrolyte deficiencies and sympathetic reflexes. Small bowel peristalsis probably returns within hours of laparotomy whereas the large bowel remains immobile for at least 1 or 2 days. Swallowed air is passed rapidly through the small bowel only to distend the atonic colon.

Adynamic ileus leads to marked loss of ECF into the distended atonic bowel. Protein exudation into the peritoneal cavity is a major additional feature of ileus due to peritonitis. Hypovolaemia and circulatory failure reflect ECF loss, and septicaemia may exacerbate circulatory problems if ileus arises as a result of infection. Gross abdominal distension poses further problems by its effect on venous return and ventilatory efficiency.

Problems in the Assessment and Management of Intestinal Obstruction

I. *Differentiation between Types of Obstruction*

Features which suggest mechanical obstruction rather than adynamic ileus include:
1. Persistence of 'ileus' for more than 3 or 4 days after abdominal surgery.
2. Absence of a recognized cause of ileus.
3. Colicky abdominal pain with increased peristaltic activity.
4. Failure to pass flatus when a patient has previously passed flatus or had bowel movements after operation.
5. Localized gas-filled loops and/or fluid levels on plain abdominal X-ray. Ileus usually produces multiple fluid levels and gaseous distension of both small and large bowel.

Clinical differentiation between simple mechanical obstruction and strangulation obstruction is notoriously difficult. Features which suggest strangulation include severe localized pain, rapid onset of shock, a tender abdominal mass with guarding, pyrexia and leucocytosis. None of these pointers is reliable and early laparotomy remains the only certain method of minimizing the occurrence and dangers of strangulation.

Adynamic ileus is suggested by gross abdominal distension, copious effortless vomiting (or copious nasogastric aspiration), constipation, failure to pass flatus and a silent abdomen. Patients usually experience abdominal discomfort rather than pain, but it is often difficult to distinguish between these two symptoms after abdominal operation. The point at issue is that patients with postoperative ileus do not require further laparotomy, whereas those with mechanical obstruction generally require further surgery and are at risk of developing strangulation.

II. *Management of Mechanical Obstruction*

Mechanical obstruction is almost invariably an indication for operation. A nasogastric tube (16 Fr) is used to keep the stomach empty. Intestinal intubation with a Miller–Abbott tube is used by some surgeons but is not recommended by us. Blood is withdrawn for grouping and cross-matching, haematocrit determination, and measurement of urea and electrolyte concentrations. A free-flowing intravenous line is established, and an additional CVP line is invaluable in the elderly and those with cardiovascular disease. Pulse and blood pressure are monitored, temperature is recorded 4-hourly, and a fluid balance chart is commenced. If the patient is shocked, a urinary catheter is inserted and hourly urine output is recorded.

In patients thought to have simple mechanical obstruction, a few hours should be spent restoring ECF volume and the patient's general condition for operation. However, resuscitation should never be dilatory as strangulation cannot be excluded clinically. The fluid infused should be normal saline with added potassium (3 g $KCl \equiv 40$ mmol K^+ per 500 ml). The amount of fluid needed is estimated by the rough guidelines mentioned above, supplemented by regular measurement of circulatory parameters.

If the patient is thought to have strangulation, resuscitation becomes a matter of urgency. In addition to the measures just outlined, blood loss is replaced, oxygen is administered (4 l/min through a well-fitting Hudson mask, equivalent to an inspired oxygen concentration of 40%), and antibiotics are commenced before operation (in our practice, gentamicin 80 mg t.i.d. and metronidazole 500 mg t.i.d., intravenous). Considerable clinical judgement is needed to determine the timing of operation and one has to balance the desire for further resuscitation against the pressing need to arrest a deteriorating intra-abdominal situation.

III. *Management of Adynamic Ileus*

Nasogastric aspiration and fluid and electrolyte replacement are the mainstays of management. Surgery is contra-indicated in the absence of a surgically correctable lesion, but the patient must be reviewed at least twice daily and a *positive decision* taken to persist with conservative therapy.[8] Mechanical obstruction must not be allowed to escape notice. Plain films of the abdomen (erect and supine) are taken each day to aid evaluation.

Most surgeons adopt an expectant attitude to adynamic ileus, checking that metabolic upsets have been corrected and that appropriate treatment for peritonitis has been instituted. Pharmacological sympathetic blockade by guanethidine (20 mg by intravenous infusion over 40 minutes while pulse and blood pressure are monitored) has been recommended, if the surgeon is convinced that there is no mechanical obstruction and the patient is in fluid and electrolyte balance. If bowel sounds return, bethanecol chloride (2·5 mg subcutaneous injection) is then given and repeated 30 minutes later if flatus is not passed.[9] In common with most surgeons, we have not employed this regime, feeling that ileus is best left to recover spontaneously.

IV. *Intestinal Pseudo-obstruction*

'Pseudo-obstruction' is an ill-understood entity in which the clinical picture of mechanical obstruction occurs in the absence of a demonstrable organic cause. Conditions with which it is associated include ventilatory failure, renal disease and head injury. The diagnosis is suspected if gaseous distension extends radiologically to the rectum but sigmoidoscopy fails to reveal an obstructing lesion. Barium enema confirms the absence of organic obstruction and allows expectant treatment. Caecostomy (undertaken if necessary under local anaesthesia) can be used as a temporary deflationary procedure if distension is so gross that caecal devitalization is feared.

ACUTE PANCREATITIS

Mortality rates following an attack of acute pancreatitis range from 10 to 20%. Persisting pain, prolonged ileus, respiratory failure, renal failure and shock indicate that a patient has severe disease and is at increased risk. Criteria used to define severity and predict outcome are shown in *Table 13.3* If three or more criteria are positive within 48 hours of admission the patient has severe pancreatitis and is more likely to need intensive care.

Table **13.3. Criteria used to define severity of acute pancreatitis**

Factor	
Pao_2	Less than 60 mmHg (7·5 kPa)
Serum albumin	Less than 32 g/l
Serum calcium	Less than 2·0 mmol/l
White cell count	In excess of 15×10^9/l
Serum transaminases	In excess of 100 units/l
Lactic dehydrogenase	In excess of 600 units/l
Plasma glucose	In excess of 10 mmol/l (in absence of diabetes)
Blood urea	In excess of 16 mmol/l (no response to i.v. fluids)
Age	Greater than 55 years

If three or more of the following nine factors are present within 48 hours of admission, the attack is considered severe.[10]

Pathophysiology of Acute Pancreatitis

Premature activation of trypsin is probably of cardinal importance in triggering 'autodigestion', although the exact mechanisms responsible are still uncertain. Such premature activation is normally prevented by storage of proteolytic enzymes in zymogen granules, by secretion of enzymes as inactive precursors to await activation in the duodenum, and by inhibitors

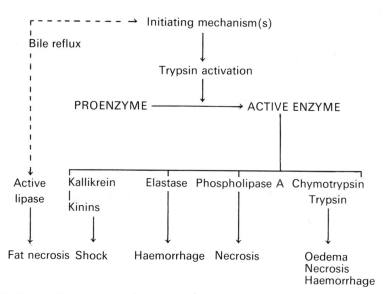

Fig. 13.3. Pancreatic enzymes and the pathogenesis of acute pancreatitis.

in pancreatic tissue and juice. Even small amounts of activated trypsin have the potential to initiate a 'cascade' phenomenon whereby other proenzymes are converted to active agents within the gland (*Fig.* 13.3). Trypsin and chymotrypsin cause proteolysis with oedema, necrosis and bleeding; elastase causes bleeding by eroding blood vessels; phospholipase A causes necrosis, and kallikrein releases kinins with local vasodilatation, increased vascular permeability and pain. Activation of the kallikrein 'kinin' system is central to the pathogenesis of shock. Exudation of plasma into the retroperitoneal tissues produces hypovolaemia, an effect compounded by escape of vasoactive agents into the systemic circulation. Adynamic ileus is usually present and hypovolaemia is accentuated as fluid and electrolytes accumulate in the distended atonic bowel.

Problems in the Management of Acute Pancreatitis

I. *Confirmation of the Diagnosis*

The clinical picture of acute pancreatitis ranges from mild abdominal pain without systemic upset to agonizing pain, prostration and circulatory collapse. A high index of suspicion is needed and acute pancreatitis should always be considered in differential diagnosis of the acute abdomen.

Hyperamylasaemia supports the clinical diagnosis of acute pancreatitis but care is needed in interpretation. The serum amylase rises 2–12 hours after the onset of pain, and approximately 5% of patients have normal amylase levels when first seen. On the other hand, 'false positive' hyperamylasaemia is found in conditions other than acute pancreatitis. The long list of conditions includes intra-abdominal catastrophes, such as perforated peptic ulcer, acute cholecystitis and intestinal strangulation, many of which may prove fatal unless treated surgically. Significant amounts of amylase are present in the salivary glands, heart, liver, intestine and kidney, and disease of these organs occasionally causes hyperamylasaemia.

Serum amylase levels in excess of 1200 units/l support a diagnosis of acute pancreatitis, whereas lesser elevations suggest conditions other than pancreatitis but do not exclude this diagnosis. Clinical vigilance cannot be relaxed even when amylase levels exceed 1200 units/l and laparotomy may have to be undertaken if there is sufficient diagnostic doubt.

Renal clearance of amylase increases during acute pancreatitis and clearance rates can be measured if serum levels are not diagnostic. Amylase-creatinine clearance ratio (ACCR) is determined on a single sample of blood (s) and urine (u) obtained simultaneously and eliminates error due to renal factors:

$$\text{ACCR } (\%) = (\text{u. amylase/s. amylase}) \times (\text{s. creatinine/u. creatinine}) \times 100$$

The ratio is normally less than 5% but rises to 5–10% in most cases of acute pancreatitis. The test is not specific and in our view has limited application.

Assays for serum lipase, trypsin and phospholipase A have been developed in an attempt to overcome the limitations of amylase measurement. Unfortunately, lipase suffers from the same drawbacks as amylase, trypsin requires radio-immunoassay; and phospholipase A measurement is still experimental.

Measurement of amylase and lipase levels in peritoneal or pleural fluid is feasible, but interpretation of results is also subject to the same considerations as interpretation of serum levels.

II. *Medical Management of Acute Pancreatitis*

There are no specific measures of proven value. Supportive measures include:

1. *Pain Relief*

Opiates are usually needed to relieve the severe pain. Morphine is said to be contra-indicated because it causes spasm of the sphincter of Oddi. Pethidine is also spasmogenic, but is the analgesic most often employed.

2. *Suppression of Pancreatic Secretion*

Pancreatic stimulation is avoided by forbidding oral intake. Nasogastric suction is used to keep the stomach empty and avoid vomiting, although controlled trials have failed to confirm its benefit in terms of outcome.[11]

There is no evidence that glucagon[12] or anticholinergics[13] rest the pancreas and we do not use them. In theory, cimetidine might rest the pancreas by reducing the amount of acid entering the duodenum. Regardless of this consideration there are grounds to support its use as a means of reducing the risk of gastrointestinal bleeding (*see below*).

3. *Countering the effects of vasoactive substances*

Aprotinin (Trasylol) is a kallikrein inhibitor which prevents or reverses shock in experimentally induced pancreatitis, but its clinical value is controversial. Early reports suggested that it was of benefit, particularly in elderly patients,[14] but this has not been confirmed.[10, 15] We do not use Trasylol.

Peritoneal lavage provides a means of removing vasoactive substances and proteolytic enzymes, and preliminary clinical results are encouraging.[16] Dialysis catheters can be placed through small mid-line incisions under local anaesthesia, and an isotonic dialysate is used. It is uncertain whether addition of Trasylol to the dialysis fluid carries any added benefit.

4. *Improvement of the pancreatic microcirculation*

Haemorrhagic pancreatitis has a worse prognosis than oedematous pancreatitis. Pancreatic blood flow is reduced in the haemorrhagic form of the disease, but is increased in oedematous inflammation. Maintenance of circulating blood volume is one of the prime aims of supportive therapy. Low molecular weight dextran, heparin and fibrinolysins improve survival in experimental pancreatitis, possibly by an effect of the pancreatic microcirculation, but their clinical role awaits definition.

III. *Prevention and Management of the Complications of Acute Pancreatitis*

Shock, respiratory failure, renal failure, metabolic upsets, haemorrhage and sepsis are the main complications which influence outcome. Much of the recent improvement in morbidity and mortality stems from the prevention and early detection of these complications.

1. *Shock*

Up to 40% of circulating blood volume may be lost in the early stages of acute pancreatitis. Pulse rate, blood pressure, CVP and urine output are monitored. Elderly patients, and those with pre-existing cardiovascular disease, pose greater problems in fluid replacement, and measurement of pulmonary wedge venous pressure (p. 377) may be considered.

Ringer lactate solution or normal saline is used for initial fluid replacement. Administration of large amounts of crystalloid promotes pulmonary oedema, and plasma or albumin should be used if more than 3–4 l of crystalloid have to be infused in the first 24 hours to maintain the circulation. Serum albumin levels are kept above 30 g/l if possible. Failure to maintain the circulation despite 'adequate' amounts of fluid replacement and satisfactory myocardial function may indicate the presence of pancreatic slough and the need for surgery (*see below*).

2. *Pulmonary insufficiency*

Pleural effusion, pulmonary oedema and atelectasis are reported in 15–55% of patients. Pleural effusions are usually left-sided and signify concomitant pleural inflammation or an internal pancreatic fistula. Respiratory insufficiency is often present without clinical or radiological evidence. In a series of 84 patients, Imrie[17] found that 38 had severe hypoxia (Pao_2 less than 60 mmHg) and 29 had moderate hypoxia, whereas only 15 patients had radiological evidence of pulmonary abnormality. Hypotension, over-infusion of crystalloid, massive tissue damage, loss of pulmonary surfactant (due to phospholipase A), decreased oxygen delivery to the tissues and abdominal distension all contribute to pulmonary impairment.

Twice-daily estimation of blood gases allows early detection of pulmonary insufficiency and the need for oxygen therapy given as 4 l/min through a well-fitting Hudson mask (equivalent to an inspired oxygen concentration of 40%) but greater flow rates and ventilatory support may be needed if Pao_2 remains low.

3. *Renal failure*

Renal failure is reported in up to 18% of patients, and carries a mortality of approximately 50%. Hourly urine output, urine osmolality, blood urea and creatinine levels are monitored to allow early recognition of renal impairment. The rate of intravenous fluid administration is adjusted to maintain a urine output of at least 30 ml/h; diuretics are only indicated if this is not achieved despite adequate fluid replacement. Dialysis is necessary if complete renal shutdown supervenes, and is usually performed by the peritoneal route to obtain the concomitant benefit of peritoneal lavage.

4. *Metabolic upsets*

Abnormalities in acid–base balance, serum electrolyte concentrations and serum calcium levels are sought routinely. Hypocalcaemia is probably secondary to a fall in serum albumin rather than calcium deposition in fat necrosis or changes involving parathyroid hormone.[18] Intravenous calcium gluconate solution (10%) is of transient benefit and it is more important to maintain circulating albumin levels.

A blood glucose level in excess of 10 mmol/l is corrected by soluble insulin in appropriate dosage.

5. *Haematological system*

Haemolysis, retroperitoneal bleeding and gastrointestinal haemorrhage may cause anaemia, and haemoglobin concentration and haematocrit are measured daily. Disseminated intravascular coagulation (DIC) with consumption coagulopathy can occur in the early stages of pancreatitis, and may be implicated in respiratory, renal and hepatic failure. A coagulation screen, platelet count and serum fibrinogen levels are assessed if hypercoagulation is suspected. Development of coagulopathy may be an early indication of pancreatic abscess or extensive slough formation.

6. *Gastrointestinal system*

Bleeding into the gut or peritoneum occurs in 5–10% of cases. Oesophageal varices, Mallory–Weiss tear, erosive gastritis or peptic ulcer may be responsible for gastrointestinal bleeding, and endoscopy is mandatory to define the bleeding point. Prophylactic cimetidine and/or antacids should be prescribed routinely in all critically ill patients.

Bleeding into the peritoneal cavity from an eroded vessel carries a high mortality and is an indication for urgent operation.

Total parenteral nutrition is necessary in those patients with a prolonged severe illness and protracted ileus, and should be instituted early.

7. *Sepsis*

Sepsis complicates pancreatitis in about 5% of cases. Sloughing of the pancreas and abscess formation are accompanied by persistent pyrexia, leucocytosis, ileus and clinical deterioration. Gastrointestinal organisms are usually responsible and coliforms are implicated in two-thirds of cases. Treatment consists of surgical drainage or resection, and appropriate antibiotic therapy. There is no evidence that 'propyhlactic' antibiotics reduce the risk of pancreatic sepsis and we do not employ antibiotics in this context.

IV. *Role of Surgery in Acute Pancreatitis*

Surgery is indicated when there is diagnostic doubt, and when a patient develops specific complications, such as pancreatic abscess, pseudocyst or major haemorrhage. The indications for emergency surgery in fulminant acute pancreatitis are more controversial. The presence of severe pain, profound shock and cardiorespiratory failure unresponsive to supportive therapy confronts the surgeon with a difficult decision. Total or subtotal pancreatic resection under these circumstances is extremely hazardous but may represent the only chance of survival. Alternatively, multiple drainage of the lesser sac may be combined with cholecystostomy, gastrostomy and jejunostomy, although there is little evidence that this approach benefits patients with extensive pancreatic necrosis and sloughing.

BILIARY TRACT DISEASE

Although biliary tract disease is common, complications needing intensive care are relatively rare. The problems to be considered here are acute cholecystitis, cholangitis, acalculous cholecystitis and the hepatorenal syndrome.

I. Acute Cholecystitis

Pathophysiology of Acute Cholecystitis

Acute cholecystitis is a common disorder which arises due to blockage of the exit from the gallbladder. Gall stones are almost always responsible and the offending stone may impact in the cystic duct or within Hartmann's pouch. Concentrated bile causes chemical irritation and mucus secretion by the gallbladder, and bacterial invasion follows unless obstruction is relieved by the stone passing onwards or falling back into the body of the gallbladder.

Unrelieved obstruction may lead to suppuration, thrombosis of mural vessels, gangrene and perforation. The inflamed gallbladder is usually walled-off by adhesions to omentum and neighbouring viscera, preventing free perforation into the peritoneal cavity. However, gangrene may supervene rapidly in the elderly and diabetic patients, allowing free perforation and biliary peritonitis before infection can be localized.

Management of Acute Cholecystitis

Conventional management of acute cholecystitis has been based on the knowledge that 90% of cases settle on a conservative regime of nil by mouth, intravenous fluids, pain relief and antibiotics. It is the 10% of patients failing to settle on this regime who may need intensive care.

Failure of conservative management is heralded by increasing pain and tenderness in the right hypochondrium, development of a palpable mass, and a rising pulse rate and temperature. Urgent cholecystectomy is the treatment of choice, but cholecystostomy followed by interval cholecystectomy may be preferred if cholecystectomy is too hazardous. These patients are frequently septicaemic and antibiotics are prescribed prior to operation (gentamicin 80 mg b.d. and ampicillin 500 mg q.i.d.), pending culture and sensitivity determinations on a specimen of bile taken at operation.

In common with many surgeons, we now recommend early operation in patients with acute cholecystitis and no longer adhere to the conventional regime of conservative management.

II. Cholangitis

Pathophysiology of Cholangitis

Obstruction of major bile ducts frequently leads to cholangitis and septicaemia. Almost 80% of patients with obstruction due to gall stones or benign stricture have significant bacterial counts in bile, whereas some 30% of those with malignant obstruction have significant counts.[19] The term 'ascending cholangitis' is misleading in that bacteria probably enter from the blood stream and do not ascend the biliary tree from the duodenum.

Management of Cholangitis

Cholangitis and septicaemia are signalled by Charcot's triad of obstructive jaundice, abdominal pain, and fluctuating pyrexia with chills and rigors. These complications are avoided, if at all possible, by prompt relief of obstructive jaundice, and by providing antibiotic cover for patients with obstructive jaundice who are about to undergo percutaneous transhepatic cholangiography (PTC), ERCP or biliary surgery.

It is our practice to cover patients with a single dose of gentamicin (80 mg i.v.) 1 hour before PTC or ERCP, and to monitor pulse, blood pressure and temperature for 12 hours following their return. Operation in the presence of obstructive jaundice is covered by intravenous administration of gentamicin (80 mg) and ampicillin (500 mg), giving three doses only, commencing with premedication. Bile is taken for culture at operation so that therapy can be adjusted in the light of sensitivity determinations, should septic complications ensue.

Development of overt cholangitis and septicaemic shock is always an indication for intensive care. Blood samples are withdrawn immediately for culture and sensitivity determination, and a therapeutic course of gentamicin and ampicillin is commenced until further bacteriological information becomes available. Pulse rate, blood pressure, urine output and CVP are monitored, and oxygen is administered. Some 85% of patients respond to these measures and further investigation can be undertaken to define the cause of their jaundice. Failure to respond is an indication for urgent operative decompression, the choice of procedure being dictated by the nature of the obstructing lesion and the patient's general condition.

III. Acalculous Cholecystitis

This uncommon but serious disorder affects patients who do not have gall stones or previous history of biliary disease. It usually follows major accidental or operative trauma associated with sepsis, and may affect young patients. Predisposing factors include prolonged dehydration and shock, sepsis, massive blood transfusion and protracted ileus. Organisms can usually be cultured from the gallbladder, and the wide range of organisms recovered suggests that haematogenous spread from a distant focus is responsible. Some believe that acalculous cholecystitis is primarily a vascular disturbance. Thompson and colleagues[20] stress that vascular insufficiency may, in itself, cause gallbladder gangrene, while an alternative explanation holds that the condition is an allergic vascular reaction to bacterial toxin (the Schwartzmann Sanerelli phenomenon).

Management of Acalculous Cholecystitis

The diagnosis should be borne in mind when pain and tenderness develop in the upper abdomen, days or weeks after major trauma. Deranged liver function is not invariable but some patients have elevated serum alkaline phosphatase and transaminase levels. Gallbladder radiology is seldom helpful. Cholecystectomy is the treatment of choice and is undertaken under antibiotic cover.

IV. The Hepatorenal Syndrome

Pathophysiology of the Hepatorenal Syndrome

Renal failure is particularly common following operation for obstructive jaundice in the presence of sepsis. The pathophysiological basis remains uncertain. There is little evidence that conjugated bile salts are directly toxic to the kidney or sensitize it to ischaemic damage. The most plausible explanation centres on the occurrence of systemic endotoxaemia in patients with obstructive jaundice.[21] Endotoxin in portal venous blood is normally removed by the hepatic Kupffer cells, and impaired Kupffer cell function in jaundice might allow endotoxin access to the systemic circulation. Endotoxins are potent renal vasoconstrictors and may further impair renal function by triggering intravascular coagulation and fibrin deposition in glomeruli.[22] All of these effects would be compounded by hypovolaemia.

Evidence of the Hepatorenal Syndrome

Intravenous fluid therapy is commenced at least 12 hours before operation to prevent hypovolaemia. Urine output is monitored hourly throughout operation and the postoperative period. The osmotic diuretic, mannitol, is used routinely by some and 20 g are given intravenously over 15 minutes in the hour before surgery, followed by 20 g during operation. This dose can be repeated on each of the first three postoperative days if urine flow rate falls despite adequate hydration. We prefer to use mannitol only if urine output falls beneath 30 ml/h and have not employed it routinely.

PERITONITIS

The majority of patients with peritonitis do not require intensive care and respond to fluid and electrolyte replacement, antibiotic therapy and timely operative intervention. In a minority, the disease process is life-threatening and intensive care is essential.

Pathophysiology of Peritonitis

The major causes of peritonitis are perforation of a hollow viscus, ischaemia of intra-abdominal organs with necrosis and gangrene, extension of infection from a neighbouring septic focus, penetrating trauma, and leakage from a gastrointestinal anastomosis. The extent and severity of infection depend on the virulence of the infecting organism, speed of onset of infection and efficacy of host defences. If infection progresses slowly, adhesions may prevent widespread dissemination and favour abscess formation. On the other hand, sudden perforation of a hollow viscus may flood the peritoneal cavity with gastrointestinal content. In general, the lower the perforation is located in the gut, the more virulent the infecting organisms. The response to peritonitis is relatively poor in the very young, the elderly and those with intercurrent disease.

The presence of gastrointestinal content, bile or bacteria in the peritoneal cavity leads to an inflammatory peritoneal reaction with serous exudation.

Paralytic ileus ensues and leads to hypovolaemia as fluid derived from ECF accumulates in the peritoneal cavity and gut lumen. Blood volume is frequently reduced by 30–40% in severe peritonitis, and greater losses are incurred if peritonitis is associated with organ strangulation. Absorption of bacteria and their toxins leads to bacteraemia, septicaemia and endo-toxaemia with deleterious effects on cardiac, pulmonary, hepatic and renal function, and impaired tissue oxygen utilization.

Management of Peritonitis

Aggressive preoperative resuscitation is of paramount importance. Consi-derable clinical judgement is needed to determine the optimal time for operation; insufficient resuscitation increases the risks of surgery whereas undue delay allows progression of the infective process. As a general rule, some 2–6 hours are needed to prepare patients with severe peritonitis for surgery.

Normal saline or Ringer lactate solution is infused intravenously but potassium is not added until an adequate urinary output has been established. The rate of fluid replacement is assessed by the state of the peripheral circulation, hourly urine output and CVP. Blood is withdrawn for grouping and cross-matching, determination of urea and electrolyte concentrations, and measurement of blood gases and acid–base status. Oxygen is administered by a Hudson mask, but abdominal distension may embarrass ventilation until distension is relieved by operation. A naso-gastric tube is passed to remove gastrointestinal secretions, avoid in-halation of gastric content, prevent further vomiting and minimize ab-dominal distension.

Blood cultures are taken on admission and antibiotic therapy is com-menced. In the first instance we prescribe gentamicin (80 mg b.d.) and metronidazole (500 mg 8-hourly) by intravenous injection or infusion, and add crystalline penicillin (1 Munit 6-hourly), if clostridial or anaerobic streptococcal infection is suspected. Gram-staining of peritoneal fluid obtained at laparotomy is used by some to select appropriate antibiotics, and specimens of infected material should be sent routinely for bacteriological culture and sensitivity determination. Antibiotic therapy in severe peritonitis should be continued for at least 5 days.

The principles of operation are to deal effectively with the primary focus of infection (e.g. close a perforation, excise gangrenous bowel), lavage the peritoneal cavity, and institute effective drainage if there are localized areas of necrotic material or frank abscesses. Most surgeons employ saline for lavage but every effort must be made to recover the instilled fluid as saline favours continued bacterial growth. Noxythiolin was once popular as an antibacterial additive but has now been superseded by tetracycline.[23]

ACUTE MESENTERIC VASCULAR ISCHAEMIA

Acute mesenteric vascular insufficiency has an annual incidence of about four cases per 100 000 population. The diagnosis is all too often delayed until the affected gut is gangrenous; the illness usually affects elderly patients and those with generalized vascular disease, and mortality rates remain around 85%. Survival depends on prompt diagnosis, aggressive resuscitation, urgent operative intervention and the highest standards of intensive care.

Pathophysiology of Acute Mesenteric Vascular Ischaemia

Ischaemia in the distribution of the coeliac axis is unusual because of the plentiful collateral supply.

The superior mesenteric artery is partially or totally occluded in almost two-thirds of individuals over the age of 55, but gradual occlusion allows development of collateral flow. Abrupt occlusion of the superior mesenteric artery is followed by disastrous consequences in that only 25–30 cm of proximal jejunum may survive while the rest of the small bowel and a variable length of proximal colon undergo necrosis.

Inferior mesenteric artery occlusion may occur without apparent ischaemia. The artery is of relatively small calibre (diameter of coeliac : superior mesenteric : inferior mesenteric $\equiv 4 : 4 \cdot 5 : 1$), but occlusion of its lumen may prove critical if flow through the superior mesenteric artery is already compromised.

Ischaemia may be due to interruption of arterial inflow, occlusion of venous outflow or failure of perfusion:

I. Arterial occlusion is most often due to atherosclerosis with superimposed thrombosis, but emboli are responsible in one-third of cases. Less common causes of arterial occlusion include dissecting aortic aneurysm, arteritis, neoplastic constriction and iatrogenic damage during operation or aortography.

II. Venous occlusion is much less common but has been reported in hepatic cirrhosis, neoplasia and patients taking the contraceptive pill.

III. Non-occlusive infarction probably accounts for some 40% of cases of midgut necrosis. The splanchnic bed is a low-priority area in shock and is denied its normal 20% of cardiac output. The combination of increased splanchnic arteriolar resistance and systemic hypotension leads readily to ischaemia and infarction.

Unrelieved ischaemia leads to progressive necrosis of all layers of the bowel wall with full-thickness gangrene and perforation. The mucosa is more susceptible than the muscle layers to ischaemia, and restoration of flow within some 6 hours may allow return to structural and functional normality. Stricture may result if ischaemic damage to a short length of bowel extends deeply into the submucosa and underlying circular muscle.

Clinical Features of Acute Mesenteric Vascular Insufficiency

Early diagnosis is difficult but essential if surgery is to restore the circulation and prevent irreversible damage. There are no specific symptoms or signs and a high index of suspicion is mandatory. A prodromal history of abdominal pain related to meals, diarrhoea and weight loss is obtained in some patients, and suspicion is heightened in patients with ischaemic heart disease, previous cerebrovascular incidents or arterial fibrillation.

Abdominal pain is the most reliable feature of the clinical presentation, but varies greatly in extent, duration and severity. Vomiting and blood-stained diarrhoea are present in some patients. Abdominal tenderness, guarding and rigidity are usually late signs which signal full-thickness necrosis and the development of peritonitis. Cardiovascular collapse is also a relatively late feature and indicates blood and plasma loss, often associated with development of septicaemia.

Aids to Diagnosis

It cannot be over-emphasized that a high index of clinical suspicion is the only key to diagnosis. Abdominal plain films are usually normal in the critical early period although aortic calcification may denote atherosclerosis. Fluid levels, gas in the gut wall and veins, and free peritoneal gas are all late signs of necrosis. Aortography can be used to confirm the diagnosis but must not be allowed to delay operation and is seldom practicable.

A leucocytosis of 20 000–30 000 cells/mm^3 is often present, and a modest elevation in serum amylase is common.

Management of Acute Mesenteric Vascular Ischaemia

I. *Resuscitation*

Vigorous preoperative resuscitation is essential and blood, plasma and crystalloid may be needed to restore and maintain the circulation. Oxygen is administered and a combination of gentamicin, metronidazole and crystalline penicillin is given prior to operation if the diagnosis of gut infarction is likely and if the patient has evidence of peritonitis. Vital signs, urine output and CVP are monitored as outlined above.

II. *Principles of operation*

Restoration of flow is the prime objective and is more likely to be successful in patients with embolic occlusion. Clot is removed from the superior mesenteric artery or flow can be supplemented by anastomosis of one of the major mesenteric tributaries to a common iliac artery.[24]

Gangrenous bowel requires resection but resection of the entire midgut is a futile exercise. In some patients, gut viability is doubtful after restoration of flow and in an attempt to avoid extensive but unnecessary resection, a positive decision may be made to close the abdomen and undertake a 'second look' some 24 hours later. A conservative approach is adopted in patients with non-occlusive infarction and gut resection is undertaken only in the presence of frank gangrene.

III. *Postoperative care*

Restoration of blood flow to ischaemic bowel is followed by profound effects on the cardiovascular system. Blood, plasma and electrolytes are lost into the bowel wall and lumen; vasoactive kinins, bacteria and bacterial toxins gain access to the blood stream; blood pressure and blood volume fall as the splanchnic bed is re-opened and metabolic acidosis is common.

Intensive care is essential and must comprise continued oxygen therapy at rates determined by periodic blood gas analysis, antibiotic cover (*see above*) and heparinization. Heparin is given by intravenous injection of 20 000 i.u. followed by infusion of 10 000–15 000 i.u. 6-hourly as indicated by results of thrombin time estimation.

Survival is virtually confined to patients in whom a defined vascular occlusion is diagnosed early and treated by prompt restoration of flow. Survival following treatment of infarction is exceptional unless only a small portion of the midgut is involved.

FISTULAE

Fistula between the skin and gastrointestinal tract, biliary system or pancreas is a relatively uncommon but potentially serious complication of alimentary disease. Mortality depends to some extent on the underlying pathological process, but has been reduced in recent years by improved standards of fluid and electrolyte balance and nutritional support.[25]

Pathophysiology of Alimentary Fistulae

I. *Cause of fistula formation*

Spontaneous fistulae arise from extension of an underlying disease process, such as Crohn's disease, diverticular disease or neoplasia.

Iatrogenic fistulae occur under the following circumstances:
1. Unrecognized operative damage to part of the alimentary tract.
2. Leakage from an anastomosis involving the gastrointestinal tract, biliary system or pancreas. Vascular insufficiency at the suture line is of paramount importance in anastomotic breakdown, while enzymatic digestion may promote leakage at anastomoses involving the pancreas. Anastomoses which include the oesophagus or distal large bowel are particularly liable to leakage and subsequent fistula formation.
3. Biopsy of an alimentary organ, notably the pancreas.
4. Drainage of an 'abscess' of the abdominal wall or perineum may complete the process of external fistula formation, particularly in patients with Crohn's disease.

II. *Consequences of fistula formation*

Frank discharge of alimentary content or secretion is usually preceded by increasing pyrexia, abdominal pain and tenderness. Wound infection may herald discharge through an abdominal wound.

The volume and appearance of discharging material depend on the site of leakage. Fluid and electrolyte loss associated with high gastrointestinal fistulae may amount to 3–4 l/day, whereas fluid loss from colonic fistula may be as little as 500 ml/day. Substantial losses of electrolytes and protein are inevitable in high output fistulae and, in the case of pancreatic or high intestinal fistulae, escape of pancreatic enzymes leads to skin excoriation and digestion.

Major nutritional problems arise because of the continuing drain of protein through the fistula, lack of adequate nutritional intake and effects of associated sepsis.

Basis of Management of Alimentary Fistulae

I. *Confirmation of fistula*

In the majority of cases, discharge of bile-stained or faecal material through a wound, 'abscess' or drain site leaves little doubt as to the true diagnosis. When there is uncertainty, a small catheter can be inserted into the skin opening and a small amount of water-soluble radio-opaque dye (Hypaque or Gastrografin) is instilled while the area is screened.

II. *Adequate external drainage*

It is most important to ensure that material escaping from the alimentary system has free egress from the abdomen. Failure to achieve free external drainage favours abscess formation, disseminated peritonitis and septicaemia. Considerable clinical judgement may be needed to determine the need for surgery in the early stages of fistula formation. It must be stressed that the aim of surgery at this stage is NOT closure of the internal site of leakage, but institution of free drainage. Suction drainage is used wherever possible, and a two-lumen 'sump' drain may be of particular value.

III. *Fluid and electrolyte balance*

An accurate fluid balance chart is established, taking care to allow for insensible losses (at least 1 litre per day) when calculating each day's fluid needs. Serum electrolytes and urea concentration are measured daily, and it may prove helpful to have periodic measurement of urinary electrolyte losses when calculating daily electrolyte replacement therapy. An intravenous line is essential. In some patients with high fistula involving the stomach, duodenum or biliary system, it may be possible to guide a naso-enteric tube beyond the fistula and so allow re-instillation of draining fistula content.

IV. *Nasogastric tube*

It is generally agreed that intubation does not reduce the volume of drainage from intestinal fistulae, when compared to simple avoidance of oral intake. On the other hand, a nasogastric tube is essential in the presence of ileus, and in patients with gastric distension and vomiting.

V. *Nutritional support*

Recognition of the need for nutritional support and the advent of parenteral nutrition have made a major impact on mortality rates. For example, Sheldon and colleagues[26] found that mortality rates fell from 45% in patients receiving less than 3000 calories, to 14% in those receiving more than this amount. It is advisable to commence parenteral feeding (c.f. Chapter 7) on diagnosis of fistula formation. In patients with low-output colonic fistula, it may prove feasible subsequently to employ elemental diets for nutritional replacement, while it may be possible to feed patients with high intestinal fistulae through a naso-enteric tube passed beyond the site of fistulation.

VI. *Exclude distal obstruction*

The majority of alimentary fistulae will close on conservative management provided there is no distal obstruction in the system involved. Contrast radiology is used to confirm the absence of such obstruction, but is usually deferred until the patient has been stabilized in terms of fluid and electrolyte balance, and nutritional support.

VII. *Skin care*

Effective suction drainage usually prevents fistula content from remaining in contact with the skin and producing excoriation. Stomadhesive and Karya gum are particularly useful in preventing damage to the skin around the external fistulous opening.

VIII. *Antibiotics*

Antibiotic therapy is not employed routinely in the management of fistulae. It should be reserved for specific indications, notably failure to control sepsis despite adequate external drainage. Culture and sensitivity determinations are imperative to select the appropriate antibiotic(s) when therapy is considered necessary.

IX. *Role of surgery*

Surgery is indicated when there is evidence of ineffective drainage with abscess formation, distal obstruction preventing fistula closure, an associated underlying disease (e.g. Crohn's), or when healing fails to occur despite adequate conservative therapy for a number of weeks. It must be emphasized that even when surgery appears inevitable from the outset, a period of 3–4 weeks conservative management may be needed to bring the patient into a condition where surgery is safe and has a reasonable prospect of success.

REFERENCES

1. MacDougall B. R. D., Bailey R. J. and Williams R. (1977) H_2-receptor antagonists and antacids in the prevention of acute gastrointestinal haemorrhage in fulminant hepatic failure, two controlled trials. *Lancet* **1**, 617.
2. Carter D. C. and Osborne D. H. (1981) In: Jirsch D. W., ed., *Horizons in General Surgery*. Lancaster, MTP Publishing.
3. Owen D. A. A., Parsons M. E., Farrington H. E. et al. (1979) Reduction by cimetidine of acute gastric hemorrhage caused by reinfusion of blood after exposure to exogenous acid during gastric ischemia in rats. *Gastroenterology* **77**, 979–985.
4. Hastings P. R., Skillman J. J., Bushnell L. S. et al. (1978) Antacid titration in the prevention of acute gastrointestinal bleeding, a controlled randomised study in 100 critically ill patients. *N. Engl. J. Med.* **298**, 1041–1045.

5. Priebe H. J., Skillman J. J., Bushwell L. S. et al. (1980) Antacid versus cimetidine in preventing acute gastrointestinal bleeding. *N. Engl. J. Med.* **302**, 426–430.
6. Cheung L. Y. and Porterfield G. (1979) Protection of gastric mucosa against acute ulceration by infusion of sodium bicarbonate. *Am. J. Surg.* **137**, 106–110.
7. Shields R. (1965) The absorption and secretion of fluid and electrolytes by the obstructed bowel. *Br. J. Surg.* **52**, 774–779.
8. Jones P. F. (1974) *Emergency Abdominal Surgery in Infancy, Childhood and Adult Life*, Chapter 3, p. 43. Oxford, Blackwell Scientific Publications.
9. Neely J. and Catchpole B. (1971) Ileus: the restoration of alimentary tract motility by pharmacological means. *Br. J. Surg.* **58**, 21–28.
10. Imrie C. W., Benjamin I. S., Ferguson J. C. et al. (1978) A single centre double blind trial of trasylol therapy in primary acute pancreatitis. *Br. J. Surg.* **65**, 337–341.
11. Naeije R., Salingret E., Clumeck N. et al. (1978) Is nasogastric suction necessary in acute pancreatitis? *Br. Med. J.* **2**, 659–660.
12. Durr H. K., Maroske D., Zelder O. et al. (1978) Glucagon therapy in acute pancreatitis. *Gut* **19**, 175–179.
13. Cameron J. L., Mehigan D. and Zuidema G. D. (1979) Evaluation of atropine in acute pancreatitis. *Surg. Gynecol. Obstet.* **148**, 206–208.
14. Trapnell J. E., Rigby C. C., Talbot C. H. et al. (1974) A controlled trial of trasylol in the treatment of acute pancreatitis. *Br. J. Surg.* **61**, 177–182.
15. MRC Multicentre Trial of Glucagon and Aprotinin (1977) *Lancet* **2**, 632–635.
16. Ranson J. H. C. and Spencer F. C. (1978) The role of peritoneal lavage in severe acute pancreatitis. *Ann. Surg.* **187**, 565–575.
17. Imrie C. W., Ferguson J. C., Murphy D. et al. (1977) Arterial hypoxia in acute pancreatitis. *Br. J. Surg.* **64**, 185–188.
18. Imrie C. W., Allam B. F. and Ferguson J. C. (1976) Hypocalcaemia of acute pancreatitis: the effect of hypoalbuminaemia. *Curr. Med. Res. Opin.* **4**, 101–116.
19. Keighley M. R. B. and Burdon D. W. (1979) Antimicrobial prophylaxis in surgery. *Gastrointestinal Surgery*, Chap. 5, p. 70. London, Pitman.
20. Thompson J. W., Ferris D. O. and Baggenstoss A. H. (1962) Acute cholecystitis complicating operation for other diseases. *Ann. Surg.* **155**, 489–491.
21. Bailey M. E. (1976) Endotoxin, bile salts and renal function in obstructive jaundice. *Br. J. Surg.* **63**, 774–778.
22. Allison M. E., Prentice C. R. M., Kennedy A. C. et al. (1979) Renal function and other factors in obstructive jaundice. *Br. J. Surg.* **66**, 392–397.
23. Stewart D. J. and Matheson N. A. (1978) Peritoneal lavage in appendicular peritonitis. *Br. J. Surg.* **65**, 54–56.
24. Marston A. (1977) *Intestinal Ischaemia* Chap. 5, p. 95. London, Arnold.
25. Himal H. S., Allard J. R., Nadeau J. E. et al. (1974) The importance of adequate nutrition in closure of small intestinal fistulas. *Br. J. Surg.* **61**, 724–726.
26. Sheldon G. F., Gardiner B. N., Way L. W. et al. (1971) Management of gastrointestinal fistulae. *Surg. Gynecol. Obstet.* **133**, 385–389.

Chapter 14

The Respiratory System

D. Campbell

The aim in intensive care, so far as the respiratory system is concerned, is essentially the same whether following a medical illness, a major surgical procedure or grave injuries, and that is to minimize interference with oxygenation and alveolar ventilation by maintaining as near normal pulmonary function as possible. *Table* 14.1 illustrates the many diseases and conditions that may lead to a degree of respiratory malfunction of such severity as to require all the supportive facilities and treatment generally only available in an intensive care unit. In a general unit of this kind, dealing with patients with medical and surgical conditions complicated by respiratory failure, the majority of patients will originate in surgical or accident units, having undergone extensive surgery or having suffered major trauma.

In the special case of cardiopulmonary bypass surgery, at one time pulmonary complications, in particular the development of 'bypass or pump lung,' were a prime cause of postoperative morbidity and mortality. Such pulmonary disturbance was probably due to many different causes, the pulmonary features in the end stage being more or less the same. Gross damage of this kind is now uncommon due to a better understanding of the causative factors and their prevention. Postoperative pulmonary insufficiency now usually can be clearly attributed to factors existing pre-operatively, such as chronic airway disease, intraoperatively to matters such as neglect to filter transfused blood or postoperatively to failure to maintain a secretion-free airway. That cardiopulmonary bypass itself has some potentially adverse effects on pulmonary function is probably true however, and histologically there is evidence of pulmonary capillary endothelial damage and damage to the alveolar epithelium with platelet and leucocyte plugging of the capillaries. There is marked degranulation of mast cells and evidence of surfactant reduction or inactivation, features

Table **14.1 Classification of respiratory failure**

Classification	Conditions
Primary infection or disease of the respiratory system	Acute pulmonary infection Chronic airways disease Asthma Emphysema Acute upper airway obstruction, e.g. *H. influenzae* infection, tumours Idiopathic pulmonary fibrosis Asbestosis Cystic fibrosis Lung tumours
Primary trauma to the respiratory system	Lung and chest-wall injuries Injuries to the airway Rupture of the diaphragm Pneumothorax, haemothorax, large pleural effusions, bronchopleural fistula Extensive pulmonary surgery Smoke inhalation in burning accidents Drowning Acid-aspiration syndrome Inhalation of foreign bodies
Congenital respiratory disease	Lung cysts Large diaphragmatic herniae Congenital airway defects, e.g. tracheo-oesophageal fistula
Secondary to other organ-systems failure or non-pulmonary disease	1. Infection: polyneuritis, tetanus, endotoxic shock 2. Thoracic cage disease: ankylosing spondylitis, burns, radiation fibrosis 3. Trauma: severe head injuries, massive intra-abdominal injury, fat and micro-embolism 4. Abdominal swelling: large tumours, ascites, obesity 5. Neurological and neuromuscular disease: polyneuritis, status epilepticus, myasthenia gravis, myopathies 6. Poisoning: paraquat (and other industrial toxic substances), sedatives and narcotics 7. Endocrine disease: pituitary and adrenal failure 8. Organ failure: myocardial and renal failure, hepatic coma 9. Anaesthesia and surgery: central nervous system depression, residual myoneural blockade, inadequate postoperative pain relief

also observed in the so-called 'shock lung' (ARDS), smoke inhalation injury and other clinical syndromes (*Fig.* 14.1). The common causative factor may be the release of vasoactive agents and lysozymes.

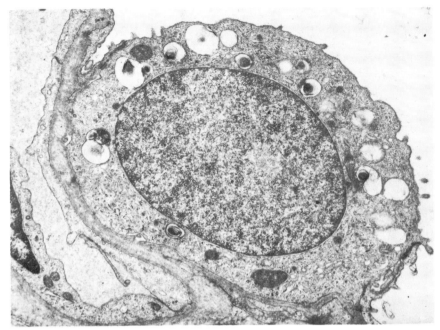

Fig. 14.1. Photomicrograph (× 17 500) of an alveolar Type 2 cell, showing clearly vesicles containing surfactant material and others which have extruded the material into the alveolus. Interference with surfactant or its precursors would appear to be a common factor in the various clinical conditions complicated by development of the adult respiratory distress syndrome (ARDS). Permission to reproduce this photograph is gratefully acknowledged to Dr Peter Toner, University Department of Pathology, Glasgow Royal Infirmary.

CONTRIBUTING FACTORS IN RESPIRATORY DYSFUNCTION

The Airway

As always in the postoperative period, meticulous attention to the patency of the airway is of prime importance in maintaining adequate pulmonary function. Retained secretions will contribute to atelectasis, maldistribution of inspired gases and predispose to pulmonary infection. Vigorous physiotherapy combined with adequate humidification of the inspired gas and frequent bronchial toilet, if necessary with the aid of a fibreoptic bronchoscope, are basic to good patient care.

The smaller airways are subject to an increase in the degree of closure which is accompanied by the reduction in total lung capacity and functional residual capacity seen after all anaesthetics for major surgery. This contributes to the ventilation perfusion disturbance already present and aggravates arterial hypoxaemia. It is apparent, therefore, that the maintenance of a clear airway by removal of secretions, controlled oxygen therapy and, in ventilated patients, the addition of a degree of positive end-expiratory pressure (PEEP) to maintain the patency of the smaller airways are fundamental to respiratory management in the immediate post-operative period. The use of PEEP is indicated also where there is evidence of pulmonary oedema.[1]

The Work of Respiration

Normally, the demand for oxygen attributable to the work of the respiratory musculature at rest is relatively small, being only about 2% of the total body oxygen consumption. This demand is greatly increased after surgery and some forms of major trauma. After median sternotomy, for instance, it has been shown that the work of respiration can be increased by as much as ten times, maximal as late as the third postoperative day.[2] In these circumstances, oxygen demand is greatly increased and cardiac output must also increase. If these demands cannot be met, cardiorespiratory failure will ensue. It is here that the argument in favour of elective postoperative ventilatory support rests, in that respiratory work is reduced and oxygen supply more likely to be guaranteed.

The Effect of Drugs

The various anaesthetic agents and other drugs used during and following surgery may also have a profound effect on respiratory function. The residual centrally depressant effects of volatile anaesthetic drugs or intravenously administered narcotic analgesics may interfere with respiratory mechanisms in various ways. Depression of the respiratory centre will lead to overall alveolar hypoventilation with carbon dioxide retention and hypoxaemia if respiration is unassisted. In addition, cough reflexes will be depressed and retention of bronchial secretions result.

There is also good evidence that many drugs employed in anaesthesia interfere with the compensatory mechanism of reflex pulmonary vasoconstriction, thus worsening the venous admixture and aggravating arterial hypoxaemia.[3] In addition it is increasingly common practice to employ vasodilator drugs to improve cardiac output by decreasing afterload. Sodium nitroprusside is widely used in this way and has been shown in some studies to reverse hypoxic pulmonary vasoconstriction and result in the redistribution of pulmonary blood flow to poorly ventilated or atelectatic areas of the lung. Although this additional shunt can increase hypoxaemia,[4] this potential disadvantage is offset by the improved circulation which follows a reduction in pulmonary vascular resistance.

Other drugs which may be used intraoperatively or postoperatively may also interfere with pulmonary function. Agents which produce release of histamine may result in bronchospasm and a dangerous reduction in alveolar ventilation. Sedative analgesics such as morphine or muscle relaxants such as curare, employed to facilitate mechanical assistance to ventilation, may trigger this mechanism. Protamine administered at the termination of cardiopulmonary bypass to reverse the effect of heparin may result in pulmonary vasoconstriction, producing pulmonary hypertension and interference with the ventilation perfusion relationship.[5]

As always, adequate reversal of muscle relaxant drugs, employed to maintain intermittent positive pressure ventilation, is of prime importance. Any residual weakness of the respiratory musculature can quickly lead to respiratory failure. It is a wise precaution to employ a peripheral nerve stimulator following pharmacological reversal to confirm the clinical assessment of its adequacy.

Alterations in Cardiac Output

The main cause of hypoxaemia in the postoperative patient is the shunting of blood across the pulmonary circulation in the following ways:
1. The continuing perfusion of unventilated or hypoventilated alveoli.
2. The bypassing of the alveoli through pulmonary arteriovenous anastomoses.
3. Low ventilation : perfusion ratios.
4. Alterations in cardiac output.

While all of these may operate at one time in any postoperative patient, the likelihood of alterations in cardiac output playing a most significant part in the process is greater in some circumstances. For instance, where the heart itself has been diseased prior to surgery or has actually been subjected to further trauma by the surgical procedure, it is likely to be less able to respond to escalating demands to improve its performance in response to an increase in respiratory work. If cardiac output postoperatively is low, or allowed to fall, a highly significant increase in shunting will occur and hypoxaemia will result. Left ventricular failure may complicate the picture further with the onset of pulmonary oedema and poorer oxygenation. This is an excellent example of the interplay of potentially adverse cardiac and pulmonary factors which may have to be recognized and dealt with expeditiously in the postoperative period if the patient is to survive.

Hypothermia

Following prolonged surgery or after resuscitation of a badly injured patient, the body core temperature is frequently subnormal, in the range 35–37 °C. While this may be expected to have a slight protective effect by reducing tissue oxygen requirements, this potential benefit is outweighed if postoperative shivering is permitted to occur and is uncontrolled.[6] Not infrequently increased oxygen demands of this nature are precisely what the patient is unable to meet, since other factors are usually operative that affect oxygen availability.

Body core temperature measurement is an essential part of patient monitoring in the intensive care unit and its usefulness is greatly enhanced by estimating continuously the core (mid-oesophageal) to skin (big toe) gradient.[7] The latter measurement gives a very good indication of the adequacy of peripheral tissue perfusion.

In addition to the causes of hypoxaemia already mentioned, the following should be considered:

1. Haemodilution may be present. If the haematocrit is less than 25–30%, oxygen carrying capacity is dangerously reduced.

2. If alkalosis is present the oxygen affinity for haemoglobin is affected.

3. As a result of stored blood transfusion, the 2,3-diphosphoglycerate content is altered, thus decreasing haemoglobin's affinity for oxygen and also resulting in a shift in the oxyhaemoglobin dissociation curve to the right. Such changes in oxygen availability may have profoundly adverse effects on the patient's haemodynamic status. For instance a 50% reduction in the oxygen carrying capacity of the blood, and a simultaneous doubling of oxygen demand for any reason, would require the cardiac output to increase by a factor of 4 to achieve full compensation.

The widespread use of sodium nitroprusside to reduce cardiac afterload carries with it a further subtle risk which may, in adverse circumstances, worsen cellular hypoxia. If an inadvertent or relative overdose is administered, for example in the presence of renal insufficiency, the accumulation of cyanide or its main toxic metabolite thiocyanate may diminish oxygen utilization at cellular level by interfering with membrane enzyme systems, producing the classic state of histotoxic hypoxia. The rate of sodium nitroprusside infusion should not be permitted to exceed 800 µg/min in a 70-kg patient if toxic blood levels are to be avoided. The formation of methaemoglobin further reduces the oxygen carrying capacity.*

Alterations in the Conscious State

The spontaneous effort of respiration postoperatively may be diminished if the vital centres have suffered any intraoperative insult. A period of inadequate cerebral perfusion or the occurrence of cerebral air embolism may so impair cerebral function as to interfere with the neuroregulation of respiration or the ability of the patient to co-operate to an adequate degree

---

*A solution of 200 mg/500 ml infused at a maximum rate of 50 ml/h is well within the safe range (editor).

with the physiotherapist. Continual assessment of the integrity of the central nervous system and the level of consciousness is an important feature of the monitoring of such patients postoperatively. A standard electroencephalogram (EEG) may be required at intervals or the continuous use of a cerebral function monitor.[8]

To summarize, therefore, it is evident that many patients following major trauma or surgery are particularly vulnerable to some degree of respiratory inadequacy. This may be a result of pre-existing respiratory disease or as a result of the cumulative effect of cardiac disease and its pulmonary sequelae or even the anaesthetic management of the patient intraoperatively.

DIAGNOSIS OF RESPIRATORY INADEQUACY

Most patients who have undergone major surgery will show some impairment of respiratory function, although this may not be of clinical significance in individual cases. This impairment is usually reflected by an alveolar–arterial gradient for oxygen in excess of 300 mmHg (40 kPa) and by varying degrees of arterial hypoxaemia. Only the most severe cases will exhibit clinical signs of carbon dioxide retention and a raised arterial carbon dioxide partial pressure. As has been discussed, the precipitating factors may be one or many and accurate diagnosis demands meticulous observation and often invasive techniques of measurement in the postoperative period. Invasive monitoring may also be essential to determine the effects of any therapy which may be embarked upon.

Blood Gas Measurement and Measurement of Shunt

Measurement of the tensions of oxygen and carbon dioxide in the arterial blood are obviously essential and routinely undertaken, usually by means of an indwelling arterial catheter. While helpful, these do not always give sufficient information regarding the degree of respiratory dysfunction, in particular the amount of intrapulmonary shunting which is present. The mixed venous oxygen tension ($P\bar{v}o_2$) is the most valuable index of oxygen demand but may only be sampled with accuracy if a pulmonary arterial catheter is in place e.g. Swan–Ganz.[9] The mixed venous tension measured in this way should be maintained above 35 mmHg (4·6 kPa) if oxygen demands are within normal limits.

Regular measurement of the degree of shunt postoperatively by the solution of the classic equation

$$Qs/Qt = \frac{C\acute{c}o_2 - Cao_2}{C\acute{c}o_2 - C\bar{v}o_2}$$

requires several assumptions and inaccuracies are inevitable.[10] Pulmonary end-capillary blood oxygen content cannot be measured directly but the capillary oxygen tension is assumed to be nearly the same as the alveolar tension which, in turn, is derived from the alveolar : air equation.[11] The oxygen contents of the mixed venous and arterial blood can, of course, be measured directly using an instrument such as the Lex-O_2-Con oxygen analyser or derived from the respective tensions by using a suitable nomogram.

It can be seen, therefore that there are two requirements if the degree of intrapulmonary shunting is to be measured frequently, one being the ability to sample pulmonary mixed venous blood via a cardiac catheter and the other to undertake the solution of the above-mentioned equation with speed and regularity. The use of programmed microprocessors has simplified the latter calculation to the extent that frequent bedside measurements can be made with sufficient speed and accuracy to guide treatment.[12]

Another problem has to be faced clinically when the attempt is made to distinguish between ventilation : perfusion mismatching and true shunting by administering an inspired oxygen concentration of 100% ($FIo_2 = 1 \cdot 0$). Normally this would be expected virtually to eliminate mismatching by increasing the alveolar oxygen tension, while a true shunt would be unaffected. However, it has been shown that respiring 100% oxygen for as little as 30 minutes can wash out alveolar nitrogen in poorly ventilated lung units and lead to patchy atelectasis and further ventilation perfusion mismatch.[13,14]

Unless these difficulties are appreciated and overcome, the clinician is forced to rely on the cruder and potentially misleading assessment of arterial oxygen and carbon dioxide tensions in the monitoring of the patient. As an example, the measurement of arterial carbon dioxide tension may be misleading when a raised level is due to increased production rather than diminished alveolar ventilation.

Measurement of Cardiac Output

Normally, the anaesthetist or clinician in the ICU assesses cardiac output changes indirectly by observing the arterial blood pressure in relation to the state of peripheral perfusion. This, while essential basic monitoring, lacks the precision required for the management of the most severely ill patients where alterations in cardiac output are likely to be the most significant contribution to shunting and arterial hypoxaemia in the absence of gross pulmonary damage. In such cases, powerful therapeutic agents may be employed, such as vasodilators of the nitroprusside type or inotropic drugs such as dopamine or isoprenaline, and their precise effect on cardiac output in the individual patient is essential information if therapy is to be rational.

Again, if in the ventilated patient it is decided to employ a positive end-expiratory pressure phase (PEEP), the possible deleterious effect on cardiac output and haemodynamics should be accurately known since it may outweigh any apparent advantages in terms of preventing premature airways closure and raising the arterial oxygen tension. Suter and his colleagues[15] described the concept of 'best PEEP' where maximum delivery of oxygen to the tissues occurs at minimum cost in terms of depression of cardiac output.

During the intravenous administration of colloids or physiological solutions, the measurement of central venous pressure in ill patients is routine. There are circumstances where this may be misleading and the measurement will not truly reflect the performance of the left side of the heart. Here, ideally, the left atrial pressure should be measured but, as this is usually impossible except after cardiac surgery, the pulmonary arterial wedge pressure (PAWP) gives a reasonable approximation (*Fig.* 14.2). Where PEEP is applied in the presence of hypovolaemia, the interference with cardiac output may be profound and close monitoring of cardiac output and the wedge pressure are essential guides to the amount of fluid replacement required and the speed with which it can be given. The potentially harmful effects of PEEP on cardiac and renal function may, to some extent, be reversed by the simultaneous use of inotropic agents such as dopamine.[16]

For these reasons there is a good case for the employment of a technique for measuring cardiac output postoperatively. This may be done by the thermal-dilution method via a triple-lumen Swan–Ganz catheter and the result computed and read out at the bedside within seconds. While probably less accurate than the classic dye-dilution technique, the thermal-dilution method has the advantage that it may be repeated many times without the limitation imposed by the accumulation of the dye.

Observation of Renal Function

The final arbiter of acid–base homeostasis in the patient will be normal or near normal renal function. Respiratory and renal function have an important inter-relationship and it is necessary to observe closely the renal performance in every case of respiratory failure. The flow of urine should be maintained at more than 30 ml/h in an average 70-kg patient and the urine/plasma osmolarity ratio should be greater than $1·2:1$ to avoid the development of acute reversible intrinsic renal failure (ARIRF or acute tubular necrosis). The measurement of serum electrolytes and creatinine, and similarly of urine electrolytes, is also mandatory if early warning of serious renal impairment is to be acquired.

Alterations in cardiac output and antidiuretic hormone activity post-operatively can have profound effects upon renal performance but respira-

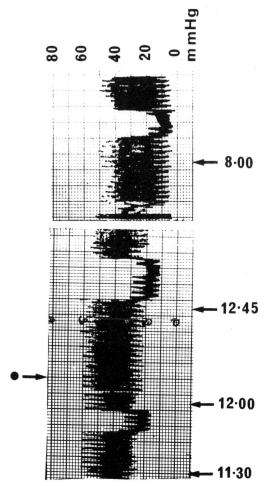

Fig. 14.2. Pulmonary arterial and pulmonary wedge pressure tracings from a male patient (age 20 years) who suffered from over-infusion of i.v. fluids following severe trauma. 11·30 a.m. Pulmonary arterial pressure 60 mmHg, mean left atrial pressure 21 mmHg. Following administration of ouabaine and frusemide, intravenously (●) there was a steady cardio-vascular improvement. 8 a.m. Pulmonary arterial pressure now 40 mmHg and mean left atrial pressure 10 mmHg. (This figure originally appeared in the *British Journal of Anaesthesia* (1977) **49**, 675. Thanks are due to the Editor and the Publishers, Macmillan Journals Ltd, for permission to reproduce this.)

tory dysfunction, either in the form of gross respiratory acidosis or low arterial oxygen levels, may also lead to depression of renal perfusion and tubular function. In the spontaneously breathing patient, metabolic acidosis resulting from renal failure can have a further depressant effect on respiratory function as well as on myocardial performance.

Powers[17] made the important point that since patients admitted to intensive care units are generally at high risk of serious complication or death 'tolerance for diagnostic and therapeutic error is reduced almost to the vanishing point. Clinical syndromes appear suddenly and progress to irreversiblity with startling rapidity.' He goes on to justify the use in critical care of very invasive monitoring techniques which could not be countenanced on a risk to benefit basis in the ordinary medical ward. There is one further important point to be considered when dealing with extremely ill patients. The technology is readily available to permit a wide range of invasive techniques and measurement but, increasingly, the problem is not one of acquiring accurate primary data quickly but of deriving secondary information speedily enough to influence clinical decisions or guide therapy accurately in an individual patient. Fortunately, the microprocessor has revolutionized bedside computing of this nature as in many other fields, and suitably programmed microprocessor-based computers can handle large amounts of data quickly and also provide indications of trends by making regular comparisons of sequential measurements in the patient. All this of course should merely be an extension of the physician's own clinical powers of observation but the new technology is invaluable when employed in a proper manner.

MANAGEMENT OF RESPIRATORY FAILURE

The proper management of respiratory failure depends first and foremost on clinical experience and 'astute observation, but secondly and increasingly on the accuracy and speed of measurement and bedside processing of large amounts of data to follow rapidly changing and complex pathophysiological processes. Essentially the questions in management are:
1. Does the patient require supplementary oxygen to breathe?
2. Is an artificial airway required?
3. Is mechanical support to ventilation required?
4. Is any specific drug therapy indicated, e.g. bronchodilators or antibiotics?

Oxygen Therapy

For the reasons that have been discussed when considering factors contributing to respiratory dysfunction and derangement of oxygen transport and utilization, oxygen therapy is always required postoperatively and following major injuries for a shorter or longer period. The question remains how much oxygen in terms of the fractional inspired concentration (FIo_2) is required and for how long? It is generally agreed that the aim should be to maintain an alveolar oxygen tension in excess of 60 mmHg (8·0 kPa) and that the FIo_2 should be adjusted accordingly but maintained at less than 1·0 and preferably not more than 0·6 to avoid the pulmonary changes resulting from oxygen toxicity.[18] Hand in hand with oxygen therapy must go efficient humidification of the dry and cold inspired gas combined with effective removal of secretions from the airway and adequate provision of pain relief.

The Artificial Airway

If the airway is in jeopardy, either due to depressed protective reflexes or continuing retention of secretions, then tracheal intubation is usually indicated. Either the nasal or the oral route may be employed, although for the short term the oral route is usually used since an airway of larger effective diameter can be introduced. The plastic one-use tubes currently employed are satisfactory from the viewpoint of tissue reaction and the critical matter is to employ a tube of the Lanz type with a cuff which is compliant with a low and controlled pressure.[19] Using this type of tube, cuff pressures of 15–25 cm water are sufficient to effect an airtight seal in most cases. This avoids the high incidence of complications, such as mucosal sloughing and tracheal stenosis, which may follow the long-term use of the conventional high pressure cuff. The presence of an artificial airway of this type avoids an excessive need for elective tracheostomy in these patients and facilitates mechanical assistance to ventilation when required.

Mechanical Assistance to Ventilation

The indications par excellence for mechanical assistance to ventilation are when excessive respiratory work is required to maintain normal blood gas values or when blood gas levels are abnormal despite the best spontaneous respiratory effort achieved by the patient. An arterial oxygen tension of less than 60 mmHg (8·0 kPa) breathing air or 80 mmHg (10·6 kPa) when breathing oxygen is an indication for assistance as is an arterial carbon dioxide tension of more than 56 mmHg (7·5 kPa).

The choice of mechanical ventilator is dictated by many factors, but the ability to alter the pattern of ventilation to maintain adequate alveolar ventilation using the lowest possible mean intrathoracic pressure is of prime importance. The ability to apply PEEP has been alluded to earlier as being necessary and the machine should ideally be capable of being adjusted to provide intermittent mandatory ventilation (IMV) during the weaning process. The ideal ventilator should have the following attributes:
I. It should be sturdy and reliable.
II. It should be easy to operate and ergonomically designed to suit nursing personnel who will often be the immediate supervisors of the patient.
III. The ventilator should be inherently safe in operation with over-pressure escape valves and alarms.

IV. It should have an adequate humidifying facility.

V. Inspired oxygen concentration (FIo_2) should be easily adjusted.

VI. The machine should have the following modes:
1. Fully controlled ventilation (IPPV).
2. Intermittent mandatory ventilation (IMV).
3. Positive end-expiratory pressure (PEEP).
4. Continuous positive airway pressure (CPAP).

VII. The ventilator must be capable of producing a wide range of tidal and minute volumes and adequate airway pressures.

VIII. The ratio of the inspiratory to the expiratory phase of respiration should be capable of adjustment independently of the rate of respiration.

Many modern ventilators now meet these requirements, but many are still unsatisfactory from the point of view of ease of regular maintenance and ease of cleansing to a bacteriologically acceptable standard. Since cross-infection is an important cause of morbidity and mortality of patients in intensive care areas, the latter point is an important one when it comes to choosing a suitable machine.[20]

The main problems which may arise during mechanical assistance to ventilation, apart from machine failure, are related to the maintenance of normal haemodynamics. If there is any occult degree of hypovolaemia then the reversal of normal intrathoracic pressures accompanying IPPV will result in an acute reduction in cardiac output. If autonomic control of peripheral resistance is interfered with by drugs, then cardiac output may be further depressed. Inadequate dosage of curariform drugs or lack of analgesia in the patient can result in 'fighting' the machine and this asynchrony of machine and patient effort can give rise to tachy-arrhythmias, gross arterial hypertension and serious interference with myocardial function. Adequate sedation in these circumstances is more effective in decreasing the afterload than an increase in the rate of administration of a vasodilator drug such as sodium nitroprusside.

There are other additional matters which require consideration when the patient with respiratory failure is ventilated mechanically. One of the classic emergencies in an ICU is the development of an acute tension pneumothorax during IPPV with or without PEEP. This leads to a catastrophic deterioration in the patient's condition with cardiovascular collapse and death, if not relieved by the rapid insertion of a pleural drain which must then be attached to a water-sealed system or Heimlich valve. A pneumothorax is particularly likely to occur where there has been a chest injury or where emphysematous bullae are present. Other forms of barotrauma, while less dramatic, are to be avoided. The injudicious use of high mean airway pressures or excessive PEEP may lead to hyperinflation of lung units and rupture of alveoli.

Considerable debate continues about some of the other effects of the use of PEEP. In particular, its effect on the extravascular lung water volume.[21] It is clear that the employment of this ventilation mode during treatment should be undertaken only where there is a clear indication, where its potentially harmful effects on the lungs and other organs and systems are understood, and where the means are available to monitor the patient very closely, if necessary using invasive techniques.

SPECIFIC DRUG THERAPY

A wide range of therapeutic agents are required in the intensive management of acute respiratory failure since the causation may be so diverse. The basic drugs employed to facilitate mechanical assistance to ventilation are common to all groups of patients and comprise sedatives such as diazepam, or others of the benzodiazepine group, narcotic analgesics such as morphine and muscle relaxant agents such as D-tubocurarine or pancuronium bromide. Drugs are administered intravenously, either in intermittent increments or increasingly by continuous infusion employing one of the many types of graduated pump or motorized syringe. Where pain is not a feature of the patient's condition, a non-analgesic sedative drug such as the steroid anaesthetic induction agent Althesin in suitable dilution or chlormethiazole may be used to produce a safe level of sedation.[22] These agents have the additional advantage, when compared with the benzodiazepines, that significant accumulation of the principal agent or any active metabolite does not occur. This enables the clinician to terminate administration in the confident expectation that, if all is well, there will be a rapid return to consciousness, thus enabling a better assessment of the cerebral state and general progress of the patient to be made. The outstanding problem is still to determine the state of awareness of the patient and whether pain is being suffered since communication is usually inadequate or absent. Reliance has often to be placed on the close observation of the autonomic responses such as lacrimation, tachycardia and peripheral vasoconstriction. It is possible that the cerebral function monitor has a useful role here.[8]

More specific therapy may be indicated, for example, where there is a need to treat cardiac failure with digitalis and diuretics or where bronchospasm is a persistent problem and where bronchodilators such as aminophylline or orciprenaline may be required. Secondary invasion by gram-negative organisms, usually accompanied by anaerobes, is an ever present danger in ICUs and may fatally complicate respiratory failure of any aetiology, if such infection is not indeed the main cause of lung failure. The clinician must ensure constant screening of the environment of the treatment area as well as the culturing of the respiratory secretions and other body fluids. The confusing numbers of antibiotics now available bewilder even the most experienced clinician at times and, as the most potent are often the most toxic, the close co-operation of an expert bacteriologist is essential and the measurement of blood levels where possible is advised. A sensible review of the position has been outlined recently by McAllister.[23]

One contentious issue requires some consideration where drug therapy is concerned, and that is the role of steroids in the management of some forms of respiratory failure. Their use is well established and quite specific where the management of the asthmatic with pulmonary failure is concerned, but is certainly less clear in the case of the adult respiratory distress syndrome (ARDS). Where there is pulmonary injury leading to this condition, the evidence in favour of the use of steroids such as methylprednisolone, usually in massive dosage, is largely based on experimental work in animals.[24] The efficacy of steroids in man is still open to question, although understandably the clinician is often persuaded to indulge in empiricism where the patient's condition is fast deteriorating despite all efforts. It is generally accepted, despite the lack of firm evidence, that the administration of steroids is justified in the adult respiratory distress syndrome accompanying endotoxic shock or resulting from direct pulmonary injury such as occurs in smoke inhalation.

Dundee and others have drawn attention to the value of the intravenous administration of doxapram in producing respiratory stimulation, particularly in the immediate postoperative period.[25] This technique of 'driving' the respiratory centre chemically is not new since other analeptics such as nikethamide have been used in this manner in the past in an effort to reverse incipient respiratory failure. While doxapram has a better therapeutic index than the older agents, it is nevertheless a non-specific central nervous system stimulant and, therefore, can produce convulsions in overdose. In addition, it is vital to accompany its administration by supplemental oxygen since this group of drugs all produce an increased oxygen demand. The indications for this type of treatment are few and generally most clinicians would opt for mechanical assistance to ventilation as a safer alternative.

When considering drug therapy it is appropriate to draw attention to the patient's energy and nutritional requirements. In addition to ensuring normal electrolyte and water balance in the patient with respiratory failure, it is vital not to lose sight of the need to provide calories, essential amino acids, vitamins and trace elements.[26] A prolonged sojourn in an intensive care unit may result in considerable loss of muscle protein since many of these patients are hypercatabolic. The extent of this may not be appreciated until an attempt is made to wean the patient from the ventilator, when muscle weakness may frustrate the process. A more subtle danger is the development of significant deficiencies in trace elements such as magnesium and zinc which may have life-threatening consequences if unrecognized and untreated. Full parenteral feeding is required, therefore, in all patients other than those whose stay in the intensive care unit is measured in hours rather than in days or weeks.

CONCLUSION

Acute respiratory failure may be the primary cause of a patient's illness or may indeed be the end stage of failure of other organs. If it is the former and is treated inadequately or inappropriately, it will inevitably have a fundamentally harmful effect on all other organ functions since the provision of an adequate oxygen supply and the efficient elimination of carbon dioxide is essential to normal cellular metabolism. The methods of treatment themselves carry inherent risks which, if not appreciated, may further prejudice the patient's recovery. Most treatment is directed to general support of respiratory function and may only buy time for more specific therapy to be effective. Having taken over the essential function of respiration by interfering with or abolishing the patient's own spontaneous effort and protective reflexes, the clinician assumes a great responsibility which can be discharged only if meticulous attention to all aspects of monitoring of vital functions and the therapy itself is assured.

REFERENCES

1. Gilston A. (1977) The effects of PEEP on arterial oxygenation. *Intens. Care Med.* **3**, 267.
2. Peters R. N., Wellows H. A. and Howe T. M. (1969) Total compliance in work of breathing after thoracotomy. *J. Thorac. Cardiovasc. Surg.* **57**, 348.
3. Sykes M. K., Arnot R. N. and Jastrzebski J. (1975) Reduction of hypoxic pulmonary vasoconstriction during Trilene anaesthesia. *J. Appl. Physiol.* **39**, 103.
4. Stone J. G., Khambatta H. J. and Matteo R. S. (1976) Pulmonary shunting during anesthesia with deliberate hypotension. *Anesthesiology* **45**, 508.
5. Branthwaite M. A. (1977) *Anesthesia for Cardiac Surgery and Allied Procedures*, p. 99. Oxford, Blackwell Scientific Publications.
6. Day J., Nunn J. F. and Prys-Roberts C. (1968) Factors influencing arterial Po_2 during recovery from anaesthesia. *Br. J. Anaesth.* **40**, 398.
7. Campbell D. (1977) Immediate hospital care of the injured. *Br. J. Anaesth.* **49**, 673.
8. Dubois M., Savege T. M., O'Carrol T. et al. (1978) General anaesthesia and changes on the cerebral function monitor. *Anaesthesia* **33**, 157.
9. Swan H. J. C., Ganz W., Forester J. et al. (1970) Catheterisation of the heart in man with use of a flow-directed balloon-tipped catheter. *N. Engl. J. Med.* **283**, 447.
10. Comroe J. H., Forster R. E., Dubois A. B. et al. (1962a) *The Lung*, p. 344. Chicago, Year Book Medical Publishers Inc.
11. Comroe J. H., Forster R. E., Dubois A. B. et al. (1962b) *The Lung*, p. 339. Chicago, Year Book Medical Publishers Inc.
12. Kenny G. N. C. (1979) Programmable calculator: a program for use in the intensive care unit. *Br. J. Anaesth.* **51**, 793.
13. Dantzker D. R., Wagner P. D. and West J. B. (1975) Instability of lung units with low V/Q ratios during O_2 breathing. *J. Appl. Physiol.* **38**, 886.
14. Suter P. M., Fairley H. B. and Schlobohm R. M. (1974) The response of lung volume and pulmonary perfusion to short periods of 100 per cent oxygen ventilation in acute respiratory failure. *Crit. Care Med.* **2**, 43.
15. Suter P. M., Farley H. B. and Isenberg M. (1975) Optimum end-expiratory airway pressure in patients with acute pulmonary failure. *N. Engl. J. Med.* **292**, 284.
16. Hemmer M. and Suter P. M. (1979) Treatment of cardiac and renal effects of PEEP with dopamine in patients with acute respiratory failure. *Anesthesiology* **50**, 339.

17. Powers S. F. (1977) In: Kinney J. M., Bendixen H. H. and Powers S. R., ed., *Manual of Surgical Intensive Care*, p. 327. Philadelphia, W. B. Saunders Co.
18. Winter P. M. and Smith G. (1972) The toxicity of oxygen. *Anesthesiology* **37**, 210.
19. McGinnis G. E., Shively J. G. and Patterson R. L. (1971) Engineering analysis of intratracheal tube cuffs. *Anesth. Analg.* **50**, 557.
20. Thorp J. M., Richards W. C. and Telfer A. B. M. (1979) A survey of infection in an intensive care unit. *Anaesthesia* **34**, 643.
21. Demling R. H., Staub N. C. and Edmunds L. H. (1975) Effects of end-expiratory pressure on accumulation of extra-vascular lung water. *J. Appl. Physiol.* **38**, 907.
22. Scott D. B., Beamish D., Hudson I. N., et al. (1980) Prolonged infusion of chlormethiazole in intensive care. *Br. J. Anaesth.* **52**, 541.
23. McAllister T. A. (1976) Recent advances in antibiotics. *Scott. Med. J.* **21**, 210.
24. Cheney F. W., Huang T. H. and Gronka R. (1979) Effects of methylprednisolone on experimental pulmonary injury. *Ann. Surg.* **190**, 236.
25. Gawley T. H., Dundee J. W., Gupta P. K., et al. (1976) Role of doxapram in reducing pulmonary complications after major surgery. *Br. Med. J.* **1**, 122.
26. Allison S. P. (1977) Metabolic aspects of intensive care. In: Norman J. and Moles M., ed., *Management of the Injured Patient*. London, Macmillan Journals Ltd.

Chapter 15

The Cardiovascular System

K. M. Taylor and W. H. Bain

PRINCIPAL PROBLEMS

Intensive medical care specifically related to cardiac pathology has developed for the most part in response to two related but distinct clinical situations:

1. Patients who have sustained acute myocardial infarction.
2. Patients undergoing open-heart surgical procedures.

The management of patients sustaining acute myocardial infarction by early transportation and admission to a specialized coronary care unit (CCU) has been associated with a greatly increased awareness of early complications, e.g. arrhythmias, and with more objective assessment of available therapies, e.g. inotropic and anti-arrhythmic agents. It is not, however, the purpose of this chapter to include detailed discussion of CCU practice, since the literature on this subject is already comprehensive. It is important to realize, however, that acute myocardial infarction may complicate the clinical course of any severely ill patient in the general intensive care unit.

This chapter will consider the approach to intensive care specifically related to cardiac pathology as encountered in the following clinical situations:

1. Routine postoperative management of cardiac surgical patients.

2. Pre- and postoperative management of severely ill cardiac surgical patients, principally those with 'low cardiac output syndrome'.

3. Cardiac pathology secondary to:

   Pre-existing shock syndromes
   Respiratory insufficiency
   Pre-existing subclinical cardiac pathology.

372

MEASUREMENT AND MONITORING

The central physiological importance of cardiac pumping in maintaining organ perfusion, and the rapidity with which disturbance or cessation of cardiac action produces irreversible pathological damage, has encouraged the development of comprehensive real-time monitoring of many indices of cardiac function. In addition to the more basic indices, derived indices of ventricular function and peripheral perfusion are increasingly employed in specialized cardiac units. Computerization of cardiac monitoring indices is being developed in several centres, both as data collection, and on-line patient management facilities.[1] The integration of monitored indices of cardiac function in clinical judgement will be further discussed below in Pathophysiological Mechanisms. In this section, the practical details of cardiac monitoring will be outlined.

I. Heart Rate

Heart rate monitoring may be accomplished electronically, either by a pulse sensor placed over a finger or toe, or by an inbuilt rate meter linked to the ECG. The simple pulse sensor is more applicable to patients without any significant cardiac dysfunction, in intermediate rather than intensive care situations. Peripheral pulse sensors may fail to pick up the pulse deficit in between cardiac rate (apical rate) and peripheral pulse rate, in rapid and haemodynamically inefficient arrhythmias, e.g. poorly controlled atrial fibrillation. ECG-linked rate monitoring is, therefore, to be preferred in the majority of intensive care situations. Ideally, the rate meter should have adjustable higher and lower alarm limits, with both visual and auditory stimuli when heart rate falls below or rises above the chosen limits.

II. Heart Rhythm

Continuous display of the ECG is the optimal method for monitoring cardiac rhythm. The ECG display unit may be linked to a paper print-out for immediate recording of any rhythm disturbances to allow accurate interpretation. More advanced monitoring systems may incorporate automatic sensing and print-out of rhythm changes, and 24-hour continuous recording of the ECG on replayable tape. For routine purposes, electrodes should be placed on both shoulders and upper thighs, to give standard leads I, II, III and leads AVr, AVl and AVf.

In addition to the continuous bedside ECG display, a complete 12-lead ECG should be recorded daily.

III. Arterial Blood Pressure

The continuous measurement of arterial blood pressure, using indwelling arterial cannulae, has become widely accepted as the optimal technique in patiens requiring intensive care. In patients undergoing open-heart surgical procedures, the arterial cannula should be inserted immediately after anaesthetic induction, and should be retained until the cardiac status has stabilized postoperatively (usually 24 hours post-operation). In severely ill patients about to undergo cardiac surgery, the arterial cannula may be inserted preoperatively under local anaesthesia, thus ensuring continuous monitoring of arterial blood pressure during anaesthetic induction, when the severely ill cardiac patient may be at risk.

The radial artery at the wrist is the preferred site for arterial cannulation, though, if necessary, the brachial, femoral and dorsalis pedis arteries may be used. Long-term cannulation of both brachial and femoral arteries is, however, less well tolerated, with a greater incidence of bleeding around the cannula and local arterial spasm. Cannulation should be performed with a pliable Teflon cannula, 18 or 20 Fr being suitable for most radial artery insertions. The cannula should be connected to a short length of monitoring line, a three-way tap connected (for arterial blood sample aspiration) and a further length of monitoring line to the pressure transducer. A constant low-flow flushing device should be included in the system, in order to maintain patency of the arterial line.

The pressure transducer should be relayed to an oscilloscope, to give a visual display of the arterial pressure waveform, and a digital read-out of systolic, diastolic and mean arterial pressure is valuable. The importance of such a system lies in the fact that the absolute level of arterial blood pressure may be misleading where significant vasoconstriction has occurred in the patient's peripheral circulation.

Normal or even supranormal levels of arterial systolic pressure may be displayed, though the narrow 'spiky' trace typical of the vasoconstricted patient will permit a more accurate assessment of the patient's cardiac status. As with heart rate meters, the blood pressure meters may be fitted with high and low level alarms.

Where the patient's cardiac status is not giving real cause for concern, non-invasive arterial blood pressure measurement may be preferred. In addition to the traditional manual determination at 15-minute intervals by sphygmomanometer, there are new devices of suitable accuracy which will

---

*Critikon, 1410 N. Westshore Boulevard, Tampa, Florida, U.S.A.

display arterial blood pressure levels using non-invasive techniques (e.g. Dinamap system*).

IV. Central Venous Pressure

The use of central venous pressure (CVP) measurement in the general intensive care situation is discussed elsewhere in this textbook. In the cardiac patient, particularly those suffering from chronic cardiac failure with cardiac valve pathology, central venous or right atrial pressure measurement, while still useful, must be interpreted with caution since the intracardiac pathology has usually influenced the absolute level of CVP which is 'normal' for that patient. For this reason, elevated levels of CVP may be encountered, and indeed required in certain cardiac patients to ensure appropriate right heart filling pressures (*Table* 15.1).

Table **15.1. CVP usually encountered in post-operative patients 6 hours after open-heart surgery**

Operation	CVP, cm H_2O	
	Mean	Range
Mitral valve replacement	12	10–15
Aortic valve replacement	10	8–12
Tricuspid valve replacement	15	12–20
Coronary vein grafts	8	5–10

Zero reference is mid-thorax.
Patients were on IPPV.
Figures taken from 880 cases.

Despite this reservation, CVP monitoring is still a valuable parameter in the management of the cardiac patient requiring intensive care.

Techniques for CVP line insertion are a source of much controversy. Some authorities, including the authors, favour insertion of CVP lines via the internal jugular vein in the triangle bounded by medical head and lateral heads of sternomastoid, and the upper border of the clavicle. The directness of this route, and its relative cleanliness, commend it for use in specialized units, though imprecise or 'multiple attempt' stabs in this area may damage the internal carotid artery, or penetrate the apical pleura. Such potentially hazardous complications have been the subject of recent reports.[2,3] Prior insertion of a fine gauge 'seeking' needle will localize the internal jugular vein and lessen the risk of trauma. Only when the vein has been accurately localized should the CVP cannula be inserted. When in situ, free flow of venous blood in the cannula and line should be ensured.

Some centres prefer subclavian vein insertion, while others utilize the more superficial external jugular vein or median cubital vein at the elbow.

These latter two sites of insertion carry a lower risk of local tissue trauma, though positioning of the cannula in the central veins or the right atrium is less assured than with the internal jugular or subclavian approaches. The femoral vein may also be used, though the cleanliness of this area is more suspect, and cannulation of the leg veins increases the incidence of deep venous thrombosis.

Accurate zeroing of the centimetre scale must be checked at intervals to ensure consistency of reference point. This may be taken as mid-thorax level in the supine patient or, if preferred, the mid-point of the clavicle. Patency of the CVP line should also be checked at frequent intervals, usually by ensuring that the characteristic respiratory excursion of the fluid column is present.

The authors' practice is to forbid use of the CVP measuring line for administration of any powerful vasoactive drugs (e.g. inotrope infusions). This avoids the risk of accidental bolus injection of vasoactive substances during manipulations of the CVP for measurement, etc.

It should be noted that non-cardiac factors may alter CVP values in the intensive care situation. The use of intermittent positive-pressure ventilation (IPPV) and also the addition of positive end-expiratory pressure (PEEP) will each raise CVP levels by 2–5 cm water.

V. Left Atrial Pressure (Direct measurement)

Direct measurement of left atrial pressure is employed in patients who have undergone cardiac surgery in whom left ventricular function is seriously impaired. In these patients, maintenance of a left atrial pressure at a level high enough to ensure optimal left ventricular filling, without overdistending the left ventricle and producing ventricular failure, is of particular importance. At the end of the operative procedure, in such cases, a cannula is inserted into the left atrium through a purse-string suture and led out through the skin to be secured on the chest wall. A pressure transducer/fluid filled line system is established and the pressure displayed on an oscilloscope. A direct left atrial pressure line is of great value in the delicate management of a severely damaged left ventricle, though great care must be taken to ensure that no air bubbles are introduced into the line, with the risk of arterial air embolism. In our experience, bleeding problems around the site of insertion in the left atrium are uncommon. When no longer required, the line is shut off, but left in situ for 5 days before removal. An alternative mode of insertion is trans-septal, passing the cannula through the right atrium, across the inter-atrial septa to the left atrium. This may reduce the risk of persistent oozing around the cannulation site.

We believe that direct left atrial pressure measurement is presently indicated in only a very small proportion of postcardiac surgery cases, and that indirect methods utilizing pulmonary artery wedge pressure, will prove to be of wider applicability.

VI. Pulmonary Artery Wedge Pressure

Inflatable balloon tip catheters, passed through the right heart, pulmonary valve and main pulmonary artery, will ultimately 'wedge' in a peripheral pulmonary artery branch. The pressure obtained, the pulmonary wedge pressure, has been shown to be an acceptably accurate reflection of left atrial mean pressure, and hence pulmonary artery wedge pressure (PAWP) measurement is an indirect method of measuring left atrial pressure.

The initial Swan–Ganz flow-directed catheters have since been further developed to incorporate thermistor sensors and proximal injection orifices to permit thermodilution cardiac output determination. PAWP measurement has been widely introduced in recent years into intensive care practice, and is likely to become an integral part of haemodynamic monitoring.

VII. Peripheral Circulation Assessment

As previously stated, assessment of the peripheral circulatory status is always necessary for an intelligent and accurate interpretation of a patient's cardiac status. Compensatory vasoconstrictor responses may allow maintenance of physiological levels of arterial blood pressure despite significant cardiac dysfuntion with substantially reduced cardiac output. Assessment of the peripheral circulatory status is considered by many to be the most accurate and sensitive indication of cardiovascular status, except in patients with severe peripheral vascular disease, or in certain phases of septic shock.

Despite its great value, assessment of peripheral circulation is principally a matter of clinical judgement, considering skin warmth, colour, degree of venous filling, and speed of capillary return after skin pressure, as indices of peripheral circulatory adequacy.

Quantifiable indices of peripheral perfusion may also be utilized. These include:

Measurement of toe temperature, or toe–core temperature differences (e.g. for 'warm up' patterns after open-heart surgery).

Urinary volume measurement (hourly) as an indirect index of renal perfusion.

Calculation of peripheral vascular resistance (PVR) and peripheral vascular resistance index (PVRI) using the standard formulae:

$$PVR = \frac{MABP - CVP}{CO} \qquad (1)$$

$$\frac{PVRI}{(\text{index units})} = \frac{MABP - CVP}{(CO/BSA)} \qquad (2)$$

where

$MABP$ = mean arterial blood pressure (mmHg)
CVP = central venous pressure (mmHg)
CO = cardiac output (l/min)
BSA = body surface area (m^2)

The normal PVRI is around 20–25 index units. Though used principally in detailed haemodynamic investigations, where cardiac output is being measured routinely, calculation of PVR values should be undertaken more frequently, particularly in view of the harmful effects of excessive degrees of peripheral vasoconstriction on left ventricular function.

VIII. Cardiac Output and Derived Indices

The facility for the accurate and repeatable measurement of cardiac output is of immense value in the assessment and management of the cardiac patient. Though still regarded by many as a research tool, routine measurement of cardiac output is increasingly employed in the haemodynamic evaluation of postcardiac surgical patients, in particular, and intensive care patients in general.

Indicator dilution techniques are usually employed for cardiac output measurement:

1. Dye Dilution

Using central venous injection of a suitable dye (e.g. indocyanine green) with continuous sampling of arterial blood through a densitometer cuvette. This standard technique is of established accuracy, though it is rather cumbersome compared to automated thermodilution techniques.[4]

2. Thermodilution

Using injection of cold solution into the circulation, with a suitably placed catheter incorporating a thermistor. In the past few years, certain balloon catheters, e.g. Swan–Ganz,[5] designed for pulmonary artery pressure monitoring have been modified to incorporate a proximal injectate orifice and a distal thermistor, thus permitting controlled thermodilution cardiac output determinations. This technique is relatively simple, and, given precise sensing of the injectate solution temperature, acceptably accurate. From the cardiac output value (each determination should ideally be performed in triplicate), the following simple indices of cardiac function may be derived:

$$\text{Cardiac index } (l \cdot m^2 \cdot min^{-1}) = CO/BSA \ (m^2)$$

$$\text{Stroke volume (ml)} = \frac{CO \times 1000}{\text{Heart rate}}$$

$$\text{Stroke volume index} \ (ml \cdot m^{-2}) = \frac{(CO/BSA) \times 1000}{\text{Heart rate}}$$

The mean values for cardiac output and cardiac index, measured in theatre immediately after open-heart surgery, are shown in *Table* 15.2.

Table 15.2. The mean (and standard deviation) values for cardiac output and derived indices from 250 patients, measured 30 minutes after cardiopulmonary bypass

Procedure	Cardiac output, $l \cdot min^{-1}$	Cardiac index, $l \cdot min^{-1} \cdot m^{-2}$	Peripheral vascular resistance, units	PVR index, units m^{-2}
Mitral valve replacement	3·92 (1·13)	2·39 (0·59)	16·6 (5·96)	26·67 (8·32)
Aortic valve replacement	5·46 (1·75)	3·04 (0·75)	12·57 (3·98)	21·66 (5·91)
Mitral and aortic valves replacement	3·79 (0·99)	2·29 (0·61)	18·17 (6·55)	30·11 (11·04)
Coronary bypass grafts	5·09 (1·37)	2·78 (0·68)	15·09 (5·29)	27·5 (9·37)

Subsequently the cardiac output usually falls during the first 4 hours after chest closure, rising again during the subsequent 12 hours to regain the preoperative value (*Table* 15.3).

IX. Blood Volume

A knowledge of the volume available to the intravascular fluid compartment is essential in the interpretation of changes in cardiac output and indices derived therefrom, such as PVR.

Table 15.3. The pattern of change in cardiac index following open-heart surgery

Cardiac index	Pre-op., %	Time
3·09	100	Pre-op.
2·63	85	0·5 hour post-bypass
2·37	77	Arrival in ICU
2·85	92	3 hours post-bypass
3·38	109	6 hours post-bypass
3·41	110	12 hours post-bypass

The plasma volume can be measured by an indicator dilution technique, and blood volume extrapolated using the haematocrit.

In practice, the intravascular volume is restored, after the patient has been weaned from heart/lung bypass, by infusing increments of 100 ml from the residual volume contained in the extracorporeal circuit until left atrial pressure, CVP, heart size and cardiac output are optimal. Subsequent loss of blood from the chest drains and gain from transfusion are charted and a positive balance of 20% of the blood lost should be achieved at 6 hours postoperatively. This 20% represents hidden losses in the form of a mediastinal haematoma or haemothorax.

The CVP or left atrial pressure (or pulmonary wedge pressure) are guides to the status of blood volume replacement. The absolute levels of these pressures, however, are also influenced by right and left ventricular function and, therefore, a change in these pressures in response to volume expansion is a more valuable guide. Thus a small rise, or no rise in CVP or LAP following the transfusion of 200 ml of blood over 15 minutes, is indicative of hypovolaemia. Where a trial transfusion of 200 ml produces rise of several mmHg in either pressure, a further increase in blood volume may be associated with a risk of precipitating pulmonary oedema unless vasodilator therapy is used concurrently.

Unexpectedly high levels of CVP or LAP will accompany cardiac tamponade in patients in whom intra-pericardial blood or clot is causing atrial compression.

X. Biochemical Monitoring

Cardiac function is very sensitive to disturbance in body biochemistry. In particular, the following simple measurements are necessary:

Arterial blood gas: Po_2, Pco_2, pH, base excess,

Plasma potassium concentration (myocardial cell excitability increases, and contractility decreases when there is a shift of intracellular K^+ into the ECF).

This 'K' shift occurs during open-heart surgical procedures, and may already be present preoperatively in patients with severe congestive cardiac failure—the so-called 'sick cell' syndrome (*see* Chapter 8).

Serum enzyme analysis for the assessment of myocardial injury is, of course, widely used in coronary care practice. The serial measurement of the myocardial-specific isoenzyme CPK-MB is recommended as the currently most accurate enzyme index of myocardial damage, and may be helpful diagnostically in the detection of peri-operative or incidental myocardial infarction. Note that this rise in serum CPK-MB occurs immediately after injury and is maximal at 2 hours.

Chart Records and Computerization of Patient Data

In addition to real-time monitoring with oscilloscope display units, permanent recording of indices of cardiovascular status and their trends are of great importance in the management of the cardiac patient.

The intensive care progress chart used in the Glasgow Cardiac Surgery units is shown in *Fig.* 15.1. This comprehensive 24-hour chart incorporates most of the parameters described in this chapter. The frequency of chart recording is varied according to the clinical status of the patient. In unstable conditions (e.g. the immediate postcardiac surgery period) observations may be recorded every 15 minutes. Once cardiovascular stability has been achieved and maintained, recordings may be made every 30 or 60 minutes. Space is provided on the chart for nursing comments and general observations, for drug administration and for arterial blood gas and electrolyte results. There is no doubt that such frequent and comprehensive recording of data is costly in terms of nursing time and concentration. The information made available is, however, of great value, particularly in interpreting trends in the clinical progress of the patient.

The availability of computerized data collection and storage offers a significant step forward in this field, while, at least theoretically, reducing demands on nursing and/or medical time. Computerization facilities may range from relatively simple input keyboards linked to an accessible data storage, to direct on-line acquisition of monitored haemodynamic and biochemical parameters, coupled not only to data handling and storage, but also to pre-programmed therapeutic intervention facilities.[6] There is little doubt that computerization of patient data will increase in intensive care unit practice, particularly with the recent developments in microprocessors.

PATHOPHYSIOLOGICAL MECHANISMS

Before considering specific clinical syndromes experienced in cardiac intensive care, it is important to gain a basic understanding of cardiac

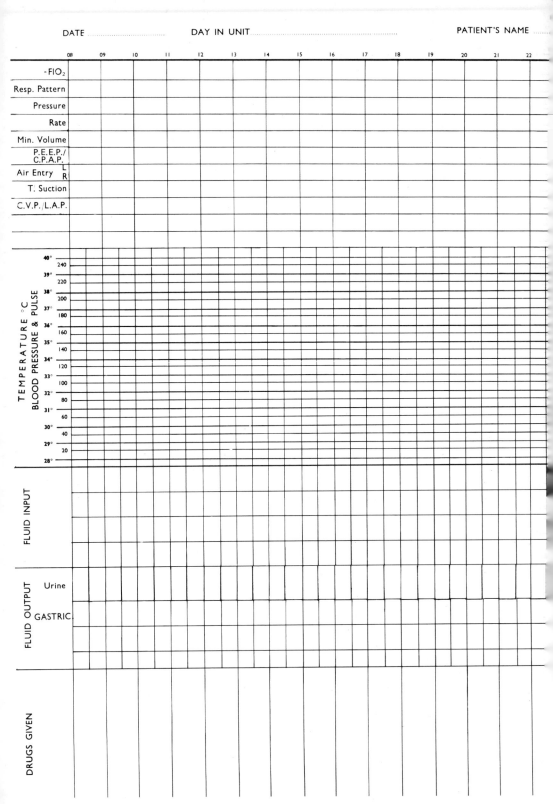

Fig. 15.1 24-hour vital function chart used in Glasgow cardiac surgery units.

Time								
Resp. Patt.								
FIO$_2$								
PO$_2$								
PH.								
Bxs.								
PCO$_2$								
P.C.V.								
K								
Na								
Cl								
Urea								
Creat.								
Ca								
Gluc.								

Time axis: 24 01 02 03 04 05 06 07 8

Temperature / pulse scale:
38° 200 37° 180 36° 160 35° 140 34° 120 33° 100 32° 80 31° 60 30° 40 29° 20 28°

FLUID BALANCE

IV 1 = ...
IV 2 = ...
IV 3 = ...
ORAL =

TOTAL   IN

URINE ....
GASTRIC ....

TOTAL   OUT

BALANCE =

Red Graph   = Core Temp.
Blue Graph = Pulse Rate
Green Graph = Skin Temp.

TRACHEAL SUCTION

1 Scanty   M = Mucoid
2 Moderate   B = Bloody
3 Profuse   P = Purulent

PUPIL SIZE

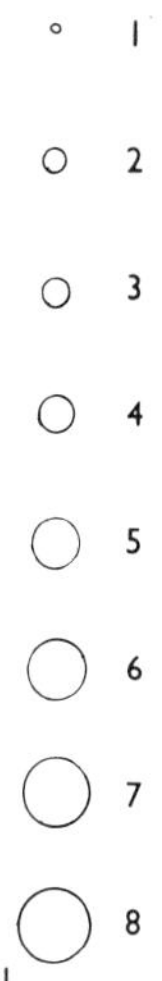

° 1
○ 2
○ 3
○ 4
○ 5
○ 6
○ 7
○ 8

Pupil scale (m.m.)

physiology, particularly in relation to those factors which affect cardiac function, and which may become disordered in pathological situations.

Concept of the Cardiac Pump

The heart is a pump, and it should never be forgotten that the aim in cardiac intensive care is the achievement and maintenance of optimal pumping efficiency. Though a specific problem may exist, e.g. an arrhythmia, its importance lies in its ability to reduce pumping efficiency, and therapy should be directed towards restoration, or at least improvement, of pumping efficiency. It is also important to remember that pumping is an energy-requiring work, and that energy supply/demand equality should always be considered. It is possible to increase cardiac output, and thus apparently improve cardiac efficiency, but if this rise in output is achieved without a balancing rise in myocardial energy supply, so that energy demand exceeds energy supply, pumping efficiency has not been improved and, indeed, serious consequences may result (e.g. myocardial ischaemia). For the purposes of considering cardiac pumping, the heart pump may be represented as the left ventricular chamber:

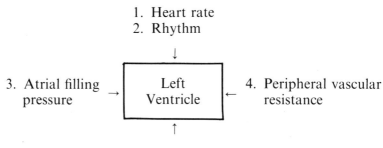

1. Heart rate
2. Rhythm

3. Atrial filling pressure → Left Ventricle ← 4. Peripheral vascular resistance

5. Myocardial contractility

1. *Heart Rate*

Cardiac output is the product of heart rate × stroke volume and thus heart rate will clearly modify cardiac output. The relationship between change in heart rate and change in cardiac output is not, however, linear, since at upper and lower extremes of heart rate, reciprocal changes in stroke volume fail to compensate.

At very low heart rates (<50–60 beats/min), the increase in stroke volume, which occurs as heart rate decreases and diastolic filling time lengthens, begins to tail off since ventricular capacity cannot increase indefinitely. At very rapid heart rates (>120 beats/min), diastolic filling time reduces to the point where it can no longer allow the degree of ventricular filling required to maintain a linear cardiac output/heart rate relationship (*Fig.* 15.2).

The diagrammatic representation of heart rate/cardiac output relationship also demonstrates that stroke volume compensation, at both high and low heart rates, will be further reduced in conditions of impaired left ventricular compliance (e.g. myocardial oedema, ischaemia or cardiomyopathies). It is clearly important, therefore, to maintain heart rate within the compensated range, particularly in patients with suboptimal cardiac function. In general terms, rates of 70–120 are considered acceptable.

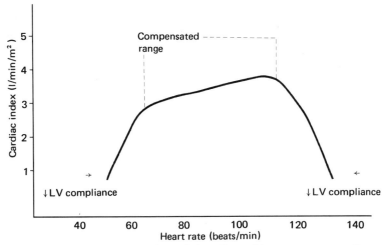

Fig. 15.2. Diagrammatic representation of the effect of heart rate on cardiac pumping efficiency.

Heart rate is also to be considered in relation to the pre-existing ventricular size, particularly in patients with longstanding valvular pathology. The valve disease may, as in the case of aortic incompetence, produce a greatly dilated ventricular cavity which requires a long diastolic filling time, and tolerates even relatively fast heart rates less well than a ventricle of normal size. Conversely, the small, rather hypoplastic ventricle, e.g. in severe mitral stenosis, tolerates slow heart rates poorly and requires a relatively rapid rate for optimal pumping efficiency.

Extremes of heart rate also affect coronary blood flow. Coronary filling occurs principally in diastole and the progressive shortening of diastole which accompanies a rise in heart rate will be associated with a reduction in coronary blood flow. Excessively slow heart rates can also compromise coronary flow, particularly in conditions of reduced ventricular compliance with a raised level of ventricular end-diastolic pressure. In these circumstances, the intramyocardial wall tension towards the end of diastole squeezes the coronary capillary bed and reduces coronary blood flow, to the further detriment of the ventricular myocardium.

II. *Rhythm*

Disturbances in cardiac rhythm may affect cardiac pumping efficiency in two ways: (1) by producing a heart rate which is outside the compensated range previously discussed, or (2) by disturbing or removing the synchronization of normal sinus rhythm, specifically the occurrence of atrial systole <0·2 seconds prior to ventricular systole. Therapy may, therefore, be directed towards restoration of normal sinus rhythm and, while this may be possible in certain situations, where sinus rhythm cannot be restored immediately, improvement may be gained in cardiac pumping efficiency by restoring heart rate to within the compensated range.

Diagnosis and management of cardiac dysrhythmias is discussed in detail in Chapter 16.

III. *Atrial Filling Pressure*

The atrial filling pressure (or 'preload') is an important determinant of cardiac pumping efficiency in relation to the stretch property of myocardial cells. As ventricular filling occurs, ventricular muscle cells are progressively stretched until ventricular systole occurs. It was Starling[7] who demonstrated that 'the energy of contraction was proportional to the initial length of the cardiac muscle fibres', that is ventricular pumping efficiency will increase as ventricular filling increases, the latter being related directly to atrial filling pressure. This phenomenon relates directly to the importance of preservation of atrial systole which can account for as much as 35% of ventricular output. Starling also found that excessive stretching of ventricular muscle led to a reduction in pumping efficiency, as occurs in cardiac failure.

As previously discussed in the section on cardiovascular monitoring, left atrial pressure measurement is a more accurate and useful parameter by which to regulate cardiac pumping efficiency, since optimalization of the left-sided filling pressure (around 10–15 mmHg) will ensure maximal efficiency of left ventricular output, i.e. the principal cardiac pumping chamber. Though right atrial pressure levels (around 5–10 mmHg) tend to move in parallel with left atrial pressure, this relationship is not always maintained. Where cardiac valve disease is present or where chamber failure occurs, atrial pressures may be abnormally elevated. In cases of right ventricular failure, or where tricuspid valve dysfunction is present, right atrial filling pressure may be greater than 25 mmHg. In the early postoperative phase in such patients, even after corrective surgery has been undertaken, elevated levels of atrial filling pressure may be required to achieve optimal cardiac function.

Despite these more complex aspects of the regulation of atrial filling pressures, the more common situation exists in relation to abnormally low levels of atrial pressure, where hypovolaemia has occurred. In this situation, low circulatory blood volume will be associated with suboptimal ventricular filling and, hence, reduced cardiac pumping efficiency. Restoration of normal levels of circulatory blood volume, and hence atrial filling pressure, will result in a corresponding improvement in cardiac output (*Fig.* 15.3).

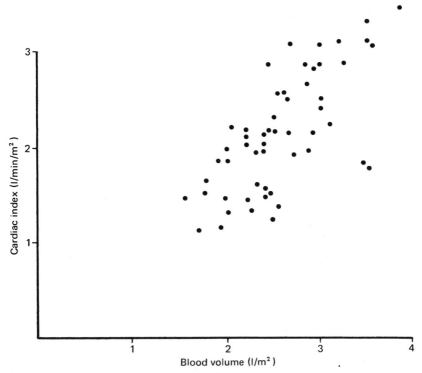

Fig. 15.3 The relationship between cardiac index and circulating blood volume, 2 hours after open-heart surgery.

In patients with severely compromised ventricular function, the danger of excessive blood or fluid replacement must always be borne in mind, and where overtransfusion has caused ventricular muscle fibres to be stretched past the point of maximal contractile response, into the downslope of Starling's curve, atrial filling pressure should promptly be reduced (e.g. by venodilators) in order to restore optimal cardiac pumping efficiency.

IV. *Peripheral Vascular Resistance*

The role of peripheral vascular resistance in modifying left ventricular performance has been recognized for many years,[8] but its clinical importance in the care of cardiac patients has only relatively recently been fully appreciated.[9] Modest elevation in peripheral resistance will be associated with increase in myocardial performance and ventricular work, where myocardial function is normal. Further elevation in peripheral resistance will, however, impose an increasing afterload on the left ventricle, with progressive reduction in cardiac pumping efficiency and fall in cardiac output. In patients with already compromised left ventricular function, even small rises in peripheral resistance above normal values (around 20 index units) may result in significant ventricular dysfunction, thus further impeding left ventricular output.

It is now widely appreciated that vasoconstriction may be a significant feature in patients with chronic cardiac failure, during cardiac surgical procedures, and particularly in the early postoperative phase following open-heart surgery. Reduction in vascular resistance levels in these varied clinical situations has been uniformly beneficial in terms of haemodynamic improvement.

The aetiology of the rise in peripheral resistance is not yet fully understood. Baroreceptor reflexes, sympathetic activity, and neuro-endocrine reflexes have variously been implicated. Activation of the renin–angiotensin system has been demonstrated, with markedly elevated plasma levels of the vasoconstrictor angiotensin II occurring during open-heart surgical procedures, and in the early postoperative period.[10] Specific angiotensin II blockade therapy has been shown to be effective in reducing inappropriately high peripheral resistance levels in cardiac surgical patients,[11,12] and in patients with chronic cardiac failure.

V. *Myocardial Contractility*

In addition to the factors affecting cardiac pumping efficiency already discussed, the contractile state of the cardiac muscle fibres themselves is a fundamental determinant of cardiac performance.

Reduced myocardial contractility may be related to temporary disturbance of myocardial cell function with anticipation of potential improvement after spontaneous recovery or appropriate therapy. Among those factors which may cause temporary reduction in myocardial contractility are: low arterial/intracellular Po_2, acidosis, low intracellular K^+/high intracellular Na^+, increased myocardial or interstitial water content, reduced tissue ionized Ca^{2+} levels, and various cardiodepressant drug effects (e.g. β-blockers, calcium antagonists, anti-arrhythmic agents). The presence of any such factor should always be considered in the management of patients with cardiac dysfunction, and appropriate corrective measures taken to optimize myocardial contractility.

Permanent reduction in myocardial contractility presents a particular problem. The underlying pathology may be myocardial fibrosis (the result of longstanding myocardial ischaemia, or previous acute myocardial infarction), or idiopathic or toxic cardiomyopathy. Unless corrective excision-type surgery is indicated, e.g. in ventricular aneurysm, or myocardial revascularization is feasible when viability of the poorly contracting ischaemic muscle is convincingly demonstrated (e.g. by nuclear imaging), management falls back on the accurate maintenance of the other factors (i.e. rate, rhythm, filling pressure and vascular resistance) at optimal levels. The vogue for using stimulating inotropic drugs to increase output from a permanently damaged ventricle is increasingly being called into question, and may well have compounded problem cases by increasing myocardial energy demand with consequent myocardial ischaemic and oxygen debt. The appropriate place for inotropic stimulation will be more fully discussed in the following section. Severe degrees of permanently reduced myocardial contractility (e.g. end-stage cardiomyopathy, or ischaemic heart disease) represent an impossible therapeutic situation and require corrective surgery if feasible, or else system replacement by cardiac transplantation.

Myocardial Energy Supply/Demand—The Coronary Circulation

As previously indicated, comprehensive assessment of cardiac pumping status must include an awareness of energy supply/demand equality. In certain clinical situations, increase in cardiac output may be possible at the expense of a myocardial energy demand which exceeds the available energy supply. Though the coronary circulation can cope with a wide physiological range of myocardial energy demand, it fails to maintain equality (1) in prolonged high output states, e.g. hyperthyroidism, arteriovenous fistulae, certain phases of sepsis or (2) where significant obstructive coronary artery disease is present.

The presence of underlying obstructive coronary disease must be assumed in a very high percentage of intensive care patients, whatever their primary pathology, in view of the prevalence in the general population. Though the coronary disease may have been subclinical, increased demand on coronary supply may produce frank coronary insufficiency. Myocardial ischaemia or even acute myocardial infarction are, therefore, frequently encountered as secondary complications in severely ill patients with possibly unrelated primary pathology. The coronary insufficiency may, however, prove to be a fatal additional pathology.

For these reasons, one should be on the lookout for evidence of previously unsuspected coronary insufficiency in severely ill patients, and the concept of maintenance of myocardial energy supply/demand equality should be an important consideration in the prophylaxis of secondary ischaemic complications. Where possible, patients at risk require particularly careful monitoring to ensure, as far as possible, that factors increasing myocardial work are minimized, e.g. vasoconstriction, tachycardias, certain inotropic drugs, even simple over-alertness and undue anxiety.

In addition, factors promoting myocardial energy supply should be optimalized, e.g. Po_2, blood sugar level, adequate aortic diastolic pressure (for diastolic coronary filling).

It may in certain cases be worth utilizing β-blocker drugs in order to reduce myocardial energy demand, even at the expense of a modest reduction in cardiac output.

PATHOPHYSIOLOGICAL MECHANISMS IN SPECIFIC CLINICAL SITUATIONS

I. Routine Postcardiac Surgery

In addition to the general principles of cardiac physiology previously discussed, certain specific pathophysiological features are involved in patients immediately following cardiac surgical procedures involving cardiopulmonary bypass (CPB). These relate to the effects of the altered mechanical perfusion of the cardiopulmonary bypass machine, and to the effects of operative stress, anaesthesia, and the possible persistence of hypothermia in the postoperative period.

It is increasingly recognized that conventional techniques of CPB are associated with significant disturbances in haemodynamics and metabolism.

The principal haemodynamic effect of conventional non-pulsatile CPB is a progressive rise in peripheral vascular resistance. The vasoconstriction commences during the period of non-pulsatile perfusion, and continues for 2–4 hours after the operation. The patients exhibit the features of cold peripheries, slow capillary refill, 'spiky' arterial waveforms, and, in a significant proportion of cases, marked systolic arterial hypertension (>150 mmHg) requiring the use of intravenous hypotensive agents. This vasoconstriction phenomenon, now well recognized, increases myocardial work and is often associated with significant falls in cardiac index.

The recent use of vasodilator therapy in such patients, e.g. with epidural anaesthesia, or sodium nitroprusside or GTN infusion, has been associated with significant improvement in cardiac index consequent upon the reduction in peripheral vasoconstriction (*Fig.* 15.4). The vasoconstriction phase is generally self terminating after 2–4 hours, with a fall in systolic BP, and progressive improvement in the peripheral circulation. During the vasoconstricted phase, levels of CVP, PWP and LAP are relatively elevated, despite the fact that most patients are hypovolaemic. As the vasoconstriction recedes, and the peripheral circulation opens up, volume replacement is necessary to maintain adequate levels of ventricular filling pressure. The aetiology of this vasoconstriction is not fully understood: catecholamines and neurogenic reflexes have been postulated. Recent studies by the authors have indicated that renin–angiotensin activation

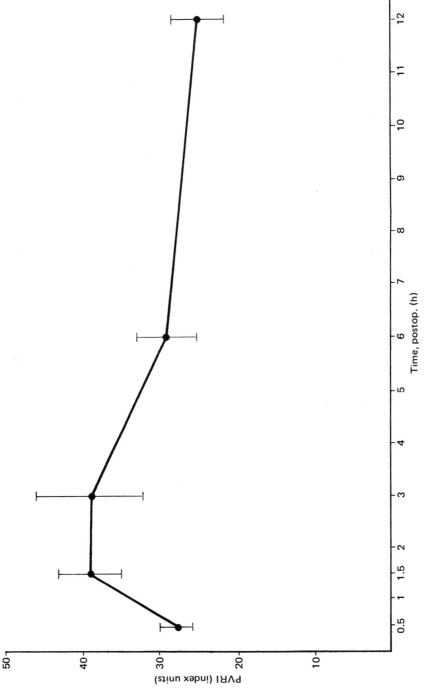

Fig. 15.4. The pattern of change in peripheral vascular resistance after open-heart surgery.

during non-pulsatile CPB appears to be of major aetiological signifi-cance.[13] Associated with the vasoconstriction is a variable degree of metabolic acidosis and cellular poassium efflux from tissues underperfused due to peripheral vasoconstriction and reduced cardiac index. Excessive degrees of acidosis and/or reduced intracellular potassium concentration may be associated with increased incidence of cardiac arrhythmias (e.g. ventricular extrasystoles, VES) and with suboptimal cardiac pumping action.[14]

Persistence of core hypothermia may also complicate and further increase vasoconstriction, and surface warming may be helpful in this regard.

In addition to the secondary effects of an elevated peripheral vascular resistance, cardiac pumping efficiency is frequently reduced after open-heart surgery as a primary consequence of myocardial cell injury sustained during the period of aortic cross-clamping. Studies have shown significant, though reversible, changes in myocardial cell ultrastructure and histo-chemistry following the cross-clamp period of myocardial ischaemia. Though great improvements in myocardial protection have occurred, par-ticularly with the use of crystalloid or cold blood cardioplegic solutions,[15,16] some degree of myocardial cell injury does occur, and this may be associated with a period of suboptimal cardiac efficiency in the post-operative period. Where myocardial oedema is present to a significant degree, reduced ventricular compliance will result.

The perfusion of vital organs (e.g. kidneys, liver, brain) has also been shown to become disordered during non-pulsatile CPB, with evidence of functional disturbances. Though full and spontaneous restoration of normal function occurs in the vast majority of patients, there is a sense in which the altered perfusion of CPB 'sensitizes' or 'primes' vital organs, rendering them more susceptible to subsequent perfusion insults. For example, the patient who undergoes an uneventful open-heart procedure may demonstrate very modest impairment in renal tubular concentration in the immediate post-perfusion period. If no further complications arise, renal function rapidly returns to normal (usually within 12–24 hours). If, however, a further perfusion insult occurs within this period, such as a cardiac arrest or a period of extreme low output, the risk of that patient developing complete renal shut down and becoming anuric is very greatly increased. Similar 'sensitization' to subsequent underperfusion has been suggested for the liver, pancreas, and brain.

II. Acute Low Cardiac Output

The patient who develops acute peripheral circulatory insufficiency as a direct result of cardiac pumping failure represents a different situation from the routine postcardiac surgery patient. Acute low cardiac output states may occur in the early postoperative period after cardiac surgery, related to myocardial ischaemia or infarction, the development of haemodynamically significant arrhythmias or, in patients whose previously compensated cardiac failure becomes decompensated, often as a result of increased peripheral vasoconstriction. Acute low cardiac output states may also occur as a result of acute myocardial infarction or haemodynamically significant arrhythmias in non-cardiac surgical patients requiring intensive care for unrelated primary pathologies.

The pathophysiological changes associated with acute low cardiac output due to cardiac pump failure include intense peripheral vaso-constriction associated with arterial hypotension, elevation in ventricular filling pressures and PWP, and under-perfusion of brain and kidney, with resultant reduction in conscious level and oliguria in severe cases. Catecholamine levels are elevated, and marked renin-angiotensin ac-tivation occurs, the high plasma levels of the vasoconstrictor angiotensin II producing further rises in peripheral resistance, and a specific constriction in subendocardial blood vessels.[17]

If uncorrected, a vicious circle of increasing vasoconstriction, increasing left ventricular work and progressive subendocardial ischaemia develops. Progressive metabolic acidosis and potassium efflux from the intracellular compartment also occur, further comprising the metabolic environment for myocardial contractility.

III. Chronic Low Cardiac Output

The pathophysiological changes associated with chronic low cardiac output secondary to longstanding cardiac disease are generally considered to reflect a combination of suboptimal left ventricular output and venous congestion. Such patients, particularly those with markedly elevated right atrial pressure due to tricuspid valve disease, may be easily detectable preoperatively. Chronic peripheral circulatory inadequacy is reflected in atrophic skin and marked peripheral cyanosis. Jugular venous pressure is elevated, hepatic congestion produces an enlarged and possibly pulsatile liver and liver function is depressed. Peripheral oedema may be present, though frequently vigorous diuretic therapy minimizes this. Renal impair-ment secondary to reduced glomerular filtration rate is often seen.

There is increasing awareness that, in such patients, cellular biochemical states become significantly disordered with the passage of time. Chronic low cardiac output appears to be associated with reduced efficiency of sodium pumping at cell membrane level. This leads to a progressive build up of intracellular sodium, and a potassium leak into the ECF and increased K^+ loss in the urine. This disturbance of intracellular Na^+/K^+ balance further compromises myocardial contractility and increases myo-cardial excitability and the risk of ventricular arrhythmias. This syndrome of inefficient sodium pumping, i.e. 'the sick-cell syndrome', is more fully discussed in Chapter 8. Patients in this category also exhibit a degree of intolerance to digoxin, exhibiting digoxin toxicity on low dosage therapy, and have a tendency to bradycardia.

These features of chronic low output may require therapy pre-operatively and, certainly, such patients often require relatively long-term biochemical and nutritional support following corrective cardiac surgery.

IV. Secondary Cardiac Pathology

A brief mention should be made of those conditions which may be of primary importance in the patient's clinical status, but which may lead to or be associated with significant secondary cardiac dysfunction.

1. *Shock Syndromes*

In addition to the peripheral circulatory failure which may accompany severe hypovolaemia and blood stream infection, it is well established that release of vasoactive substances in shocked patients may produce direct depression of myocardial contractility.[18] The different circulatory patterns associated with hypovolaemic and septic shock are discussed in detail elsewhere. (*See* Chapter 9.)

2. *Respiratory Failure and Cor Pulmonale*

Severe chronic lung disease, particularly chronic obstructive airways disease, may be associated with progressive right-heart failure. Pulmonary hypertension, eventual right ventricular failure and venous congestion produce similar features to the chronic venous congestion of low cardiac output. In cor pulmonale, however, retention of carbon dioxide will be associated with a hyperdynamic vasodilated circulation, with central cyanosis if significant hypoxaemia is present. The high output cardiac failure syndrome in such patients may be further compromised if injudicious use of bronchodilator sympathomimetics induce marked tachycardia, further increasing cardiac work in a hypoxaemic environment.

3. *Pre-existing Subclinical Cardiac Pathology*

In the general intensive care situation, it should not be forgotten that many patients who have subclinical cardiac disease may be precipitated into a decompensated phase if myocardial energy supply/demand equality is

disturbed as a consequence of their primary pathology. Though particularly likely in the case of asymptomatic coronary artery disease, subclinical
chronic valve disease patients may be unable to cope with the increased
circulatory demands of a serious illness.

THERAPY

It has been stated previously in this chapter that the principal aim in
cardiac intensive care is the achievement and maintenance of optimal
cardiac pumping efficiency. In the authors' opinion, the greater the
understanding of the pathophysiology operative in any individual patient,
the more likely is the choice of therapy to be appropriate and, therefore,
effective. Therapy in cardiac intensive care may be considered as:
Primary therapy—directed towards optimalization of cardiac pumping
efficiency.
Secondary therapy—directed towards compensation or protection of vital
organs from the pathological consequences of underperfusion.

PRIMARY THERAPY

The principal areas of primary therapy are detailed in *Table* 15.4.

Table **15.4. Points of intervention in primary cardiac therapy in
cardiac intensive care**

1.↑ *Cardiac output*	Rate
	Rhythm
	Atrial filling pressure
	Myocardial contractility
2.↓ *Vascular resistance*	Sedation
	Vasodilators
3.↑ *Myocardial energy supply*	Coronary vasodilators
	Glucose and insulin

Therapy Directed Towards Increasing Cardiac Output

I. *Modification of Heart Rate*

Where heart rate falls outside the 'compensated range', cardiac output
may be improved by increasing or decreasing heart rate, as appropriate (*see
Table* 15.5). Rates in excess of 120 beats/min are generally due to
supraventricular tachycardia or atrial flutter/fibrillation, though sinus
tachycardia may occur, especially in patients following coronary artery

Table 15.5. **Drugs commonly used to modify heart rate after cardiac surgery**

Condition	Drug	Amount, mg
Tachycardia (>120 beats/min)	Ouabain	0·125 i.v.
	Digoxin	0·25 i.v.
	Practolol	2–4 i.v.
Bradycardia (<60 beats/min)	Atropine	0·2 i.v.
	Isoprenaline 2 mg in 500 ml 5% dextrose, infused at 5–10 ml/h	
	Demand ventricular or atrial pacing	

surgery procedures. In non-sinus tachycardias, intravenous administration of 0·125 mg ouabain or a digoxin preparation (e.g. 0·25 mg Lanoxin or 0·1 mg Medigoxin) may be given and the dose repeated 2-hourly until the heart rate falls below 120/min. Digoxin preparations should be used in reduced dosage in patients already receiving maintenance digoxin therapy, until serum digoxin levels are obtained. Sinus tachycardias may not respond to a digoxin preparation, but practolol, given by slow intravenous injection in a dose of 2–4 mg may be effective, the injection being stopped when ECG signs of rate reduction are seen. Where the occurrence of a supraventricular tachyrhythmia is followed by clinical or measured evidence of a significant fall in cardiac output (i.e. with blurring of consciousness, vomiting, peripheral vasoconstriction and oliguria) more urgent therapy is indicated and electrical cardioversion should be considered. (It should be remembered that certain patients, typically those with the small volume left ventricle, e.g. in severe pure mitral stenosis, require a relatively higher than average heart rate, in order to achieve maximal cardiac output. In such patients, heart rates of 120 beats/min may be indicated.)

Bradycardia, i.e. heart rate 60 beats/min, may be temporarily corrected using intravenous atropine 0·2 mg though usually longer-term therapy is required. Chronotropic agents (e.g. isoprenaline, dopamine) may be used, isoprenaline being given as an intravenous infusion (2 mg isoprenaline in 500 ml of 5% dextrose or Ringer lactate), adjusting the infusion rate by an infusion pump, to achieve the required elevation in heart rate. Artificial temporary pacing may also be used in patients with significant bradycardia.

Temporary pacing wires are sutured to the heart before chest closure in the following categories of patients:
1. Patients with intraoperative bradycardia.
2. Patients with evidence of persisting A–V block in the post-bypass ECG.
3. Patients with calcific aortic valve disease requiring aortic valve replacement.
4. Patients requiring tricuspid valve surgery.

5. Patients with preoperative bradycardia related to long-term digoxin therapy.

Where ventricular pacing has been set up, pacing should be used as a second-line therapy in patients with sinus bradycardia, since the chronotropic effect of isoprenaline, for example, will be achieved without the loss of atrial systole. (It should be remembered that certain patients, typically those with the large volume, dilated left ventricle, e.g. in severe aortic incompetence, require a relatively lower than average heart rate in order to achieve maximal cardiac output. In such patients, heart rates of 60 beats/min may be acceptable.)

II. *Restoration of Heart Rhythm*

The therapy of cardiac arrhythmias is discussed in detail in Chapter 16.

In general terms, apart from the life-threatening arrhythmias (ventricular tachycardia, ventricular fibrillation, cardiac asystole), therapy for arrhythmia may be directed either towards restoring a more efficient pumping rhythm (e.g. sinus rhythm for atrial fibrillation), or simply towards modifying an excessively slow or fast heart rate associated with the arrhythmia. Patients who go into atrial fibrillation after cardiac surgical procedures may, for the majority, be left in atrial fibrillation, controlling the rate with digoxin until spontaneous reversion to sinus rhythm occurs, or until cardioversion is carried out.

The commonest rhythm disturbance after cardiac surgery is the development of ventricular extrasystoles (VES). When frequent (more than 15/min or 1/ECG monitor sweep), cardiac pumping efficiency may be significantly impaired. VES may be abolished by administration of potassium chloride (10–20 mmol/h by burette infusion, or by a stat injection of 5 mmol given into a central vein over 5 minutes). Intracellular K^+ depletion is likely to be the aetiology of the myocardial irritability in the majority of cases. Continuing VES, or multifocal VES, may be diminished or abolished by the infusion of lignocaine, given by infusion pump, controlling drug infusion rate according to response. This drug exerts some degree of myocardial depressant effect, and should be used with caution in patients with impaired left ventricular function.

VES may simply be associated with excessive bradycardia, in which case an increase in heart rate will reduce their frequency or even abolish their occurrence.

III. *Adjustment of Atrial Filling Pressures*

As indicated in the section on pathophysiology, cardiac muscle contracts more vigorously with increasing fibre stretch up to a critical point, beyond which further stretch produces a diminishing contractile response.

It is clear, therefore, that cardiac pumping efficiency will be reduced at both subnormal and supranormal levels of atrial filling pressure.

The optimal levels of atrial filling pressure vary to a considerable extent, dependent on the particular cardiac abnormality present, as outlined previously.

Where filling pressures are excessively low, volume replacement is indicated. The choice of volume expander depends largely on the haematocrit level in the post cardiac surgery period, and the nature of continuing blood or fluid losses. The authors' preference is to use whole blood, or packed red cells, according to haematocrit, failing which, gelatin-based solutions, e.g. Haemaccel.

Excessively high levels of atrial filling pressure may occur in patients who have been over-transfused or who suffer significant impairment of ventricular function in the early postoperative period. In such cases, overstretching of ventricular muscle produces reduced myocardial contractility and ventricular ejection. This is a potentially serious haemodynamic situation, and therapy should be directed promptly towards reduction in atrial filling pressures, either by removing a volume of blood from the circulation, e.g. from the arterial line, or by venodilator therapy to increase the capacity of the venous system and reduce atrial filling. Drugs such as sodium nitroprusside and hydralazine have been used in this situation, though they also produce a similar dilatation effect on the arterial side of the circulation, with consequent fall in arterial blood pressure. The nitrates (isosorbide and GTN) or pentolinium have been shown to be more specific and more effective venodilator agents, and are, therefore, of particular use in the reduction of elevated atrial filling pressure levels. (Elevated atrial filling pressures will also be encountered in cardiac tamponade from excessive postoperative bleeding. Prompt re-opening of the chest and relief of the tamponade is indicated.)

IV. *Improvement in Myocardial Contractility*

Only when the preceding factors are rendered optimal can therapy directed towards increasing myocardial contractility be sensibly undertaken. There is little doubt that inotropic agents have been used extensively in recent years, possibly to a greater extent than conditions warranted, but there is a developing awareness of the correct clinical situations in which inotropic agents may be safely and effectively used. Disorders of myocardial contractility may be classified as: temporary or permanent (*Table* 15.6).

Temporary reduction in myocardial contractility may occur in conditions of hypoxia and acidosis, where appropriate correction of arterial Po_2 and pH will be associated with improved cardiac output. Electrolyte imbalance may also reduce contractility, particularly where sodium pump function is suboptimal and intracellular sodium concentration rises as intracellular potassium concentration falls. Therapy for this 'sick-cell' syndrome, e.g. glucose–insulin–potassium regimes, are discussed in detail in Chapter 8. Where serum calcium levels are low, restoration of normal serum calcium levels will improve cardiac output. Temporary reduction in myocardial contractility may also be the result of a drug effect, e.g. with β-blockers, or anti-arrhythmia agents such as lignocaine, and the use of these drugs in patients with compromised ventricular function must be closely controlled.

Table 15.6 **The common causes of impairment of myocardial contractility**

Myocardial contractility	*Causes*
Temporary	Hypoxia
	Acidosis
	Electrolyte imbalance (e.g. Na^+, K^+, Ca^{2+})
	Drug effect (e.g. β-blockers, lignocaine, etc.)
	Vasodepressor substances (septic shock)
Permanent	Cardiomyopathies
	Ischaemic heart disease: previous infarction
	or dyskinetic ischaemic myocardium

Where cardiac output remains low despite adjusting heart rate, rhythm, filling pressures and correcting any temporary reduction in contractility, the possibility of some permanent disorder in myocardial contractility must be considered. Fortunately, such patients represent the minority of cardiac surgical patients. Therapy in most cases consists of the addition of an inotropic agent to the programme of measures already discussed in order to increase the contractile force of the myocardium. In using inotropic therapy, it must be remembered that myocardial work is being increased, and that unless myocardial energy supply is correspondingly increased, an energy supply–demand inequality will be produced. In low output states, however, it may be that increased cardiac output will be associated with increased coronary blood flow, and that both supply and demand will improve.

The choice of inotropic agent tends to be a matter of personal preference, though the effect of the agent on heart rate must be taken into consideration, depending on the patient's existing heart rate. The various agents commonly used as inotropes in cardiac surgical patients are detailed in *Table* 15.7.

The authors' preference is to use adrenaline (5 mg/500 ml) given by infusion pump at 5–30 ml/h as the first line inotropic agent within the first 24 hours of the cardiac operation. Though adrenaline infusion may be continued up to and beyond 48 hours postoperatively, its continued use may be associated with increased peripheral vasoconstriction. Adrenaline has, in most patients, little effect on heart rate, in contrast to isoprenaline, which may be considered as a principally chronotropic agent. The drugs dopamine and dobutamine are inotropic and chronotropic, and tend to be more useful in longer-term inotropic support, since their use is generally not associated with peripheral vasoconstriction.

Table 15.7. **The dominant receptor sites and dosage schedules of inotropic agents**

Inotropic agent	*Dose,* $\mu g\,kg^{-1}\,min^{-1}$	*Receptor site*			
		Beta 1	*Beta 2*	*Alpha*	*Dopamine*
Adrenaline	0·06–0·18	+ +	+ +	+ – + +	0
Dopamine	1–30	+ +	0	+ – + +	+ +
Isoprenaline	0·02–0·18	+ +	+ +	0	0
Dobutamine	2–40	+ +	+	+	0

From Tinker J.[21]

When inotropic agents are in use, dosage and concentration are adjusted according to haemodynamic response and fluid balance requirements. Where peripheral vasoconstriction remains a problem, a peripheral vaso-dilator such as sodium nitroprusside should be given concomitantly.

In most cardiac surgical patients, even in those with persistent disorders of myocardial contractility, the increased haemodynamic demands of the operative and early post-operative period place increased demands on cardiac pumping efficiency. If therapy safely sees the patient through this phase, progressive improvement thereafter is the norm.

V. *Therapy Directed Towards Reducing Vascular Resistance*

Awareness of the potentially harmful effects of vasoconstriction has led to the widespread use of vasodilator therapy to reduce elevated levels of peripheral vascular resistance and so improve cardiac output. As previously indicated, increased vasoconstriction is a most frequent finding in patients in the immediate postoperative phase after open-heart surgery. Haemodynamic studies have demonstrated a consistent rise in cardiac output in response to reduction in elevated PVR levels.[19] Before discussing vasodilator drugs, it should be noted that inadequate sedation may be associated with vasoconstriction, and that patients, particularly those on IPPV, must be adequately sedated in order that they do not fight the ventilator.

Vasodilator agents in common use in cardiac surgery patients include sodium nitroprusside, glyceryl trinitrate, chlorpromazine and certain intra-venous hypotensive drugs such as hexamethonium, diazoxide, etc. The authors' preference is to use a controlled infusion of sodium nitroprusside (200 mg in 500 ml 5% dextrose) starting with 5 ml/h and increasing the infusion rate according to haemodynamic response. Where vasodilatation is achieved, atrial filling pressures and systemic arterial pressures will fall, and volume replacement is indicated. Nitroprusside infusion may be controlled satisfactorily since its effect is both rapid in onset, and short in duration. Induced vasodilatation using other agents mentioned, except GTN, is longer acting and, therefore, less easy to control. The use of nitroprusside infusion requires protection of the infusion bottle from light, its frequent replacement with fresh solution in long-term infusions, and the administration of parenteral vitamin B_{12} in the long-term infusion situation (> 24 hours). Nitroprusside, and the other agents described, are non-specific vasodilators. Early work with specific blockers of angiotensin II (angiotensin converting enzyme inhibitors) suggest that they may prove to be of even greater value in this area of therapy.[20]

VI. *Therapy Directed Towards Increasing Myocardial Energy Supply*

Cardiac pumping efficiency is not solely related to cardiac output, but also to energy supply to the myocardium. Though little work has yet been carried out in this area, there is evidence to suggest that specific coronary vasodilatation may in certain patients be associated with an overall improvement in myocardial performance. Certain drugs already discussed have been shown to exert some degree of coronary vasodilatory effect, e.g. nitroprusside, and angiotensin inhibitors. More specific coronary effects will, however, be achieved with glyceryl trinitrate and the longer-acting nitrates such as isosorbide dinitrate.

SECONDARY THERAPY IN CARDIAC INTENSIVE CARE

Secondary therapy is that which is directed towards the protection of vital organs from the pathological consequences of underperfusion. It assumes, therefore, that maximal primary therapy is already in progress, but that full achievement of optimal cardiac pumping efficiency has not been possible.
    In this section, only the kidney and brain will be considered.

I. Secondary Therapy Protecting Renal Function

The kidney is physiologically relatively well protected from moderate degrees of underperfusion. Where cardiac output is particularly low, however, renal perfusion becomes significantly impaired and oliguria develops, leading to anuria and acute renal failure if uncorrected. Selective preservation of renal blood flow has been demonstrated with the drug dopamine, and infusion of this drug may restore adequate urinary volumes (> 30 ml/h) in addition to its myocardial inotropic effect.

Functional preservation of the renal tubules may be accomplished by a mannitol infusion (100 ml of 20% solution) and/or intravenous diuretic therapy. If subsequent early improvement in cardiac output is anticipated, these short-term methods may satisfactorily preserve urinary flow during the underperfusion period.

II. Secondary Therapy Protecting Cerebral Function

Preservation of cerebral cellular function in the presence of underperfusion is largely limited to the reduction in or prevention of cerebral oedema which may either lead directly to permanent brain cell injury, or compound and increase the pathological effects of reduced cerebral perfusion. In patients on IPPV, hyperventilation to maintain arterial P_{CO_2} in the range 30–35 mmHg may be undertaken, with the caveat that excessive reduction in arterial P_{CO_2} will increase peripheral vasoconstriction. Administration of intravenous dexamethasone, 6–8 mg stat and 4 mg q.i.d., is recommended and infusion of mannitol (100 ml, 20% solution) may also be used. Recent studies suggest that intravenous barbiturate administration may protect the brain from continuing underperfusion.

SYSTEM REPLACEMENT IN CARDIAC INTENSIVE CARE

In severe cardiac pump failure, full therapeutic measures may be insufficient to maintain cardiac output at a level consistent with patient survival. In such circumstances, some form of system replacement must be considered.

I. Circulatory Assist Devices

Mechanical devices are available, and in clinical use, which provide some means of circulatory assistance to the failing heart. These include:
1. Intra-aortic balloon pump (IABP).
2. Left ventricular assist devices (LVAD).
3. Artificial heart.
The IABP is widely used in major cardiac surgical units as a proven means of partial circulatory assistance. A balloon catheter is positioned in the descending aorta, just below the aortic arch. The catheter is connected to a pneumatic system (vacuum pump and compressor) which alternately inflates and deflates the balloon. Balloon inflation/deflation is triggered from the patient's ECG or arterial pressure waveform to produce a synchronized counterpulsation effect. Balloon inflation occurs during diastole, and increases diastolic aortic arch pressure and hence diastolic

coronary artery filling. Balloon deflation occurs at ventricular ejection, reducing aortic arch pressure and 'off loading' the failing ventricle, allowing increased stroke volume without increasing left ventricular work. A typical arterial pressure waveform from a patient on IABP counter-pulsation is shown in *Fig.* 15.5. IABP circulatory assistance may be used:

1. In weaning patients off cardiopulmonary bypass after cardiac surgical procedures.
2. In patients who sustain postoperative pump failure, e.g. from acute myocardial infarction.
3. In preoperative patients with severe pump failure.

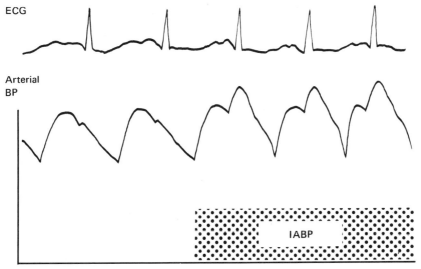

Fig. 15.5. Radial artery blood pressure trace showing diastolic augmentation of pressure trace using a synchronized intra-aortic balloon pump.

Left Ventricular Assist Devices

These devices are still largely experimental, although they have been used clinically in some centres. The devices vary in detail of construction, but basically consist of a valved pumping chamber receiving input blood from the left atrium or left ventricle and returning the blood to the ascending or descending aorta. The device may be within the chest cavity or can be external. Pumping is often pneumatically driven, and is synchronized to the patient's own cardiac action. At the present time, prevention of blood clotting and the occurrence of blood stream infection constitute significant problems, but further refinements in LVADs are inevitable, and they offer, in output terms, a greater pumping capacity than IABP assistance.

Complete take-over of cardiac pumping by an artificial heart remains an experimental possibility at the present time, though animal studies have proved most encouraging. The use of such devices, both LVAD and artificial heart, assumes that the patient's own cardiac function will improve sufficiently to take over the circulation within a matter of days.

II. Corrective Surgery

The ultimate means of system replacement, for intractable and progressive cardiac pump failure, is cardiac transplantation. Improved methods of immunological management may increase the clinical applicability of this surgically possible procedure. Results from the few centres which have experience in cardiac transplantation indicate that appreciable survival times and a satisfactory quality of life are seen in suitable patients. Future application in the management of inoperable congenital cardiac anomalies is also a possibility.

At present, however, corrective surgery has a more limited, but nevertheless successful, role in certain patients. After myocardial infarction, mitral valve incompetence may be produced from ischaemic rupture of papillary muscle apparatus. Infarcts involving the interventricular septum may produce septal rupture and a ventricular septal defect. In such patients, the haemodynamic insult of valve incompetence or ventricular septal defect (VSD) shunt in addition to the initial effect of the myocardial infarction may produce cardiac pump failure and a life-threatening situation. Surgical replacement of the mitral valve or closure of the VSD may be life-saving in such patients. Though immediate operation may be imperative, if possible surgery should be deferred until the infarct area has undergone some degree of fibrous replacement (ideally 4–6 weeks post-infarct) when the tensile strength of the tissues is more amenable to surgery. IABP circulatory support is often used in severe cases to maintain the circulation until surgery is performed.

REFERENCES

1. Robicsek F., Masters T. N., Reichertz P. L. et al. (1977) 3 years' experience with computer-based intensive care of patients following open-heart and major vascular surgery. *Coll. Works Cardiopulm. Dis.* **21**, 48.
2. Cook T. L. and Dueker C. W. (1976) Tension pneumothorax following internal jugular vein cannulation and general anaesthesia. *Anesthesiology* **45**, 554–555.
3. Apps M. C. P. (1980) How to cannulate the internal jugular vein. *Br. J. Hosp. Med.* **24**, 74.
4. Hamilton W. F. (1962) Measurement of the cardiac output. Handbook of physiology 2. *Circulation* **1**, 551–584.
5. Swan H. J. C., Ganz W., Forester J. et al. (1970) Catheterisation of the heart in man with use of a flow-directed balloon-tipped catheter. *N. Engl. J. Med.* **283**, 447.
6. Sheppard L. C., Kirklin J. W. and Kouchoukos N. T. (1974) Computer controlled interventions for the acutely ill patient. *Comput. Biomed. Res.* **4**, 125.
7. Starling E. H. (1918) *The Law of the Heart Beat.* New York, Longmans.

8. Sonnenblick E. H. and Downing S. E. (1963) Afterload as a primary determinant of ventricular performance. *Am. J. Physiol.* **204**, 604.
9. Taylor K. M., Bain W. H. and Morton J. J. (1980) The role of angiotensin II in the development of peripheral vasoconstriction during open-heart surgery. 1. *Am. Heart. J.* **100**, 935–937.
10. Taylor K. M., Morton J. J., Brown J. J. et al. (1977) Hypertension and the renin–angiotensin system following open-heart surgery. *J. Thorac. Cardiovasc. Surg.* **74**, 840.
11. Taylor K. M., Cassals J., Morton J. J. et al. (1979) The haemodynamic effects of angiotensin blockade after cardiopulmonary bypass. *Br. Heart J.* **41**, 380.
12. Roberts A. J., Niarchos A. P., Subramanian V. A. et al. (1978) Hypertension following coronary artery bypass graft surgery. Comparison of haemodynamic responses to nitroprusside, phentolamine, and converting enzyme inhibitor. *Circulation [Suppl. 1]* **58**, 43.
13. Taylor K. M., Brannan J. J., Bain W. H. et al. (1979) The role of angiotensin II in the development of peripheral vasoconstriction during cardiopulmonary bypass. *Cardiovasc. Res.* **8**, 269.
14. Flear C. T. G. (1970) Electrolyte and body water changes after trauma *J. Clin. Pathol. Suppl.* **4**, 16–31.
15. Bretschneider H. J., Gebhard M. M. and Preusse C. J. (1981) Reviewing the pros and cons of myocardial preservation within cardiac surgery. In: Longmore D. B., ed., *Towards Safer Cardiac Surgery*, pp. 21–53. Lancaster, MTP.
16. Nayler Winifred G. (1981) Preservation of the myocardium: some biochemical considerations. In: Longmore D. B., ed., *Towards Safer Cardiac Surgery*, pp. 627–647. Lancaster, MTP.
17. Gavras H., Kremer D., Brown J. J. et al. (1975) Angiotensin- and norepinephrine-induced myocardial lesions: experimental and clinical studies in rabbits and man. *Am. Heart J.* **89**, 321.
18. Lefer A. M., Glenn T. M., O'Neill T. J. et al. (1971) Inotropic influence of endogenous peptides in experimental haemorrhagic pancreatitis. *Surgery* **69**, 220–228.
19. Stinson E. B., Holloway E. L., Derby G. C. et al. (1977) Control of myocardial performance early after open-heart operations by vasodilator treatment. *J. Thorac. Cardiovasc. Surg.* **73**, 523.
20. Taylor K. M., Casals J., Morton J. J. et al. (1979) The haemodynamic effects of angiotensin blockade after cardiopulmonary bypass. *Br. Heart J.* **41**, 380.
21. Tinker J. (1979) A pharmacological approach to the treatment of shock. *Br. J. Hosp. Med.* **21**, 26.

Chapter 16

Cardiac Arrhythmias

I. Hutton

Arrhythmias are abnormalities of cardiac rhythm in a *patient* and are of particular relevance when they result in hypotension or cardiac failure. Arrhythmias should never be interpreted in abstract from the electrocardiogram but always in the context of a rhythm abnormality in a patient where information about the physiological and biochemical status is vital. A precise diagnosis is essential before embarking on any form of anti-arrhythmic therapy and definition of the various cardiac arrhythmias and conduction problems is therefore necessary.

SINUS NODE PROBLEMS

I. *Sinus bradycardia* is defined as a heart rate less than 60 per minute. It occurs in healthy individuals during sleep and in trained athletes, and is the normal reaction to vagal stimulation such as the Valsalva manoeuvre, carotid sinus massage and the 'diving reflex'. Drugs which produce sinus bradycardia include digoxin and β-adrenoreceptor blocking drugs. Pathological sinus bradycardia can occur after acute inferior myocardial infarction or result from sinus node dysfunction as part of the tachycardia–bradycardia syndrome.[1, 2] Sinus bradycardia is usually asymptomatic and requires no treatment but if there is haemodynamic disturbance with cardiac failure and hypotension, temporary cardiac pacing is indicated in order to increase heart rate and cardiac output.

II. *Sinus tachycardia* is defined as a heart rate greater than 100 per minute. When the heart rate approximates to 140 per minute there should be suspicion of atrial flutter with A–V block. Only when there is a single P wave for each QRS complex can sinus tachycardia be identified. Sinus tachycardia is usually a physiological response to exercise, emotion or

406

infection. Increase in heart rate may be used to maintain cardiac output in the event of cardiac failure, hypotension or pulmonary infarction. Drugs which increase heart rate include synthetic catecholamines, such as isoprenaline or dopamine. Treatment should be directed at the underlying pathological process responsible for the tachycardia rather than the tachycardia itself, but sedation can be of value.

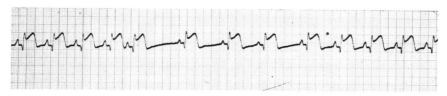

Fig. 16.1. Sinus arrest. No. P wave is identified and there is a pause before next normally conducted sinus beat.

III. *Sinus arrest* occurs when no sinus impulses are generated and P waves cannot be identified on the electrocardiogram, resulting in a pause usually interrupted by an escape beat which may be A–V junctional or ventricular in origin (*Fig.* 16.1) Sinus arrest is found in the elderly with degenerative disease of the conduction system, complicating acute inferior myocardial infarction and as a result of digoxin toxicity. Treatment consists of the intravenous administration of atropine or by temporary or even permanent cardiac pacing. Sinus arrest may be part of the 'sick sinus syndrome' described above. When a sinus beat is absent sino-atrial block is the underlying mechanism if the subsequent pause equals two normal sinus cycles (*Fig.* 16.2).

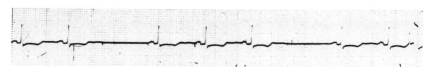

Fig. 16.2. Sino-atrial block. The P wave is absent and the pause from the one normally conducted sinus beat to the next equals 2 normal sinus cycles.

ATRIAL TACHYARRHYTHMIAS

I. *Atrial ectopic beats* are found not infrequently in normal individuals and are often associated with exercise, alcohol, tobacco and caffeine ingestion. Pathologically these are often found in patients with pulmonary hypertension secondary to chronic lung disease or mitral valve disease. The atrial ectopics can be recognized on the ECG by the premature and abnormal P waves as compared with the preceding sinus P wave. The premature P wave when conducted is followed by a QRS complex which is usually normal but may be prolonged as a result of aberrant conduction. An additional means of recognition is the fact that the pause following a conducted atrial ectopic is generally less than the full compensatory pause found after a ventricular ectopic beat. Usually no specific therapy is required.

II. *Atrial tachycardia* is a supraventricular tachycardia with an atrial rate of between 150 and 250 beats/min. Atrial tachycardia may be conducted on a 1 : 1 basis producing a ventricular rate of 150–250 per minute. The P wave will have a bizarre configuration but is often hidden in the QRS complex. Aberrant conduction may take place and slurring and broadening of the QRS complex will be found. Atrial tachycardia frequently has an abrupt onset and termination when the term paroxysmal atrial tachycardia is used. Paroxysmal atrial tachycardia is found in young people, usually females, with no obvious underlying cardiac pathology (*Fig.* 16.3). This atrial

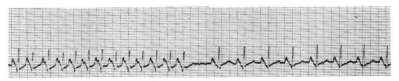

Fig. 16.3. Atrial tachycardia. The initial part of the tracing shows paroxysmal atrial tachycardia at a rate of 180 per minute, reverting to sinus rhythm at a rate of 100 per minute.

tachyarrhythmia can also be found in patients who have ventricular pre-excitation associated with the Wolff–Parkinson–White syndrome, (*Fig.* 16.4). The underlying mechanism is re-entry at the A–V junctional level and thus treatment is directed at interruption of the re-entry mechanism either by simple means such as vagal stimulation, or by drugs which slow A–V conduction, such as digoxin, verapamil and β-adrenoreceptor blocking drugs. Agents which depress excitability and automaticity are also useful, such as quinidine, procainamide or disopyramide.

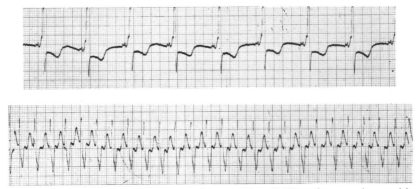

Fig. 16.4. Wolff–Parkinson–White syndrome. The ECG of a patient with the Wolff–Parkinson–White syndrome. The upper panel shows lead 2 with the short P : R interval, the slurring of the upstroke of the QRS—the delta wave and ST : T wave change. The bottom panel shows atrial tachycardia, frequently found in such patients.

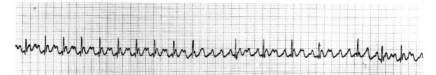

Fig. 16.5. Atrial flutter. This shows atrial flutter with varying atrial ventricular block. The arrows indicate the atrial activity.

III. *Atrial flutter* is a supraventricular tachycardia with an atrial rate of 200–350 per minute (*Fig.* 16.5). The flutter or F waves have a characteristic saw-tooth appearance particularly in the inferior leads of the ECG. Atrial flutter is usually associated with a degree of A–V block, most commonly 2 : 1 A–V block but the block may be variable. The QRS complexes are regular and usually resemble the QRS complex of the preceding sinus conducted beat. Caution should always be exercised in the analysis of heart rates between 140 and 160 per minute. Flutter waves may not be obvious but alteration of ECG paper speed or carotid sinus massage may help to make the flutter wave more evident. Atrial flutter invariably leads to haemodynamic deterioration and prompt treatment is necessary. Verapamil and disopyramide may correct the atrial flutter to sinus rhythm and digoxin will increase the A–V block and reduce ventricular rate. Electrical cardioversion at energy levels of 20–30 Ws is normally the treatment of choice. Overdrive atrial pacing is the other definitive therapeutic alternative. This arrhythmia is found not infrequently after cardiac surgery particularly in patients who have had mitral valve replacement.

IV. *Atrial fibrillation* is characterized by rapid totally irregular fibrillation waves and an irregular ventricular response (*Fig.* 16.6). The atrial rate is

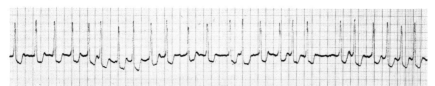

Fig. 16.6. Atrial fibrillation. The P waves are absent, and the R : R interval varies. The ST changes would be consistent with digitalis effects.

commonly between 350 and 500 beats/min with a varying ventricular response depending on whether or not the patient is being treated with cardiac glycosides. Clinical deterioration occurs rapidly, and results from a combination of loss of atrial transport function and the rapid ventricular rate. In addition the patient is at risk from systemic emboli even in the absence of mitral valve obstruction. The treatment of choice is digoxin to slow the ventricular rate by increasing the degree of A–V block. Beta-adrenoreceptor blocking drugs may be added if the ventricular rate is difficult to control despite adequate digoxin therapy. Electrical cardioversion should certainly be considered in the postoperative situation but is likely to be unsuccessful in chronic atrial fibrillation, especially in association with mitral valve disease, where there is significant left atrial enlargement.[3] In the acute situation, anticoagulation, in an attempt to prevent systemic embolism, is unnecessary, unless there is a history of previous embolization. The use of a prophylactic anti-arrhythmic agent such as amiodarone or disopyramide has been shown to decrease the incidence of recurrence of the arrhythmia.[4, 5]

V. *A–V junctional rhythms* arise from a focus in the A–V node with acceleration of its basic rate of impulse formation (*Fig.* 16.7). This may be

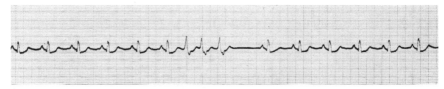

Fig. 16.7. A–V junctional rhythm. The three complexes in the middle of the tracing arise from a focus in the proximity of the A–V node. The P wave can be identified after the QRS complex and the abnormal QRS represents aberrant conduction.

an escape rhythm in the context of sinus arrest or S–A block. The P wave, if identified, may precede or be superimposed on the QRS complex. The PR interval is usually less than 0·12 seconds and the P wave is inverted in leads II, III and AVF due to retrograde activation of the atria from the A–V junctional pacemaker. This abnormality of rhythm is usually transient and active therapy is rarely indicated. A–V junctional rhythms may be digitalis induced and are best treated with β-adrenoreceptor blocking drugs or diphenylhydantoin.[6]

VENTRICULAR TACHYARRHYTHMIAS

1. Ventricular Ectopics

Ventricular ectopics or premature beats are initiated by ectopic foci in either ventricle. Ventricular ectopics are recognized by the fact that the beat is premature and the QRS complex is wide, slurred and often notched. The ectopic beat is followed by a full compensatory pause and unifocal ventricular ectopics will have a fixed coupling interval to the preceding normally conducted QRS complex (*Fig.* 16.8). Ventricular ectopics arising from the right ventricle will resemble the QRS morphology of a left bundle branch block pattern. Bigeminy is characterized by a ventricular ectopic following each normal sinus beat in a repetitive fashion and is a common finding in digitalis toxicity (*Fig.* 16.9). An interpolated ventricular ectopic is a premature beat that occurs immediately between two normal beats with no compensatory pause. A ventricular fusion beat is found when normal sinus and abnormal ectopic impulses arrive more or less simultaneously in

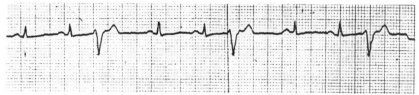

Fig. 16.8. Unifocal ventricular ectopic beats. The premature broad splintered QRS complexes indicate ventricular ectopic beats. There is a compensatory pause after each ectopic beat and there is a fixed coupling interval between the normally conducted sinus beat and the ventricular ectopic beat.

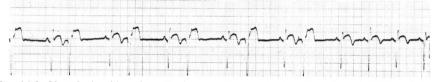

Fig. 16.9. Ventricular bigeminy. Each normally conducted sinus beat is followed by a ventricular ectopic beat. There is a fixed coupling interval between the sinus beat and the ventricular ectopic beat. A common finding in digitalis toxicity.

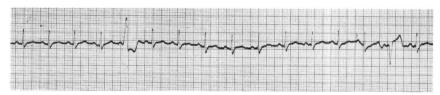

Fig. 16.10. A ventricular fusion beat and an interpolated ventricular ectopic. The first ventricular ectopic noted in the tracing is a fusion beat, a combination of the sinus beat and ectopic complexes. The second ventricular ectopic beat in the tracing is a premature beat that occurs midway between two normal beats and there is no compensatory pause.

the ventricles (*Fig.* 16.10). The QRS configuration will be a combination of the ectopic and sinus beat complex and is therefore called a fusion beat. The presence of fusion beats should raise the suspicion of ventricular parasystole. A parasystolic ventricular focus is a premature beat which bears a fixed relationship not to the preceding sinus beat but to subsequent premature beats (*Fig.* 16.11). The parasystolic pacemaker is of much less prognostic significance than other premature ventricular ectopics because it is probably a region of unidirectional conduction and cannot be prematurely discharged by sinus impulses as they spread through the ventricular myocardium.

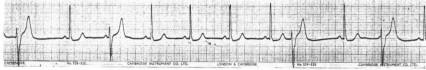

Fig. 16.11. Ventricular parasystole. The ventricular ectopic beats bear a fixed relationship to each other and not to the preceding sinus beat.

Ventricular tachyarrhythmias may arise from a focus of abnormal automaticity or from a re-entrant circuit which may involve the myocardium. Ventricular tachyarrhythmias are potentially more dangerous than atrial or A–V junctional tachycardias. In addition to the underlying cardiac pathology the role of digitalis toxicity, hypokalaemia and hypotension must be emphasized.

In the context of acute myocardial infarction there is now controversy as to the significance and relevance of the ventricular ectopics initiating ventricular tachycardia and ventricular fibrillation. In the postoperative intensive care situation, it would seem prudent to suppress ventricular ectopics which are close to the apex of the T wave, the so-called R on T phenomenon (*Fig.* 16.12) and repetitive forms of ectopics and couplets (*Fig.* 16.13). These forms of ventricular premature ectopics are associated with the greatest probability of developing ventricular tachycardia or ventricular fibrillation. The parenteral administration of lignocaine is the treatment of choice.

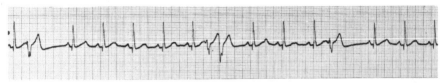

Fig. 16.12. R on T phenomenon. Ventricular ectopic beats which fall on the T wave, resulting in couplets.

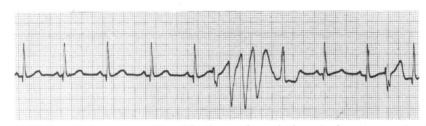

Fig. 16.13. R on T phenomenon. Repetitive forms of ventricular ectopics consequent on the R on T phenomenon.

II. Ventricular Tachycardia

This is a maintained ventricular ectopic rhythm with a ventricular rate usually between 150 and 200 beats/min. The QRS complex is broad, slurred and notched, and the P wave is usually hidden in it (*Fig.* 16.14). Ventricular tachycardia may be confused with paroxysmal atrial tachycardia with bundle branch block or aberrant conduction and every attempt should be made to identify the P wave which will have a fixed relationship with the

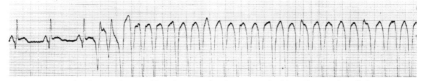

Fig. 16.14. Ventricular tachycardia. A ventricular ectopic hits the peak of the T wave and ventricular tachycardia ensues. Note the broad, slurred QRS complex. P waves are absent.

QRS complex in the latter. Additional means of identification include slowing of the heart rate in atrial tachycardia by carotid sinus pressure (*Fig.* 16.15), irregularity of the P–R interval in ventricular tachycardia and appropriate identification of any preceding ectopic beat. This form of ventricular tachycardia rapidly leads to hypotension and cardiac failure and although sinus rhythm may be restored by a blow to the sternum, the administration of anti-arrhythmic agents in the context of hypotension is dangerous and electrical conversion is preferred.

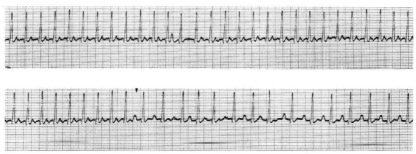

Fig. 16.15. Carotid sinus pressure as a means of identifying arrhythmias. The arrow indicates the application of carotid sinus pressure with reversal of a supraventricular tachycardia to a sinus tachycardia.

A more benign form of ventricular tachycardia is 'slow ventricular tachycardia' or accelerated ventricular rhythm or idioventricular tachycardia. These terms are used synonymously to describe an ectopic ventricular rhythm with a rate of less than 100 beats/min (*Fig.* 16.16). Some authors recommend the use of atropine to increase sinus activity with a prophylactic pacemaker in situ but as the prognosis is good and haemodynamic disturbance is rare an expectant policy can be adopted.

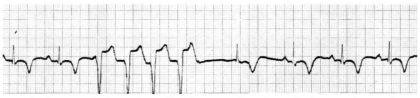

Fig. 16.16. Slow ventricular tachycardia. Shows a salvo of ventricular ectopic complexes at a rate of less than 100 per minute.

III. Ventricular Fibrillation

This is characterized by irregular waves of ranging amplitude and configuration and occurring at a rate of 250–500 beats/min (*Fig.* 16.17). This arrhythmia must be corrected immediately and defibrillation by d.c. shock is the only effective therapy. Defibrillation with the least energy minimizes the risk of myocardial damage and it is recommended that the first shock be 200 Ws. If this is unsuccessful 400 Ws should then be used. If, however, metabolic acidosis has occurred sodium bicarbonate is required to correct this. Further failure may be corrected by the use of lignocaine or mexiletine, followed by defibrillation.

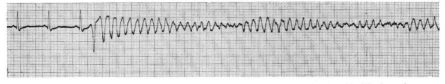

Fig. 16.17. Ventricular fibrillation. Consequent on R on T, ventricular fibrillation characterized by irregular waves of amplitude and configuration is noted.

ATRIOVENTRICULAR BLOCK

The ECG appearances of A–V block are determined by the level of block or delay, the degree of block and the origin of the escape rhythm. In recent years intracardiac recording techniques[7] have clarified the underlying pathophysiology of A–V conduction disorders. By recording atrial, His bundle electrocardiograms and the scalar ECG the site of delay can be localized to the A–V node or His–Purkinje system.[8]

I. First Degree A–V Block

First degree A–V block with prolongation of the P–R interval on the electrocardiogram to greater than 0·22 seconds, indicates underlying pathology of A–V nodal structures.[9] There is no indication for active therapy but first degree A–V block in association with the acute development of left bundle branch block usually indicates bifascicular block and is an indication for the insertion of a temporary pacemaker.

II. Second Degree A–V Block

There are two types of second degree A–V block, Mobitz type I which is the more common, better known as the Wenkebach phenomenon, and Mobitz type II block.

Mobitz type I is characterized by prolongation of the P–R interval from complex to complex until finally the atrial complex is not conducted to the ventricles and there is a pause with either an escape A–V junctional beat or resumption of a similar cycle (*Fig.* 16.18). The Wenkebach phenomenon usually indicates disease of the A–V nodal structures[9] and the QRS complex will be normal. Digitalis toxicity should always be suspected in patients with type II A–V block especially in association with calcific aortic valve disease, either pre- or postcardiac surgery. Temporary pacing is rarely necessary as this type of conduction defect does not usually lead to haemodynamic disturbance. The introduction of intracardiac electrograms has allowed a more precise definition of the site of block. In 90% of cases of 2 : 1 A–V block the impulse will be blocked at the level of the A–V node.

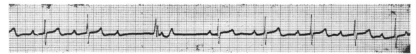

Fig. 16.18. Mobitz I. Mobitz I, or the Wenkebach phenomenon, demonstrates the prolongation of the PR interval from complex to complex until finally the P wave is not followed by a normal sinus beat and an escape A–V junction beat is noted.

In Mobitz type II the A–V block is a consequence of block below the His bundle and is characterized by broadening of the QRS complex. Mobitz type II block is recognized by intermittently blocked P waves without preceding progressive P–R prolongation (*Fig.* 16.19). It is important to distinguish Mobitz I from Mobitz II block as the latter is of graver prognostic significance and temporary pacing is recommended. Depending on the underlying pathology a permanent pacemaker should be considered and the available evidence suggests that the incidence of syncope and sudden death can be reduced in asymptomatic patients.[10]

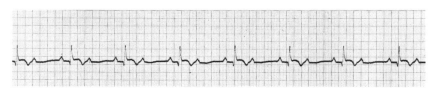

Fig. 16.19. Mobitz II. This is a form of the Mobitz type II block showing intermittent P waves not followed by a conducted beat.

III. Complete Heart Block

Complete heart block indicates failure to conduct atrial impulses to the ventricles and the presence of a totally independent pacemaker rhythm at rate of 30–40 beats/min. If the QRS complexes are of normal appearance the pacemaker controlling the ventricles is in the region of the His bundle[11]

(*Fig*. 16.20). When the QRS complex is broad and distorted the pacemaker site is in the distal His–Purkinje system[12] (*Fig*. 16.21). Even in the congenital form of complete heart block with the narrow QRS complexes although the risk of syncope is small, permanent pacing is recommended. In the other form, usually due to degenerative disease of the intraventricular conduction system,[13–15] permanent pacing is indicated.

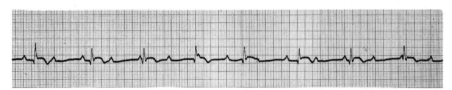

Fig. 16.20. Congenital complete heart block. There is no relationship between the P wave and QRS complex. The QRS complexes are of relatively normal appearance.

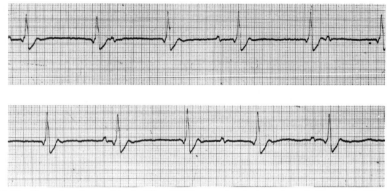

Fig. 16.21. Complete heart block. The QRS complex is broad and distorted. There is no relationship between P wave and QRS complex. This is the more common form of complete heart block and is usually due to degenerative disease of the intraventricular conducting system.

Complete heart block must be distinguished from A–V dissociation where conduction through the A–V node is still possible. A–V dissociation will be found if either the sinus rate slows to be less than the intrinsic rate of the A–V node or if A–V junctional or ventricular pacemakers accelerate to a rate faster than the prevailing sinus rate (*Fig*. 16.22). A–V dissociation is often transient and active intervention is rarely required.

Fascicular block or bundle branch block in acute situations rarely calls for active therapy but in the chronic situation with underlying cardiac

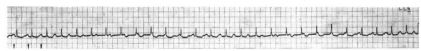

Fig. 16.22. A–V dissociation. There is no association between the P wave and QRS complexes but occasionally a normally conducted sinus beat is found, indicating that conduction through the A–V node is still possible.

pathology bifascicular disease may be a percursor of complete heart block.[16]

THE ELECTROPHYSIOLOGICAL BASIS FOR ARRHYTHMIAS

Automaticity is the capacity to form an electrical impulse and is the normal property of the specialized conducting tissue in the cells of the sino-atrial node, specialized atrial fibres, the atrio-ventricular node and the fibres of the His–Purkinje system. These pacemaking cells are under the external control of influences such as the sympathetic nervous system mediated through β-receptors in the cells and circulating catecholamines which will increase the speed and frequency of conduction through the A–V node. Parasympathetic nervous activity exerts the opposite effect of slowing the heart rate. Arrhythmias may therefore be generated by changes in the normal automatic mechanism or by a focus of abnormal automaticity resulting from myocardial ischaemia or damage, hypokalaemia, hypocalcaemia and hypoxia.

The alternative mechanism for the genesis of arrhythmias is a re-entry mechanism. Re-entry occurs as a result of an imbalance between conduction and refractoriness in cardiac tissue so that a small cardiac impulse on reaching refractory tissue is deflected and re-enters adjacent areas of myocardium by dual conduction pathways.[17] These re-entry pathways are found in sites which demonstrate very slow conduction such as the A–V node. Re-entry can be produced by conditions which shorten refractoriness or alter the boundary between Purkinje fibres and normal ventricular myocardium or which slow conduction.[18]

THE MANAGEMENT OF CARDIAC ARRHYTHMIAS

The need for treatment of arrhythmias is usually dictated by their haemodynamic consequences and knowledge of their prognostic significance. It is inappropriate to consider the management of arrhythmias in other intensive care situations as similar to that of acute myocardial infarction. Anti-arrhythmic therapy need not be used if the underlying cause of the arrhythmia can be successfully treated. This dictum is particularly relevant in the context of electrolyte imbalance, such as hypokalaemia or hypocalcaemia, acidosis, hypoxia, digoxin toxicity, congestive cardiac failure or pulmonary thrombo-embolism. Not only is it important to control or treat the underlying cause for the arrhythmia but anti-arrhythmic therapy may well be unsuccessful unless the underlying cause is removed—hypokalaemia is the obvious example in the context of ventricular arrhythmias.

The aims of anti-arrhythmic therapy are to:
1. Terminate the arrhythmia and restore sinus rhythm.
2. Abolish ectopic beats which may be responsible for the initiation of the tachycardia.
3. To slow the heart rate either directly or indirectly in atrial tachycardias by slowing conduction through the A–V node.

ANTI-ARRHYTHMIC DRUGS

Anti-arrhythmic drugs are best classified by reference to their clinical application. Agents which work principally on atrial tachyarrhythmias include quinidine, procainamide and disopyramide. Those which are effective on A–V junctional rhythms include digoxin, verapamil and β-adrenoreceptor blocking drugs and those which act specifically on ventricular arrhythmias include lignocaine and mexiletine. Procainamide and disopyramide will also act on ventricular arrhythmias as will the newer anti-arrhythmic agents, amiodarone and tocainide.

Quinidine, procainamide and disopyramide have membrane stabilizing effects and will depress contractility of cardiac muscle. They act principally on the fast sodium channel which causes rapid depolarization, particularly in Purkinje and ventricular tissue. Thus automaticity will be suppressed or abolished in the His–Purkinje system and this action will combat arrhythmias generated by enhanced pacemaker activity. There is little effect on the normal S–A node. Another effect is to prolong the effective refractory period relative to action potential duration. There is a linear relationship between plasma concentration and effect.

Digoxin will prolong A–V nodal conduction and delay recovery. Beta-adrenoreceptor blocking drugs act by competitive blockade of the β_1 cardiac receptors leading to slowing of the S–A node and prolonged A–V conduction by reducing automaticity in the His–Purkinje system. Verapamil is a calcium antagonist which has a profound effect on the A–V node but no effect on atrial and ventricular muscle or the His–Purkinje system.

Lignocaine, mexiletine and diphenylhydantoin are of particular value in ventricular arrhythmias by suppressing or abolishing automaticity in the His–Purkinje system. They also have a quinidine-like action in prolonging the effective refractory period compared with the action potential duration. Diphenylhydantoin is used exclusively in the therapy of digoxin-induced ventricular arrhythmias particularly in the presence of hypokalaemia.

In the context of intensive care situations, where parenteral therapy will be used almost exclusively, it seems appropriate to consider some of the newer anti-arrhythmic drugs which may be given parenterally followed by oral therapy if indicated. A detailed list of dosage schedules will be found in *Table* 16.1.

Lignocaine is accepted as the standard parenteral agent for suppression of ventricular arrhythmias associated with acute myocardial infarction and cardiac surgery, and will control 85–90% of ventricular arrhythmias. Lignocaine is rapidly metabolized by the liver and the effect of a single bolus lasts for 4–5 min only. Standard therapy is a loading dose of 70–100 mg intravenously. The infusion regime should be 2 mg/min for a 70-kg adult. Some authors suggest 3–4 mg/min.[19-21] but the higher dosages can result in a significant incidence of serious side effects including drowsiness, paraesthesia, muscle twitching and convulsions. Higher plasma concentrations can cause respiratory arrest. A reduced dosage should be used in patients with hepatic dysfunction.

Procainamide was formerly used in the management of lignocaine-resistant ventricular arrhythmias and has been shown to be effective,[19] but has been largely superseded by the newer anti-arrhythmic agents, disopyramide and mexiletine.

Mexiletine is similar in its structure to lignocaine but is not as rapidly metabolized by the liver. Mexiletine should only be used for lignocaine-resistant ventricular arrhythmias. The drug is given as a bolus of 200 mg over 3 minutes followed by a somewhat complicated dosage schedule of 3 mg/min for 1 hour, followed by 1·5 mg/min for 3 hours and then 1 mg/min subsequently.[22] The drug has also been used orally in both the acute and post-myocardial infarction patients and a significant reduction in ventricular arrhythmias has been demonstrated.[23,24] Side effects are frequent, particularly during initiation of therapy and are mainly gastrointestinal and neurological including tremor, diplopia, paraesthesia and confusion. Hypotension and bradycardia have also been reported.[25]

Disopyramide is very similar to quinidine and procainamide in its actions but there are subtle differences, and it has been shown to be effective in the treatment of ventricular arrhythmias when quinidine has been unsuccessful.[26] It is of particular value in the treatment of the atrial arrhythmias associated with the Wolff–Parkinson–White syndrome, where there is an anomalous atrioventricular connection in addition to the usual pathway through the A–V node and His bundle. Disopyramide has also been shown to be effective in the treatment of lignocaine-resistant ventricular arrhythmias.[27] Excessive caution should be exercised in the use of disopyramide in patients with left ventricular dysfunction since there is a risk of precipitating cardiac failure.[28] Anticholinergic side effects include dry mouth, urinary retention, constipation and blurred vision.[5]

Disopyramide is absorbed well orally and protein binding is concentration dependent. The drug is metabolized in the liver but some 40% is excreted unchanged in the urine. The dose should be reduced in patients with renal impairment. In the emergency treatment of arrhythmias 2 mg/kg is given over 5 minutes the maintenance dose is 100–150 mg 6-hourly. Orally the loading dose is 300 mg followed by 100 mg q.i.d.

Like quinidine and procainamide, disopyramide can slow conduction in

Table **16.1. Administration, metabolism and excretion of anti-arrhythmic drugs**

Drug	Dosage	Effective plasma concentration, μg/ml	Half-life in plasma, hours	Metabolism/ excretion
Lignocaine	*i.v.* 70–100 mg bolus. Can be repeated every 5 minutes to a total of 300 mg Then 2·0–3·0 mg/min by constant infusion	1–5	1·5–2	Hepatic
Mexiletine	*i.v.* 200 mg bolus 3 mg/min, for 1 hour 1·5 mg/min for 3 hours 1 mg/min infusion *Oral* Loading dose 600 mg 200 mg t.i.d.	1–2	10	Hepatic
Disopyramide	*i.v.* 2 mg/kg over 5 minutes *Constant infusion* 0·4 mg/kg/h *Oral* 300 mg—loading 200 mg—8-hourly	2–4	6	Renal
Procainamide	*i.v.* 100 mg every 2 minutes to a total of 1000 mg *Constant infusion* 2–6 mg/min	3–10	3–4	Hepatic
Diphenyl-hydantoin	*i.v.* 100 mg every 5 minutes to a maximum of 1000 mg *Oral* Loading dose 1000 mg *Maintenance* 400 mg daily	5–18	20–30	Hepatic
Digoxin	*i.v.* 0·5 mg–bolus 0·25 mg 6-hourly for 24 hours. *Oral* Digitalizing dose— 1·5 mg *Maintenance* 0·25–0·5 mg	1–2	36	Renal

Table **16.1** (cont.)

Drug	Dosage	Effective plasma concentration, µg/ml	Half-life in plasma, hours	Metabolism/excretion
Propranolol	*i.v.* 1 mg/min to a total of 5 mg	30–50 ng/ml	3–4	Hepatic
Practolol	*i.v.* 10–20 mg slowly	1·5–5	7–11	Renal
Verapamil	*i.v.* 5–10 mg at 1 mg/min *Oral* 40–120 mg 8-hourly	—	3–7	Hepatic

all parts of the heart and precipitate automatic behaviour in ectopic sites. Thus potentially fatal conduction problems and arrhythmias can occur. Careful scrutiny of the ECG is indicated for evidence of QRS prolongation and increase in the QT interval.

Verapamil is a calcium antagonist which was first introduced as an antianginal agent but is now used principally in the management of A–V junctional tachyarrhythmias.[29] Verapamil acts by slowing conduction in the A–V node and blocks the re-entry circuit found in most A–V junctional tachyarrhythmias, but is of no value in the treatment of ventricular arrhythmias. Verapamil invariably causes a fall in blood pressure and although this is usually transient, cardiac failure or left ventricular dysfunction is an absolute contraindication to its use. The intravenous dosage is 5–10 mg over a 2-minute period. Although verapamil can be given by continuous infusion the author prefers to use a bolus dose to correct the arrhythmia to sinus and then use an alternative therapy parenterally. The other principal use of verapamil is in the Wolff–Parkinson–White syndrome where verapamil will slow A–V nodal conduction and block re-entry tachycardias. Unlike disopyramide there is no effect on the accessory pathway. The major side effect is myocardial depression and verapamil should not be used if the patient is receiving digoxin or β-adrenoreceptor blocking therapy. Verapamil should not be used if there is evidence of sinus node dysfunction.[30]

Digitalis is of considerable value in the management of A–V junctional tachyarrhythmias particularly in the context of cardiac failure. The digitalis glycosides have a narrow toxic–therapeutic ratio and digitalis toxicity has been reported in as many as 20% of a hospital population.[31] Digitalis acts indirectly through autonomic mechanisms and also directly on the A–V node and thus A–V nodal conduction is prolonged since the refractory period is increased and conduction velocity diminished. In atrial flutter and atrial fibrillation the ventricular response will be controlled by prolongation of A–V nodal recovery. Digoxin is recommended in a dosage of 0·25 mg i.v. followed by 0·25 mg 6-hourly i.v. until control of the ventricular rate is achieved or sinus rhythm established. Intramuscular digoxin is not recommended because of the variability of absorption and because of severe pain at the injection site. Hypokalaemia must always be corrected and after the 'digitalizing' dose is administered, maintenance therapy can be dictated by plasma levels of digoxin and by the patient's renal function. Digoxin should always be used with caution in the elderly.[32]

Digitalis toxicity can result in any form of cardiac arrhythmia but generally results in depression of conduction or increased automaticity by ectopic pacemakers. Measurement of plasma digoxin levels, particularly if in the toxic range, can be of value but must always be interpreted in the clinical context.[33] The first line of treatment of digitalis toxicity is to correct hypokalaemia, if present. The drugs of choice for digitalis-induced automaticity problems are diphenylhydantoin and β-adrenoreceptor blocking drugs. High grade A–V block should be treated by intravenous pacing. If in doubt about digitalis toxicity and a further digitalis effect appears to be indicated, a small intravenous dose of ouabain can be used since its effect will be apparent within 30 minutes.

With the introduction of newer anti-arrhythmic drugs, β-adrenoreceptor blocking drugs have only a limited role in the management of cardiac arrhythmias and should be limited to patients with digitalis toxicity and in the operative and postoperative onset of arrhythmias caused by increased catecholamines (e.g. phaeochromocytoma). They are of value in atrial tachyarrhythmias; beta-blockade will result in slowing of the sino-atrial node, prolongation of A–V conduction and decreased automaticity in the His–Purkinje system. The greatest clinical experience relates to propranolol,[34] but in the intensive care environment, intravenous practolol is now used more frequently in a dosage of 5–10 mg for the correction of atrial tachyarrhythmias.[35,36]

Amiodarone must be mentioned although only available in oral preparation. This is a unique anti-arrhythmic agent widely used in the continent of Europe. Amiodarone is effective against both supraventricular and ventricular arrhythmias including ventricular fibrillation. It prolongs the action potential duration and increases the refractory period. It has no membrane depressant action and can be used in cardiac failure.[37] It should be used in the treatment of resistant arrhythmias and is of particular value in the Wolff–Parkinson–White syndrome.[38] Amiodarone is very slowly eliminated and has a half-life of 30 days. The usual dose is 200–800 mg daily. The major side effect is the development of corneal deposits which usually do not interfere with vision but may upset corneal metabolism.

Cardiac pacing can be a very effective therapy particularly when atrial pacing is used. An increase in heart rate can suppress ventricular arrhythmias irrespective of whether the mechanism is re-entry or automaticity: so-called 'overdrive suppression.' The use of an appropriately timed stimulus can interrupt the re-entrant pathway by depolarizing the atrium. Arrhythmias can also be terminated by short bursts of rapid stimulation.[39] The use of intracardiac stimuli in the treatment of arrhythmias has been excellently reviewed by Haft.[40]

Acknowledgements

The author wishes to thank Dr A. C. Tweddel for providing the excellent illustrations.

REFERENCES

1. Ferrer M. I. (1973) The sick sinus syndrome. *Circulation* **347**, 635–641.
2. Kaplan M. B., Langendorff R., Lev M. et al. (1973) Tachycardia–bradycardia syndrome (so-called sick sinus syndrome). *Am. J. Cardiol.* **31**, 497–508.
3. Resnekov L. (1973) Present status of electroversion in the management of cardiac dysrhythmias. *Circulation* **47**, 1356–1363.
4. Sodermark T., Edhag O., Sjögren A. et al. (1975) Effect of quinidine in maintaining sinus rhythm after conversion of atrial flutter or atrial fibrillation. *Br. Heart J.*, **37**, 486–492.
5. Heel R. C., Brogden R. N. and Speight T. M. (1978) Disopyramide: a review of its pharmacological properties and therapeutic use in treating cardiac arrhythmias. *Drugs* **15**, 331–338
6. Smith T. W. and Haber E. (1973) Digitalis (I). *N. Engl. J. Med.* **289**, 945–952.
7. Schlerlag B. J., Lau S. H., Helfant R. H. et al. (1969) Catheter technique for recording His bundle activity in man. *Circulation* **39**, 13–18.
8. Narula O. S., Schlerlag B. J., Sanet P. et al. (1971) Atrioventricular block, localisation and classification by His bundle recordings. *Am. J. Med.* **50**, 146–165.
9. Spear J. F. and Moore E. M. (1973) In: Dreyfus L. S. and Ukoff W. O., ed., *Cardiac Arrhythmias: The 25th Hahnemann Symposium*, p. 293. New York, Grune & Stratton.
10. Dhingra R. C., Denes P. Wu D. et al. (1974) The significance of second degree atrioventricular block and bundle branch block. *Circulation* **49**, 638–646.
11. Kelly D. T., Bordsky S. J., Mirowski M. et al. (1972) Bundle of His recordings in congenital complete heart block. *Circulation* **45**, 277–281.
12. Rosen K. M., Loeb H. S., Chuquima R. et al. (1970) Site of heart block in acute myocardial infarction. *Circulation* **42**, 925–933.
13. Lenegre J. (1964) Aetiology and pathology of bilateral bundle branch block in relation to complete heart block. *Prog. Cardiovasc. Dis.* **6**, 409–444.
14. Davies M. J. (1976) *Pathology of the Conducting Tissue of the Heart.* London, Butterworths.
15. Sowton E., Henrix G. and Roy P. (1974) Ten-year survey of treatment with implanted cardiac pacemaker. *Br. Med. J.* **3**, 155–160.
16. Kulbertus H. E. (1973) The magnitude of risk of developing complete heart block in patients with LAD-RBBB. *Am. Heart J.* **86**, 278–280.
17. Cranefield P. F., Wit A. L. and Hoffman B. F. (1973) Genesis of cardiac arrhythmias. *Circulation* **47**, 190–204.

18. Hoffman B. F. and Cranefield P. F. (1964) The physiological basis of cardiac arrhythmias. *Am. J. Med.* **37**, 670–684.
19. Wyman M. G. and Hammersmith L. (1974) Comprehensive treatment plan for the prevention of primary ventricular fibrillation in acute myocardial infarction. *Am. J. Cardiol.* **33**, 661–667.
20. Lie K. I., Wellens H. J., Van Cadell F. J. et al. (1974) Lidocaine in the prevention of primary ventricular fibrillation. *N. Engl. J. Med.* **291**, 1324–1326.
21. Campbell N. P. S., Kelly J. G., Adgey A. J. J. et al. (1979) Observations on haemodynamic effects of mexiletine. *Br. Heart J.* **41**, 182–186.
22. Campbell N. P. S., Pantridge J. R. and Adgey A. J. J. (1977) Mexiletine in the management of ventricular dysrhythmias. *Eur. J. Cardiol.* **6**, 245–258.
23. Campbell R. W. F., Talbot R. G., Dolder M. A. et al. (1975) Comparison of procainamide and mexilitine in prevention of ventricular arrhythmias after acute myocardial infarction. *Lancet* **1**, 1257–1260.
24. Chamberlain D. A. (1980) Oral mexiletine in high risk patients after acute myocardial infarction. *Proc. VIII European Congress of Cardiology*, 2654 p. 217.
25. Chew C. Y. C., Collett J. and Singh B. N. (1979) Mexiletine: a review of its pharmacological properties and therapeutic efficacy in arrhythmias. *Drugs* **17**, 161–181.
26. Vismara L. A., Vera Z., Miller R. R. et al. (1977) Efficacy of disopyramide phosphate in the treatment of refractory ventricular tachycardia. *Am. J. Cardiol.* **39**, 1027–1034.
27. Sbarbaro J. A., Rawling D. A. and Fozzard H. A. (1979) Suppression of ventricular arrhythmias with intravenous disopyramide and lidocaine: efficacy comparison in a randomised trial. *Am. J. Cardiol.* **55**, 513–520.
28. Podrid P. J., Schoeneberger A. and Lown B. (1980) Congestive cardiac failure caused by oral disopyramide. *N. Engl. J. Med.* **307**, 614–617.
29. Singh B. N., Ellrodt G. and Peter C. T. (1978) Verapamil: a review of its pharmacological properties and therapeutic use. *Drugs* **15**, 169–197.
30. Mangiardi L. M., Hariman R. J. and McAllister R. G. (1977) Electrophysiological and haemodynamic effects of verapamil. Correlation with plasma drug concentrations. *Circulation* **57**, 366–372.
31. Smith T. W. and Haber E. (1973) Digitalis II. *N. Engl. J. Med.* **289**, 1010–1015.
32. Dall J. L. C. (1970) Maintenance digoxin in elderly patients. *Br. Med. J.* **2**, 705–706.
33. Shapiro W. (1978) Correlative studies of serum digitalis levels and the arrhythmias of digitalis intoxication. *Am. J. Cardiol.* **41**, 852–859.
34. Gibson D. G. and Sowton E. (1969) The use of beta-adrenergic blocking drugs in dysrhythmias. *Prog. Cardiovasc. Dis.* **12**, 16–39.
35. Jewitt D. E., Mercer C. J. and Shillingford J. P. (1969) Practolol in the treatment of cardiac dysrhythmias due to acute myocardial infarction. *Lancet* **2**, 227–230.
36. Gibson D. G., Balcon R. and Sowton E. (1968) Clinical use of practolol as an antidysrhythmic agent in heart failure. *Br. Med. J.* **3**, 161–163.
37. Rosenbaum M. B., Chiale P. A., Halpern M. S. et al. (1976) Clinical efficacy of amiodarone as an antiarrhythmic drug. *Am. J. Cardiol.* **38**, 934–944.
38. Rosenbaum M. B., Chiale P. A. Ryba D. et al. (1974) Control of tachyarrhythmias associated with the Wolff–Parkinson–White syndrome by amiodarone hydrochloride. *Am. J. Cardiol.* **34**, 215–223.
39. Wellens H. J. J. (1978) Value and limitations of programmed electrical stimulation of the heart in the study and treatment of tachycardias. *Circulation* **57**, 845–851.
40. Haft J. I. (1974) Treatment of arrhythmias by intracardiac electrical stimulation. *Prog. Cardiovasc. Dis.* **6**, 539–568.

Chapter 17

The Nervous System

J. Douglas Miller

Intensive monitoring and care has only recently expanded into the area of brain resuscitation and the management of coma. This is related to several factors. With the development of electronic transducers and compact display devices came increasing demand for specialized areas for respiratory and cardiac care with facilities for continuous monitoring of blood pressure, heart rate and ECG. It was at first considered that such facilities had little to offer the unconscious brain-damaged patient, for how could the complex and subtle function of the nervous system be reduced to a numerical value or a waveform on a cathode-ray oscilloscope? As understanding of the physiology of cerebral blood flow, intracranial pressure and the effects of brain distortion produced by intracranial mass lesions increased, it became clear that secondary haemodynamic and hydrodynamic disturbances formed the basis of dramatic neurological deterioration in patients with a wide variety of primary neurological disorders.

Awareness has been growing of the importance of the 'second insult' as a significant source of mortality and morbidity in patients with head injury, intracranial haemorrhage and ischaemic stroke. By this is meant the superimposition of a systemic or cerebral ischaemic or hypoxic insult to the already damaged brain (*Table* 17.1). This may be produced by an episode of arterial hypotension, intracranial hypertension, low haematocrit, respiratory obstruction or pulmonary dysfunction. If, to these insults, are added the effects of epileptic seizures and intracranial or systemic infection, then much of the in-hospital morbidity and mortality of comatose patients can be accounted for. In a study of 116 patients who had talked at some time after sustaining a head injury, but then deteriorated and died in hospital, Rose and his colleagues[1] found that death was due to avoidable secondary factors in more than half of these fatalities. Miller[2] found that the significant secondary insults of arterial hypotension, hypoxaemia and anaemia were present on admission to hospital in 44 of a series of 100 consecutive comatose head-injured patients. These secondary insults contributed significantly to an increase in mortality and severe morbidity.

Table 17.1. **Secondary insults to the injured brain**

Systemic insults	Intracranial insults
Hypoxaemia	Intra- or extracerebral haemorrhage
Hypotension	Brain swelling/oedema
Anaemia	Raised intracranial pressure
Hypercapnia	Cerebral vasospasm
Hyponatraemia	Intracranial infection
Pyrexia	Epilepsy

In the comatose patient there appears, therefore, to be a strong case for monitoring even the basic systemic variables of arterial blood pressure and blood gases. Over the past 10 years the benefits of continuous monitoring of intracranial pressure have been acknowledged. There has also been increasing readiness to rely upon continuous physiological monitoring as a guide to the progress of the comatose patient and to increase the use of muscle relaxants and central nervous system depressants in the management of patients with severe brain damage.

In considering methods of continuous monitoring in the intensive care unit, Griffith and Becker[3] have described first, second and third generation monitoring systems. In the case of monitoring systems for central nervous system (CNS) disorders, almost all current systems are of the first generation variety in which the data displayed is an unprocessed direct record of the pressure which is being measured. Second generation systems employ a degree of data reduction or measure the results of controlled perturbations of the physiological variable. Intracranial pressure monitoring systems are now reaching this second generation stage. Data may be automatically displayed as various mathematical derivatives of the original pressure and measurements of intracranial compliance can be made. The third generation stage has not yet been reached. At this stage, for example, data obtained from intracranial pressure monitoring would be employed to regulate the administration of therapy for intracranial hypertension.

In this chapter, the special problems of monitoring function and dysfunction in the craniospinal axis will be surveyed, citing both available and developing techniques of CNS monitoring. Pathophysiological mechanisms for the production of primary and secondary brain damage will be summarized and, based upon these mechanisms, the principles and practice of therapy for the comatose patient in the intensive care unit will be discussed briefly.

SPECIAL PROBLEMS OF MONITORING BRAIN FUNCTION IN THE INTENSIVE CARE UNIT

I. The Clinical Assessment of CNS Function

Without question the most effective way to assess the integrity of cerebral, spinal cord and nerve function has been, and continues to be, the neurological examination. This subtle evaluation requires the patient to respond in a certain way to auditory, visual and tactile stimuli. In the comatose patient much of this process is impossible. Until 1965 the neurological evaluation of the comatose patient was usually restricted to those parts of the traditional neurological examination which could still be carried out, the pupil light response, tendon reflexes and the plantar responses. This provided little useful information. Plum and Posner[4] addressed this problem directly in their landmark book *Diagnosis of Stupor and Coma* in pointing out the role of brain stem dysfunction in the genesis of coma and ways of testing this effectively at the bedside.

Another problem in the assessment of the unconscious patient has been the terminology of varying degrees of coma. Numerical systems based upon a single scale of descriptive terms have not proved useful or reliable because much of the terminology remains subjective. Furthermore, the correct constellation of signs of dysfunction does not often coexist so that it can frequently be difficult to place the patient at a single appropriate point on a unidimensional coma scale.

Teasdale and Jennett[5] developed in Glasgow what is now the most widely used coma scale. It is based on three separate simple scales for eye opening, motor response and verbal response to standardized stimuli (*Table* 17.2). The terminology used was selected after testing as that which

Table 17.2. The Glasgow coma scale

	Eye opening		*Motor response*		*Verbal response*
4	Spontaneous	6	Obeys commands	5	Orientated
3	To command	5	Localizes pain	4	Disorientated
2	To pain	4	Flexor withdrawal	3	Words
1	Nil	3	Abnormal flexor	2	Sounds
		2	Extensor	1	Nil
		1	Nil		

yielded the lowest degree of inter-observer variability among both English speaking and non-English speaking personnel. The Glasgow coma scale has now been adopted in many countries and is strongly recommended here.

If one poses the question 'how valuable is bedside neurological examination in a comatose patient?' the answer today must be that the

examination remains extremely valuable provided one uses correct terminology and performs the correct tests of CNS function.[6] These will be
described in the following section. Useful though the clinical examination
can be, it still does not provide a continuous record of CNS function, but is
limited to the frequency with which clinical examination can be performed.
Furthermore, the administration of paralytic or sedative drugs will vitiate
the examination. Hopes have been raised that some form of continuous
monitoring of electrophysiological function may become a feasible
alternative.

II. Problems of Electrophysiological Monitoring of CNS Function

Until recently, the problems involved in recording brain electrical activity
as a means of continuously monitoring brain function in comatose patients
in the ICU were so great as to make the project impossible. Continuous
recording of the EEG over long periods of time raises immense problems of
data handling and analysis. In addition, the origin and significance of many
of the waveform patterns seen on EEG remains controversial. Measurement of evoked potentials would be a better approach because this would
test the integrity of certain pathways in the nervous system. Dysfunction in
those pathways could be analysed quantitatively in terms of waveform
latency and amplitude. Until recently, the degree of amplification required
to discern the small evoked response amid the sea of electrical interference
in the intensive care unit and the artefact produced by movement in the
comatose head-injured patient made this an impossible goal. With the
advent of sophisticated filtering systems and compact computing equipment to average the responses obtained from 500 to 1000 stimuli, it is now
possible to identify the constant evoked response because the random
electrical activity is averaged out. By using different stimuli, it is possible to
measure in the same patient visual, auditory and somatosensory evoked
potentials.[7] The equipment is expensive, however, and at this stage it still
requires a long time (more than 2 hours) to make a complete set of
recordings in a comatose patient. For the present, therefore, this and other
neurophysiological techniques must be considered as research projects
rather than practical tools for clinical management.

III. The Vulnerability of the CNS to Ischaemic Hypoxic Damage

As Plum has eloquently pointed out, if uraemia indicates renal failure, then
coma means brain failure with all the urgency and gravity which that term
implies. Time is of the essence in moving toward a definitive diagnosis to
explain coma. Sadly, this is not always appreciated in the general medical
or surgical ICU. There is often a tendency to provide only airway and

systemic support for the comatose patient while the chances of treating a potentially reversible lesion ebb steadily away.

In thinking about the extreme vulnerability of the brain to ischaemic insults, the phrase which comes to mind is 'so little leeway, so little time'. If the blood supply to the brain is completely and abruptly cut off, neurological function ceases in 12 seconds and within 10 minutes irreversible structural brain damage has occurred. In the comatose patient who is already showing decerebrate rigidity, even the slightest further neurological deterioration will manifest itself by complete loss of all motor activity and usually by loss of the pupil light response and all respiratory activity.

For this reason, in seriously ill comatose patients, the monitoring system must be continuous, rapid and able to detect even small changes in factors which will adversely affect neurological function. Clinical surveillance is crucial but can be interfered with by drugs. Continuous electrophysiological surveillance is not yet a practical reality. For this reason, it is important to supplement the systemic monitoring system which is measuring blood pressure, heart rate and body temperature with some index of intracranial events. Possibilities include continuous monitoring of intracranial pressure (ICP) and measurements of cerebral blood flow and brain energy metabolism.

IV. Monitoring of Cerebral Hydrodynamic and Haemodynamic Variables

The advent of continuous ICP monitoring into clinical practice has been a major step forward in the management of the comatose patient. The difference between arterial and intracranial pressure is equivalent to cerebral tissue perfusion pressure[8]. Elevation in ICP can herald the development of intracranial haemorrhage, oedema or brain swelling and signals the failure of treatment. However, the procedure of measuring ICP is not without risk of infection or haemorrhage. Technical problems of fluid leakage or catheter blockage can result in serious underestimation of the true degree of elevation of ICP.

By performing controlled manipulations of CSF volume, it is now possible to obtain useful estimates of the rates of CSF production and outflow resistance. The bulk compliance of the intracranial contents can also be estimated. This latter measurement anticipates the increase in intracranial pressure which might result should an additional volume be added to the craniospinal contents in the form of blood volume during cerebral vasodilatation, brain water due to brain oedema or of extraneous mass due to expansion of a haematoma or cyst.[9] The estimation of bulk compliance can therefore be regarded as a way of anticipating problems. These deliberate perturbations of CSF volume do, however, carry some increased risk of intracranial infection and they cannot be undertaken lightly. The physiological basis for compliance measurements and, indeed,

for some increases in intracranial pressure is still not completely understood and, for the most part, these second generation monitoring studies of
intracranial pressure are currently used more for clinical research than for
routine patient management.

Cerebral blood flow can be measured only sporadically in the human and
it is not, therefore, a useful mode of continuous monitoring of brain
circulatory function. It does, however, yield important information which
is unobtainable by other means. At this time, cerebral blood flow
measurement is available only in certain centres as a research tool.

V. Intracranial Contrast Studies

The methods used for monitoring the function of the CNS and its
supporting circulation do not yield information on structural abnormalities. This requires other studies that include CT scanning (computerized
axial tomography), angiography, ventriculography or air encepha-
lography. The performance of such intracranial contrast studies requires
that the patient be moved out of the ICU and detached from most of his
monitoring equipment. Clearly, in a critically ill patient this is a time of
great risk but the information from these studies may be crucial. One role
of continuous monitoring of brain function in the ICU should be to
determine if and when an intracranial contrast study is indicated, for
example when significant neurological deterioration has occurred, when
ICP has become elevated or when there has been no neurological
improvement after a finite period of observation and treatment. In such
circumstances it may be considered that the risks of moving the patient
temporarily out of the ICU are now outweighed by the risks of not having
the information which the intracranial contrast study will provide. This
important type of risk balancing process is a continuing challenge to the
physician who is managing a comatose patient in the intensive care unit.[10]

MONITORING CNS FUNCTION IN
THE INTENSIVE CARE UNIT

I. Neurological Assessment of the Comatose Patient at the Bedside

A working definition of coma is a crucial starting point for any discussion
on the evaluation of the comatose patient. Coma is a sleep-like state in
which the patient gives no indication of awareness of the environment but,
unlike sleep, from which he or she cannot be aroused. In more practical and
objective terminology, Jennett and his colleagues define coma as failure to
open the eyes or to utter recognizable words in response to verbal or
painful stimuli, coupled with inability to obey simple commands. Thus

'coma' is signified by a score equal to or less than E1 M5 V2 on the Glasgow coma scale (*Table* 17.2).

The many causes of coma all share the common mechanism of impairing the function of the centrally located reticular activating system of the brain stem, either directly or by interfering with its input and outflow. This may be due to distortion of the brain stem secondary to supratentorial mass lesions or to strategically placed damage within the brain stem, caused usually by haemorrhages or infarcts. Alternatively, diffuse cerebral involvement by trauma, anoxia, ischaemia, infection or toxins (endogenous or exogenous) can interfere sufficiently with functions of the reticular core to induce coma.

Serial neurological evaluation of comatose patients is extremely important, both to determine the anatomical location of neurological dysfunction and to record improvement or deterioration in the patient's condition. There are five main areas of interest in the neurological evaluation: the conscious level, the pattern of respiration, the size and reaction of the pupils, eye movements and motor function. From these factors the examiner aims to answer three key questions: 'What is the present level of responsiveness to standard stimuli and how has it changed from previous assessments? Is there brain stem dysfunction? Is there focal cerebral hemisphere damage?.'

Conscious Level

While the Glasgow coma scale is useful for describing patients who are deeply unconscious, it is less effective in describing return to wakefulness. Lack of eye opening as an index of coma is valid only in the first three days following the ictus. At a variable time thereafter some patients who remain otherwise unresponsive and vegetative will develop spontaneous eye opening, although their eyes still may not open in response to verbal or painful stimuli. The motor scale is the most important of the three. The main problem in its use in the comatose patient is that the most important pathophysiological distinction, between 3 and 4 (normal and abnormal flexion), is also the hardest to make at the bedside. The presence of wrist flexion and pronation and tucking of the thumb into the palm are important clues to the presence of abnormal flexor posturing or decortication. This motor abnormality signifies a very much greater degree of motor system dysfunction than normal flexor withdrawal of the upper limb to a painful stimulus. In recording the motor response to define conscious level, the better response of the two sides tested is used.

It is possible to add the three scores obtained for the Glasgow coma scale and to express the result as a single number. The advantages of this type of data reduction are more apparent than real, however, and inevitably entail some loss of information as the same total score can be obtained under different physiological circumstances. When the patient is aphasic, has a tracheostomy or endotracheal tube in place or has bilateral periorbital swelling, it may not be possible to assess certain parts of the coma scale. This does not vitiate use of the scale. The functions which can be tested are recorded and those which cannot are simply omitted.

Respiratory Pattern

While it is true that many comatose patients have abnormal respiration and apnea is the common mode of death in progressive brain compression, hopes that recording the type of respiratory abnormality would reliably indicate loci of cerebral dysfunction have not been realized in practice. Comatose patients may hyperventilate or have Cheyne–Stokes, ataxic or apneustic respiration. Any or all of these abnormalities may be present at different times in the same patient. The only clear correlation between respiration and brain damage that emerged from an extensive study of 227 patients by North and Jennett[11] was that all patients with medullary lesions had abnormal respiratory patterns and many patients with cerebellopontine and midbrain lesions had irregular breathing also.

The practical conclusion from such studies is that comatose patients frequently have abnormal respiration, but that recording the precise pattern is not of sufficient diagnostic value that it should override the need for establishing adequate ventilation using a respirator.

Pupil Size and Reaction

Abnormalities in the size of the pupil and in its response to light or other stimuli may be produced by peripheral lesions affecting the second and third cranial nerves or by central lesions which interrupt the integrative pathways in the brain stem.

Clearly the first priority is to establish whether an abnormality is peripheral or central in origin. When a pupil abnormality is unilateral, comparison of the direct and consensual light reflexes in both eyes will distinguish between an optic nerve or oculomotor nerve lesion. Bilateral absence of the pupil reaction to light is nearly always a sign of impairment of brain stem function, paricularly if the pupils are irregular or small. Maximally dilated and fixed pupils are an accompaniment of severe and usually preterminal global brain ischaemia. When bilateral fixed dilated pupils are seen and yet relatively normal neurological function is present one should suspect that mydriatic agents have been instilled in the eye as an aid to fundoscopy. When the central and peripheral third nerve and sympathetic pathways are intact, pinching on the side of the neck should result in dilatation of the ipsilateral pupil, the ciliospinal reflex. When this response is absent and there is no reason to suspect peripheral nerve damage, it is an additional sign of brain stem dysfunction.

Ocular Movements

Comatose patients may have disturbances of the resting position of the eyes, abnormal spontaneous eye movements, or disturbance of reflexly produced eye movements. It is crucial to distinguish between peripheral ocular motor palsies and central lesions which impair the integrated function of eye movements. The patient with an oculomotor (third nerve) palsy will have outward deviation of the affected eye due to unopposed action of the abducent (sixth) nerve. Patients with sixth nerve palsy will show medial deviation of the affected eye. When there is skew deviation of the eyes in a vertical direction, the causal lesion is located centrally in the brain stem, affecting the medial longitudinal fasciculus which is responsible for integrating the functions of the third, fourth and sixth cranial nerve nuclei.

Comatose patients may exhibit spontaneous roving eye movements and, on occasion, these may be dysconjugate without indicating structural brain stem damage. This becomes of significance when the eyes become dysconjugate in a vertical direction as this does indicate brain stem dysfunction. Conjugate deviation of both eyes to one or other side may be produced by either of two mechanisms. A destructive lesion in the frontal pre-motor (eye-field) area will produce deviation of the eyes to the side of the affected hemisphere. This is commonly seen in stroke patients who are also hemiplegic and the rule is that the patient with a frontal lesion looks away from the hemiplegic side. The opposite effect occurs when the frontal lesion is irritative rather than destructive as occurs in an epileptic focus. During seizures the patient looks away from the affected hemisphere towards the affected arm and leg if they too are involved in the seizure. This is known as an adversive seizure.

Pontine lesions also produce a conjugate deviation of the eyes, in this case away from the affected side. Since these lesions are also commonly associated with hemiplegia, the rule is that with this type of brain stem lesion the patient's eyes deviate towards the affected side. These spontaneous deviations of the eyes are by no means present in all cases and, even when present, may only last for some hours after the ictus. In most patients it is necessary to induce reflex eye movement in order to test the integrative function of the brain stem centres for controlling eye movement.

Reflex eye movements my be elicited in either of two ways. The doll's head manoeuvre in which the head is passively rotated to one side and then to the other through 90° tests the oculocephalic reflex. Instilling iced water into the external auditory meatus stimulates the oculovestibular reflex. The latter is the more powerful stimulus and, when assessing patients for a neurological definition of brain death, reflex eye movements must never be declared absent unless full oculovestibular testing has been tried in both ears.[12]

In an awake patient the normal response to head turning is that the eyes move in the direction that the head is turned and reflex movement is suppressed. In the comatose patient with intact ocular pathways, the eyes remain in the vertical orientation and thus, when the head is turned to the left, the eyes move to the right so as to remain apparently looking towards the ceiling. Similarly, when the head is turned rapidly to the right side the eyes move leftward to remain vertically orientated. An abnormal response occurs when the oculocephalic test induces dysconjugate eye movements and yet there is no evidence of a peripheral cranial nerve lesion. This finding suggests a lesion affecting the medial longitudinal fasciculus. The other type of abnormality, seen in deep coma with brain stem impairment, is lack of any response so that the eyes move with the head and show no tendency to reassume the vertical orientation.

In testing the oculovestibular response it is important that the patient's head be raised 30° above the horizontal so that maximum stimulation of the lateral semicircular canal can be obtained. Approximately 20 ml of iced water should be gently syringed into the ear after ensuring that the tympanic membrane is accessible and intact. In a conscious patient this manoeuvre would result in violent nystagmus, but in the comatose patient who has intact ocular pathways within the brain stem and intact cranial nerves, the normal response is tonic conjugate deviation of both eyes towards the side of the irrigated ear. Abnormal responses indicating brain stem dysfunction consist of either dysconjugate movements or lack of any movement at all. In every test both ears should be irrigated with iced water. If it is not possible to do this because of local damage to one ear, it is possible to induce eye movement in the direction opposite to the irrigated ear by instilling warm water onto it. About 20% of patients with absent oculocephalic responses prove to have a response to oculovestibular testing. For this reason, brain stem reflexes can never be declared absent unless oculovestibular testing has been carried out.

Motor Function

Assuming that the patient is comatose, there will be no response from the motor system to verbal stimuli and painful stimuli need to be applied. In assessing motor function the stimuli should be located so that each limb and the face can be tested separately for the motor response to pain. In this way not only will the best response be obtained but evidence of unilateral facial or limb weakness will be elicited. To produce a motor response in the face, firm supraorbital pressure can be applied. In testing the limbs the most satisfactory stimulus is heavy pressure with a hard object such as a pencil across the nail bed of the fingers or toes. This provides a strong stimulus without producing unsightly and distressing bruising. To compare the motor response in the arms, sternal pressure should also be applied and it may also be useful to provide a painful stimulus to the proximal portions of the limbs to elicit the motor response.

All of the information should be entered on a clinical flow sheet, an example of which is shown in *Fig.* 17.1.

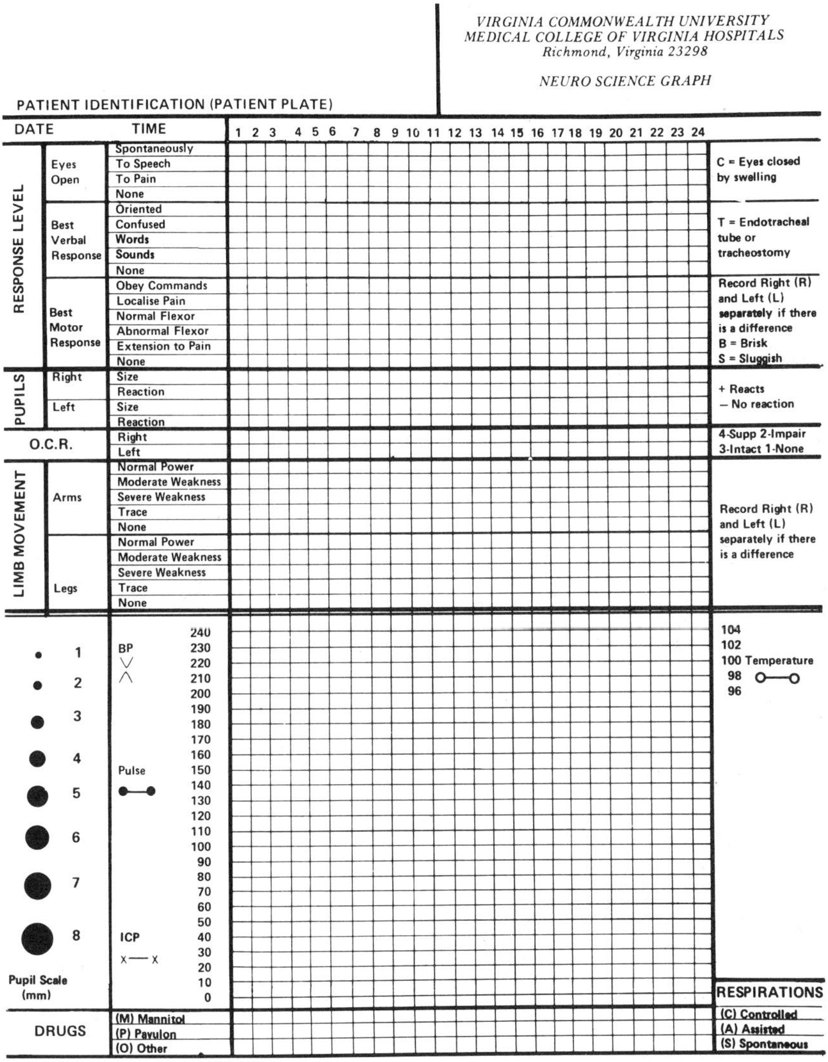

VIRGINIA COMMONWEALTH UNIVERSITY
MEDICAL COLLEGE OF VIRGINIA HOSPITALS
Richmond, Virginia 23298

NEURO SCIENCE GRAPH

Fig. 17.1. A clinical flow sheet for use in a neurosurgical ICU. Data on the Glasgow coma scale are entered on the top half of the sheet, together with information about pupil size and reaction, oculocephalic reflexes (OCR) and motor power. On the bottom half of the sheet vegetative functions and ICP are entered. On the reverse of the sheet (not shown here) is a fluid balance chart. This has been adapted from a sheet developed in Glasgow by Teasdale and Jennett. [15]

Brain Death

It is appropriate at this point to clarify the definition of brain death. This is a clinically defined state and does not depend legally upon electronic or other technical aids. Brain death is present when there is no evidence of brain stem function and the best motor response elicitable in the face or limbs is a reflex in the lower limbs. There should be no spontaneous respiration even when the patient is disconnected from the ventilator and the arterial P_{CO_2} allowed to rise while maintaining diffusion oxygenation by passing oxygen into the airway. In addition to apnoea, absence of brain stem function means that there should be no pupil light reflex, no gag reflex, no corneal reflex, no oculovestibular reflex, no ciliospinal reflex. This clinical status should be verified by two physicians and the presence of apnoea must be recorded on two occasions separated by at least 1 hour. Finally, even in the presence of all of the above signs, brain death can be declared present only when the patient is known to be free from the effects of hypothermia and drugs and when the cause of the neurological dysfunction is known as, for example, in cases of head injury and subarachnoid haemorrhage.

Effects of Drugs on Assessment of Neurological Function

Many comatose patients are managed in intensive care units with artificial ventilation in order to preserve the airway. In most cases this means that the patient receives muscle relaxants. Even when these are withheld for some time it becomes difficult to know whether the patient is still partially under the influence of these agents. Even more of a problem is the mounting use of barbiturates for 'brain protection' because, in such cases, much longer periods of time are required before one can be assured that the patient is free from the sedative influence of this agent. There is a poor correlation between the effects of barbiturates and the levels in the blood.[10] Not only is clinically assessed neurological activity depressed in the patient receiving barbiturates but brain electrical function is also depressed. The EEG may be almost entirely flat and evoked potentials are largely abolished. The early waves on the somatosensory and auditory evoked potentials, which indicate brain stem function are, however, preserved to some extent (Greenberg R. P., personal communication).

II. Neurophysiological Aids to Patient Monitoring

The EEG

For the EEG to be useful as a patient monitoring system in comatose patients, considerable data reduction is required. This has been done in the form of the cerebral function monitor and, also, in various types of computer-processed data handling in which the dominant frequencies in sequential time periods are displayed as histograms. Though such techniques are useful for detecting seizures in a paralysed patient, they have proved less valuable for monitoring the depth of coma since the EEG is so sensitive to the effects of drugs.

Evoked Potentials

It is now possible to record somatosensory, auditory and visual evoked potentials in the same patient. Somatosensory potentials, obtained by stimulating the median or sciatic nerves, ascend in the posterior columns of the spinal cord, pass through the brain stem to reach the thalamus and cerebral cortex. Auditory potentials enter the brain stem via the eighth cranial nerve and ascend through a precisely defined pathway in the brain stem with known neuronal stations before reaching the auditory cortex. The visual evoked potential, on the other hand, traverses the cerebral hemispheres via the lateral geniculate body and does not pass through the brain stem before reaching the occipital cortex. Combination of these evoked potentials permits a distinction to be drawn between lesions which involve the hemispheres and lesions which involve the brain stem.[7] This distinction can be further sharpened when the early individual waves of the auditory and somatosensory responses are examined closely. This is because each positive and negative wave in this early phase reflects passage of the neuronal impulse through known brain stem nuclei.

The Direct Cortical Response

A clear and reproducible waveform can be produced by stimulating the surface of the cerebral cortex and recording from adjacent cortical surface. The amplitude of this direct cortical response is very closely related to the adequacy of the cerebral circulation, failing completely when cerebral blood flow is reduced to less than 40% of control values.[13] This form of electrophysiological monitoring has been used to assess the adequacy of cerebral cortical perfusion during induced hypotension in the course of intracranial aneurysm surgery. The drawback of the method is that the stimulating and recording electrodes have to be introduced into the cranial cavity on the surface of the brain, unlike the electrodes used for the recording of evoked potentials which are simply mounted on the intact scalp. The recording of the direct cortical response is limited to information obtained from the immediate vicinity of the electrodes and there is no guarantee that the rest of the cerebral cortex is behaving in the same way.

III. Haemodynamic and Hydrodynamic Measurements

Intracranial Pressure Monitoring

The most reliable measurement of CSF pressure in patients with brain damage is yielded by direct measurement from the cranial cavity. In the presence of intracranial space-occupying lesions, there is progressive blockage of the CSF pathways which communicate between the supratentorial and infratentorial compartments and the spinal canal.[14,15] When such blockage becomes complete, CSF pressure measured from a lumbar puncture fails to reflect the intracranial CSF pressure. Furthermore, subsequent leakage of CSF through the small tear in the dura and arachnoid produced by the spinal needle, will further lower the spinal CSF pressure and magnify any pressure gradient which has developed between the cranial and spinal compartments. In this way tentorial and tonsillar herniation can be exacerbated.

The most widely used technique of monitoring intracranial pressure, at the present time, is the placement of a catheter in the frontal horn of the lateral ventricle and connection of this fluid-filled catheter with a standard arterial pressure transducer mounted at the patient's bedside.[16] The height of the transducer is adjusted to be level with the foramen of Monro to avoid any hydrostatic pressure difference between the patient and transducer (*Fig.* 17.2). An arterial range pressure transducer is most frequently used because, in patients with brain damage, intracranial pressure may quite frequently exceed 40 or even 60 mmHg. When the lateral ventricles are too small to be punctured with safety, the dura mater is opened and a tightly fitting screw is placed into the drill hole in the skull.[17] The rest of the arrangement is the same as for the ventricular catheter assembly. Other methods have been used which employ transducers in the subdural or the epidural space.[18] These may be connected with the exterior via wire cable or in some cases the device is implanted and uses a telemetric system. The problem with most implanted devices is that should the system fail or become inaccurate there is no way of determining the extent of the error, other than by invading the subarachnoid or ventricular CSF space to obtain a direct hydrostatic pressure measurement.

The resting level of ICP is important both as an absolute value and in relation to arterial pressure.[9] Because intracranial venous pressure and CSF pressure rise and fall in parallel, the difference between arterial and intracranial pressure is very nearly equivalent to the cerebral perfusion pressure.[8] Normal ICP should be less than 10 mmHg. Levels up to 20 mmHg are commonly seen, however, and would not be considered definitely abnormal. Persisting levels of mean ICP (diastolic plus one-third of pulse pressure) of more than 20 mmHg are unequivocally abnormal.[19] Levels in excess of 25 mmHg should be treated. There is now a wealth of evidence that levels of ICP above 40 mmHg are always deleterious, particularly in the patient with head injury or intracranial haemorrhage, in

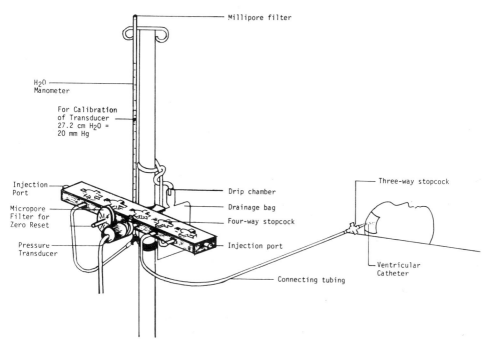

Fig. 17.2. Diagram showing a method for establishing ICP monitoring at the bedside using a multiport manifold clamped to an intravenous drip stand. This system permits recalibration and CSF drainage with minimum exposure of CSF to external contamination. The entire system may be easily varied in height to remain level with the patients brow.

whom such pressures are invariably associated with neurological and neurophysiological dysfunction. In patients with benign intracranial hypertension and hydrocephalus elevated ICP does not appear to cause such dramatic neurological sequelae. There is, however, a high correlation between intracranial hypertension and papilloedema, which if unchecked will result in optic atrophy.[20]

Another manifestation of raised ICP is waves of increased pressure, so that ICP varies widely when recorded over a period of time. ICP is more frequently elevated at night.[21] This emphasizes the importance of continuous monitoring. Spot measurements of short duration may record the ICP when it is at the lower limit of what is in fact a widely fluctuant range.[22,23] Two principal types of abnormal ICP wave are of significance.[16] The first is the plateau or 'A' wave in which ICP abruptly increases from a relatively normal level to more than 50 mmHg, remains elevated for 5–20 minutes or, on some occasions, even longer and then abruptly descends to normal (*Fig.* 17.3). Plateau waves are often accompanied by transient worsening of neurological status, e.g. emergence of decerebrate rigidity or vegetative effects such as flushing of the face, sweating and changes in respiration. Simultaneous measurements of cerebral blood flow have shown that, during the period of high ICP, there is the paradox of cerebral vasodilatation with increased cerebral blood volume, yet reduced cerebral blood flow. Cerebral blood flow returns towards normal if the pressure wave ends spontaneously but, if ICP is abruptly decreased in the middle of a wave by aspiration of CSF, cerebral blood flow remains low. Plateau waves are considered to result from cerebral vasomotor instability and loss of tone produced by brain stem dysfunction coupled with decreased compliance in the craniospinal axis and obstruction of venous flow into the dural venous sinuses.

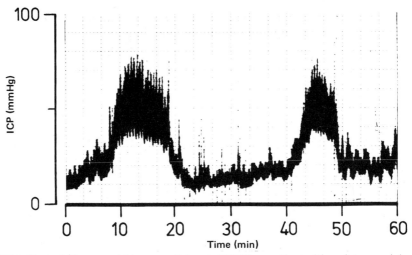

Fig. 17.3. Typical plateau or 'A' waves of elevated ICP in a patient with an intracranial mass lesion prior to therapy with dexamethasone. 24 hours after therapy had begun these waves had disappeared.

The second important ICP wave is the sharply peaked B wave which rises to 25–50 mmHg and is usually associated with changes in respiration (*Fig.* 17.4). In this case the respiratory changes are thought to be the cause and not the result of the ICP wave. A period of hypoventilation causes hypercarbia, cerebral vasodilation and elevated ICP. An abrupt increase in respiratory minute volume then reduces ICP.

As ICP increases so also does the magnitude of the CSF pulse pressure (*Fig.* 17.5). The ratio between the height of the mean ICP and the magnitude of the pulse pressure bears some relationship to cerebral vasomotor tone.[24] This is presently under investigation and it is too early to use the information in routine clinical practice.

Monitoring of Arterial and Cerebral Perfusion Pressure

Since cerebral perfusion pressure is derived from the difference between arterial and intracranial pressure, critical reductions of perfusion pressure

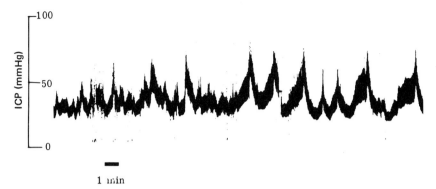

Fig. 17.4 Typical 'B' waves of elevated ICP in a patient with head injury. These were associated with periodic fluctuations in respiratory depth and frequency.

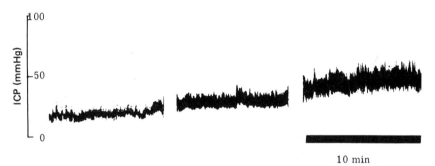

Fig. 17.5. Three sequences of ICP separated by 30-minute intervals in a patient with rising ICP, to show the relationship between intracranial pulse pressure and the height of mean ICP.

may result either from a fall in arterial pressure or from increased ICP which is not accompanied by an adequate increase in arterial pressure. In the management of the comatose patient with brain damage, arterial hypotension is always to be avoided because of a high association with ischaemic brain damage. Elevations in ICP can also be associated with ischaemic brain damage. Elevated ICP is somewhat better tolerated than haemorrhagic arterial hypotension, because the latter is associated with increased sympathetic discharge and some narrowing of the inflow vessels to the brain.[8] Arterial hypertension is also to be avoided because this increases the risk of intracranial haemorrhage, increases the rate of production of brain oedema and makes the brain stiffer, less compliant, and more liable to severe intracranial hypertension.[25]

In the patient with severe brain injury, elevation of arterial pressure may be secondary to intracranial hypertension, the well-known Cushing response.[26] In this event, the best way of managing the blood pressure is to attempt to lower ICP. To reduce blood pressure in such a case would cause a drastic reduction in cerebral perfusion pressure and lead to severe ischaemic brain damage. If the ICP can be reduced there is nearly always a satisfactory secondary reduction in arterial pressure.

Measurement of Cerebral Blood Flow and Derived Indices

Although single measurements of cerebral blood flow cannot be considered in the same light as continuous monitoring of arterial or intracranial pressure and, although the measurements are complex and not widely available, the information is important and unique. The flow and volume of blood in the cerebral circulation is important for support of neurological function and for regulating ICP and CSF physiology. In the damaged brain blood flow is often not homogeneously distributed. Areas of hyperaemia and ischaemia may coexist. The key measurement is of blood flow and volume in the cerebral microcirculation at its interface with the tissues.

Several methods are available for assessing the cerebral circulation, each with its advantages and disadvantages. Cerebral angiography provides an accurate morphological assessment of the larger cerebral vessels at one point in time. Because of the extensive potential cross-circulation available in the cerebral vascular bed, this anatomical information is of limited value in assessing blood flow. When the circulation time of contrast is unduly prolonged this is associated with low cerebral blood flow.[27] Methods have been described for measuring the transit time of tracers across the cerebral vascular bed following intravenous injection, but these provide limited information about the behaviour of the cerebral circulation on a regional basis. Measurement of regional cerebral blood flow following intravenous injection or inhalation of ^{133}Xe solution using multiple externally placed counters, is currently the best accepted method in patients.[28] With this technique, it is possible to detect areas of hyperaemia and ischaemia, as well as measure mean cerebral blood flow, expressed in millilitres of blood flowing through 100 g of brain tissue per minute. When this information is combined with cerebral perfusion pressure, cerebral vascular resistance can be calculated. When blood flow measurements are combined with measurements of the cerebral arteriovenous differences for oxygen, glucose, lactate or other metabolites, then cerebral metabolic uptake or production rates for these substances can be calculated.

In patients who are in coma, cerebral blood flow may be low, normal or occasionally increased. The cerebral metabolic rate for oxygen and glucose is, however, invariably decreased often to less than half of the normal value in the comatose patient.[29]

With the advent of positron emission transverse tomography and the availability of short-lived cyclotron-produced isotopes, it is now possible to examine cerebral metabolism in different regions of the brain in vivo. The equipment is extremely expensive and available only at a small number of centres, but already there are indications that this technique will greatly enhance our understanding of the genesis of areas of brain dysfunction and damage in many types of traumatic, vascular and metabolic brain disorder.[30]

When it is possible to carry out more than one measurement of cerebral blood flow at a single session, it becomes possible to test the response of the cerebral circulation to physiological stimuli. The most common functions tested are the responses to changes in arterial blood pressure or arterial P_{CO_2}. The normal response to a moderate change in arterial blood pressure is little or no change in blood flow. Since there is a change in perfusion pressure, but no change in flow, this indicates a change of cerebral vascular resistance consistent with dilatation of cerebral vessels when blood pressure falls or constriction of resistance vessels when blood pressure rises. The normal response to changes in arterial P_{CO_2} is vasoconstriction when P_{CO_2} is reduced from 40 towards 20 mmHg but no further constriction beyond that point. When arterial P_{CO_2} is increased cerebral vessels dilate and blood flow increases up to arterial P_{CO_2} levels between 80 and 100 mmHg. Beyond that, maximum values are reached and blood flow and vascular calibre do not alter further. In patients with regional brain damage, isolated areas of impaired reactivity to blood pressure and P_{CO_2} are commonly found. Thus in head-injured patients, areas of unresponsive circulation in the frontal and temporal areas correspond well with the distribution of severe surface contusions. In patients with unilateral stroke there is fairly good correlation between the area of dysfunctional brain and regional disturbances of cerebral vascular response.[31] Less commonly, cerebral vascular responsiveness is disturbed on a global rather than a regional basis. This is usually seen only in severely ill patients.

The importance of these findings is that following a primary ischaemic, haemorrhagic or traumatic insult to the brain, the cerebral circulation becomes much more vulnerable to a secondary insult such as hypoxia, hypotension or raised ICP. Normally, these latter insults would provoke protective vasodilatation, but in the damaged brain this does not occur. There follows a fall in oxygen carriage and ischaemic/hypoxic brain damage.

Other Measurements of Importance in Comatose Patients with Brain Damage

Body temperature must be carefully monitored. Elevated temperature is associated with cerebral vascular dilatation, increase in cerebral blood volume and elevation of ICP. The rate of formation of vasogenic brain oedema, where fluid is leaking from damaged vessels into the cerebral white matter, is increased when body temperature is raised and decreased when body temperature is lowered.[32]

Central venous pressure or, better still, pulmonary artery and pulmonary capillary wedge pressures are important to monitor when comatose patients are experiencing problems with respiratory gas exchange or are being treated with barbiturates. In the patient who is already volume-depleted, administration of even small doses of barbiturate may cause an undesirable and dangerous reduction in arterial blood pressure. Neurogenic pulmonary oedema is an elusive, rare, but very dramatic complication of brain damage and may be much better assessed and managed when central pressure measurements are available.

Electrolytes and fluid balance are important in any patient in the intensive care unit. The particular danger for the comatose patient with brain damage is a reduction of serum sodium levels. Falls below 120 mmol/l are commonly associated with exacerbation of brain oedema and dramatic elevations of ICP.

PATHOPHYSIOLOGY OF PRIMARY AND SECONDARY BRAIN DAMAGE

I. Concepts of Primary and Secondary Brain Damage

The entire thrust of intensive care management of the brain-damaged patient is related to the importance of the second insult in causing further brain damage in an already critically ill patient. In patients with head injury, intracranial haemorrhage and ischaemic stroke, local disruption or infarction of brain tissue is followed by perifocal swelling of the brain. The actual lesion itself may also expand due to haemorrhage or to absorption of water. The lesion, together with the expanding perifocal area may soon constitute a sizeable intracranial mass lesion which leads to distortion and shift of the brain and to elevation in ICP. These lead, in turn, to further brain damage which may be located in areas remote from the original lesion. Other deleterious processes, such as cerebral vasospasm or intracranial infection, may also be set in train by the initial injury or haemorrhage. These processes will be briefly described in this section with the aim of indicating how secondary brain damage may arise and may be avoided.

Intracranial Mass Lesions and Brain Shifts

Brain tissue is a viscoelastic substance. When it is indented or compressed it tends to flow away from the distorting force. When the force is removed it takes some time before the indentation of the brain disappears. The brain is snugly contained, not only within the skull, but also within the membranous confines of the falx cerebri and tentorium cerebelli. Following expansion of a unilateral supratentorial mass there is a predictable and important series of events.[33] With first expansion of the mass brain begins to take up the available room in the subarachnoid space which was previously occupied by CSF (*Fig.* 17.6). The ventricle on the side of the compressing lesion becomes smaller, and the brain as a whole begins to move downwards in an axial direction through the tentorial hiatus. The midbrain is actually pushed downward. In addition, parts of the cerebral hemisphere are also propelled through the tentorial hiatus depending upon the location of the expanding lesion. If it is in the temporal lobe the medial part of the temporal lobe is forced down through the tentorial hiatus alongside the midbrain producing side-to-side compression of the midbrain and obliterating the local CSF space, the cisterna ambiens. If the expanding lesion is frontal or occipital, brain tends to herniate through the posterior part of the tentorial hiatus above the quadrigeminal plate.

The clinical consequences of this process are depression of the conscious level due to impairment of the function of the central reticular formation of

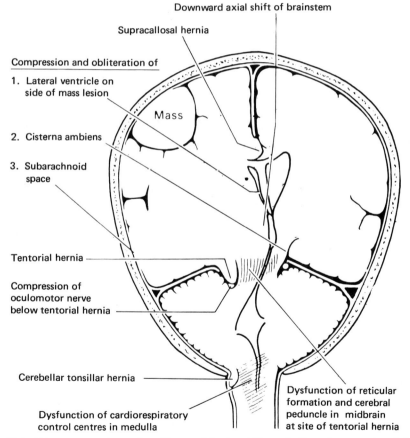

Fig. 17.6. Diagram to show the effects of brain shift and distortion produced by a supratentorial expanding mass lesion. Reproduced by permission from Jamieson and Kay's *Textbook of Surgical Physiology,* 3rd ed., Churchill Livingstone, Edinburgh, 1978.

the brain stem, and contralateral hemiparesis followed by cerebrate rigidity affecting the contralateral limbs due to interruption of the cortical spinal tract in the cerebral peduncle. The motor disturbance may be bilateral and related to impingement of the opposite peduncle on the free edge of the tentorium, as the midbrain is not only pushed downward but laterally. The third cranial nerve is often involved, in tentorial herniations, caught between the posterior cerebral and superior cerebellar arteries. This produces dilatation of the ipsilateral pupil, ptosis and outward deviation of that eye due to unopposed action of the sixth nerve. When the herniating process is posteriorly located, there is failure of upward gaze due to distortion of the superior colliculi.

If downward axial herniation of the brain stem continues, downward herniation of the cerebellar tonsil through the foramen magnum will follow. There is also stretching of the perforating branches of the basilar artery. These processes impair medullary function. This is associated with elevation of arterial pressure and slowing of the pulse rate, the well-known Cushing response, and interference with the control of respiration which may be manifest variously as Cheyne–Stokes respiration, ataxic respiration or, finally, apnoea.[26, 11] This process may occur rapidly. By the time the patient is decerebrate with changes in blood pressure and heart rate, apnea is not far away.

The presence of CSF in the subarachnoid space is one means by which pressures can become equally distributed throughout the craniospinal axis. During the process of expansion of a mass lesion, as the subarachnoid space is encroached upon, so also is the capacity for equalizing pressures. By the time the subarachnoid space over the affected hemisphere has disappeared and the cisterna ambiens has been blocked, a sizeable pressure gradient can build up across the tentorium. This gradient acts as a further propulsive force in increasing the degree of brain herniation and downward axial shift of the brain stem.[34]

The Genesis and Effects of Raised Intracranial Pressure

Under normal conditions, cerebral spinal fluid pressure remains in the range of -5 to $+10$ mmHg throughout the craniospinal axis. Pressures recorded from the epidural and subdural space are also in this range under normal conditions.[22] This pressure is being recorded within a dynamic fluid system which has regulated inflow and outflow of CSF and blood. One cause of elevated ICP is an increase in CSF outflow resistance such that the CSF pressure must rise higher before an adequate amount of fluid can be absorbed from the system. Other causes of raised ICP arise from outside the CSF space. These have in common that they represent an increase in volume of some other compartment, extraneous, as in the case of an extra-axial blood clot or brain tumour, intrinsic by addition of fluid to the extracellular space in brain oedema or by expansion of the volume of the cerebrovascular compartments.[9] These processes reduce the volume of the CSF space and change the equilibrium for balanced production and absorption of fluid so that this must be reset at a higher CSF pressure.[35] One or more of these mechanisms may be operative in patients with brain injury or haemorrhage and it is not surprising that elevated ICP is exceedingly common. In comatose patients with head injury or intracranial haemorrhage elevated ICP occurs in over 40% despite prompt evacuation of mass lesions and artificial ventilation.[19]

The effects of raised ICP are essentially two-fold. Pressure gradients within the craniospinal axis aggravate brain shift and herniation, which in turn cause neurological dysfunction either directly by tissue distortion or indirectly by strangulation of the blood supply. The second mechanism by which raised ICP produces ill effects is by reducing cerebral perfusion pressure. When the difference between arterial and intracranial pressure falls below 40 mmHg, cerebral ischaemia will occur even under normal conditions.[18] In chronic arterial hypertension or in patients with ischaemic, haemorrhagic or traumatic brain damage, much higher perfusion pressures may be required to perfuse the brain adequately.[36] High intracranial pressure does not, by itself, damage neurological function. If there is no brain shift or herniation nor any maldistribution of pressure, and, if cerebral perfusion pressure is maintained, then high levels of ICP may be tolerated without evidence of neurological deterioration. These conditions are seldom fulfilled. A notable exception is benign intracranial hypertension in which patients may sustain elevations of ICP of over 40 mmHg without loss of consciousness.[20]

General aims of therapy are therefore to maintain adequate perfusion pressure (80–100 mmHg) and to ameliorate any brain distortion or shift by evacuation of the causative mass lesion if at all possible.

Ischaemic and Hypoxic Brain Damage

In patients who die from head injury or intracranial haemorrhage, a striking amount of additional ischaemic/hypoxic brain damage is frequently encountered.[37, 38] This takes the form of scattered infarcts located in the basal ganglia, hippocampus and cerebral cortex.

In the patient who has sustained primary brain damage or haemorrhage, such secondary changes can be explained by several different mechanisms. In the multiply-injured patient reduced blood pressure or impaired pulmonary function with hypoxaemia will reduce the perfusion pressure and the effective delivery of oxygen to the brain. Raised intracranial pressure will likewise reduce cerebral perfusion pressure. Cerebral arterial vasospasm occurs not infrequently in head injury and intracranial haemorrhage. Vasospasm increases cerebral vascular resistance in the territory of the affected vessel and may be responsible for ischaemia in their distribution.[39] Cerebral vasospasm is usually identified angiographically. Angiograms show only larger cerebral vessels, but cerebrovascular resistance is largely determined by changes in the calibre of much smaller vessels. Cerebral vasospasm probably has a more profound effect when it involves such distal resistance vessels.

Brain oedema in which the white matter of the brain is expanded by fluid, is associated with a reduction in cerebral blood flow. At the present time there is debate as to whether the apparent cerebral ischaemia seen in areas of brain oedema is a dilution artefact produced by relative expansion of the oedematous tissue while blood vessels remain constant.

Infection and Brain Damage

Intracranial infection has a devastating effect on the damaged brain.[40] Even when meningitis or encephalitis is successfully treated by antibiotics, profound neurological deficits may remain. It is thought that infections promote vasculitis and superficial cerebral infarction. This effect is more pronounced when the brain is already damaged as in head injury, intracranial haemorrhage or stroke. When the patient is already unresponsive to verbal stimuli, the onset of intracranial infection is difficult to detect. Any fall in conscious level which cannot be explained on the basis of changes in blood pressure, intracranial pressure or respiratory function, should lead the clinician to suspect intracranial infection as a possible cause and consider lumbar puncture.

PRINCIPLES OF THERAPY IN THE COMATOSE PATIENT

Respiratory Function

There is increasing acceptance of the benefits of artificial ventilation of comatose patients even though neurological function is difficult to assess because the patient must usually be paralysed for satisfactory ventilation. Most comatose patients who have sustained brain damage, hyperventilate if left alone and arterial P_{CO_2} will reduce to less than 20 mmHg. It is the goal of management in the intensive care unit to provide good oxygenation, but such severe hyperventilation is not desirable.[41] Most patients are artifically ventilated with a large tidal volume and relatively slow rate to maintain arterial P_{CO_2} around 30 mmHg. Induction of muscular paralysis can save the patient a great deal of the energy which is expended in violent hyperventilation and spontaneous abnormal motor movements. This is an aid to the reduction of body temperature and caloric requirements. Mechanical ventilation with muscular paralysis will often reduce ICP even before arterial P_{CO_2} is reduced below normal (*Fig.* 17.7).

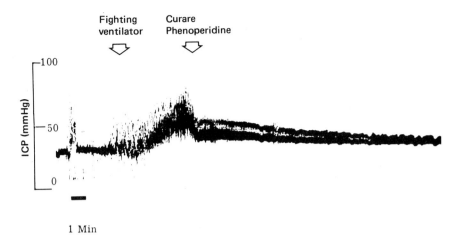

Fig. 17.7. Record from a patient with a head injury in whom muscle relaxant had worn off showing the rise in ICP as the patient resisted artificial ventilation and the fall in ICP as muscle relaxation and sedation were re-established. End-tidal CO_2 did not change appreciably during this period of recording.

Patients who are in coma with brain damage may quite often be hypoxaemic, despite an adequate inspired oxygen fraction, minute volume and arterial Pco_2.[42] Addition of PEEP is desirable to raise arterial Po_2 but concern is often expressed about the effects of PEEP on ICP. End expiratory pressures up to 10 cm H_2O seldom cause an increase in ICP, but higher levels of PEEP may sometimes be associated with marked increases in ICP, particularly in patients whom ICP is high to begin with and intracranial compliance is poor.[42,43]

Management of Raised Intracranial Pressure

If ICP rises above a predetermined level (25–30 mmHg mean) or if a lesser rise in ICP is associated with neurological deterioration, a well-rehearsed series of steps should be taken. The position of the patient should be checked relative to the height of the transducer and for possible jugular compression. The airway should be checked for obstructions. Blood gases should be drawn, blood pressure checked and the transducer system re-zeroed and checked. If there is still intracranial hypertension and the patient is not hypercarbic or hypoxic, the next step is to ensure that the patient has not developed an intracranial mass lesion. This can be most effectively done by CT scanning.

   When the basic cause of intracranial hypertension is an intracranial expanding lesion, the method of choice of reducing ICP is surgical removal of the mass lesion. This not only achieves a reduction in ICP but ameliorates the brain shift and distortion associated with the presence of the mass. When there is much perifocal swelling, surgical decompression may produce only a temporary reduction in ICP. This is commonly the case in patients with very severe head injury. Following removal of an intracranial haematoma, about half of these patients require further measures to reduce ICP to normal.

Not all cases of intracranial hypertension are associated with intracranial mass lesions. In many cases there is no brain shift or distortion, and other non-surgical measures are required to deal with the problem. In this section the commonly used and some newer therapies for intracranial hypertension will be reviewed briefly.

Hyperventilation produces cerebral vasoconstriction and a reduction in intravascular pressure downstream from the resistance vessels with a consequent reduction in cerebral blood volume. These factors produce a fall in ICP of about 30%. The effect is immediate and can be sustained for several hours, although there is some tendency for the effect to diminish with time. The usual practice is to reduce arterial P_{CO_2} to about 20 mmHg.[16] The effectiveness of hypocapnia depends upon retention of cerebrovascular responsiveness to changes in arterial P_{CO_2}. This may be lost in certain areas of the brain, but it is unusual to find complete global loss of CO_2 reactivity.[28] Therefore this technique of lowering the ICP should always be tried first.

When ICP is being monitored by means of a catheter placed in the lateral ventricle, it is possible to control elevated intracranial pressure by *CSF drainage* through the catheter. It is important that the pressure against which drainage occurs be quite high, 15–20 mmHg (200–250 mmH₂O). If too low a drainage pressure is used the ventricle will simply collapse, no further CSF drainage will occur and the pressure recording will also be lost.[19] This method of controlling intracranial pressure is most useful in patients who have normal or enlarged ventricles. When the ventricles are extremely small and shifted, the technique is not as effective.

Administration of intravenous infusions of mannitol or other *hyperosmolar agents*, such as urea or glycerol, have been widely employed in the control of intracranial pressure.[44] The common principle is that plasma osmolarity is abruptly increased by rapid infusion of the solution and this favours withdrawal of fluid from the brain as the tissue is perfused by the hyperosmolar blood. The effectiveness of this technique depends upon a relatively intact blood–brain barrier, so that the osmotic gradient can be maintained and water can be drawn out of brain tissue without large scale passage of the osmotic agent into the tissue. This does occur, but to a relatively small extent. Urea penetrates more readily into the grey matter of the brain than mannitol or glycerol and this may account for briefer duration of effect. Some consider, however, that hypertonic urea produces greater pressure reduction than other agents. A much quoted problem in osmotherapy is the occurrence of 'rebound'. As the effectiveness of the osmotic agent wears off, ICP returns not only to the level it was at prior to administration of the agent but rises considerably beyond this point. This has been attributed to penetration of the osmotic agent into the brain and reversal of the passage of water so that tissue becomes even more engorged with water. This appears to be a largely theoretical consideration. With the most widely used agent, mannitol, rebound phenomena are unusual. A more likely explanation for any further increase of ICP is that, in a lesion where the blood–brain barrier is not intact, there is little osmotic withdrawal of brain water and the process of swelling continues locally despite a reduction of ICP due to withdrawal of water from normal brain elsewhere.[45] As this process finishes the status quo is restored, but now the lesion and perifocal swelling are larger than before and ICP rises accordingly.

Mannitol should be administered as a rapid infusion of 1 g/kg body weight given over 10 minutes. This will produce a reduction of ICP within ten minutes and the effect should last for three or four hours. If mannitol has been extremely effective, when the next dose is required, a smaller dose 0·25 or 0·5 g/kg body weight can be tried. The principle should be to give the smallest load of osmotic agent that produces a therapeutic effect. The reason for this is that when frequent osmotherapy is required plasma osmolarity increases progressively and if osmolarity is more than 340 mosmol/l prior to administration of the next dose, there is an extremely high risk that the patient will develop severe renal and metabolic problems.[46] It is our policy to use mannitol in a dose of 1 g/kg body weight for emergency purposes, such as the transfer of a sick patient with intracranial hypertension to the operating room or to the X-ray department. When osmotherapy is required in the intensive care unit, it is used only where hyperventilation and CSF drainage have failed, its effect is measured on ICP, and the smallest effective dose of mannitol that can be employed is used.

Corticosteroid therapy has been widely advocated in the control of intracranial hypertension with varying success in different groups of patients, ranging from dramatic improvement in patients with peritumoural oedema to no effect whatsoever in patients with severe posthypoxic intracranial hypertension. The indications for steroid therapy were clearly put by Maxwell et al.[47] and the description remains true today. Steroids are most effective where oedema is focal and due to a chronic process such as a tumour or brain abscess. Steroids are least effective where brain swelling is global and the process is acute such as hypoxia, ischaemia or trauma. Cortical steroids are normally administered in the form of dexamethasone 4 mg 4 times daily or methylprednisolone 40 mg 4 times daily. Some have advocated the use of higher dosage regimes for short periods of time in patients with severe head trauma using dexamethasone 100 mg per day.[48,49] The results of high dose steroid therapy are controversial and no clear benefit has been demonstrated on intracranial hypertension in severely head injured patients.[50,51]

Barbiturate therapy is finding increasing favour at the present time as a means of controlling intractable intracranial hypertension. Barbiturates reduce cerebral blood flow and metabolism. Administration of pentobarbitone in dosages sufficient to produce burst suppression on the EEG (50–100 mg/h) often renders control of ICP easier. In some cases no other form of therapy is required.[52] Not all cases of resistant intracranial hypertension will respond, however, and administration of barbiturates may provoke dangerous reductions in arterial pressure. It is essential that the patient is not suffering from volume depletion prior to the administration of barbiturates. Central venous pressure monitoring is not entirely adequate for this and it is the policy in several centres where barbiturates are used freely to insert a Swan–Ganz catheter to monitor central pressures prior to administration of barbiturates. This is not a therapy to be lightly undertaken.[53]

Management of Brain Oedema

The term 'brain oedema' is often used erroneously in the context of the comatose patient with severe brain damage. Brain oedema is an increase in the water content of the brain with an increase in tissue volume. In many cases of head injury or intracranial haemorrhage, the brain is swollen but the cause of the swelling is not an increase in brain water but engorgement of cerebral blood vessels. In these cases the most appropriate treatment is to control the cerebrovascular resistance. Hyperventilation and possibly barbiturates are the most effective ways of doing this. In the zone of viable brain around brain tumours, haematomas and cerebral infarcts there is, however, an increase in tissue water content. The rate of formation of this oedema fluid is increased by cerebral vasodilatation and an increase in intra-arterial pressure.[54] Once the fluid enters the extracellular space, it percolates through the white matter of the brain and eventually reaches the ventricular system where it is absorbed. This movement of fluid through the brain is affected by brain tissue compliance. When the compliance is high, tissue can swell, fluid can pass easily and will eventually be absorbed in the ventricles. Where tissue compliance is low and intracranial pressure is high, the process is slowed down and fluid tends to remain in the tissues.[55]

In addition to employing mannitol and steroids other aspects of management of cerebral oedema can be based upon physiological principles. The arterial blood pressure should not be allowed to rise to a very high level because this favours the increased production of oedema. Similarly, cerebral vasodilatation should be controlled either by inducing hypocapnia or by administering barbiturates. It is helpful to reduce ICP as this favours passage of oedema fluid out of the brain into the ventricular system. It is important to control body temperature as pyrexia favours the production of oedema fluid. Hypothermia can be employed to slow this process.[56] In general, measures used to control raised ICP are also effective in the control of brain oedema.

Management of Cerebral Vasospasm

Vasospasm is another loosely employed term which is often used to explain clinical deterioration in a patient without verification. It is important to establish by angiography whether or not vasospasm is present because of the methods of therapy that must be employed to control it. Despite the enormous amount of research in this area on the role of neurotransmitters, blood products and prostaglandins in the genesis and exacerbation of cerebral vasospasm, its exact cause in patients with cerebral haemorrhage and head trauma is not yet known. Treatment has been empirically based and, to date, no uniformly successful method of therapy has emerged. Local, intravenous and intra-arterial infusions of alpha-adrenergic blockers or papaverine have had their advocates but have not been of proven value. The most promising regime to date has been the employment of vigorous hydration of the patient coupled with elevation of arterial pressure.[57] Clearly, this is a procedure which has many possible drawbacks. In a patient with subarachnoid haemorrhage due to a ruptured cerebral aneurysm, it can be safely used only after verified clipping of the aneurysm. In patients with severe head trauma it can be used only when there is no problem with elevated ICP.

CONCLUSIONS

In the aftermath of a severe primary insult to the brain, be it ischaemic, haemorrhagic or traumatic, a certain population of neurons are irrevocably destroyed yet the patient may survive, and often with a minimal or tolerable neurological deficit. At the same time, however, much larger areas of the central nervous system are in a precarious situation. If optimal conditions of oxygenation and perfusion are provided, the area of primary brain damage is minimized. If they are not, ischaemia, necrosis and oedema spread into surrounding areas or develop in distant zones, thus magnifying the total burden of CNS damage.

The goal of intensive care of the brain-damaged patient is to avoid, or to detect and treat, secondary insults to the injured brain which can extend the original zone of brain damage. In this chapter, attention has been focused on a scheme of bedside monitoring in the intensive care unit which is aimed at detecting changes in conscious level and neurological function, in respiratory gas exchange, fluid and electrolyte balance, and in arterial and intracranial pressure. This type of vigilance demands a smooth well-practised multidisciplinary team of physicians, nurses, technicians and many other ancillary staff.

The principles of care of the acutely brain damaged patient in the ICU need to be applied as soon as possible after the ictus, at the roadside and in transit and need to be extended long into the follow-up period. In the patient with severe brain damage, each remaining neuron is very precious and its loss represents one more little defeat for medical care. Its preservation is a minor triumph which is often not appreciated at the time. The recovery process is slow but after 3–6 months the results may be remarkable. One of the most heartening sights for the staff of a neuro-intensive care unit is to see some of their patients 6 months later.

Acknowledgements

J. D. Miller was supported by NIH Grant NS12587.

REFERENCES

1. Rose J., Valtonen S. and Jennett B. (1977) Avoidable factors contributing to death after head injury. *Br. Med. J.* **2**, 615–618.
2. Miller J. D., Sweet R. C., Narayan R. et al. (1978) Early insults to the injured brain. *JAMA* **240**, 439–442.
3. Griffith R. L. and Becker D. P. (1979) Physiological monitoring of the head injury patient. *Advances in Neurology* **22**, 51–72.
4. Plum F. and Posner J. B. (1966) *The Diagnosis of Stupor and Coma*, p. 197. Philadelphia, Davis.
5. Teasdale G. and Jennett B. (1974) Assessment of coma and impaired consciousness. A practical scale. *Lancet* **2**, 81–84.
6. Bates D., Caronna J. J., Cartlidge N. E. F. et al. (1977) A prospective study of non-traumatic coma: methods and results in 310 patients. *Ann. Neurol.* **2**, 211–220.
7. Greenberg R. P., Mayer D. T., Becker D. P. et al. (1977) Evaluation of brain function in severe human head trauma with multimodality evoked potentials. *J. Neurosurg.* **47**, 150–170.
8. Miller J. D., Stanek A. and Langfitt T. W. (1972) Concepts of cerebral perfusion pressure and vascular compressions during intracranial hypertension. In: Meyer J. S. and Schade J. P., ed., *Progress in Brain Research*, Vol. 35, pp. 411–432. Amsterdam, Elsevier.
9. Miller J. D. (1975) Volume and pressure in the craniospinal axis. *Clin. Neurosurg.* **22**, 76–105.
10. Bruce D. A., Gennarelli T. A. and Langfitt T. W. (1978) Resuscitation from coma due to head injury. *Crit. Care Med.* **6**, 254–269.
11. North J. B. and Jennett S. (1974) Abnormal breathing patterns associated with acute brain damage. *Arch. Neurol.* **31**, 338–344.
12. Teasdale G. and Smith J. (1975) Eye movements and brain stem dysfunction after head injury. *J. Neurol. Neurosurg. Psychiatry* **38**, 822–829.
13. Teasdale G., Rowan J. O., Turner J. et al. (1977) Cerebral perfusion failure and cortical electrical activity. *Acta Neurol. Scand. [Suppl. 64]* **56**, 430–431.

14. Langfitt T. W. (1969) Increased intracranial pressure. *Clin. Neurosurg.* **16**, 436–471.
15. Kaufmann G. E. and Clark K. (1970) Continuous simultaneous monitoring of intraventricular and cervical subarachnoid cerebrospinal fluid pressure to indicate the development of cerebral or tonsillar herniation. *J. Neurosurg.* **33**, 145–150.
16. Lundberg N. (1960) Continuous recording and control of ventricular fluid pressure in neurosurgical practice. *Acta Psychiatr. Neurol. Scand.* [*Suppl.* 149] **36**, 1–193.
17. Vries J. K., Becker D. P. and Young H. F. (1973) A subarachnoid screw for monitoring intracranial pressure. *J. Neurosurg.* **39**, 416–419.
18. Levin A. B. (1977) The use of a fiber optic intracranial pressure monitor in clinical practice. *Neurosurgery* **1**, 266–271.
19. Miller J. D., Becker D. P., Ward J. D. et al. (1977) Significance of intracranial hypertension in severe head injury. *J. Neurosurg.* **47**, 503–516.
20. Johnston I. and Paterson A. (1974) Benign intracranial hypertension II, CSF pressure and circulation. *Brain* **97**, 301–312.
21. Marshall L. F., Smith R. W. and Shapiro H. M. (1978) The influence of diurnal rhythms in patients with intracranial hypertension: implications for management. *Neurosurgery* **2**, 100–102.
22. Langfitt T. W. (1969) Increased intracranial pressure. *Clin. Neurosurg.* **16**, 436–471.
23. Johnston H. and Jennett B. (1973) The place of continuous intracranial pressure monitoring in neurosurgical practice. *Acta Neurochir. (Wien)* **29**, 53–63.
24. Avezaat C. J. J., Van Eijndhoven J. H. M. and Wyper D. J. (1979) Cerebrospinal fluid pulse pressure and intracranial volume-pressure relationships. *J. Neurol. Neurosurg. Psychiatry* **42**, 687–700.
25. Leech P. J. and Miller J. D. (1974) Intracranial volume/pressure relationships during experimental brain compression in primates. II, Effects of induced changes in arterial pressure. *J. Neurol. Neurosurg. Psychiatry* **37**, 1099–1104.
26. Cushing H. (1903) The blood pressure reaction of acute cerebral compression, illustrated by cases of intracranial hemorrhage. *Am. J. Med. Sci.* **125**, 1007–1044.
27. Greitz T. (1956) Radiologic study of brain circulation by rapid serial angiography of the carotid artery. *Acta Radiol.* [*Suppl*] **140**, 1–123.
28. Obrist W. D., Gennarelli T. A., Segawa H. et al. (1979) Relation of cerebral blood flow to neurological status and outcome in head injured patients. *J. Neurosurg.* **51**, 292–300.
29. Shalit M. N., Beller A. J., Feinsod M. et al. (1970) The blood flow and oxygen consumption of the dying brain. *Neurology* **20**, 740–748.
30. Grubb R. L. Jr, Raichle M. E., Eichling J. O. et al. (1977) Effects of subarachnoid hemorrhage on cerebral blood volume, blood flow and oxygen utilizations in humans. *J. Neurosurgery* **46**, 446–453.
31. Fieschi C., Agnoli A., Battastihi N. et al. (1968) Derangements of regional cerebral blood flow and of its regulatory mechanisms in acute cerebrovascular lesions. *Neurology* **18**, 1166–1179.
32. Clasen R. A., Pandolfi S., Laing L. et al. (1974) Experimental study of relation of fever to cerebral edema. *J. Neurosurg.* **41**, 576–581.
33. Miller D. and Adams H. (1972) Physiopathology and management of increased intracranial pressure. In: Cirtchley M., O'Leary J. L. and Jennett B., ed., *Scientific Foundation of Neurology*, pp. 308–324. London, Heinemann.
34. Fitch W. and McDowall D. G. (1971) Effect of halothane on intracranial pressure gradients in the presence of intracranial space-occupying lesions. *Br. J. Anaesth.* **43**, 904–912.
35. Miller J. D. and Sullivan H. G. (1979) Management of severe intracranial hypertension. *Int. Anesthesiol. Clin.* **17**, 19–75.
36. Miller J. D., Garibi J., North J. B. et al. (1975) Effects of increased arterial pressure on blood flow in the damaged brain. *J. Neurol. Neurosurg. Psychiatry* **38**, 657–665.
37. Graham D. I. and Adams J. H. (1971) Ischemic brain damage in fatal head injuries. *Lancet* **1**, 265–266.

38. Graham D. I., Adams J. H. and Doyle D. (1978) Ischemic brain damage in fatal non-missile head injuries. *J. Neurol. Sci.* **39**, 213–234.

39. MacPherson P. and Graham D. I. (1978) Correlation between angiographic findings and the ischemia of head injury. *J. Neurol. Neurosurg. Psychiatry* **41**, 122–127.

40. Miller J. D. (1976) Infection in head injury. In: Vinken P. J. and Bruyn W. W., ed., *Handbook of Neurology*, In: Braakman R., ed., *Injuries of the Brain and Skull*, Part II, Vol. 24, pp. 215–230. Amsterdam, North-Holland.

41. Froman C. (1968) Adverse effects of low carbon dioxide tensions during mechanical over-ventilation of patients with combined head and chest injuries. *Br. J. Anaesthesia* **40**, 383–386.

42. Frost E. A. M. (1977) Respiratory problems associated with head trauma. *Neurosurgery* **1**, 300–306.

43. Shapiro H. M. and Marshall L. F. (1978) Intracranial pressure responses to PEEP in head injured patients. *J. Trauma* **18**, 254–256.

44. Cottrell J. E., Robustelli A. and Post K. (1977) Furosemide and mannitol-induced changes in intracranial pressure and serum osmolality and electrolytes. *Anesthesiology* **47**, 28–30.

45. Pappius H. M. and Dayes L. A. (1965) Hypertonic urea—its effects on the distribution of water and electrolytes in normal and edematous brain tissues. *Arch. Neurol.* **13**, 395–402.

46. Becker D. P. and Vries J. K. (1973) The alleviation of increased intracranial pressure by the chronic administration of osmotic agents. In: Brock M. and Dietz H., ed., *Intracranial Pressure: Experimental and Clinical Aspects*, pp. 309–315. Berlin, Springer-Verlag.

47. Maxwell R. E., Long D. M. and French L. A. (1972) The clinical effects of a synthetic gluco-corticord used for brain edema in the practice of neurosurgery. In: Reulen H. J. and Schurmann K., ed., *Steroids and Brain Edema*, pp. 219–232. Berlin, Springer-Verlag.

48. Faupel G., Reulen H. J., Muller D. et al. (1976) Double blind study on the effects of steroids on severe closed head injury. In: Pappius H. M. and Feindel W., ed., *Dynamics of Brain Edema*, pp. 337–343. Berlin, Springer-Verlag.

49. Gobiet W., Bock W. J., Liesegang J. et al. (1976) Treatment of acute cerebral edema with high dose of dexamethasone. In: Beks J. W. F., Bosch D. A. and Brock M., ed., *Intracranial Pressure III*, pp. 231–235. Berlin, Springer-Verlag.

50. Gudeman S. K., Miller J. D. and Becker D. P. (1979) Failure of high dose steroid therapy to influence intracranial pressure in patients with severe head injury. *J. Neurosurg.* **51**, 301–306.

51. Cooper P. R., Moddy S., Clark W. K. et al. (1979) Dexamethasone and severe head injury: a prospective double blind study. *J. Neurosurg.* **51**, 307–316.

52. Rockoff M. A., Marshall L. F. and Shapiro H. M. (1979) High-dose barbiturate therapy in man. A clinical review of sixty patients. *Ann. Neurol.* **6**, 194–199.

53. Miller J. D. (1979) Barbiturates and raised intracranial pressure. *Ann. Neurol.* **6**, 189–193.

54. Klatzo I. (1967) Neuropathological aspects of brain edema. *J. Neuropathol. Exp. Neurol.* **26**, 1–14.

55. Reulen H. J., Tsuyama M., Tack A. et al. (1978) Clearance of edema fluid in cerebrospinal fluid. *J. Neurosurg.* **48**, 754–764.

56. Shapiro H. M., Wyte S. R. and Loeser J. (1974) Barbiturate-augmented hypothermia for reduction of persistent intracranial hypertension. *J. Neurosurg.* **40**, 90–100.

57. Kosnick E. J. and Hunt W. E. (1976) Post-operative hypertension in the management of patients with intracranial arterial aneurysms. *J. Neurosurg.* **45**, 148–154.

Chapter 18

The Hepatic System

J. M. Hood

The liver is the largest organ in the body, weighing approximately one-fiftieth of the total body weight. Its great size reflects its importance in fulfilling many functions crucial to the maintenance of homeostasis. Its functions can be classified broadly into synthetic and metabolic. Among the very many substances which are synthesized in the liver are albumin, many of the clotting factors, α_1-antitrypsin, etc. The metabolic functions include a fundamental role in the metabolism of carbohydrates, fats and proteins and, as a by-product of the latter, the formation of urea. Many drugs and toxins are metabolized in the liver and excreted either into the bloodstream or the bile.

Consequently when liver malfunction develops the effects are extremely widespread and variable and are also, to some extent, dependent upon the cause of dysfunction and its rate of development. Furthermore, it is convenient to separate hepatocellular dysfunction from biliary, although this of course is somewhat artificial. Probably one of the more common manifestations of liver dysfunction is the onset of jaundice but, in addition, liver failure can result in any combination of the following: defective haemostasis, portal hypertension, ascites, renal failure and coma. Each of these will be discussed in considerable detail later in this chapter.

Liver failure is usually the outcome of some underlying disease process and whether failure occurs a short time after the onset of the illness, i.e. acute fulminant hepatic failure, or as a final outcome of a chronic underlying disease such as alcoholic cirrhosis, depends upon many factors, the most important being the aetiology itself. Hepatic failure of the acute fulminant variety manifests itself in quite a different way to the decompensation of a chronic hepatic disease process.

It is difficult to obtain figures as to the incidence of either variety of hepatic failure, but it is known that liver and biliary tract disease is the fifth leading cause of death in the U.S.A. being surpassed only by cardio-vascular disease, malignancy, accident and respiratory disease. The incidence of fulminant hepatic failure complicating chronic liver disease is low.

In all studies of acute fulminant liver failure, viral hepatitis accounts for the largest number of cases but, of those patients who develop viral hepatitis, less than 1% go on to develop the syndrome of fulminant hepatic failure,[1] while approximately 5% develop progressive liver disease and the remainder resolve completely with no residual liver damage.

There is now little doubt that halothane does cause a hepatitis which may be of a fulminant nature associated with a high mortality rate.[2] It is also accepted that the mechanism whereby halothane brings about liver damage is of an immunological type probably altering liver cell components.[3,4] The incidence of fulminant hepatitis increases with repeated exposure[5] and in the U.S. National Halothane Study the incidence of hepatic necrosis for patients with multiple exposure was 0·7 per 1000.[4] Other risk factors which have been identified so far are obesity[6] and the female sex. In those who recover there is no residual hepatic lesion.[7]

Drugs rarely cause damage by a direct action on the liver cell and one or two mechanisms are usually involved. In the first, the damage is mediated by a metabolite-related substance which combines covalently with cell proteins and in the second an immunological reaction to the drug renders a constituent of the liver cell antigenic. An example of the first type is paracetamol and the second halothane.

Carbon tetrachloride ingestion results in jaundice within 48 hours. Renal failure is also common. Related substances such as trichloroethylene or glue containing toluene act similarly, as does DDT.

Paracetamol is not uncommonly used as a suicide agent and here jaundice develops on the third or fourth day. The overall mortality of 201 patients admitted with paracetamol overdose to a district general hospital was 3·5%. Mortality is dose related.[8] Chronic ingestion of paracetamol can result in chronic liver damage.

Methotrexate toxicity usually results from long-term therapy and does not usually cause fulminant hepatic failure.[8]

Isoniazid, especially when combined with rifampicin can result in fulminant hepatitis and, here, orientals are especially at risk. A mortality rate of 12% has been reported when overt liver damage develops.[8]

Amanita phaloides is now one of the more important causes of fulminant failure due to toxins.[9]

Fulminant hepatic failure is best defined as in the Fulminant Hepatic Failure Surveillance Study[10] as the clinical syndrome associated with massive necrosis of liver cells or with sudden severe impairment of hepatic function. A further requirement is that it should occur within 8 weeks of the onset of symptoms and that previous liver function is assumed to be normal.

The syndrome is extremely variable in its outcome and the prognosis is dependent upon many factors. Among those of importance are:

I. *Aetiology*. Hepatitis of both type A and B can cause fulminant failure in approximately 1% of cases. Here the mortality rate, as found in the survey, was 17 and 19% for A and B, respectively. Halothane had a survival rate of only 4% whilst in other drug-induced cases, a mortality of 50% was reported.

II. *Stage of coma*. This is best defined as in the manner of Adams and Foley in 1949[11] and, not unexpectedly, mortality is highest in Stage IV (82·4%), and thereafter mortality declines to (52%) in Stage III and 33% in Stage II.

III. *Age*. Mortality increases with age and in the Surveillance Study the mortality of those patients in Stage IV coma under 15 years of age was 66% and in those aged 15–44 years it was 78%, whilst in those older than 45 years it was as high as 95%.

IV. *Alpha-fetoprotein levels*. In a study of 64 patients in fulminant hepatic failure it was found that the alpha-fetoprotein level was elevated in 23% of the survivors but in only 9·8% of the fatal cases. The rise in alpha-fetroprotein was found early after the development of Stage IV coma and was thought to constitute an encouraging prognostic sign when other tests were unhelpful.

Measurement and Monitoring

There are many different means whereby liver function can be assessed to aid in the general management of a patient with liver failure. These can be divided into biochemical, haematological and radiological investigations.

Biochemical Tests of Liver Function

These offer perhaps the most readily available and most widely used assessment of liver function. Standard biochemical tests will measure the total serum bilirubin and this may be elevated for a number of reasons. In general the highest levels will be obtained in obstructive jaundice and here the bilirubin will be predominantly conjugated. In primary hepatocellular jaundice, intermediate levels will be encountered and here unconjugated bilirubin will be largely responsible for the rise. In haematological jaundice, the bilirubin does not generally attain high levels and it will be usually conjugated in form. At present, the emphasis in differentiating the cause of jaundice on the basis of the direct and indirect bilirubin estimations is not as important as in the past, partly because of the unreliability of the tests and in many centres only the total level is now estimated. Before leaving the subject of elevated bilirubin levels[12] attention should be paid to some of the syndromes which result in an elevated level resulting from a congenital defect. These include the Dubin–Johnson syndrome[13] and the Crigler–Najjar syndrome.[14]

The liver enzymes normally measured are L-alanine aminotransferase and aspartate aminotransferase, although gamma-glutamyl transpeptidase and pseudocholinesterase are also not infrequently determined. In general, in liver failure due to a primary hepatocellular failure, the level of liver enzymes becomes markedly elevated but it should be realized that, in the terminal stages, the levels once more return towards, or actually attain, normal values. This is a bad prognostic sign. In obstructive jaundice, the enzyme levels either remain within normal limits or only become slightly elevated, providing that no complications intervene such as cholangitits which can result in an elevation of the enzymes. Normal levels of L-alanine aminotransferase and aspartate aminotransferase are 10–45 and 10–40 i.u., respectively.

Serum gamma-glutamyl transpeptidase (γGT) is an enzyme which is found mainly in the kidney, but lower levels are found in the liver and, to a lesser extent, the pancreas. Although elevated levels occur in severe renal disease the enzyme is a good indicator of liver cell dysfunction. γGT does not rise and fall in association with the aminotransferases. Normal levels are 7–34 i.u.

The third part of a standard liver function test is the alkaline phosphatase level. This is an enzyme which is present in many tissues including bone, intestine, placenta, leucocyte and kidney, in addition to liver, although serum levels are mainly derived from bone, intestine and liver. The liver does not excrete alkaline phosphatase into the bile. In biliary tract obstruction, for some ill-understood reason, alkaline phosphatase enters the systemic circulation. The normal adult range is 1·5–4·0 Bodansky units, 3–15 King–Armstrong units or 20–85 i.u. Higher levels occur in children and in late pregnancy. The liver alkaline phosphatase can be identified from the other isoenzymes by electrophoresis on starch gel. It is also heat stable, as opposed to bone alkaline phosphatase. A simple means of ensuring that an elevated alkaline phosphatase is of liver origin, is to measure the 5-nucleotidase level. 5-Nucleotidase is an enzyme which resides mainly in the hepatic microvilli and, if this is elevated, is presumed to be of liver origin. Pollock et al.[15] showed the serum 5-nucleotide phosphodiesterase level (5-NPD) to be a better indicator of the presence of hepatic metastases than liver scan, carcino-embryonic antigen, alpha-fetoprotein, aspartate aminotransferase, bilirubin or alkaline phosphatase levels. They found the accuracy of the test to be 84% and the predictive value 75%. Highest levels of alkaline phosphatase are seen in complete biliary tract obstruction. Intermediate levels occur in cholestatic jaundice and also in liver infiltrations most commonly due to secondary neoplastic deposits.

Blood ammonia is mentioned mainly for historical interest. It used to be routinely estimated to predict the onset of impending hepatic encephalopathy but, its correlation with increasing degrees of encephalopathy, is not as good as octopamine levels and in many centres it is no longer estimated. Normal levels should not exceed 1 μg/ml. One situation in which it is still of some value is in Reye's syndrome where hyperammonaemia forms an important part of the syndrome.

Serum proteins are often used as estimates of the severity of chronic liver disease. Total protein levels are normally 6–8 g/dl of which albumin constitutes approximately 4–6 g. In severe liver disease hypoalbuminaemia is frequently encountered and is often accompanied by an elevation in serum globulins. Hypoalbuminaemia, in the absence of other aetiological factors such as poor dietary intake and abnormal losses from the kidney, usually indicates a loss of functioning hepatocytes.

α_1-Globulin deserves special mention since α_1-antitrypsin accounts for a substantial part of the α_1-globulin fraction and a readily available screening test in suspected cases of α_1-antitrypsin deficiency is to estimate the α_1-globulin level. If it is low then α_1-antitrypsin deficiency may be present and an estimation of α_1-antitrypsin itself can then be made.

Alpha-fetoprotein is a normal fetal protein synthesized by embryonal liver and yolk sac cells. During normal gestation alpha-fetoprotein levels rise early and drop to 50 mg/dl in the newborn. It has been shown that, in a high proportion of primary hepatocellular carcinomas, an elevation of alpha-fetoprotein occurs. It is also interesting to note that, in hepatocellular tumours associated with the oral contraceptive pill, alpha-fetoprotein usually remains within normal limits.[16]

Haematological Tests

Prothrombin is an essential clotting factor synthesized in the liver and its synthesis is dependent upon vitamin K. Before a bleeding tendency develops the level must be depressed to approximately 10% or less of normal level. This is why spontaneous bleeding is rare in obstructive jaundice, but in terminal liver failure it is not unusual.

Fibrinogen is also manufactured in the liver and again in severe liver failure its levels become appreciably depressed. Platelet and leucocyte levels may also be measured and both tend to fall in the presence of severe portal hypertension and splenomegaly. The lack of platelets together with low levels of clotting factors tend to increase the risk of a bleeding tendency and increase the hazards of any surgical procedure in such patients.

Radiology

Oral cholecystography is the simplest X-ray test, but is of little value in advanced degrees of liver disease since gallbladder visualization depends on normal liver function. Likewise, intravenous cholangiography is of little use in hepatic failure.

Percutaneous transhepatic cholangiography is a very valuable test and was first described by French and Vietnamese physicians in Hanoi in 1937.[17] Early problems were associated with the use of relatively large needles. The major breakthrough came in 1974 when Professor K. Okuda of Chiba University, Japan introduced the thin needle technique now associated with his name. A very fine needle is introduced into a radicle of the bile duct and after fluoroscopic screening to ensure puncture of a duct, contrast is introduced. This gives high quality pictures of the biliary tree and, since then, many reports of good results with this technique have been published.[18,19] Visualization rates of 80–93% with dilated ducts and 60–80% with normal calibre ducts are not unusual.

Complications occur in about 6·5% of patients and the commonest is cholangitis. This is most common in the presence of calculous disease or benign stricture whilst, in the presence of malignant disease, it is uncommon.[20] Major bleeding problems are rare as is biliary peritonitis which was not unusual with the larger older needles.

The technique has been taken further and it is now possible to decompress an obstructed bile duct by, first, locating a duct with a Chiba needle and then passing a fine polyethylene cannula into the duct. The cannula can then be advanced past the bile stricture and on into the duodenum. This then allows free drainage of bile into the duodenum. If the stricture cannot be negotiated with the catheter the bile can be drained externally.

The value of percutaneous catheterization of the bile duct lies in relieving jaundice by non-surgical means in cases where surgery would merely be palliative and in improving the general condition of patients when surgery may be curative. It has been shown that prior biliary decompression reduces subsequent surgical risk, in that infective and anastomotic complications are less common.

High quality venograms of the portal system can also be obtained using a Chiba needle. Percutaneous transhepatic portal venography is now tending to replace older methods of portal venography, such as injection of the contrast material into the splenic pulp. This technique was first described by Bierman in 1952 and was technically refined by Wiechel in 1971. It has since been used in the investigation of portal hypertension by several authors[21,22] and its value in localizing the site of insulinomas has also been noted.[23]

The other method of investigating the biliary system in the presence of jaundice is by means of endoscopic retrograde cholangiography. Here, a side-viewing fibreoptic duodenoscope is passed and the ampulla of Vater identified. It is then possible to insert a catheter into the ampulla and inject radiographic contrast material so outlining the distal bile duct. In a typical large series reported by Ligours et al.,[24] the bile duct was outlined in 206 of

278 patients and infectious reactions occurred in 20 of 295. The procedure has a low morbidity rate, but the occurrence of fatal cholangitis has been reported.[25]

Selective angiography of the coeliac axis is of value in delineating abnormal circulation within the liver and a venous phase can be obtained to give some information about the portal vein, but with the exception of these two applications angiography is not of great value in the investigation of advanced liver disease. Ultrasonic scanning of the liver is a non-invasive and relatively inexpensive method of investigation which, with operator experience, can yield much useful information. Its value in jaundice has been shown by many authors.[26,27] Ultrasonography is also of value in diagnosing the presence of liver metastases.[28]

Computerized axial tomography has a place in the investigation of liver disease, but it is not as specific as ultrasound and its poorer resolution renders it unable to pick up very small lesions in the liver.

Radioisotope techniques are valuable in several respects in investigation of hepatobiliary disorders. Technetium sulphur colloid scans are those most often used and their main value is in the demonstration of space-occupying lesions, such as liver metastases. Some indirect evidence as to the state of liver function can also be obtained with this scan, for normally the liver should take up a higher concentration of isotope than the spleen or bone marrow, but in patients with moderate to severe degrees of hepato-cellular dysfunction the normal is reversed and the liver takes up less isotope.

The newer isotope of technetium, diethyl iminodiacetic acid (DIDA), is taken up by the hepatocytes and secreted into the bile so that extrahepatic biliary obstruction can be more easily differentiated from hepatocellular causes of jaundice. It is also of value in the diagnosis of acute cholecystitis for here the gallbladder is non-functioning and so no isotope enters it or at least it fails to concentrate it.[31]

Radioisotope methods have also been used in recent years to evaluate the portal circulation. One of the methods used has been to use $^{99}Tc^{m}O_4$, 10 mCi of which was instilled per rectum and scintigrams were then taken of the portal area. Satisfactory visualization of the portal vein was thus obtained.[32]

When considering the consequences of liver failure there are two completely separate entities which should be thought of. First, the clinical consequence of acute liver failure and secondly, chronic liver decompensation, when the picture of portal hypertension is dominant.

Considering acute failure, here the effects of liver failure can be seen acting on many of the systems of the body. In the central nervous system the consequences become manifest as hepatic encephalopathy, on the renal system the hepatorenal syndrome may develop, on the clotting–fibrinolytic system abnormal bleeding is seen. In addition, ascites is often present. The pathophysiology of each of these entities will be discussed in more detail below.

HEPATIC ENCEPHALOPATHY

Hepatic encephalopathy is one of the common and obvious manifestations of the later stages of hepatic failure. The syndrome is characterized by mental and neuromuscular abnormalities which, in turn, are secondary to a metabolic defect which arises as a consequence of hepatic failure. Although much has been learnt recently about these biochemical abnormalities much remains as yet unknown.

The syndrome itself is characterized in its earliest stages by a simple psychomotor stage which progresses with varying rapidity to fully established coma and eventually death. There are many factors which are known to precipitate the patient, who is on the brink of hepatic encephalopathy, into this state and, clearly, when considering the management of such patients due regard should be given to these.

The best known factor is an excess nitrogenous load due either to an excessive dietary intake of protein secondary to an upper gastrointestinal bleed. It is known that patients in liver failure have an increased risk of upper gastrointestinal bleeding which can either be secondary to oesophageal varices or to a bleeding peptic ulcer,[33] the incidence of which is increased in liver disease. Any other causes of an increased nitrogenous load can also result in hepatic encephalopathy.

The second category of precipitating causes is the indiscriminant use of medication and here two types of drug are particularly liable to produce hepatic coma: diuretics of almost all types and those narcotics which rely on the liver for their metabolism.

Hepatic encephalopathy can also be brought on by the coincident development of a systemic infection, either viral or bacterial. The development of a spontaneous or primary peritonitis is especially liable to occur in patients with established ascites who are already approaching the terminal stage of liver failure.

Lastly, and by no means least, surgical causes of hepatic encephalopathy should be mentioned. Here the most obvious are shunt surgery and, in particular, portacaval shunts,[34] although other varieties of shunt, such as the distal splenorenal shunt, are by no means immune from precipitating hepatic encephalopathy. Any surgical procedure which reduces the blood flow to a severely decompensated liver can precipitate hepatic coma.

Many biochemical abnormalities have been noted in hepatic coma such as an increased level of ammonia, glutamine and alpha-ketoglutarate in muscle, brain and spinal fluid, increased levels of fatty acids and mercaptans, etc. However, the two abnormalities which seem to be of greatest practical importance are the occurrence of false neurotransmitters and the abnormal pattern of amino acids. Both of these will be discussed in more detail.

In 1971, Fischer and Baldessarini[35] suggested that the occurrence of false neurotransmitters was the most important pathophysiological process to

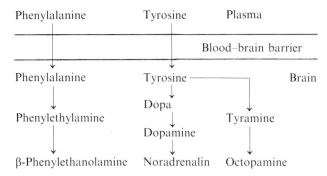

Fig. 18.1. The production of false neurotransmitters in the aetiology of hepatic coma.

account for hepatic coma, in particular octopamine was thought to be of significance (*Fig.* 18.1).

It has been suggested that octopamine competes with the normal neurotransmitter dopamine at a central level, so interfering with the normal brain functions. Lam et al.[36] found serum and urinary levels of octopamine to be elevated in all of the 25 patients with hepatic encephalopathy and they also found that there was a statistically significant correlation between the degree of encephalopathy and the serum and urine octopamine levels. Manghani et al.[37] studied 17 controls and 33 patients with hepatic encephalopathy and 13 patients with liver disease and no encephalopathy. Here abnormal levels were found only in the presence of hepatic encephalopathy and, when liver disease was present but encephalopathy was absent, the levels did not differ from those of controls. Serum levels were found to be more reliable than urinary. Lloyd et al.[38] showed that in Reye's syndrome, octopamine levels were also elevated and Block et al.[39] showed that, in an experimental situation, octopamine levels also corresponded with the level of consciousness.

Rossi-Fanelli et al.[40] produced further clinical evidence for a possible role of octopamine in the pathogenesis of hepatic encephalopathy. They found a significant association between encephalopathy and an elevated level of octopamine, but they could not distinguish effectively between grades 3 and 4. They have further shown a negative correlation between octopamine and ammonia suggesting that the levels of these two substances varied independently. They went on to show that the correlation between either ammonia or octopamine and the level of hepatic encephalopathy is not as good as it is with the CSF glutamine level.

Despite this positive evidence there has been some recent contradictory experimental evidence. In a study in rats, Zieve and Olson depressed brain dopamine content by 92% and noradrenaline by 88% using intraventricular infusion of octopamine without affecting the alertness of the rats. Extremely high levels of brain octopamine were achieved.

Amino acid abnormalities have been noted to occur in hepatic en-cephalopathy for many years. In 1962, Richmond[41] reported that high levels of methionine and phenylalanine occurred in patients with liver disease and that these were cleared more slowly from the plasma than normal. In the same year, Guroff et al.[42] reported that elevated levels of phenylalanine occurred, and he suggested that perhaps this may interfere with the uptake of tyrosine which is an essential precursor of several of the brain's neurotransmitters.

It is now generally agreed that, in hepatic coma, high levels of aromatic and sulphurated amino acids occur and that the level of branched-chain amino acids is decreased.[43] The blood urea concentration rises in up to 80% of patients with terminal liver failure. Two broad categories of renal failure are seen in association with liver failure. In the first, which is otherwise called functional renal failure, there is a reduction in the glomerular filtration rate, the ability to handle a water load is diminished and blood urea and creatinine concentration rise. A concentrated urine with a low sodium concentration (less than 10 mmol/l) and high osmolality is produced. The urine : plasma osmolality ratio rises to over 1 : 1·1. The second type is characterized by evidence of renal tubular damage and hence the urinary sodium concentration is above 12 mmol/l and the osmolality of the urine is low. Histological changes are apparent early in contrast to the functional type, although the functional variety can proceed to this type in its later stages when there may be evidence of secondary tubular damage.

It is the first type which is more properly labelled 'hepatorenal syndrome' and here the pathophysiology is very complicated, but among the factors responsible is a definite impairment in the ability to handle sodium which the kidney then retains. Whether sodium retention is a secondary or primary phenomenon is still unknown, but evidence tends to support the fact that it is primary.

Many factors may precipitate the onset of the hepatorenal syndrome and among the better known are gastrointestinal haemorrhage, abdominal paracentesis, over-vigorous use of diuretics, use of nephrotoxic antibiotics and mesangiocapillary glomerulonephritis with IgA and complement deposits in the kidney. The latter is found more commonly in cirrhotics.[44] Another standard abnormality which has been noted is a renal deposition of lipid which was found by Hovig et al.[45] in four patients with hepatorenal syndrome. This deposit may represent large-molecular-weight, low density lipoprotein and that the mechanism from the deposition may be similar to that which occurs in familial lecithin : cholesterol acyltransferase deficiency.

Accepting that abnormal sodium retention is one of the important manifestations of the syndrome, much speculation has gone into the possible causes of this. One possibility is a lack of effective intravascular volume and work with total body immersion, which acts as a central volume stimulus without having to actually give fluid, has shown that a marked natriuresis occurs even in cirrhotics.[46] Other possible causes include hepatic venous obstruction and this in turn may act in several ways:[47]

1. Increased formation of hepatic lymph.
2. Decreased hepatic blood flow with impairment of hepatic degradation of aldosterone.
3. The release of a hepatic humoral factor which is capable of stimulating the renin–angiotensin system with resultant increased secretion of aldosterone.
4. Levy has shown that selective hepatic venous outflow block has resulted in significant sodium retention which is independent of hyperaldosteronism, portal venous pressure, decrement of filtered sodium load or of neural changes.

The excessive retention of sodium seems to result from the renal standpoint in an excessive reabsorption of sodium rather than in an alteration in the filtered load. Although glomerular filtration rate may be decreased in advanced liver disease it does not seem to be the primary factor responsible. Among the suggested causes of the increased sodium retention are:

1. Hyperaldosteronism
2. Alteration in intrarenal blood flow distribution. It has been shown that there is a redistribution of the renal blood flow away from the renal cortex towards the medulla.[48]
3. Increased sympathetic activity
4. Alterations in the endogenous release of prostaglandins by the kidney
5. Changes in the kallikrein kinin system
6. Possible role of humoral natriuretic factor, perhaps released from the liver
7. Vasoactive intestinal polypeptide

It seems unlikely that hyperaldosteronism is responsible because a dissociation between plasma aldosterone levels and sodium excretion has been shown and spontaneous natriuresis has been seen without alteration in the aldosterone levels. Conversely, the administration of aminoglutethimide which is a substance which decreases the plasma aldosterone level, has failed to achieve a natriuretic effect.

No matter what the precise cause of the hepatorenal syndrome may turn out to be, from a therapeutic standpoint the most effective form of treatment has been liver transplantation. It is now well established that even those patients who have required dialysis prior to liver transplantation achieve complete reversal of their renal failure after successful liver transplantation. This was first shown by Iwatsuki et al.[49] in 1973 and has subsequently been confirmed on many occasions. This would seem to suggest that failure of the liver must play a crucial role in the pathophysiology of the hepatorenal syndrome and, when this is successfully reversed, then the renal function will return to normal.

PORTAL HYPERTENSION

Normally portal vein pressures should be 5–10 mmHg or a wedged hepatic venous pressure of 4 mmHg. Intrasplenic pressure should not normally be above 17 mmHg. Portal hypertension is classified according to the sites of obstruction and some of the more common causes are shown in *Table* 18.1.

Table **18.1. Classification of portal hypertension**

I. *Prehepatic*
   1. Portal vein obstruction
     a. Congenital anomalies
     b. Infective—portal pylephlebitis secondary to sepsis in the abdomen, e.g. appendix
     c. Tumour—encroachment of adjacent malignancies
     d. Haematological diseases, e.g. polycythemia rubra vera

II. *Hepatic*
   1. Cirrhosis of any type
   2. Advanced polycystic disease of the liver
   3. Infiltrative diseases, e.g. sarcoid or Gaucher's disease

III. *Post-hepatic*
   1. Hepatic venous occlusion (Budd–Chiari syndrome)
     a. Idiopathic
     b. Secondary—tumour invasion from either primary or secondary liver tumour or adjacent neoplasms, oral contraceptives, membranous obstruction of the vena cava

Hepatic causes are the most common in the adult and the cirrhotic group is the largest. In the U.S.A. and South Africa, alcoholic cirrhosis is most common, in the United Kingdom cryptogenic cirrhosis and in parts of Africa schistosomiasis is the cause. The role of hepatitis B in causing cirrhosis is becoming increasingly recognized.

Pre-hepatic causes are uncommon in the adult but they constitute the most important group in children where portal venous occlusion is the commonest cause of portal hypertension.

Post-hepatic obstruction (the Budd–Chiari syndrome) is a less common type and is usually idiopathic but, of late, the role of oral contraceptives in causing hepatic venous occlusion has been recognized.[50]

Theoretically portal venous hypertension can be due to an increased flow through the portal vein or to an increased resistance to flow. As can be seen from the list of common causes, in the clinical situation it is almost invariably the latter which causes the condition. As a consequence of this, there is a decreased portal venous perfusion of the liver and collaterals open in an attempt to reduce portal venous pressure. It is the development of these collaterals which results in oesophageal varices. The sites where collaterals develop can be listed as follows:

1. Lower oesophagus between the coronary vein (portal) and the azygos vein (systemic)

2. Rectal submucosa between the middle and superior haemorrhoidal veins (portal) and the inferior haemorrhoidal vein (systemic)
3. Para-umbilical between the left portal vein and the epigastric veins
4. Parietal peritoneum between veins of Retzius (portal) and the veins of Sappey (systemic)
5. Left renal vein between splenic vein (portal) and the left renal vein.

The effect of the collaterals, in addition to helping to lower portal venous pressure, is to divert products of digestion which have been absorbed from the alimentary tract, from the liver. This is one of the causes which attributes to the development of hepatic encephalopathy.

The Liver and Haemostasis

The liver plays a central role in red cell breakdown and subsequent metabolism of the products thereof, in addition to its crucial role in coagulation. Abnormalities result from both of these aspects as the liver fails.

The effects of liver failure on coagulation and, to a lesser extent, fibrolysis are the most important haematological consequence of acute liver failure. The coagulation 'cascade' (*Fig.* 18.2) is believed to be set in action either by the intrinsic pathway whereby exposed subendothelial collagen sets in process a series of events resulting in the activation of Factor XII, or, alternatively, tissue thromboplastins, released as a result of tissue damage, set in sequence a process whereby Factor VII is activated. As a result of this process the end result is the formation of a stable clot.

Fibrinogen is synthesized almost exclusively in the liver by the parenchymal cells. It is present in the circulation at levels of 2–4 g/1 and is a relatively stable substance having a half-life of 5 days.

The vitamin-K-dependent factors, i.e. Factors II, VII, IX and X, are all synthesized by the liver and their production is dependent upon an adequate supply of vitamin K and on the normal functioning of the liver cells. The liver initially synthesizes the basic precursors or proteins of Factors II, VII, IX and X and the role of vitamin K has recently been shown to be that it directs the insertion of a second carboxyl group into the carbon of the glutamic acid residues. This results in the formation of carboxyglutamic acid which confers coagulant activity on the precursor proteins, so enabling them to bind calcium and, hence, actively promote coagulation.[51]

Factor VIII is probably synthesized in the liver as well as in other parts of the reticuloendothelial system and Factor XIII is, likewise, probably synthesized in the liver as well as in the megacaryocytes.

In liver failure, deficiency of vitamin-K-dependant Factors II, VII, IX and X effects both the extrinsic and intrinsic pathways and results in a

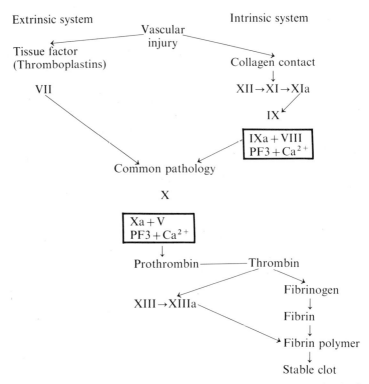

Fig. 18.2. A schematic representation of the coagulation process. PF3 = platelet function 3; a = activated function.

prolongation of the prothrombin time (PT) and in the partial thrombo-plastin time (PTT), respectively. The PT is considered by many to be the best screening test for coagulation defects occurring in liver disease.[52] Assays of the factor with the shortest half-life (Factor VII, approximately 6 hours), have been shown to be of prognostic benefit in acute hepatic failure. It has been shown that when the level of this factor falls below 9% the prognosis is poor.[53]

The evaluation of bleeding in liver disease can be a complex process which is usually initiated by bleeding from a local cause such as gastritis, duodenal ulceration or oesophageal varices. The patient may be deficient in Factors II, VII, IX and X and have thrombocytopenia and abnormal platelet function. All of this can be further aggravated by intravascular coagulation and a consumptive coagulopathy.

Thrombocytopenia is very common in liver disease and is generally attributed to portal hypertension and the subsequent hypersplenism. Normally, one-third of the total circulating platelet mass resides within the spleen and, although the total platelet mass is not decreased in thrombo-cytopenia secondary to splenomegaly, the increased size of the spleen results in more platelets being trapped within the spleen. Splenectomy often improves the thrombocytopenia as does a portacaval shunt.[54]

A further factor which is responsible for thrombocytopenia in some forms of liver disease is alcohol which is known to decrease the platelet count.[55]

As mentioned previously the fibrinolytic system may also be adversely affected in liver function. *Fig.* 18.3 shows a schematic representation of this system.

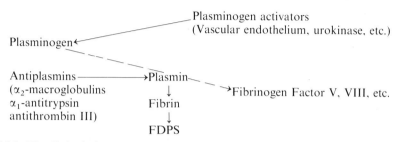

Fig. 18.3. The fibrinolytic system.

The central role of the liver is evidenced by the fact that it is probably the site of production of plasminogen.[56]

Increased fibrinolytic activity is thought to occur in cirrhosis,[57] following liver resection and after liver transplantation,[58] while decreased activity has been noted in acute hepatic failure and obstructive jaundice. Although much of the evidence as to precisely what happens to the fibrinolytic system in hepatic failure is not clearly established, it would probably be fair to say that, at the present time, it is believed that primary fibrinolysis occurs in situations of acute liver trauma and surgical stress, whilst intravascular coagulation with secondary fibrinolysis is a complication of chronic hepatocellular failure.

Therapy

In considering the management of a patient with portal hypertension and its secondary consequences, the problem of most concern to the clinician is bleeding from oesophageal varices. This manifests itself as an upper gastrointestinal haemorrhage with haematemesis and malaena and one of the first aims after appropriate restoration of blood volume, is to establish the source of the bleeding. The fact that a patient is suffering from cirrhosis is not, in itself, sufficient to allow one to assume that the cause of the bleeding is oesophageal varices. It is well known that patients with liver failure have a higher incidence of both duodenal ulceration and gastric erosions, and hence the simplest means of establishing a definitive cause for the bleeding is to perform an upper gastrointestinal endoscopy with a flexible fibreoptic duodenoscope. This will not only allow the presence of varices to be identified, but will establish if they are the cause of the bleeding or if it is due to other pathology in the stomach or duodenum.

If the site of bleeding is a duodenal ulcer or gastric erosion, then the treatment will initially take the form of antacids and cimetidine together with appropriate resuscitation with fluid and blood. If a duodenal ulcer continues to bleed then surgery may be indicated.

Where oesophageal varices are the cause of the haemorrhage, then the initial step is to try the effects of a vasopressin infusion. Vasopressin has an effect on the portal circulation which results in a fall in portal venous pressure. In a study by Swan et al.[59] hepatic wedged venous pressure in a group of 25 patients with bleeding oesophageal varices was 30 ± 2 mmHg and an infusion of vasopressin (0.01 units $\cdot$ kg$^{-1} \cdot$ min^{-1}) resulted in a fall to 20 ± 3 mmHg within 10 min of commencing infusion. At operation portal venous pressure was 41 ± 2 cm H$_2$0 and with a similar dose of vasopressin, the pressure fell to 31 ± 2 cm H$_2$O. Vasopressin also has a direct effect on the lower oesophageal sphincter which results in an increase in pressure.[60] This action, together with its effects of portal venous pressure, acts synergistically to help stop the bleeding from oesophageal varices and this beneficial effect has been shown by several groups.[61,62]

A new pharmacological method which has been shown to be helpful in stopping bleeding varices is the use of somatostatin. Tyden et al.[63] reported the results of treatment of one patient with a dose of 250 μg i.v./h. This resulted in the cessation of bleeding while the infusion was running, but as soon as it was stopped bleeding recommenced. The patient was later shunted and, at operation, the effect of somatostatin on portal venous pressure was studied and it was found to reduce the pressure by approximately 35%.

If vasopressin infusion fails to control the haemorrhage then the next step is to pass a Sengstaken–Blakemore tube. In some centres this tube has gained a very unfavourable reputation and mortality rates as high as 20% have been described in association with the usage of the tube.[64] With careful attention to detail this high mortality rate can be avoided.

First, instead of the conventional 3-lumen tube, a 4-lumen tube should be used. The fourth lumen provides for aspiration of the oesophagus above the level of the oesophageal balloon and this helps to prevent overflow or spill or saliva into the trachea. To aid passing the tube, it is helpful to have it well chilled, preferably in the ice compartment of a refrigerator. This gives a certain stiffness to the tube which facilitates its passage. The gastric balloon is inflated with 200 mls of air. The addition of contrast material to the gastric balloon enables the position of the tube to be checked with greater confidence. Having inflated the gastric balloon the oesophageal balloon is then inflated to a pressure of 30–40 mmHg. The latter pressure should never be exceeded, as this can damage the oesophagus and lead to its eventual necrosis. The pressure should be checked regularly. Finally it is essential that a patient with an inflated Sengstaken–Blakemore tube in situ, should be carefully nursed preferably in an intensive care unit. With these simple precautions the tube should not be dangerous. Pitcher[65] showed that in a series of 50 patients, a 92% initial success rate in stopping the bleeding could be achieved with the Sengstaken–Blakemore tube.

The tube should be left inflated for 24–36 hours then deflated. It is convenient to leave it in situ for a further 12–24 hours and, if no further bleeding occurs, it can then be removed. Should further bleeding develop, then the balloon can be reinflated for a further period which should not exceed 24 hours.

While control of bleeding has been obtained by either vasopressin or the Sengstaken– Blakemore tube, the question of what to do with the patient next should be considered. If only temporary control is gained, then an emergency procedure will be required to stop the bleeding. *Fig* 18.4 shows a suggested management plan.

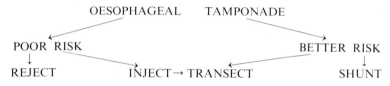

Fig. 18.4. The plan of management for patients with bleeding oesophageal varices.

Those who are considered to be a poor risk on the grounds of severely compromised liver function, age or complicating systemic disease should either be managed by conservative means alone or subjected to sclerotherapy.[66, 67]

The idea of direct transoesophageal ligation of varices dates back to the work of Boerema in 1949 and Crile in 1950 and since then the method has undergone various modifications of technique with equally variable results. The mortality rate however, generally lies somewhere between 22%[68] and 55%.[69] A newer modification of the method has been reported by Johnston[70] in which the autosuture stapler (SPTU) gun has been used. He has reported a series of 30 patients with an overall mortality rate of 10% and a recurrent bleeding rate of 10%. All of these patients were considered to be unsuitable for shunting for one reason or another. This, at least, seems to be an interesting new modification to the old idea of direct oesophageal transection.

As direct surgical attack on bleeding varices carries a high mortality, other methods of control have been sought and one of the other non-surgical methods worthy of mention is transhepatic coronary vein occlusion using either autogenous clot or Gelfoam. The technique, which at first thought may seem attractive, is not free of complications and in a series of 43 patients reported by Bengmark et al.[71] there was a 35% incidence of rebleeding and in 2 patients control of bleeding was not achieved. Of the 43 patients, 5 developed portal vein thrombosis within 2 months of the procedure and this resulted in 2 deaths.

Emergency shunting has a high mortality and if it can be avoided it should be. The mortality rate will be influenced considerably by the patient's liver function and, if it is good, then acceptable survival figures can be obtained, but, in those patients with poor function, very high mortality rates have been reported. The mortality rate is also adversely affected by increasing age and with other systemic diseases, such as diabetes. Even in the best series such as that of Orloff et al.[72] the mortality rate has been 52%.

In patients whose bleeding has been initially controlled by other means and whose liver function is good, a shunting procedure may be considered. Having decided that a patient is suitable for shunting, it remains to decide which form of shunt is preferable. The major criticism of standard end-to-side portacaval shunt is that the blood flow to the liver is reduced and that liver function suffers as a consequence of this. Furthermore, the incidence of hepatic encephalopathy remains rather high and so several techniques have been developed whose aim has been to minimize any reduction in hepatic blood flow which might occur. One technique to achieve this is to add an arterialization procedure to the standard end-to-side portacaval shunt. Adamson et al.[73] reported the use of a saphenous vein graft from the right gastroepiploic artery to the stump of the portal vein. This was carried out in 18 patients. There was one early postoperative death and the remainder were followed for a mean of 15·4 months. None required restriction of dietary protein intake and liver function remained good. There were two late occlusions of the fistula and the only episode of hepatic encephalopathy occurred in one of these.

The distal splenorenal shunt or Warren shunt is considered to be more selective than any other type of shunt. Recently Maillard et al.[74] studied the haemodynamics of the shunt.

A comparison of splenorenal and portacaval shunts was made by Busuttil and Tompkins,[75] 17 patients being randomly allocated to either type of shunt. Those with splenorenal shunts had significantly less postoperative encephalopathy and hepatic failure and a larger survival than those with portacaval shunts. In another study by Warren's group,[76] 26 splenorenal shunts were compared to 29 non-selective shunts (composed of 18 mesorenal, 6 mesocaval and 5 others). There were three operative deaths in each group. There was no difference in hepatic function between the two groups preoperatively, but postoperatively there was a significant difference, the splenorenal shunts fairing better. At 3–6 years follow-up there was no difference in total cumulative mortality, shunt occlusion or recurrent variceal haemorrhage, but there was significantly less hepatic encephalopathy with the Warren shunt.

The other type of shunt which is popular in the treatment of portal hypertension is the mesocaval or interposition shunt.[77, 78] In one of the larger series of mesocaval shunts in recent years, Dowling[79] reported the results of 137 mesocaval shunts over a 10-year period. The shunt patency rate was, as expected, high at 85%, encephalopathy occurred in 19% and rebleeding after shunting occurred in 12%. A comparison of mesocaval shunt and distal splenorenal shunt was made by Reichle et al.[80] and, in this prospective trial, they found that the distal splenorenal shunt had a significantly lower rate of post-shunt encephalopathy, but that the meso-caval was better at controlling the bleeding in an emergency situation.

The management of upper gastrointestinal bleeding can be summarized as follows. After adequate resuscitation precise diagnosis is important. Treatment then depends upon initial control of bleeding either by vasopressin or by Sengstaken–Blakemore tube. If this fails or if haemorrhage recurs, then further treatment depends upon the condition of the patient. Poor risk patients do better with sclerotherapy and better risk by transection preferably with an autosuture staple gun. Finally in the group where bleeding is controlled and where liver function is adequate, these may be considered to be candidates for one of the various shunt procedures, (*Fig.* 18.5).

Treatment of patients with the Budd–Chiari syndrome presents a special problem worthy of discussion. Here, as mentioned above, the problem lies at the level of the hepatic veins and so conventional shunting will not

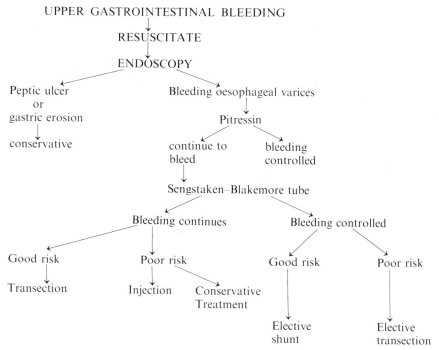

Fig. 18.5. Management plan for upper gastrointestinal bleeding associated with portal hypertension.

control the portal hypertension. Orloff and Johansen[81] recently proposed that side-to-side portacaval shunting is an adequate means of treatment. This theory is based on the use of the portal vein as an outflow tract rather than an inflow as is its normal use. In an initial study in dogs, its efficacy was established and it was then applied to 6 patients, 5 of whom did well and were followed from 8 months to 7 years. Ascites and portal hypertension were both well controlled.

Other types of shunt have been proposed, such as that by Fonkalsrud et al.[82] who used a Teflon graft from the splenic vein to the left lower lobar branch of the pulmonary artery. Chapman and Ochsner[83] treated a 33-year-old female with idiopathic Budd–Chiari syndrome by means of a shunt from the right common iliac vein to the right atrium of the heart with a side arm to the superior mesenteric vein. This received a satisfactory result.

The patient with ascites which is refractory to the usual treatment with diuretics and medical means has always presented a difficult problem. Within recent years the Le Veen shunt has been introduced to treat such a problem. Basically, the shunt consists of a Silastic tube from the peritoneal cavity to the internal jugular vein and, along its course, is a valve to encourage flow from the peritoneal cavity to the vascular system. The shunt is not only beneficial in alleviating severe intractable ascites, but is also of benefit in improving the renal function of patients either with established hepatorenal syndrome or those on the verge thereof. Several studies have demonstrated improvement in renal function following the insertion of the Le Veen shunt.[84–86]

Although the shunt is effective in both reducing and controlling ascites and in improving renal function, it is not without complications, and the commonest problem has been the development of a coagulopathy. In a prospective study of 15 patients by Schwartz,[87] a consumptive coagulopathy was demonstrated after insertion of the Le Veen shunt in 11 patients.

SYSTEM REPLACEMENT

The liver, as opposed to many other organs in the body, possesses a remarkable ability to regenerate after a loss of up to 80% of its cell mass. This loss can either be due to surgical resection or to the effects of the various disease processes. It is known that 20% of the original liver mass is adequate to support life and over the course of the next several weeks regeneration will take place. When a loss of more than 80% occurs or when the remaining tissue is already diseased then the phenomenon of liver failure, which has been described earlier, occurs.

The object of liver support systems is to tide the failing liver over until the regeneration process becomes well established. Many different approaches have been made to the solution of this problem and each of these will be briefly outlined.

Steroids

The role of steroids in the treatment of fulminant hepatic failure has recently been clarified by the report from the European Association for the Study of the Liver (EASL)[88] and the current consensus of opinion would now seem to weigh heavily against the use of steroids in fulminant hepatic failure.

Exchange Transfusion

As early as 1958, Lee and Tink reported the survival of a patient with acute hepatic failure treated by exchange tranfusion. Since then, there have been a large number of publications on the subject, but to date there is no agreement as to whether the treatment is of benefit or not.

Perhaps the best data come from Redecker et al.[89] who have published the results of the only controlled trial on exchange transfusion versus conservative therapy for patients with fulminant hepatitis and Stage IV coma. They had 28 patients in the trial and 15 were allocated randomly to exchange transfusion, the remainder were in the control group. There was a higher mortality in the exchange transfusion group than in the control group, but the criticism of this study is that, of the 15 selected for exchange transfusion, only 8 were indeed exchanged and all of these died. Currently this treatment modality is going out of vogue although, in selected cases, it may be of some benefit.

Extra-corporeal Liver Perfusion

This method of treatment consists basically of connecting the patient to an isolated but functioning animal liver, usually pig. The method was developed in several centres in the late 1960s and early 1970s but despite the usual early enthusiastic reports[90] and the fact that coma can be reversed, the long-term survival figures have been very disappointing.

The best result obtained has been by Abouna et al.[91] who kept a 23-year-old man with hepatic coma from liver necrosis alive for two and a half months with 16 perfusions using pigs on 10 occasions, baboons on 3, calf once and one human. The patient also had 20 exchange transfusions.

Haemoperfusion and Membrane Haemodialysis

Haemodialysis has no appreciable clinical value in the treatment of hepatic failure.[92] Toxins which are as yet incompletely elucidated build up in hepatic failure and these are not dialysable through conventional cellophane membranes. It is theoretically possible to remove these substances by haemoperfusion through adsorbents or ion-exchange resins, but a number of possible side effects may occur:
  1. Adsorption or disruption of formed blood elements
  2. Embolization of resin material into the circulation
  3. Removal of vital substances from the blood
  4. Addition of toxic substances to the blood.
With these theoretical and practical problems in mind there is a continuing search for the ideal exchange resin. Several different resins have been developed and tested in both the experimental and clinical situation:
  1. Albumin–colloidian encapsulated charcoal: this has been developed by Chang et al.[93]
  2. Poly-hydroxyethyl methacrylate (polyhema) encapsulated charcoal: several groups have worked with this including Andraiti,[94] Fennimore et al.[95] and Gazzard et al.[96] at King's College Hospital
  3. Use of co-polymers and cellulose: this is the basis of the Strathclyde group work and Thysell[97]
  4. Encapsulated petroleum pitch charcoal: this method was pioneered in Japan by Ohta's group.[98]
It is not known which of the absorbed factors are responsible for the recovery of consciousness, but a significant fall in the arterial levels of phenylalanine, methionine and tyrosine occurred during the haemoperfusion and, as these are closely involved in the metabolism of cerebral neurotransmitters, it is possible that the therapeutic effect is achieved by this means, although this is by no means certain.

In view of the damage to the formed elements of the blood in passing it over adsorbents, a new approach was developed which entails separation of the cellular elements from the plasma by means of a microporous membrane and then passing the plasma over an adsorbent column. This method has not, as yet, undergone any extensive clinical trials but early results of animal research are promising.[99]

In view of this apparent failure of haemoperfusion, emphasis shifted back to haemodialysis and although dialysis with the conventional cuprophane membrane does not result in any clinical benefit,[92] it was shown that the use of the more permeable polyacrylonitrile membrane was advantageous. Benefit appears to be in the prolongation of survival rather than in achieving higher final survival figures.

Sixty-five patients have now been treated in this manner at King's College Hospital[100] and 20 of these (30·8%) have survived to go home. This compares to a 15% survival figure on conservative treatment alone from the same institution. The King's College Hospital figures differ from those of Opolon in that, in the former group, those who recovered consciousness remained well and returned home.

Of all forms of liver support which have been tried to date, short of liver transplantation, haemodialysis and haemoperfusion seem to offer the best future. Adsorbent resins currently available all have some shortcomings, the most important of which is the inefficiency with which they remove protein bound substances, but more efficient resins are being developed to overcome these problems.

LIVER TRANSPLANTATION

Liver transplantation, in selected cases, probably offers the best form of treatment to patients with advanced progressive liver failure. The history of liver transplantation is longer than many people realize. The first successful auxiliary liver transplant was performed in dogs and was reported by Welch in 1955[101] and within a short period of time two groups, one from Harvard and one from North Western University in Chicago, were able to report on successful experimental homotransplantation in dogs. In March 1963, Starzl performed the first human orthotopic transplant.[102] Following this, some of the early human transplants were performed with auxiliary livers such as those by Absolom[103], but since that time the orthotopic site has been that generally preferred although there has been some renewed interest of late in the auxiliary site.[104]

As liver transplantation is an operation which involves many technical problems in addition to the usual problems of rejection common to all forms of vascularized organ transplantation, patient selection is clearly of crucial importance. In the Denver series, patients older then 45 years of age were usually rejected as the mortality has been shown to rise steeply with increasing age. Furthermore, transplantation for primary hepatic malignant neoplasms is not now undertaken because of the prohibitively high recurrence rate.

In considering candidates for transplantation, the group can be divided into adults and children. In the adult group, probably the commonest indication is terminal stages of chronic aggressive hepatitis whether HBsAg (hepatitis B surface antigen) positive or negative although clearly the latter type is preferable. The only successful attempt to clear the HBsAg marker from the serum of a liver transplant recipient for a prolonged time has come from the Cambridge–King's College group.[105] Other indications in the adult include primary biliary cirrhosis, alcoholic cirrhosis, secondary biliary cirrhosis, sclerosing cholangitis and the Budd–Chiari syndrome. Clearly any patient in the above group of diseases has to be nearing end stage before such a major undertaking as transplantation can be considered. In the paediatric age group, the commonest indication is primary biliary atresia followed by α_1-antitrypsin deficiency disease.[106] Other indications include inborn errors of metabolism in which the primary defect resides in the liver, such as Wilson's disease, congenital tyrosinaemia and type IV glycogen storage disease.

In the early experience of both the Denver group and the Cambridge group, technical problems were the major cause of mortality and rejection accounted for less than 20% of the deaths. Of the many technical problems, the most important has been the establishment of suitable and adequate biliary drainage. Of the first 93 patients transplanted in Denver, bile fistula formation occurred in 30% and almost always led to death. At this time the usual means of biliary drainage was cholecystoduodenostomy.[107] In addition to biliary fistula, this means of biliary drainage resulted in a high incidence of cholangitis and subsequent revision of the biliary drainage system was often required. There was also a high incidence of duodenal fistula. The ideal means of achieving primary biliary drainage is now considered to be a direct duct-to-duct anastomosis performed over a T-tube splint usually introduced through the donor cystic duct. This tube is left in place for up to 2 years. In cases where primary duct-to-duct anastomosis is not possible, for example where the recipient has sclerosing cholangitis then the preferred means of drainage is via cholecystojejunostomy to a Roux-en-Y loop of jejunum. This latter method has not been totally free of problems which result either from the development of an enteric fistula in the early postoperative period, or at a later stage the development of obstructive jaundice due to the blockage of the cystic duct by sludge.

Calne has preferred the use of the donor gallbladder as a type of common chamber to which both the donor and recipient common duct are anastomosed.[108] This anastomosis is then stented with a T tube.

The results of liver transplantation have steadily improved from the early years and this is again well illustrated by Starzl's results. Of the first 15 transplants only 5 one-year survivors resulted (30%). Among the last reported group of 30 there were 15 (50%). It is also informative to look at the subsequent fate of these one year survivors. Of the 31 who survived for 1 year and were transplanted during the period, March 1963 to July 1976, 14 were still alive at a follow-up of 3–9 years. Of the 15 one-year survivors of the period August 1976 to December 1977, 13 were still alive after $1-2\frac{1}{2}$ years. It was not an unreasonable generalization to say that those who survive to 1 year and are well are likely to achieve prolonged survival.[109]

A further hope for the future lies in the better means of immuno-supression which has recently been applied clinically. The first is the utilization of thoracic duct cannulation and the discarding of the lymphocytes in the fluid[110] and the second is the use of the immunosuppressive drug cyclosporin A.[111] With further advances in patient selection, patient management, surgical technique and immunosuppression, it is hoped that results of liver transplantation can be further improved to the stage when it will no longer be looked upon as an experimental technique.

REFERENCES

1. Cossart Y. E. (1977) *Viral Hepatitis and Its Control,* p. 5., London, Baillière Tindall & Cox.
2. Inman W. H. and Mushin W. W. (1978) Jaundice after repeated exposure to halothane: a further analysis of reports to the Committee on the Safety of Medicine. *Br. Med. J.* **2**, 1455–1456.
3. Vergani D., Eddleston A. L. W. F., Tsantoulas D. et al. (1978) Sensitization to halothane altered liver components in severe hepatic necrosis after halothane anaesthesia. *Lancet* **2**, 801–803.
4. Sherlock S. (1978) Halothane hepatitis. *Lancet* **2**, 364–365.
5. Schlippertt W. and Anoras S. (1978) Recurrent hepatitis following halothane exposures. *Am. J. Med.* **65**, 25–30.
6. Walton B., Simpson B. R., Strunm L. et al. (1978) Unexplained hepatitis following halothane. *Br. Med. J.* **1**, 1171–1176.
7. Miller D. J., Dwyer J. and Klatskin G. (1978) Halothane hepatitis: benign resolution of a severe lesion. *Ann. Intern. Med.* **89**, 212–215.
8. Sherlock S. (1979) Progress report: hepatic reactions to drugs. *Gut* **20**, 634–648.
9. Wauter S. J. P., Rossel C. and Farquet J. J. (1978) *Amanita Phalloides* poisoning treated by early charcoal haemoperfusion. *Br. Med. J.* **2**, 1465.
10. Trey C. (1972) The fulminant hepatic failure surveillance study: brief review of the effects of presumed aetiology and age on survival. *Can. Med. Assoc. J.* **106**, 525–527.
11. Adams D. and Foley T. (1949) Neurological changes in more types of severe liver disease. *Trans. Am. Neurol. Assoc.* **74**, 217–219.
12. Killenberg P. G., Stevens K. D., Wilderman R. F. et al. (1980) The laboratory as a variable in the interpretation of severe bilirubin fractionation. *Gastroenterology* **78**, 1011–1015.
13. Seliggohn V. and Shani M. (1977) The Dubin–Johnson syndrome and pregnancy. *Acta Hepatogastroenterol (Stuttg.)* **24**, 167–169.
14. Wolkoff A. W. (1979) Clinical conference. Crigler–Najjer syndrome (type 1) in an adult male. *Gastroenterology* **76**, 840–848.
15. Pollock T. W., Mullen J. L., Tsou K. L. et al. (1979) Serum 5-nucleotide phosphodiesterase as a predictor of hepatic metastases in gastrointestinal cancer. *Am. J. Surg.* **137**, 22–25.
16. Littlewood E. R., Barrison I. G., Murray-Lyon I. M. et al. (1980) Cholangiocarcinoma and oral contraceptives. *Lancet* **1**, 310–311.
17. Huard P. and Do Xuan Hop (1937) La ponction transhépatique des camaux biliaires. *Bull. Soc. Med.-Chir. De l'Indochine* **15**, 1090–1100.
18. Berry M., Norendranathon M., Rojaini M. et al. (1978) Chiba needle cholangiography in hepatobiliary diseases. *Australas. Radiol.* **22**, 139–144.
19. Rogos V. R., Rupha C. and Schaefer L. (1979) Perkutane transhepatische cholangiographie mit dunner nader. *Aetschft fur die Gesamte Inner Medzin* **34**, 97–101.
20. Jain S., Long R. G., Scott J. et al. (1977) Percutaneous transhepatic cholangiography using the Chiba needle—80 cases. *Br. J. Radiol.* **50**, 175–180.
21. Simert G., Lunderquist A., Tylen V. et al. (1978) Correlation between percutaneous transhepatic portography and clinical findings in 56 patients with portal hypertension. *Acta Clin. Scand.* **144**, 27–34.
22. Musha H., Takayasu K., Rakojima Y. et al. (1978) Percutaneous transhepatic portography III. Clinical significance of intrahepatic shunt index measured by this technique. *Acta Hepatol. Jap.* **19**, 871–879.
23. Kallio H. and Suranta H. (1979) Localization of occult insulin secreting tumours of the pancreas. *Ann. Surg.* **189**, 49–52.
24. Liguros C., Goubrou H., Chavy A. et al. (1974) Endoscopic retrograde cholangiopancreatography. *Br. J. Surg.* **61**, 359–362.

25. Lam J. K., Wong K. P., Chan P. K. W. et al. (1978) Fatal cholangitis after endoscopic retrograde chalangiopancreatogram in congenital hepatic fibrosis. *Aust. N.Z. J. Surg.* **45**, 199–202.
26. Vallon A. G., Lees W. R. and Cotton P. B. (1979) Grey scale ultrasonography in cholestatic jaundice. *Gut* **20**, 51–54.
27. McKay A. J., Duncan J. G., Lam P. et al. (1979) The role of grey scale ultrasonography in the investigation of jaundice. *Br. J. Surg.* **66**, 162–165.
28. Cosgrove D. O. and McCready :V. R. (1978) Diagnosis of liver metastases using ultrasound and isotope scanning techniques. *J. R. Soc. Med.* **71**, 652–657.
29. Morris A. I., Fawcett R. A., Wood K. et al. (1978) Computerised tomography. Ultrasound and cholestatic jaundice. *Gut* **19**, 685–688.
30. Raskin M. M. (1978) Hepatobiliary disease: a comparative evaluation by ultrasound and computed tomography. *Gastrointest. Radiol.* **3**, 267–271.
31. Pastakia B. (1980) Hepatobiliary imaging with ^{99m}Tc-labelled compounds. *Lancet* **1**, 153–154.
32. Kuroki T., Minowa T., Kawa M. et al. (1978) Evaluation of per rectal portal scintigraphy in hepatic cirrhosis. *Acta Hepatol. Jap.* **19**, 669–684.
33. Phillips M. M., Ramsby G. R. and Conn H. O. (1975) Portacaval anastomosis and peptic ulcer. *Gastroenterology* **68**, 121–131.
34. Conn H. O. (1973) Complications of portacaval anastomosis: by-products of a controlled investigation. *Gastroenterology* **59**, 207–220.
35. Fischer J. E. and Baldessarini R. J. (1971) False neurotransmitters and hepatic failure. *Lancet* **2**, 75–79.
36. Lam K. C., Tall A. R., Goldstein G. B. et al. (1973) Role of a false neurotransmitter, octopamine, in the pathogenesis of hepatic and renal encephalopathy. *Scand. J. Gastroenterol.* **8**, 465–472.
37. Manghani K. K., Lunzer M. R., Billing B. H. et al. (1975) Urinary and serum octopamine in patients with portal systemic encephalopathy. *Lancet* **2**, 943–946.
38. Lloyd K. G., Davidson L., Price K. et al. (1977) Catecholamine and octopamine concentrations in brains of patients with Reye's syndrome. *Neurology* **27**, 985–988.
39. Block P., Delorme M. C., Rapin Jr et al. (1978) Reversible modifications of neurotransmitters of the brain in experimental acute hepatic coma. *Surg. Gynecol. Obstet.* **146**, 551–558.
40. Rossi-Fanelli F., Cangiano C. and Attili A. (1976) Octopamine plasma levels and hepatic encephalopathy: a reapraisal of the problem. *Clin. Chim. Acta* **67**, 255–261.
41. Richmond J. and Girdwood R. H. (1962) Observations on aminoacid absorption. *Clin. Sci.* **22**, 301–314.
42. Guroff G. and Udenfriend S. (1962) Studies on aromatic aminoacid uptake by rat brain in vivo. *J. Biol. Chem.* **237**, 803.
43. Cascino A., Cangiano C., Calcaterra V. et al. (1978) Plasma aminoacid imbalance in patients with liver disease. *Dig. Dis.* **23**, 591–598.
44. Rodes J. (1978) *Symposium on Hepatorenal Syndrome.* 14th Congress of Internal Medicine. Rome, October 15–19.
45. Hovig T., Blornhoff J. P., Holme R. et al. (1978) Plasma lipoprotein alterations and morphologic changes with lipid deposition in the kidney of patients with the hepatorenal syndrome. *Lab. Invest.* **38**, 540–549.
46. Epstein M. (1979) Deranged sodium homeostasis in cirrhosis. *Gastroenterology* **76**, 622–635.
47. Sherlock S. (1978) *Water and Salt Metabolism in Liver Diseases.* 14th Congress of Internal Medicine. Rome, October 15–19.
48. Rosoff L., Williams J., Moult P. et al. (1979) Renal haemodynamics and the renin-angiotensin system in cirrhosis: relationship to sodium retention. *Dig. Dis. Sci.* **24**, 25–32.

49. Iwatsuki S., Popoutzer M. M., Cormann J. L. et al. (1973) Recovery from 'hepatorenal' syndrome after orthotopic liver transplantation. *N. Engl. J. Med.* **209**, 1155–1159.

50. Clubb A. W., and Giles C. (1968) Budd–Chiari syndrome after taking oral contraceptives. *Br. Med. J.* **1**, 252–253.

51. Stenflo J. (1974) Vitamin K and the biosynthesis of prothrombin. IV, Isolation of peptides containing prosthetic groups for normal prothrombin and corresponding peptides from dicoumarol-induced prothrombin. *J. Biol. Chem.* **249**, 5527–5535.

52. Koller F. (1973) Theory and experience behind the use of coagulation test in the diagnosis and prognosis of liver disease. *Scand. J. Gastroenterol. [Suppl 8]* **19**, 59–61.

53. Dymock I. W., Tucker J. S., Woolf I. L. et al. (1975) Coagulation studies as prognostic index in acute liver failure. *Br. J. Haematol.* **29**, 385–395.

54. Sullivan B. H. Jr, Tuner K. J. (1961) The effect of portacaval shunt on thrombocytopenia associated with portal hypertension. *Ann. Intern. Med.* **55**, 598–603.

55. Cowan D. J. (1973) Thrombokinetic studies in alcohol-related thrombocytopenia. *J. Lab. Clin. Med.* **81**, 64–76.

56. Roberts H. R. and Lederbaum A. I. (1972) The liver and blood coagulation: physiology and pathology. *Gastroenterology* **63**, 297–330.

57. Fletcher A. P., Biederman D., Moore D. et al. (1964) Abnormal plasminogen–plasmin system activity (fibrinolysis in patients with hepatic cirrhosis. *J. Clin. Invest.* **43**, 681–695.

58. Von Kaulla F. N., Kaye H., Von Kaulla E. et al. (1966) Changes in blood coagulation before and after hepatic transplantation in dogs and man. *Arch. Surg.* **92**, 71–79.

59. Swan K. G., Howard M. M., Rocko J. M. et al. (1980) Operative vasopressin and mesocaval shunting for portal hypertension. *Surgery* **87**, 46–51.

60. Miskowiak J. (1978) How the lower oesophageal sphincter affects submucosal oesophageal varices. *Lancet* **2**, 1284–1285.

61. Mallory A., Schaefer J. W., Cohen J. R. et al. (1980) Selective intra-arterial vasopressin infusion for upper gastrointestinal tract haemorrhage. *Arch. Surg.* **115**, 30–32.

62. Arousen K. F., Bjorkman I., Lindstrom K. et al. (1979) The mechanism of lysine-vasopressin haemostasis in bleeding oesophageal varices. *Acta Chir. Scand.* **145**, 231–234,

63. Tyden G., Samnegard H., Thulin L. et al. (1978) Treatment of bleeding oesophageal varices with somatostatin. *N. Engl. J. Med.* **299**, 1466–1467.

64. Conn H. O. and Simpson J. A. (1968) A rational programme for the diagnosis and treatment of bleeding oesophageal varices. *Med. Clin. North Am.* **82**, 1457.

65. Pitcher J. L. (1971) Safety and effectiveness of the modified Sengstaken–Blakemore tube: a prospective study. *Gastroenterology* **61**, 291.

66. Johnstone G. W. and Rodgers H. W. (1973) Experience in the use of sclerotherapy in the control of acute haemorrhage from oesophageal varices. *Br. J. Surg.* **60**, 797–800.

67. Terblanche J., Northoven J. M. A., Bornman P. et al. (1979) A prospective evaluation of injection sclerotherapy in the treatment of acute bleeding from oesophageal varices. *Surgery* **85**, 239–245.

68. Kirby R., Burke F. D. and Jones J. D. T. (1975) Emergency and elective surgical treatment of portal hypertension: a review of 23 years experience. *Ann. R. Coll. Surg.* **57**, 148–158.

69. Pugh R. N. H., Murray-Lyon I. M., Dawson J. L. et al. (1973) Transection of the oesophagus for bleeding oesophageal varices. *Br. J. Surg.* **60**, 646–649.

70. Johnston G. W. (1978) Simplified oesophageal transection for bleeding varices. *Br. Med. J.* **1**, 1288–1291.

71. Bengmark S., Borgesson B., Hoevels J. et al. (1979) Obliteration of oesophageal varices by PTP: a follow-up of 43 patients. *Ann. Surg.* **190**, 549–554.

72. Orloff M. J. (1967) Emergency portacaval shunt: a comparative study of shunt, varix ligation and non-surgical treatment of bleeding oesophageal varices in unselected patients with cirrhosis. *Ann. Surg.* **166**, 456.

73. Adamson R. J., Britt K., Iyer S. et al. (1978) Portacaval shunt with arterialization of the portal vein by means of a low flow arteriovenous fistula. *Surg. Gynecol. Obstet.* **146**, 869–876.

74. Maillard J. N., Flamont Y. M., Hay J. M. et al (1979) Selectivity of the distal splenorenal shunt. *Surgery* **86**, 363–371.

75. Busuttil R. W. and Tompkins R. K. (1979) Ramdomised control study of distal splenorenal and portacaval shunts in the treatment of bleeding oesophageal varices. *Am. J. Surg.* **138**, 62–67.

76. Warren W. D. (1978) A randomized controlled trial of the distal splenorenal shunt. *Ann. Surg.* **188**, 271–282.

77. Rosenthal D., Deterling R. A., O'Donnell R. F. et al. Interposition grafting with expanded polytetrafluoroethylene for portal hypertension. *Surg. Gynecol. Obstet.* **148**, 387–390.

78. Cameron J. L., Auiderman G. D., Smith G. W. et al. (1979) Mesocaval shunts for the control of bleeding oesophageal varices. *Surgery* **85**, 257–262.

79. Dowling J. B. (1979) Ten years experience with mesocaval shunts. *Surg. Gynecol. Obstet.* **149**, 518–522.

80. Reichler F. A., Fahrey W. F. and Golsorkhi M. (1979) Prospective comparative clinical trial with distal splenorenal and mesocaval shunts. *Am. J. Surg.* **137**, 13–21.

81. Orloff M. J. and Sohansen F. H. (1978) Treatment of Budd–Chiari syndrome by side-to-side portacaval shunt: experimental and clinical results. *Ann. Surg.* **188**, 494–512.

82. Fonkalsrud E. W., Kinde L. M. and Longuine W. P. (1966) Portal hypertension from idiopathic superior vena caval obstruction. *J. Am. Med. Assoc.* **196**, 129–139.

83. Chapman J. E. and Oshsner J. L. (1978) Iliac-mesenteric atrial shunt procedure for Budd–Chiari syndrome complicated by inferior vena caval thrombosis. *Ann. Surg.* **188**, 642–646.

84. Wapnick S., Grosberg S., Kinney M. et al. (1978) Renal failure in ascites secondary to hepatic, renal and pancreatic disease. Treatment with a Le Veen peritoneovenous shunt. *Arch. Surg.* **113**, 581–585.

85. Berkowitz H. D., Mullen J. L., Miller L. D. et al. (1978) Improved renal function and inhibition of renin and aldosterone secretion following peritoneovenous (Le Veen) shunt. *Surgery* **84**, 120–126.

86. Ausley J. D., Bethel R. A., Bowan P. A. et al. (1978) Effect of peritoneovenous shunting with the Le Veen valve on ascites renal function and coagulation in six patients with intractable ascites. *Surgery* **83**, 181–187.

87. Schwartz M. L., Swainn W. R. and Vogel S. B. (1979) Coagulopathy following peritoneovenous shunting. *Surgery* **85**, 671–676.

88. Report from the European Association for the Study of the Liver (1979) Randomised trial of steroid therapy in acute liver failure. *Gut* **20**, 620–623.

89. Redeker A. G. and Yamahiro H. S. (1973) Controlled trial of exchange transfusion therapy in fulminant hepatitis. *Lancet* **1**, 3–6.

90. Parbhoo S. P., Kennedy J., James I. M. et al. (1971) Extra-corporeal pig-liver perfusion in treatment of hepatic coma due to fulminant hepatitis. *Lancet* **1**, 659–664.

91. Abouna G. M., Serrov B., Boehmeg H. G. et al. (1970) Long-term hepatic support by intermittent multispecies liver perfusions. *Lancet* **2**, 391–396.

92. Opolon D., Huguet C. L., Bidallier M. et al. (1976) Haemodialysis versus cross haemodialysis in experimental hepatic coma. *Surg Gynecol. Obstet.* **142**, 845–854.

93. Chang D. (1972) *Artificial Cells.* Springfield, Illinois, U.S.A., Thomas.

94. Kolff W. J. (1971) Coated adsorbents for direct blood perfusion: haema/activated charcoal. *Trans. Am. Soc. Artif. Intern. Organs.* **17**, 222–228.

95. Fennimore J., Watson P. A., Munro G. D. et al. (1974) The design and evaluation of a convenient carbon haemoperfusion system. *Proc. Eur. Soc. Artif. Organs* 1, 90–99.
96. Gazzard B. G., Portmann B., Weston M. J. et al. (1974) Charcoal haemoperfusion in the treatment of fulminant hepatic failure. *Lancet* 1, 1301–1307.
97. Thysell H., Lindholm T., Heinegard D. et al. (1976) A haemoperfusion column using cellophane coated charcoal. *Proc. Eur. Soc. Artif. Organs* 2, 212–215.
98. Amano I., Kano H., Saito A. et al. (1976) Efficacy of petroleum charcoal haemoperfusion and acetate free dialysate in 10 patients with hepatic coma. *Proc. Eur. Dial. Transplant. Assoc.* 13, 262–272.
99. Castino F., Scheucher F., Malchesky P. S. et al. (1976) Microemboli-free blood detoxification utilizing plasma filtration. *Trans. Am. Soc. Artif. Intern. Organs* 22, 637–645.
100. Williams R. (1979) Trials and tribulations with artificial liver support. *Gut* 19, 578–583.
101. Welch C. S. (1955) A note on transplantation of the whole liver in dogs. *Transplant. Bull.* 2, 54–55.
102. Starzl T. E., Marchioro T. L., Von Kaulla K. N. et al. (1963) Homotransplantation of the liver in humans. *Surg. Gynecol. Obstet.* 117, 659–676.
103. Absolom K. B., Hagihara P. F., Griffen W. O. Jr et al. (1965) Experimental and clinical heterotopic liver homotransplantation. *Rev. Int. Hepatol.* 15, 1481–1490.
104. Crosier J. H., Immelman E. J., Van Hoorn-Hickman R. et al. (1980) Cholecystojejuno-cholecystostomy: a new method of biliary drainage in auxiliary liver allotransplantation. *Surgery* 87, 514–523.
105. Calne R. Y., McMaster P., Portmann B. et al. (1977) Observations on preservation bile drainage and rejection. *Ann. Surg.* 6, 282–290.
106. Hood J. M., Koep L. J., Peters T. L. et al. (1980) Liver transplantation for advanced liver disease with alpha-1-antitrypsin deficiency. *N. Engl. J. Med.* 302, 272–274.
107. Starzl T. E., Porter K. A., Putnam C. W. et al. (1976) Biliary complications after liver transplantation with special reference to the biliary cast syndrome and techniques of secondary duct repair. *Surgery* 81, 213–221.
108. Calne R. Y. (1976) A new technique for biliary drainage in orthotopic liver transplantation utilizing the gallbladder as a pedicle graft conduit between donor and recipient common bile ducts. *Ann. Surg.* 184, 605–609.
109. Starzl T. E., Koep L. J., Schorter G. P. J. et al. (1979) The quality of life after liver transplantation. *Transplant. Proc.* 11, 252–256.
110. Starzl T. E., Koep L. J., Halgrimson C. G. et al. (1979) Liver transplantation 1978. *Transplant. Proc.* 11, 240–246.
111. Calne R. Y., McMaster P. and Evans D. B. (1980) Cyclosporin A and the media. *Br. Med. J.* 1, 43.

Chapter 19

The Renal System

M. E. M. Allison and A. C. Kennedy

'Bones can break, muscles can atrophy, glands can loaf, even the brain go to sleep, without immediately endangering our survival, but when the kidneys fail . . . neither bone, muscle, gland nor brain can carry on.'

H. W. Smith, 1943

Failure of the kidneys to fulfil their essential function is an ever present threat to any patient requiring intensive care. At least five essential factors are required for successful kidney action (*Table* 19.1); disturbance or loss of one or more of these results in renal insufficiency. At the outset, it is important to have a brief account of terms commonly used in clinical practice in dealing with patients with acute renal failure.

Table **19.1. Factors essential for normal renal function**

1. Sufficient numbers of functioning nephrons
2. Adequate renal blood flow, correctly distributed throughout kidney
3. Normal glomerular permeability
4. Intact tubule cell structure and function
5. No obstruction to outflow of urine from the kidney

Potential acute renal failure is particularly common in the critically ill patient in association with a number of high risk factors (*Table* 19.2). In these situations the initial changes in renal function are often easily understandable in physiological terms and potentially reversible, if appreciated and dealt with expeditiously. This situation has been termed pre-renal failure.

Established acute renal failure should be defined simply as a rise in

486

Table 19.2. **Patients at risk of acute renal failure**

Surgical	1. Hypotension (trauma, endotoxins)
	2. Hypovolaemia (haemorrhage, burns)
	3. Infection (endotoxaemia, peritonitis)
	4. Jaundice
Medical	1. Hypotension (cardiac failure)
	2. Nephrotoxins (aminoglycosides, radiocontrast agents, *cis*-platinum, methotrexate, uric acid)
	3. Infection (pneumonia)
	4. Respiratory failure and hypoxia
Obstetric	1. Hypotension and hypovolaemia (antepartum and postpartum haemorrhage)
	2. Eclampsia
	3. Infection (septic abortion)

endogenous serum creatinine concentration above normal in a patient with previously good renal function and which persists despite absence or correction of adverse haemodynamic or obstructive factors. This rise in the level of nitrogenous waste products in the blood is due to the sudden decrease in whole kidney glomerular filtration rate (GFR) and is generally associated with oliguria (< 400–500 ml urine per day). It is still commonly referred to as acute tubular necrosis. However, non-oliguric or high output acute renal failure is also a significant problem and probably occurs more frequently than is generally recognized.[1-3] In a recent prospective study, Anderson[2] observed that 54 out of 92 patients with progressive azotaemia, had urine volumes in excess of 600 ml per day. In 80% of these patients urine volumes exceeded 1 litre per day. While the morbidity and mortality in this group were lower than in oliguric patients, non-oliguric acute renal failure can be difficult to manage clinically and often frustrates clinicians in charge of intensive care units. Thus it is misleading simply to measure daily urine volumes since this does not reflect whole kidney GFR or renal concentrating ability, both of which are impaired in all forms of acute renal failure.

Acute-on-chronic renal failure should be defined as a sudden progressive rise in serum creatinine concentration in a patient known to have longstanding renal impairment and hence a low GFR. In clinical practice, serum creatinine concentration is an acceptable indicator of GFR, although some transtubular transport of creatinine undoubtedly occurs and endogenous creatinine production is dependent on muscle mass. However, as the GFR falls serum creatinine concentration will rise exponentially (*Fig.* 19.1). In the patient with chronic renal failure any further small fall in GFR due, for example, to haemorrhage or hypotension, will cause a steep rise in serum creatinine concentration. These patients, therefore, form a special risk category.

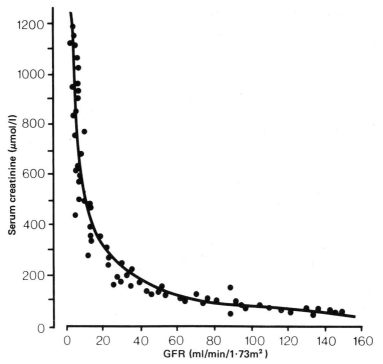

Fig. 19.1. Dependence of serum creatinine concentration (μmol/l) on GFR (ml per min per 1·73 m²) in patients with a wide range of renal function. A fall in GFR (glomerular filtration rate) of 50%, approximately doubles the serum creatinine concentration. Thus a 'small' rise in serum creatinine concentration (e.g. 100 → 200 μmol/l) indicates an approximate 50% fall in whole kidney function.

INCIDENCE

Published figures on the incidence of acute renal failure from large medical centres in Europe and North America over the last 15 years are remarkably consistent, most reporting an incidence in adults of 20–40 patients per year requiring dialysis.[4–6] *Table* 19.3 gives the figures from the Renal Unit of

Table **19.3 Number of patients with acute renal failure managed in Glasgow Royal Infirmary**

	1959–70	*1976–80*
Surgical	133 (53·8%)	103 (53%)
Medical	56 (22·7%)	87 (44%)
Obstetric	62 (23·5%)	6 (3%)
Total	251	196
Average incidence	23 per year	40 per year

Glasgow Royal Infirmary over an initial 11-year period (1959–70) and more recently for a further 5 years (1976–80). Three groups of patients have been distinguished, surgical, medical and obstetric, based on the nature of the precipitating incident (*Table* 19.2). Despite advances in intensive care, the overall incidence of acute renal failure over these years has not changed greatly, the major exception being the virtual disappearance of acute renal failure due to abortion since 1976. The increased number of patients with a 'medical' cause during 1976–80 was due to a rise in the ingestion of dangerous nephrotoxins, such as paraquat and paracetamol, and to an increase in the incidence of acute renal failure related to infection.

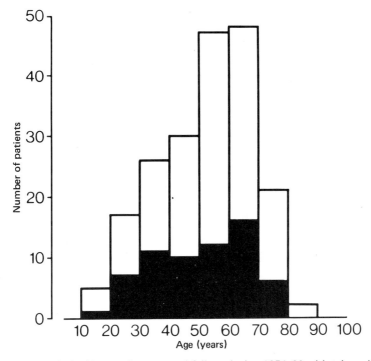

Fig. 19.2. Increase in incidence of acute renal failure during 1976–80 with advancing years, peak incidence being in the 60–70 year age group. This trend is still present, although not so obvious, in patients with respiratory failure (■) who subsequently developed acute renal failure.

The incidence of acute renal failure increases with increasing patient age (*Fig.* 19.2) and is particularly high in certain situations. Thus, patients with pre-existing respiratory failure being managed in a respiratory intensive care unit have a 10% incidence of acute renal insufficiency[7] while the incidence in 2191 patients admitted to a general trauma unit in the United States during 1973–77 was only 1·5%.[3]

PATHOPHYSIOLOGICAL MECHANISMS IN
ACUTE RENAL FAILURE

Pathology

Changes in function of an organ or its component cells might be expected to be reflected in changes in structure. Acute renal failure is no exception. Reported alterations vary from gross necrosis of proximal tubule cells, easily visible on light microscopy or microdissection, to minute changes in the electron microscopic appearance of the glomerular capillary wall. In addition, progress in cell biology now permits the study of enzyme function of intracellular structures. Thus, subtle changes in mitochondrial structure and function have been detected within 24 hours of injection of folic acid, a known nephrotoxic agent, into rats.[8]

Historically, the Second World War tragically provided considerable opportunity for the study of the pathological changes which accompany acute renal failure. Thus the victims of air raids, dying after severe crushing injury and associated shock, often had acute renal insufficiency despite absence of direct kidney damage. Histological examination of their kidneys at autopsy showed degenerative changes in the tubules and the presence of numerous intratubular casts.[9] Both the precise nature and the pathogenesis of these lesions, however, remained in dispute until 1951. In that year Dr Oliver published his monumental microdissection studies of these and other kidneys from patients dying with acute renal failure and from experimentally-induced nephrotoxic and ischaemic renal failure in animals.[11]

Two basic defects were described. First, the so-called nephrotoxic lesion, with widespread generalized necrosis of renal tubule cells. This was found primarily after ingestion of specific nephrotoxins, such as mercuric chloride.

Second, the ischaemic lesion which he called 'tubulorhexic'. This lesion consists of localized destruction of the entire tubule wall and, while it can be found in any part of the nephron, the ascending limb of the loop of Henlé and distal tubule are its most frequent sites. It should be emphasized that both types of lesion frequently occur together in a single patient. Thus ingestion of a nephrotoxin with generalized tubule necrosis is often followed by a period of shock and ischaemia and thus tubulorhexis. In addition to these lesions, all kidneys examined showed evidence of intratubular casts and peritubular inflammatory reaction.

Dr Oliver felt that 'the situation is much too complex to be covered by any meaningful term' since it is impossible to 'find a phrase that covers everything and describes nothing'. Today the term 'acute tubular necrosis' is often used to describe these pathological changes. In fact, extensive necrosis of tubular epithelial cells is an uncommon finding on renal biopsy of patients during acute renal failure. Thus, a recent examination of 57 renal biopsies from patients with acute renal failure[12] showed that, while necrosis of individual tubular epithelial cells does occur, by far the most common lesion is an absence of the proximal tubular brush border. Interestingly, kidney material from patients with non-oliguric acute renal failure was remarkably similar to that from patients with oliguric renal impairment.

Regeneration of normal epithelium after severe toxic or ischaemic injury in the rat is complete within four weeks. Recovery is probably even quicker in man, although it has been observed that peritubular inflammatory changes can persist well into the recovery phase long after the cells themselves have returned to normal.[12]

The glomeruli are usually described as showing few structural abnormalities in acute renal failure, although deposition of fibrin and platelets corresponding to intravascular thrombosis has been described, especially after endotoxic shock.[13] Recently endothelial and epithelial cell swelling and distortion of foot processes have been described on electron microscopy of glomeruli from animals with experimental acute renal failure due to norepinephrine or mercuric chloride. As yet these have not been reported in human acute renal failure and their relationship to changes in glomerular permeability remains speculative.[14]

Pathophysiology

The relatively simple clinical definition of established acute renal failure given at the beginning covers a complex multitude of changes in kidney physiology. Advances in our understanding of these have, of necessity, been made largely from studies of a wide variety of animal models of renal impairment (*Table* 19.4).

Table 19.4. Animal models of acute renal failure

Primarily nephrotoxic	Mercuric chloride
	Aminoglycosides
	Uranyl nitrate
	Uric acid
	Folic acid
	Uranium
	Lead
	cis-Platinum
Primarily vasomotor	Clamp renal artery for 1 hour
	Infuse norepinephrine into renal artery
	Haemorrhage and retransfusion
	Intramuscular glycerol
	Intravenous endotoxin

Four basic mechanisms have been accepted as occurring in all of them: renal vasoconstriction, tubular obstruction, a fall in glomerular ultra-filtration coefficient and back leakage of filtrate across damaged tubular epithelium. The pathogenesis of acute renal failure has been the subject of several excellent recent reviews.[15-18] *Fig.* 19.3 summarizes our knowledge and is adapted from Stein et al.[15] and Schrier et al.[18] The relative significance of each mechanism varies both with the model studied and with the time course of the development of the acute renal failure; there is no single unifying concept of acute renal failure.

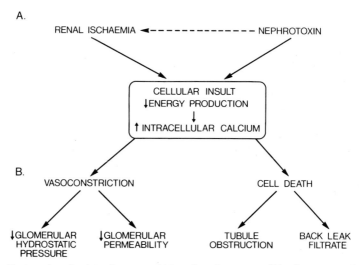

Fig. 19.3. Factors involved in the onset (A) and maintenance (B) of acute renal failure.

While some of the animal models studied are of questionable direct relevance to the human situation, two models have been particularly useful to the clinician, namely, the ischaemic kidney and the effect of aminoglycosides.

An experimentally induced severe and reproducible model of ischaemic acute renal failure can be produced in the rat by cross-clamping the renal artery for one hour.[16,17] The presence of the contralateral kidney ensures the survival of the animal and allows sequential observations of the recovery phase to be made. The course of renal failure in this model can be divided into three phases: an initial phase, a maintenance phase and an early and late recovery phase.

In the initial 24 hours after release of the clamp, there is a profound fall in urine flow rate, a reduction in GFR to less than 2% of control values and a fall in renal blood flow of 20–50%. Despite this fall in renal blood flow, however, glomerular capillary hydrostatic pressure is within the normal range; urine flow rate falls due to obstruction of each nephron by sloughing of brush border microvilli and their subsequent impactment in straight segments of the proximal tubule. Very high intratubular hydrostatic pressures can be measured above the block. Restoration of renal blood flow to control values by volume expansion with isotonic sodium chloride does not improve the situation.

Twenty-four hours after removal of the clamp, renal failure is maintained by a further fall in renal blood flow due to a marked increase in preglomerular vascular resistance. Glomerular capillary hydrostatic pressure then falls and single nephron filtration capability declines markedly. In addition, there is also evidence of back leakage of glomerular filtrate across the damaged tubular epithelium.

Interestingly, less severe ischaemia results in a high output type of non-oliguric renal impairment. This is presumably due to continued filtration in nephrons without severe cell damage and hence obstruction, but which are still unable to reabsorb the filtered load. High dose levels of barbiturates given in conjunction with the ischaemic episodes can convert a potential non-oliguric to an oliguric renal impairment, presumably due to reduction in metabolic requirements of tubular cells under the influence of these drugs.

Recovery occurs in a biphasic manner over the following 1–4 weeks. First there is regeneration and repair of tubular epithelium with a decrease in transtubular leakage and a loss of intratubular casts. Later there is progressive vasodilatation, a rise in glomerular hydrostatic pressure and a return of glomerular filtration towards normal. There is some evidence that a high salt intake during this recovery phase may be beneficial in hastening the improvement in filtration rate.

In contrast, the factors involved in the induction of renal impairment during administration of the aminoglycoside antibiotic gentamicin are somewhat different. This substance is now widely used in intensive care units, but it is capable of direct nephrotoxic damage in experimental animals even at doses considered to be safe in clinical practice. Serious nephrotoxic side effects are reported in man,[19] often in the form of non-oliguric acute renal failure.

Two phenomena have been found to account for this impairment. First, there is extensive necrosis of tubule cells, most marked on the tenth day of injection in rats, when 75–90% of the outer cortical tubules are necrotic. Surprisingly, microinjection studies have revealed no evidence of transtubular leakage and full recovery of these lesions eventually occurs despite continued administration of high doses of gentamicin.

Second, and more interestingly, there is a fall in single glomerular nephron filtration rate due to a marked fall in the glomerular capillary ultrafiltration coefficient. This factor can now be measured directly in surface glomeruli of a certain strain of rats. The ultrafiltration coefficient is determined by the surface area available for filtration and the hydraulic conductivity of the glomerular capillary wall. A decrease in ultrafiltration coefficient has also been noted with the nephrotoxic agent uranyl nitrate.

In the experimental animal, gentamicin nephrotoxicity rarely results in uraemic deaths unless intravascular volume is depleted, either by dietary salt restriction or frequent phlebotomy. This is of obvious relevance to the clinical situation where maintenance of correct fluid balance is of primary importance in the management of acute renal failure.

The precise mechanisms by which these changes in renal vascular resistance, renal blood flow and glomerular permeability occur remain speculative. A rise in angiotensin II production, with subsequent afferent arteriolar vasoconstriction and a fall in glomerular capillary ultrafiltration coefficient, or a defect in prostaglandin production have been suggested, but not proven. Schrier et al.[18] have recently emphasized the critical role of intracellular calcium, anoxia or nephrotoxic damage resulting in a rise in cytosolic calcium and subsequent cell death (*Fig.* 19.3).

MANAGEMENT

All patients requiring intensive care should be considered as potential candidates for developing acute renal failure. The basic objectives of their management can be considered under four headings, depending on the stage of evolution of their illness.

1. Recognize early those at Particular Risk

While all patients requiring intensive care are at risk of developing acute renal failure, it is well recognized that the incidence of this problem is increased in specific situations (*Table* 19.2). These patients merit even more scrupulous attention to continuous monitoring of fluid balance state and renal function. In addition to routine measurements of serum creatinine, electrolytes and urinary sodium excretion, repeated clinical examination for evidence of hypovolaemia, electrolyte imbalance or infection is absolutely essential. It has been shown that the main aetiological factors precipitating renal failure in the intensive care unit are gastrointestinal bleeding, leading to hypovolaemia and shock, sepsis, drug nephrotoxicity (especially aminoglycosides) and hypotension; these four problems accounted for 78% of the cases of renal failure reported between 1974 and 1977 in a respiratory intensive care unit. In addition there is an increased susceptibility to acute renal failure in patients with liver impairment in whom administration of intravenous mannitol and saline, before and during surgery, has been shown to reduce the incidence of this complication.[20]

II. Analyse the Significance of Oliguria

Oliguria due to potentially reversible prerenal factors must be differentiated from oliguria due to established acute renal failure (acute tubular necrosis). This is extremely important and often presents the inexperienced physician with undue difficulty. Differentiation is based on several factors derived from the history, clinical examination and simple biochemical measurements. In some patients an intravenous pyelogram may also be useful.

Careful clinical examination is essential to detect evidence of hypovolaemia, hypotension or cardiac failure. Acute or acute-on-chronic extrarenal obstructive uropathy should be suspected if the patients become virtually anuric, if there is swelling or tenderness of the kidneys or if there is any clinical or radiological suspicion of bladder, ureteric or pelvic obstruction.

Table 19.5. Significance of oliguria

	Pre-renal oliguria	Acute renal failure
Urine osmolality, mosmol/kg	> 500	< 350
Urine/plasma osmolality ratio	> 1·2	< 1·05
Urine sodium, mmol/l	< 20	> 40
Urine/plasma creatinine	> 40	< 20
Fractional excretion sodium*	< 1	> 1
Not helpful: Proteinuria, urine microscopy, height of blood urea		

$$* FE_{Na} = \frac{(U/P) \text{ sodium}}{(U/P) \text{ creatinine}} \times 100.$$

Table 19.5 lists the simple biochemical measurements which can be made on initial evaluation of the problem. It should be emphasized that urine samples must obviously be obtained as fresh as possible and before the administration of diuretics or mannitol. At first, a high urine osmolality and a high urine-to-plasma osmolality ratio are of great help since this generally indicates reasonably intact kidney physiology and a 'normal' physiological response to hypovolaemia, etc. These patients thus require immediate attention to prerenal factors such as correction of fluid and electrolyte deficits and not the administration of inappropriate diuretics. Espinel and Gregory[21] compared the usefulness of these various measurements in achieving the correct diagnosis in a series of 87 patients with acute renal failure. The fractional excretion of sodium was identified as the single most effective non-invasive test, a value greater than one indicating acute tubular necrosis or urinary tract obstruction and less than one being associated with prerenal oliguria or acute glomerulonephritis.

High-dose intravenous pyelography[22] can be useful in patients in whom there is no apparent reason for acute renal failure. It is helpful in establishing whether obstruction is the cause and may help to distinguish between acute tubular necrosis (an early persisting nephrogram) and unsuspected chronic renal disease (an early but faint persisting nephrogram with kidneys usually reduced in size).

III. Consider the Use of Mannitol, Frusemide or Dopamine Hydrochloride

The concept behind the use of these drugs is that the development of acute renal failure may be prevented or attenuated in the early stages by the promotion of a solute diuresis (mannitol or frusemide), by renal vaso-dilatation (mannitol or dopamine) or by alterations in cellular metabolism.

Mannitol

Isotonic or hypertonic mannitol was the earliest drug used[23, 24] and has proved to be the best substance currently available for the prophylaxis of acute renal failure in high risk situations, by virtue of its ability to increase solute excretion and raise intratubular hydrostatic pressure and hence flow rate. In addition, it may help to prevent cell swelling due to anoxia and reduce the associated rise in intracellular calcium which precipitates cell death.[18] Thus jaundiced patients undergoing surgery or those having major aortic surgery should receive mannitol together with adequate intravenous saline replacement before and during operation.[20] It should be given therapeutically for the immediate treatment of nephrotoxins such as myoglobulin, uric acid or low-molecular-weight dextran, all of which cause very significant intratubular obstruction. Careless or inappropriate use of mannitol, however, may cause pulmonary oedema or dangerous hypo-natraemia, especially when used in large quantities in those with incipient cardiac failure.

Frusemide

The use of this diuretic (and others such as bumetanide or ethacrynic acid) has been widely advocated in the early stages of potential acute renal failure, when 250–1000 mg are given intravenously as a single dose or by infusion. A rise in solute excretion and intratubular pressure usually follows. The use of daily high dose frusemide has been claimed to shorten the duration of the oliguric phase of acute renal failure,[25] but this has not been confirmed by others.[26]

Indiscriminate use of high dose frusemide is dangerous. Serious hypovol-aemia may result in an already compromised patient, unless adequate fluid replacement is given. There is evidence that the drug can potentiate the nephrotoxicity of various antibiotics and temporary or permanent deafness can occur, especially if gentamicin has also been given. Repeated high dose use of this drug in the management of acute renal failure, is, therefore, not advocated.

Dopamine

Henderson et al[27] have reported favourably on the use of a low dose dopamine hydrochloride infusion ($1\mu g \cdot kg^{-1} \cdot min^{-1}$ for 12 hours) in acutely oliguric patients who had not responded to 250 or 500 mg frusemide. The majority of patients produced an increased volume of urine which lessened the problems of management and may have reduced dialysis requirements. Although promising, the study was uncontrolled and further experience will be required. However, Henderson et al. noted that the dosage of dopamine was low, that they found it easy to use and free from side effects, such as nausea, vomiting, tachycardia and arrhythmias and no dependence developed allowing withdrawal of the drug without recurrence of oliguria.

Table 19.6. Management of potential, early acute renal failure

1. Treat primary ischaemic or toxic event
2. Restore effective circulatory blood volume—plasma
3. Catheterize and measure hourly urinary indices: volume, osmolality, sodium excretion, before diuretics or dopamine
4. If (3) indicates pre-renal oliguria continue and/or increase fluid infusion and increase cardiac output
5. If (3) indicates possible acute renal failure but U/P osmolality ratio still >1.05 and duration of oliguria is <48 hours with no cardiac failure, give 100 ml 20% mannitol over 15 minutes, up to twice
6. If as (5) but with gross cardiac failure or pulmonary oedema, no nephrotoxin exposure, give frusemide 250–1000 mg i.v. over 10–30 minutes
7. If hypotensive despite plasma consider dopamine 1 μg per kg body weight per minute, probably in conjunction with mannitol or frusemide

Table 19.6 outlines our general approach to the problem of an oliguric patient with potential acute renal failure. In experimental animals, mannitol and frusemide are most effective when given before the insult used to initiate acute renal failure, when the degree of protection is directly proportional to the rate of solute excretion produced by the drug. All agree that, after an insult, treatment must be very prompt to achieve success. Some patients go through an early stage when mannitol may produce a diuresis and rise in GFR. We found that these patients could often be predicted on the basis of the U/P osmolality ratio ($> 1·05$) and the short duration of oliguria (< 48 hours) provided shock had been corrected.[24]

Other Drugs

A variety of other substances have been used both in experimental animals and in man to attempt prevention or reversal of acute renal failure, but have either not proved very successful or have failed to gain acceptance in clinical practice. These include prostaglandins (PGE_2), angiotensin inhibitors, adrenergic blocking agents and hydralazine. A recent exciting development has been the observation that the prevention of a rise in intracellular calcium by the drug verapamil, which blocks the cellular uptake of calcium, can greatly attenuate the acute renal failure produced in experimental animals by intrarenal infusion of norepinephrine. [28] Further studies on the intracellular mechanisms involved in the onset of acute renal failure are awaited.

IV. Apply Effective Management for Established Acute Renal Failure

The principles of management for established acute renal failure are control of fluid balance, control of electrolytes, especially potassium, provision of adequate calories and amino acids, control of infection, provision of adequate dialysis, and continuing attention to the underlying cause and careful scrutiny for developing complications.

1. Fluid Balance

The basic daily requirement is 600 ml plus replacement of measured fluid losses (urine, gastric aspirate, diarrhoea, fistula drainage, etc.) and correction of any continuing fluid deficit. It is essential to avoid dehydration which can only prejudice recovery of renal function and also to avoid over-hydration with its attendant dangers of acute left ventricular failure. The patient must be examined daily, noting tissue turgor and the presence or absence of oedema. Serum albumin concentration should be measured frequently. If possible the patient should be weighed daily. Central venous pressure measurements are invaluable in critically ill patients or if the clinician has any doubts about fluid balance in individual patients.

2. Diet

It is essential to provide adequate calories, protein and amino acids to minimize the patient's own tissue breakdown and to encourage healing. The route of administration is dictated by the clinical situation but there is good evidence that those patients able to take an adequate balanced diet by mouth do best and this should be encouraged at all times.[29] An intake of 0·25 g of protein per kg body weight can be associated with normal nitrogen balance, provided calorie intake is high and essential amino acids are given. The role of intensive intravenous feeding in improving the mortality rate in those patients unable to eat or severely hypercatabolic is still debated. Details of parenteral nutrition are given elsewhere (Chapter 7). In acute renal failure it has been proposed that provision of essential L-amino acids and adequate calories as glucose could improve nitrogen balance and decrease urea production rate.[30] This remains unproven. Uraemia, per se, is associated with the development of peripheral insulin resistance and hence it is recommended that blood sugar is checked frequently and insulin added as required to the amino acid and glucose regime.

3. Electrolytes

The general rule is restriction of sodium and potassium, unless there is biochemical or clinical evidence of depletion or losses from the various body fluids. Hyperkalaemia (plasma potassium concentration over 6·0 mmol/l) is the main danger and can be treated as an emergency for a few hours by intravenous soluble insulin (20 units) and glucose (25 g). In addition, correction of acidosis, which promotes movement of potassium from serum into the cells and administration of intravenous calcium gluconate (20 ml, 10%), which has a cardio-protective effect are also worthwhile. In the long term, ion-exchange resins are used (e.g. sodium or calcium resonium, 30 g twice daily). Dialysis is very effective in removing potassium.

4. Infection

Infection is very commonly present or develops in patients with acute renal failure in intensive care units. There is experimental evidence that acute uraemia per se is detrimental to immunological function. Wherever possible, vigorous attempts should be made to identify the organism, or organisms, responsible, identify drug sensitivities, and monitor the dosage of antibiotics by frequent estimations of blood levels. Further details of management of infection are given in Chapter 9.

5. *Dialysis*

Dialysis should be commenced early in patients with established acute renal failure, particularly if they are hypercatabolic, when there is good evidence that intensive 'prophylactic' dialysis is beneficial in improving morbidity and mortality.[31] In addition it should enable better nutritional support. No patient with acute renal failure should be permitted to die from uraemia or from electrolyte imbalance; if death does occur, it should only be because of the development of progressive and unmanageable complications such as infection or because of continuation of the basic problem such as respiratory or cardiac failure.

Both haemodialysis, using either an arteriovenous shunt or a veno-venous route via a large central vein, or peritoneal dialysis are available. Peritoneal dialysis is simple to perform and certainly has a significant role to play in the management of chronic renal failure. However, in acute renal failure, especially in hypercatabolic states, it is much less satisfactory. Relative contra-indications to peritoneal dialysis include paralytic ileus or recent abdominal surgery. Respiratory problems may be precipitated by peritoneal dialysis because of impairment of diaphragmatic movement and the patient can find it painful and tiring. Haemodialysis is generally preferable, especially for hypercatabolic acute renal failure patients, but may be technically difficult in those with persisting hypotension, which renders extracorporeal circulation difficult, if not impossible, and severe cardiac failure. Rarely, a haemorrhagic state makes heparinization for haemodialysis hazardous.

Dialysis also enables fluid removal as well as removal of end products of nitrogenous metabolism. This is very useful as it permits a more liberal fluid intake and easier provision of calories, etc.

6. *Gastrointestinal Bleeding*

The use of H_2-receptor antagonists appears to have reduced the incidence of gastrointestinal haemorrhage in established acute renal failure.

7. *Recovery Phase*

The duration of oliguria in most series is around 10–12 days, but occasionally may be much longer, for 30 or more days. Thereafter, daily urine volumes rise rapidly and carefully controlled fluid replacement is essential. Urinary potassium losses are high, and potassium supplements may be required.

PROGNOSIS

Figures published on the mortality rate of patients with acute renal failure make grim reading, ranging from 37%[6] to 85%.[32] Distressingly, despite advances in intensive care, these figures have not improved over recent years. Thus, in Glasgow Royal Infirmary, during 1959–70, we reported an overall mortality rate of 44%,[5] while our mortality rate for 1976–80 is 58%.

Prognostic index scoring systems have been devised by several groups.[6, 33] Six factors are apparent which obviously influence prognosis: age, infection, respiratory failure, liver impairment, gastro-intestinal bleeding and the underlying cause of the acute renal failure. Thus, acute pancreatitis complicated by the problem carries almost 100% mortality, while renal failure complicating respiratory failure or severe jaundice has a mortality rate of approximately 80%[7, 32]. These factors are considered in *Table* 19.7. However, it should be emphasized that recovery is still possible even with a combination of several adverse features and prediction of a lethal outcome in any one patient is impossible.[6, 34] We, therefore, believe that if any of these are present or develop during the course of acute renal failure, therapy should be intensified rather than lessened or withdrawn.

Table **19.7. Prognostic indices**

Mortality	Patients
High	Age >60 years; peritonitis or other infection; acute pancreatitis; pre-existing liver impairment (jaundice); on assisted ventilation
Intermediate	Age <50 years, but with infection or other complications
Low	Age <50 years; not infected; specific nephrotoxins (e.g. aminoglycosides); methaemoglobulinuria; acute hypovolaemia quickly corrected (e.g. postpartum haemorrhage); non-oliguric acute renal failure of any age
BUT—Recovery still possible even with combination of several adverse features	

RENAL FUNCTION AFTER RECOVERY

In contrast to the high immediate mortality rate, the long-term outlook for the patient who recovers from acute renal failure is excellent, at least in respect of renal function. Knowledge of this makes management of the uncomplicated patient extremely satisfying. The patient almost always is restored to normal blood urea and electrolyte values. Detailed study carried out at least one year after an episode of acute renal failure in 50 patients showed that in 87%, the glomerular filtration rate exceeded 50 ml/h.[35] Long-term regular dialysis therapy is not generally required, unless the episode has been one of acute-on-chronic renal failure.

REFERENCES

1. Levinsky N. G. and Alexander F. A. (1976) Acute renal failure. In: Brenner B. M. and Rector F. C. Jr, eds. *The Kidney*, pp. 806–837. Philadelphia, W. B. Saunders.
2. Anderson R. J., Linas S. L., Berns A. S. et al. (1977) Nonoliguric acute renal failure. *N. Engl. J. Med.* **296**, 1134–1138.
3. Shin B., MacKenzie C. F., McAslan T. C. et al. (1979) Postoperative renal failure in trauma patients. *Anesthesiology* **51**, 218–221.
4. Stott R. B., Cameron J. S., Ogg C. S. et al. (1972) Why the persistently high mortality in acute renal failure ? *Lancet* **1**, 75–79.
5. Kennedy A. C., Burton J. A., Luke R. G. et al. (1973) Factors affecting the prognosis in acute renal failure. *Q. J. Med.* **42**, 73–86.
6. McMurray S. D., Luft F. C., Maxwell D. R. et al. (1978) Prevailing patterns and predictor variables in patients with acute tubular necrosis. *Arch. Intern. Med.* **138**, 950–955.
7. Kraman S., Khan F., Patel S. et al. (1979) Renal failure in the respiratory intensive care unit. *Crit. Care Med.* **7**, 263–266.
8. Kirschbaum B. B. (1979) Alterations in mitochondrial properties in folate nephropathy. *Nephron* **24**, 297–301.
9. Bywaters E. G. L. and Beall D. (1941) Crush injuries with impairment of renal function. *Br. Med. J.* **2**, 427–432.
10. Dunn J. S., Gillespie M. and Niven J. S. F. (1941) Renal lesions in two cases of crush syndrome. *Lancet* **1**, 549–552.
11. Oliver J., MacDowell M. and Tracy, A. (1951) The pathogenesis of acute renal failure associated with traumatic or toxic injury. Renal ischemia, nephrotoxic damage and the ischemuric episode. *J. Clin. Invest.* **30**, 1307–1439.
12. Solez K., Morel-Maroger L. and Sraer J. D. (1979) The morphology of 'Acute Tubular Necrosis' in man. Analysis of 57 renal biopsies and a comparison with the glycerol model. *Medicine* **58**, 362–376.
13. Wardle E. N. (1975) Endotoxin and acute renal failure. *Nephron* **14**, 321–332.
14. Stein J. H. (1977) The glomerulus in acute renal failure. *J. Lab. Clin. Med.* **90**, 227–230.
15. Stein J. H., Lifschitz M. D. and Barnes L. D. (1978) Current concepts on the pathophysiology of acute renal failure. *Am. J. Physiol.* **234**, F171–F181.
16. Finn W. F. (1980) Postischemic acute renal failure: initiation, maintenance and recovery. *Investigative Urology* **17**, 427–431.
17. Finn W. F. (1977) The renal system. In: Earley L. E. and Gottschalk C. W., ed., *Acute Renal Failure in Strauss and Welt's Diseases of The Kidney*, 3rd ed., pp. 167–210. Boston, Little, Brown & Co.
18. Schrier R. W., Burke T. J., Conger J. D. et al. (1981) Newer aspects of acute renal failure. *Proceedings of 8th International Congress of Nephrology*, pp. 63–69.
19. Kahn T. and Stein R. M. (1972) Gentamicin and renal failure. *Lancet* **1**, 498.
20. Allison M. E. M., Prentice C. R. M., Kennedy A. C. et al. (1979) Renal function and other factors in obstructive jaundice. *Br. J. Surg.* **66**, 392–397.
21. Espinel C. H. and Gregory A. W. (1980) Differential diagnosis of acute renal failure. *Clin. Nephrol.* **13**, 73–77.
22. Cattell W. R., McIntosh C. S., Moseley I. F. et al. (1973) Excretion urography in acute renal failure. *Br. Med. J.* **2**, 575–578.
23. Eliahou H. E. (1964) Mannitol therapy in oliguria of acute onset. *Br. Med. J.* **1**, 807–809.
24. Luke R. G., Briggs J. D., Allison M. E. M. et al. (1970) Factors determining response to mannitol in acute renal failure. *Am. J. Med. Sci.* **259**, 168.
25. Cantarovich F., Galli C., Benedetti L. et al. (1973) High dose frusemide in established acute renal failure. *Br. Med. J.* **1**, 449–450.

26. Kleinknecht D., Ganeval D., Gonzalez-Duque L. A. et al (1976) Frusemide in acute oliguric renal failure. A controlled trial. *Nephron* **17**, 51–58.
27. Henderson I. S., Beattie T. J. and Kennedy A. C. (1980) Dopamine hydrochloride in oliguric states. *Lancet* **2**, 827–828.
28. Burke T. J., Arnold P. E. and Schrier R. W. (1981) A role for intracellular calcium in the pathogenesis of norepinephrine (NE)-induced acute renal failure. *Abstracts of 8th International Congress of Nephrology*, p. 222.
29. Leonard C. D., Luke R. G. and Siegel R. R. (1975) Parenteral essential amino acids in acute renal failure. *Urology* **6**, 154–157.
30. Abel R. M., Beck C. H., Abbott W. M. et al. (1973) Improved survival from acute renal failure after treatment with intravenous essential L-amino acids and glucose. *N. Engl. J. Med.* **288**, 695–699.
31. Conger J. D. (1975) A controlled evaluation of prophylactic dialysis in post-traumatic acute renal failure. *J. Trauma* **15**, 1056–1063.
32. Amerio A., Campese V. M., Coratelli P. et al. (1981) Prognosis in acute renal failure accompanied by jaundice. *Nephron* **27**, 152–154.
33. Cullen D. J., Civetta J. M., Briggs B. A. et al. (1974) Therapeutic intervention scoring system: a method for quantitative comparison of patient care. *Crit. Care Med.* **2**, 57–60.
34. Routh G. S., Briggs J. D., Mone J. G. et al. (1980) Survival from acute renal failure with and without multiple organ dysfunction. *Postgrad. Med. J.* **56**, 244–247.
35. Briggs J. D., Kennedy A. C., Young L. N. et al. (1967) Renal function after acute tubular necrosis. *Br. Med. J.* **3**, 513–516.

Chapter 20

The Peripheral Vascular System

A. J. McKay and J. G. Pollock

The concept of intensive care for the critically ill or injured patient has only become a practical reality within the last two decades. Over approximately the same period of time peripheral vascular surgery has emerged as a specialist branch of surgery in its own right.[1] The growth of the specialty has stemmed from improvements in arterial prostheses together with advances in anaesthetic and resuscitative techniques.

Applying the principles of intensive care to patients requiring peripheral vascular surgery has led to a progressive reduction in operative mortality, so that an elective aortic bifurcation graft should now be performed with an operative mortality of not more than 2%.[2]

The need now is for careful selection of cases requiring intensive care within a specialist unit, so that expensive facilities can be used to maximum efficiency.[3]

The use that vascular surgery patients make of intensive care facilities will vary from hospital to hospital. In many vascular units both elective and emergency cases are managed in a general ward where nursing and medical staff are familiar with the intensive monitoring these patients require. This is particularly appropriate where peripheral vascular surgery is performed exclusively in a unit which does not also undertake general surgery. In other centres lack of such expertise or limitation of trained nursing staff may make it advisable for these patients to be managed, at least initially, in an intensive care unit.

In this chapter we shall highlight the need for careful case selection, preoperative assessment, intraoperative monitoring and intensive postoperative care in vascular patients. The chapter may conveniently be divided into three sections:

    I. Elective vascular surgery
   II. Emergency vascular surgery
  III. Vascular incidents arising within an intensive care unit

I. ELECTIVE VASCULAR SURGERY

We shall use a case of aortic bifurcation graft to detail the relevant points of management.

On admission to hospital, as well as routine preparation for major surgery, a fairly rigid ward discipline is enforced. A very careful search is made for any source of nasopharyngeal or skin sepsis. The nursing and physiotherapy staff begin to teach the patient the techniques that will be used post-operativly to prevent deep venous thrombosis. For example, the patient is taught simple leg exercises to prevent pooling of venous blood in the calf sinuses. Prolonged periods of pre-operative bed rest are rigorously avoided and early mobilization following surgery encouraged. Antibiotic prophylaxis is given routinely in the form of cloxacillin, 500 mg 6-hourly, this being used for 24 hours before surgery and continued for 5 days post-operatively.

Despite the evidence favouring the use of 'mini-heparin' in the prevention of deep venous thrombosis and pulmonary thrombo-embolism in many other branches of surgery,[4] we do not recommend its routine use in vascular surgery. This follows our own experience of its use in a trial situation when the incidence of haemorrhagic complications was unsatisfactorily high and the trial had to be abandoned. In addition, other workers have shed some doubt on the efficacy of low dose heparin in preventing pulmonary embolism in patients undergoing abdominal surgery.[5]

We do make use of a heel pad to keep the calves off the operating table but other peroperative anti-thrombotic measures, such as anti-embolectomy stockings and inflatable leg cuffs, are clearly inappropriate where surgery is frequently undertaken to distal vessels.

Intraoperative Monitoring

The responsibility for much of this aspect of care will rest with the anaesthetist. If at all possible, two anaesthetists should be available at the critical stages of the procedure and at all times close co-operation is required between the anaesthetic and surgical teams. The following monitoring techniques are employed in every patient.

Electrocardiogram

In addition to standard limb leads, the use of a V5 chest lead is now routine to assist in the detection of subendocardial ischaemia as revealed by ST segment depression on this lead.[6] Continuous visual monitoring allows early detection of cardiac arrhythmia.

Central Venous Pressure

This is usually measured via an internal jugular vein catheter though the choice of site for placement of the central line is often dependent on the personal preference of the anaesthetist. In particular, central venous pressure monitoring allows assessment of the patient's tolerance of a deliberate fluid load.

These patients are particularly susceptible to a low junctional rhythm during anaesthesia, and characteristic 'Cannon' V-waves assist in establishing this diagnosis.

Arterial Pressure

The radial artery can be cannulated with very little risk to the patient and this allows continuous visualization of the arterial waveform on an oscilloscope. In addition, beat-to-beat monitoring of stroke volume is possible, as well as continuous monitoring of arterial pressure. Furthermore, arterial blood gas analysis is thus made readily available at any time during the procedure.

Urinary Output

All patients should have a urinary catheter in situ. The urinary output is controlled by maintenance of a satisfactory central venous pressure and diuretics are not generally required. However, when the level of aortic occlusion is proximal to the origin of the renal artery, then mannitol 20 g is given routinely prior to cross-clamping the aorta. It is rare for such suprarenal clamping to last longer than ten minutes and significant renal ischaemia is not a practical problem. In a small number of patients with suprarenal lesions, more prolonged renal ischaemia is inevitable and the kidneys may be protected not only by the use of mannitol but also by the use of regional anticoagulants and cooling.

Other Monitoring Methods

Pulmonary artery and 'wedge pressures' can be measured using the Swan–Ganz balloon-tipped pulmonary artery catheter.[7] Although it is not our routine practice to make use of this catheter, it undoubtedly provides a more sensitive indicator of left ventricular dysfunction particularly in patients with arterial hypertension and coronary artery disease. Recently, we have found that in selected patients it may make a useful contribution to management, for example, in a patient who has suffered from previous left ventricular failure but requires urgent major arterial surgery such as excision of an abdominal aortic aneurysm. It is our feeling, however, that the central venous pressure measurement of right heart function is adequate for most cases.

Cardiac output, if thought desirable, can be measured using a dye dilution or thermal dilution methods.

Operative Considerations

Several stages in the management of a patient undergoing ABG require special mention.
1. Induction of anaesthesia—these patients often have associated myo-cardial and cerebral ischaemia and will not tolerate significant hypotension for any period of time. Such hypotension inevitably occurs with induction of anaesthesia but techniques should be modified to minimize the risks involved.
2. Cross-clamping of the aorta may be associated with sub-endocardial ischaemia and, at this point, the patient is particularly prone to develop left ventricular failure.
3. On completion of the first of the lower anastomoses, the aortic clamp is released and hypotension occurs as the limb circulation is re-opened. It is essential that the patient is in positive fluid balance prior to this stage, perhaps by as much as 500 ml. In addition, an inevitable acidosis occurs and should be measured. The actual level of acidosis is very variable, but the appropriate dose of bicarbonate should be given to correct it. Similarly, on opening the second limb of the graft a more minor episode of hypotension should be anticipated. It is worth noting that, in the elderly patient with an aortic aneurysm, no collateral distal circulation will have developed and so the risk of such hypotension is much greater than in the patient with distal occlusive disease and extensive collateral circulation.
4. Intraoperative anticoagulation: in common with the majority of vascular surgeons we routinely make use of systemic heparin therapy in the elective situation (5000 units of heparin intravenously after pre-clotting of the prosthesis). Some surgeons, in addition, make use of regional heparinized saline. We recommend the routine use of systemic anticoagulation with full reversal of heparin at the end of the procedure. Although a recent report suggested that the peroperative use of normal saline may render the patient hyper-coagulable,[8] we have found no evidence that this occurs in our heparinized patients.

Postoperative Monitoring

The first and essential 'postoperative' measurement in these patients is to assess the adequacy of their surgery. No patient should be allowed to leave theatre if the patency of the graft is in question. There is no doubt that clinical observation of limb colour, venous filling, temperature and the presence of peripheral pulses are inadequate in this context. Several ancillary aids are now available and their use will undoubtedly become more widespread and reduce the need for subsequent surgery due to graft failure. Three methods are particularly worthy of mention.

Electromagnetic Flow Meters

It is known that pulsation of an artery is not an accurate assessment of the adequacy of blood flow. The use of an electromagnetic flowmeter probe applied around the aorta distal to the graft will confirm adequacy of the anastomoses.

Peroperative Arteriography

This is of particular value following the completion of difficult distal anastomoses after embolectomy and in the post-traumatic limb. In addition, there is evidence that its routine use leads to a detection of the more common causes of technical failure and their subsequent elimination.[9] It has been clearly demonstrated in limb salvage surgery that angiography must show at least one vessel reaching the pedal arch or reconstructive surgery will be unsuccessful.

Non-invasive Techniques

1. *Doppler ultrasound*

In the postoperative situation, this allows objective detection of peripheral pulses and in the more modern machines a waveform print-out can be produced. The value of a simple Doppler probe with a sphygmomanometer to measure ankle pressures intraoperatively has previously been reported.[10]

2. *Pulse volume recorder (PVR)*

This segmental air plethysomograph is perhaps the most significant development in the field of per and postoperative assessment of graft patency. It has the singular advantage that the print-out on the strip chart recorder can be easily read by both nursing and medical staff when the patient returns to the ward. If the PVR is available peroperatively then an inadequate anastomosis can readily be detected.

Intensive nursing and medical care is essential for at least 24 hours postoperatively. The period immediately following extubation is particularly dangerous. The anaesthetist or respiratory technician must be on hand to record the adequacy of postextubation ventilation. If this is considered inadequate an early decision to continue with assisted ventilation must be made.

After a relatively lengthy operation, body temperature must be maintained and we routinely make use of a 'space-blanket' together with conventional bedding. Indeed, some surgical units go so far as to employ artificial heating aids during operation, together with electric blankets postoperatively.

One unhappy product of the modern unidirectional flow theatre is the inevitable patient cooling which occurs and it is not unusual for the postoperative patient's temperature to be around 34 °C. This level of hypothermia is associated with acidosis, peripheral vasoconstriction and an increased incidence of cardiac arrhythmias. In addition to the measures outlined above, we occasionally make use of the alpha-blocking agent droperidol and have also made use of chlorpromazine, both for its peripheral vasodilatory effect and to prevent the patient from shivering (cf. the use of nitroprusside in this context).

On return to bed, patients are nursed with, at most, one pillow. The pulse, blood pressure and central venous pressure are initially recorded every 15 minutes. The arterial line remains in situ to allow easy access to arterial blood samples for blood gas analysis. Oxygen is given to maintain an arterial Po_2 greater than 100 mm Hg. Recent evidence[11] suggests that analgesia is best given in the form of a continuous morphine infusion. This is an important aspect of postoperative care and the patient should not be deprived of adequate sedation since excessive pain may overstimulate the sympathetic nervous system and produce hypertension and tachycardia together with peripheral vasoconstriction. However, it is clearly necessary to strike a balance between adequate sedation and the danger of respiratory depression.

Operative blood loss will normally have been replaced before the patient leaves theatre and, if that is the case, then the intravenous fluid requirements are adjusted according to the central venous pressure and urinary output, which is monitored hourly. A total of 3 l of clear fluid (Ringer lactate; 1 N saline; 5% dextrose) in the first 24 hours after surgery is usually adequate to maintain a urinary output of not less than 30 ml/h. Should such a level not be maintained, then additional intravenous fluid, often in the form of plasma-protein solution, is used, using the central venous pressure as the guide to level of hydration. Only in the face of a rising CVP but continuing lack of diuresis, should the use of diuretics be considered. In general, their use is to be deprecated since they merely confuse the correct assessment of fluid balance.

Arterial blood gas analysis should be performed within four hours of surgery and urea and electrolytes measured. It is particularly important that serum potassium be maintained in the normal range to prevent cardiac arrhythmias during this critical phase. The peripheral pulse pattern is noted as soon as the patient returns to the ward and thereafter checked on a regular basis. Any change in this pattern or alteration in limb perfusion must be treated as a matter of extreme urgency and, if re-exploration is required, this should be undertaken without delay.

As mentioned above the use of the pulse volume recorder or limb pressures assessed by Doppler ultrasound both provide objective means of assessing the adequacy of the peripheral circulation.

On the immediate postoperative day, if all parameters are stable, the CVP line, nasogastric tube and urinary catheter are removed and ECG monitoring discontinued. Although the theoretical fear of gastric dilation has led to the routine use of a nasogastric tube, some recent work in our department has suggested that its use could safely be discontinued.[12] Oral fluid is started initially at 25 ml/h and active chest physiotherapy is instituted. Simple leg and foot exercises to prevent venous thrombosis are commenced and, by the second postoperative day, the patient is allowed out of bed for a short time. Monitoring of temperature, pulse and blood pressure continues throughout the entire hospital stay, together with regular review of peripheral pulse pattern. With several arterial anastomoses having been undertaken, the possibilty of postoperative bleeding should never be neglected. In this regard the abdomen and groins are regularly inspected for the possible development of an expanding haematoma and a rise in pulse rate and falling blood pressure which does not respond to adequate fluid replacement as monitored by CVP, should make one suspicious of intra-abdominal bleeding.

Some specific postoperative complications are worthy of mention.

a. Intestinal Ileus

Since modifying surgical technique some years ago, we rarely find prolonged intestinal ileus to be a significant clinical problem. We no longer place the small intestine in a plastic bag during aortic dissection and take considerable care to return the loops of small bowel in an orderly fashion following repair of the posterior peritoneum. Similarly the greater omentum is carefully replaced as near its original position as possible. Ileus does occasionally occur but usually responds to conventional therapy of nasogastric aspiration and intravenous fluids with restriction of oral intake. The occasional patient who develops a prolonged ileus without mechanical obstruction soon becomes severely catabolic. It may become necessary to make use of parenteral feeding in order to achieve nitrogen balance and reversal of the catabolic state. The insertion of a central venous line for feeding purposes must be performed under scrupulously aseptic conditions, since infection of the arterial prosthesis must not occur.

It is important not to assume that gastrointestinal hold-up is due to ileus and not mechanical obstruction. The extensive nature of the surgery and, in particular, mobilization of the duodenum renders these patients at risk of developing an obstruction consequent on adhesion formation. If this is suspected and the patient does not respond to a trial of 'drip and suck', then surgery should not be delayed since such mechanical kinks rarely settle spontaneously. If the diagnosis is considered then the use of a lateral decubitus film will be helpful in its confirmation.

b. Renal Failure

If adequate fluid balance is maintained the acute tubular necrosis syndrome should be a very rare occurrence. When acute renal failure is suspected, however, urinary and plasma osmolarity should be measured and a review made of the entire fluid and electrolyte balance since surgery. The management of established acute tubular necrosis does not differ in patients following aortic bifurcation graft (ABG) from that in other situations with initial therapy being restriction of intravenous fluids to 500 ml plus measured losses. Electrolyte imbalance must, of course, be corrected as required. If renal dialysis is contemplated then such a decision must be made after consultation between the surgeon, renal physician and cardiologist involved, bearing in mind that elective ABG would not have been performed had the outlook of the patient not been considered good.

c. Intestinal Ischaemia

When an inlay ABG is inserted the inferior mesenteric artery is divided. The marginal colonic arterial anastomosis is almost always adequate to maintain colonic blood flow, but occasionally intestinal ischaemia occurs postoperatively. The presence of bloodstained diarrhoea together with a pyrexia and leucocytosis should alert one to this possibility. Initial management is conservative with restriction of oral fluids and use of broad-spectrum antibiotics together with metronidazole. Most cases will settle with this management although a mucosal cast may be passed around the tenth postoperative day. The diagnosis can be confirmed by sigmoidoscopy or colonoscopy and, on the rare occasion when a barium enema is also necessary, the colonic appearance may be strikingly similar to that of end-stage ulcerative colitis with a 'hose-pipe' colon appearance. Only in the severely ill patient who fails to respond to the above regime should laparotomy be considered.

d. Diabetes Mellitus

With so many diabetic patients undergoing major arterial surgery, detailed knowledge of the control of diabetes is clearly required. We have made use routinely of a sliding scale to control insulin requirement in the post-operative period, but occasionally seek the help of a diabetic physician for the difficult case. The ready availability and relative inexpense of the new glucose meters may aid this aspect of management with 'spot' glucose estimations made possible.

e. Prevention of Infection

Although the development of a wound infection, urinary tract infection or respiratory tract infection is considered serious and treated appropriately, the lethal infection associated with vascular surgery which must be prevented is graft infection. To this end staphylococcal infection is actively looked for by the routine use of nasal and perineal swabs taken from every patient and from the theatre staff on a regular basis. Cross-infection in the ward is prevented by rigid ward discipline and the detection of any source of infection would preclude surgery.

Careful nursing has an important role to play in preventing postoperative complications. While the patient is recovering from surgery, nursing staff maintain the patient's oral hygiene, assist with chest physiotherapy and apply established nursing techniques to prevent pressure sores. As well as lengthening the period of hospitalization, such sores may provide a focus for infection. These nursing measures are of particular importance in the amputee in whom the development of a penetrating os calcis ulcer on the surviving limb can be nothing short of a disaster. In such patients, very early ambulation is to be encouraged and we have recently made use of inflatable limb splints to provide more adequate protection for the stump.

This rigorous regime, together with careful skin preparation at the time of surgery, should result in a very low incidence of graft infection and all patients are, of course, covered by appropriate antibiotics. A further possible source of infection is the groin incision and surgical technique should be such that the incidence of groin lymph fistula is kept to an absolute minimum.

Postoperative care is naturally directed towards the prevention of known complications of major vascular surgery. It is vital that medical, nursing and paramedical staff all encourage the patient in the early postoperative period. The environment of an intensive care unit or area may seem hostile to a patient who is likely to be already apprehensive and under considerable strain. The importance of simple regular human communication, must not be underestimated.

Although we have concentrated on the patient having an aortic bifurcation graft, those who undergo limb salvage surgery require particular mention. These patients are frequently severely ill with all the features of widespread atherosclerosis often in association with chronic obstructive airways disease and the typical small vessel and neurological changes of diabetes. Improvements in arterial graft materials, e.g. expanded polytetrafluoroethylene (PTFE) and gluteraldehyde-tanned umbilical veins have made it technically possible for the distal limb of a graft to reach small calibre tibial vessels. Making use of these grafts has greatly reduced operative time since dissection and preparation of the long saphenous vein is unnecessary. As surgical techniques improve, such very ill patients will increasingly undergo surgery and their postoperative intensive care will constitute a major clinical challenge.

Carotid Endarterectomy, Subclavian/Carotid Shunts: Aortic Arch Surgery

We will deal only with the most commonly performed, namely, carotid endarterectomy (CEA).

The preoperative assessment and care of these patients in other respects does not materially differ from that outlined for the patient with aorto-iliac disease.

Operative Considerations

Care is required in placing the patient on the operating table since hyperextension of the neck may damage the vertebral arteries and, in the presence of carotid artery disease, vertebrobasilar insufficiency is also likely.

Intraoperative monitoring should include central venous pressure, arterial pressure and ECG tracing, as for ABG patients. For some years several means have been used to protect cerebral function during CEA. These include induced hypertension, hypercapnia, hypocapnia, temporary intraluminal bypass shunts, EEG monitoring, or combinations of these measures.[13,14] Our policy is to use general anaesthesia with the blood pressure maintained a little above the normal for the patient. Acid base and blood gas monitoring is routine but we do not use alteration in Pa_{CO_2} levels to protect cerebral circulation. Prior to cross-clamping of the common carotid we do use systemic heparinization, together with a local injection of 1% lignocaine to the carotid sinus tissue. We routinely measure end-stump carotid pressure, but only if this pressure is significantly higher than the 50 mmHg considered safe by many authors[15,16] would we not use an intraluminal shunt. We agree with the opinion[13] that routine use of the shunt does not constitute a major technical handicap.

It must be noted that the above principles of treatment are those practised in our unit, but many eminent vascular surgeons have published excellent long-term results without using transluminal shunts on any patient.[21]

Postoperative Care and Complications

The intensive care of these patients includes monitoring of the cardio-vascular parameters previously mentioned when dealing with aorto-iliac disease. The following specific points relate to the patient who has undergone CEA:

1. Ventilation must be closely observed and may become inadequate despite an apparently straightforward anaesthetic.
2. Postoperative arterial hypertension is a common occurrence in the immediate postoperative period and systolic pressures of up to 200 mmHg are not uncommon. Such hypertension will usually respond to routine antihypertensive agents and we have recently used a nitroprusside infusion in this context.
3. Headache. Severe headache is a common postoperative occurrence and should be treated with appropriate analgesia but nursing and medical staff must be alert to the possibility of cerebral oedema.
4. Bleeding. Despite meticulous technique, haematoma formation may occur and, even in the presence of suction drains, respiratory embarrassment may develop due to tracheal compression. For this reason regular inspection of the wound must be undertaken.
5. Cranial nerve damage. Both the vagus and hypoglossal nerves may be damaged during surgery, but an awareness of their exact anatomical location should prevent permanent damage. Temporary neuropraxia may occur if either nerve is inadvertently grasped between the blades of a controlling arterial clamp. While a temporary deviation of the tongue is very noticeable, it is a much less severe complication than respiratory upset due to laryngeal muscle palsy.

Long-term Results

With the combination of careful case selection, meticulous surgical technique and intraoperative monitoring, excellent long-term results can be achieved. Overall mortality should be not more than 1%.[13,16] The incidence of stroke after operation should be not more than 2%.

II. EMERGENCY VASCULAR SURGERY

1. Aneurysm
   a. Thoracic aorta
   b. Abdominal aorta

      c. Visceral, e.g. splenic, renal

      d. Elsewhere, e.g. carotid, subclavian

2. Arterial embolism

      a. Peripheral

      b. Mesenteric

3. Trauma

      a. Sharp or blunt trauma

      b. Iatrogenic

4. Deep venous thrombosis

5. Drug overdosage, e.g. ergotamine

6. Other, e.g. hypothermia, frostbite

While patients with arterial or venous damage from any of the above conditions may require emergency vascular surgery, we will highlight those cases who most require application of intensive care principles in their management.

1. Ruptured Abdominal Aortic Aneurysm

Without surgery the mortality from a ruptured aortic aneurysm is virtually 100%. In patients who survive long enough to reach an operating theatre, the mortality ranges from 40 to 50%[17, 18] and in our own hospital it is 44%. Although one recent series reported the significantly reduced mortality figure of 14·8%,[19] even at their best these figures are worthy of contrast with the pattern in elective aneurysm surgery where mortality figures have been ever diminishing.[20, 21] Indeed in the last 100 elective cases done in the Royal Infirmary, Glasgow, the mortality has been 2%.

Emergency aortic aneurysm surgery is arduous, expensive and time-consuming. It is rare for surgery to be impossible for technical reasons alone, but experience has shown that the 50% of these patients who die do so from renal and myocardial disease. Frustratingly, this multisystem failure causes death despite the continuing patency of the arterial prosthesis.

Knowing these figures, preoperative assessment of these patients should be all the more thorough. In our experience, there is seldom need to rush straight to theatre from the casualty department. A careful ordered assessment of the patient's general condition and likely operative outcome should be made and the following factors must be considered.

i. Age

While physiological age is more important than chronological age in this context, the patient over 80 years old has to be exceptional before surgery is justified.

ii. Time from Rupture

Often these patients are transferred from district general hospitals to a specialist unit, thus prolonging the time of cardiovascular instability. This aspect of care should be improved. It has been shown that there is benefit in providing a custom-built transfer ambulance together with a medical 'shock' team who will stabilize the patient prior to transfer then establish suitable monitoring during the journey between hospitals.[3] Others have recommended the use of a G-suit which can be applied prior to transfer, offering preoperative stability during the often difficult time of transfer.

Sadly these facilities are at present not widely available and hurried transfer to the central unit, often without a medical officer in attendance, is commonplace. It is all the more important then that time be taken to assess the patient adequately. Especially important is the degree of hypotension and the length of time this has been present. Related to this is the measurement of urinary output from the time of rupture. The patient who has produced little or no urine and has not established a systolic blood pressure of at least 100 mmHg for more than four hours, is less likely to recover renal function following emergency surgery.

iii. Myocardial Ischaemia

As mentioned earlier, all patients with peripheral vascular disease have myocardial ischaemia but a specific history of previous myocardial infarction or sustained angina is obviously a relative contraindication to major emergency surgery.

iv. Distal Vessel Run-off

Happily, most abdominal aortic aneurysms are limited to the aorta between the renal arteries and aortic bifurcation. A proportion of patients, however, will have absent distal pulses due either to associated peripheral disease, embolism from the aneurysmal sac or thrombosis due to cardiogenic shock. Evidence of distal vessel involvement again implies more severe disease and the chances of full recovery following surgery are correspondingly lowered.

The preoperative assessment indicated above can be made carefully but fairly swiftly. If surgery is decided upon then all the monitoring facilities previously outlined for elective aortic replacement should be available. In some cases time will be critical and the patient may require to proceed to surgery urgently. On such occasions the delay required for central venous and arterial lines to be inserted is unacceptable. Ten units of blood should be cross-matched, the patient anaesthetized without muscle relaxant and the operation commenced. The single most important aspect of such a patient's care is control of the source of bleeding.

The incidence of infected aortic aneurysms is a matter of some controversy. While infection was not found by one group of workers after routine culture,[22] others have found infection in up to 20% of ruptured aneurysms.[23] We routinely take a bacteriology swab from the aneurysmal sac, its value being that when an unsuspected organism is grown it can be treated with the most appropriate antibiotic if post-operative infection is a problem. After insertion of the prosthesis, the residual aneurysmal sac can usefully be used to separate the graft from the peritoneal contents.

The postoperative care is identical in all respects to that offered to the elective aortic graft patient although, of course, after a ruptured abdominal aortic aneurysm, the cardiovascular trauma is considerably greater and patients are, therefore, more critically ill and potentially unstable.

2. Arterial Embolism

a. Peripheral

The clinical pattern of this sudden vascular emergency is well known and documented in every clinical textbook. The common source for embolus is thrombus on the endocardium, either following myocardial infarction or in the presence of rheumatic valvular disease or due to an arrhythmia such as atrial fibrillation. The precipitating episode immediately prior to embolization is often a sudden transient alteration in heart rhythm. More unusually, embolus may consist of a platelet aggregation or a fragment of atheromatous plaque which has become dislodged from a proximal stenotic or aneurysmal lesion. The common site of impaction of the embolus in the upper limb, is the third part of the axillary artery or the brachial bifurcation. In the lower limb impaction commonly occurs at the bifurcation of the aorta ('saddle' embolus) at the common femoral artery bifurcation or at the popliteal artery. Management of arterial embolism is emergency embolectomy using the Fogarty catheter,[24] surgery usually being performed under local anaesthetic. Systemic heparinization is instituted as soon as the diagnosis is established (5000 units stat).

Although it has been traditionally taught that embolectomy is only successful if performed within 10–12 hours of the acute event, in common with other vascular surgeons, we have often undertaken this procedure many hours after this time has elapsed. It may be possible to partly clear distal vessels and thus sufficiently improve limb viability to allow a more distal level of amputation. However, in the late embolectomy, two additional factors need to be considered. First, sudden reperfusion of ischaemic tissues can cause severe acidosis with possible renal failure, the so-called myonephropathic metabolic syndrome.[25] Secondly, whenever there is any suggestion of increased intracompartmental tension in the affected limb, there should be no hesitation in performing adequate fasciotomy in at least two compartments.

b. Mesenteric

The cause of acute intestinal ischaemia is non-occlusive in 40% of cases and occurs following a reduction in cardiac output due to myocardial infarction, congestive cardiac failure or hypovolaemia due to sudden loss of volume in the intravascular compartment. Arterial embolism accounts for 30% of cases, the most commonly affected vessel being the superior mesenteric artery. In 20% of patients the cause of ischaemia is arterial thrombosis and in the remaining patients ischaemia is due to a variety of causes, such as venous thrombosis, arteritis or aortic dissection.

The mortality in acute intestinal ischaemia is widely reported at around 85%,[26, 27] although one recent paper did show an overall mortality of 46%.[28] The authors of that work claimed that, by having a high index of suspicion and making use of selective arteriography, such a reduction in mortality should be possible in most centres.

The clinical presentation of patients with acute intestinal ischaemia follows a fairly standard pattern. Surprisingly, shock may not be a prominent feature in the early stages although it always develops in time. More than half have a white blood cell count of greater than 20 000 white blood cells per ml. Severe pain is always present. When a superior mesenteric artery embolus occurs, the artery is occluded in the middle of its course in 80% of cases, whereas in those where thrombosis has caused occlusion, 90% will have obstruction at the origin of the vessel. Treatment, when possible, is by embolectomy.

Where localized infarction has occurred resection must, of course, be undertaken with preservation of as great a length of viable small bowel as possible. If any doubt exists as to the viability of bowel, then a deliberate decision to undertake a second look laporotomy 24 hours later should be taken.

After revascularization, there is evidence that a period of parenteral nutrition lasting approximately 2 weeks from the time of the episode may contribute to a reduction in the high mortality. Inevitably these patients are severely ill and postoperatively require full supportive care, particularly with reference to fluid balance. They are especially sensitive to cardiac arrhythmias and anti-arrhythmic agents are often required.

3. Trauma

i. General

The vascular surgeon will become involved with cases of trauma in many situations. Arterial damage is classically associated with such long bone fractures as supracondylar fracture of the humerus and fractures of the tibia and fibula. Arterial damage may occur with or without associated venous disruption in dislocation without fracture of the knee or shoulder joints.[29]

Patients with multiple injuries and multi-organ involvement will often require long-term intensive care and their management may well involve several medical and surgical disciplines. The initial resuscitative measures required are dealt with elsewhere in this book, but the vascular complications raise several important management issues. When major vessel damage, either venous or arterial is suspected, early expert assessment is required. Arterial reconstruction must take precedence, for example, over fixation of fractures unless this can be carried out speedily. Arteriography is of considerable value both in establishing the exact nature of the injury and also to confirm the efficacy of vascular reconstruction. All necrotic tissue must be excised aggressively since growth of anaerobic organisms will almost inevitably mean major limb amputation. Such growth should be assumed in all major trauma when vascular damage is found and appropriate antibiotic therapy instituted. (Penicillin 1000 000 units; cloxacillin 500 mg 6-hourly.) When major debridement has been undertaken primary wound closure will be the exception. As mentioned with regard to embolectomy, compartmental tension especially in the lower limb may rise to surprisingly high levels after any prolonged period of ischaemia and the use of adequate fasciotomy is to be encouraged.

There has been a tendency for some surgeons involved in the early management of trauma cases to consider inadequate distal limb perfusion to be due to 'arterial spasm'. This concept is dangerous and should be viewed with suspicion. In almost all such situations 'spasm' should be interpreted as occlusion and treated appropriately.

ii. Specific Vascular Trauma

The ever-increasing use being made of invasive investigative and monitoring techniques has led to an inevitable rise in the number of cases of iatrogenic vascular trauma.

Central venous lines

Improvements both in technique and catheter construction have meant that complications from the insertion of central venous pressure and parenteral feeding lines are now less frequent but these do still occur. While internal jugular or subclavian vein lines are convenient for long-term parenteral nutrition, they are both associated with a small but significant morbidity.[30] When the requirement for CVP monitoring is expected to be relatively short term, most anaesthetists favour the internal jugular vein. This route is favoured not only for the ease of access, but also because a direct effect can be obtained for any urgently required drugs.

Despite possible damping of the true central venous pressure level, an antecubital fossa vein remains the safest means of inserting the central catheter in the absence of specific expertise. Often, of course, patients requiring this monitoring are gravely ill and may have been hospitalized for a long period so that such a vein is not available. However, it should be possible to use this route in many patients and there is a danger that the internal jugular or subclavian route will unnecessarily become the site of choice. It should not be forgotten that many patients can be fed for long periods using a fine bore enteral tube, thus precluding the requirement for vascular access.

Arteriography

Translumbar aortography, aortic arch arteriography and carotid arteriography are now widely available and being used more and more frequently. While they are remarkably safe procedures in expert hands they remain invasive and are inevitably associated with a morbidity and, rarely, mortality. Patients require to be monitored following these investigations and, where there is doubt about limb viability or a change of peripheral pulse pattern occurs, a vascular surgeon's opinion should be sought. Familiarity should not lead to carelessness and a regular review of these patients is essential if the occasional tragedy is to be prevented. It is sound clinical practice to document both the pre- and post-angiogram pulse pattern clearly in the case sheet.

Multiple arterial puncture

While several studies have shown that multiple punctures of the same artery for blood gas analysis can be safely performed, occasionally damage will occur either in the form of thrombosis or false aneurysm formation. The practical lesson is that such arterial sampling should be performed carefully with adequate compression after puncture. If repeated sampling is anticipated, a permanent arterial line is probably less hazardous than multiple direct punctures.

4. Deep Venous Thrombosis

The debate on how best to prevent the formation of clot in the deep venous sinuses of the lower limb continues. As already stated in our experience the incidence of complications from the routine use of prophylactic heparin is unacceptably high to commend its use in elective vascular surgery. We place considerable emphasis on aggressive physiotherapy and early patient mobilization, together with specific measures already mentioned. Like others, we await with interest the results of several studies which are attempting to identify those patients most at risk of developing deep venous thrombosis. Such a study is at present underway in our own hospital and, as has been suggested by other workers, it will hopefully become possible in the future to select patients who will most benefit from prophylaxis.

The diagnosis of deep venous thrombosis is frequently made but all too rarely confirmed. It is known that clinical examination alone is a poor means of assessing venous occlusion and the time-honoured clinical signs are all too often inaccurate.[31] The use of a portable Doppler ultrasound machine will confirm the presence of a venous occlusion but gives no information as to the nature of the thrombosis. The use of isotopically labelled fibrinogen is becoming more widespread and is undoubtedly a more sensitive means of detecting clot in the leg veins.[32] The value of bilateral ascending venography has been established in this context.[33] However, in less expert hands this technique may not visualize the important proximal venous channels, i.e. the iliofemoral segment. Direct femoral vein puncture, selective cross-over catheter or pertrochanteric venography can overcome this deficiency.[34] We would recommend that, whenever deep venous thrombosis is suspected, emergency bilateral venography should be immediately arranged since this investigation alone will allow identification of the nature and site of any dangerous loose clot.

Much has already been written on whether the detection of such loose clot should lead to treatment by heparin or streptokinase[35] or whether surgery is the treatment of choice. Each clinical case requires to be treated carefully on its merits but, when the exact nature of the thrombosis has been detected radiologically, a more logical treatment regime can be established. Furthermore, when routine venography is used a surprising proportion of patients will be found to have bilateral thrombosis and a significant number of pelvic vein anomalies will be detected.[33]

When loose clot has been detected and multiple embolization is occurring, surgery is required. It is rarely necessary to do more than ligate the superficial femoral vein in the groin on both sides, following an adequate iliofemoral thrombectomy confirmed radiologically. Venous drainage of the affected limb continues through the cleared profunda femoris vein. The operation of caval ligation for iliofemoral thrombosis should virtually never be performed and plication of the vein to divide it into small channels which allow continuation of flow but prevent passage of major thrombus is safe and effective. Ingenious filters have been introduced for impaction in the inferior vena cava but these have a significant incidence of caval damage in use.

In the great majority of cases bed rest with adequate lower limb elevation together with passive leg exercises will prevent the necessity for surgery. It is worth noting that all too often such elevation is entirely inadequate with the lower limb held at a level below that of the inferior vena cava.

III. VASCULAR INCIDENTS ARISING WITHIN AN ICU

As vascular surgeons, we are asked to deal with a relatively large number of problems which have arisen within an intensive care unit. These are briefly summarized below.

1. Inadequate Perfusion due to Pump Failure—'Cardiac Gangrene'

This is characterized by symmetrical ischaemic changes usually affecting both legs, but the changes may also involve the upper limbs. The affected extremities are cold and cyanotic but peripheral pulses may be present. Pain may not be a prominent feature. Sensory loss is limited to the ischaemic areas. The treatment consists of improving cardiac output (where that is possible) and instituting local measures to overcome stasis in the peripheral vessels. Passive movements of toes, ankles and knees should be carried out for 5 minutes in every half hour for 36–48 hours. This simple treatment may either prevent the formation of gangrene or allow demarcation of healthy tissue to occur at such a level that subsequent limited amputation of digits is all that is required.[36]

2. Arterial Embolus—Peripheral or Mesenteric

These topics have already been covered in detail but both occur more frequently in patients requiring intensive care. Peripheral emboli are especially common in the coronary care unit due to antecedent myocardial infarction or cardiac arrhythmia. It is worth emphasizing that peripheral arterial embolectomy is a relatively minor procedure usually performed under local anaesthesia. Rarely would a patient be too ill to undergo this operation. Early referral for surgery is essential if the best long term results are to be achieved.

3. Deep Venous Thrombosis

Again, non-ambulant patients in intensive treatment units are especially prone to develop deep venous thrombosis and regular examination of the calves must be performed together with intensive nursing care and physiotherapy. Ascending venography may not be possible and so the diagnosis must be confirmed by the use of Doppler ultrasound and isotope scanning.

4. Iatrogenic Arterial Damage

The widespread use that is made in intensive treatment units of venous and arterial catheter lines inevitably means that the complications associated with their use will occur. Central lines must be inserted under strictly aseptic conditions if septicaemia is to be prevented. Peripheral pulse patterns must be documented before and after the insertion of arterial lines. Potentially toxic drugs must not be injected intravenously without adequate dilution.

REFERENCES

1. Debakey M. E. (1979) The development of vascular surgery. *Am. J. Surg.* **137**, 697–738.
2. Thompson J. E. and Garrett W. V. (1980) Peripheral arterial surgery. *N. Engl. J. Med.* **302**, 491–503.
3. Ledingham I. (1977) *Recent Advances in Intensive Therapy I.* Edinburgh, Churchill Livingstone.
4. Kakkar V. V., Corrigan T. P., Fossard G. T. et al. (1977) Reappraisal of results of international multicentre trial. *Lancet* **1**, 567–569.
5. Immelman E. J., Jeffery P., Benatar S. R. et al. (1979) Failure of low-dose heparin to prevent significant thromboembolic complications in high-risk surgical patients: interim report of prospective trial. *Br. Med. J.* **1**, 1447–1450.
6. Blackburn H., Taylor H. L., Okamoto N. et al. (1967) Standardisation of the exercise electrocardiogram. A systematic comparison of chest lead configurations employed for monitoring during exercise. In: Karvonen M. J. and Barry A. J., ed., *Physical Activity and the Heart.* Springfield, Charles C. Thomas.
7. Swan H. J. C., Ganz W., Forrester J. et al. (1970) Catheterisation of the heart in man with use of a flow directed balloon tipped catheter. *N. Engl. J. Med.* **283**, 447–451.
8. Janvrin S. B., Davies G. and Greenhalgh R. M. (1980) Postoperative deep vein thrombosis caused by intravenous fluids during surgery. *Br. J. Surg.* **67**, 690–693.
9. Dardik H., Ibrahim I. M., Koslow A. et al. (1978) Evaluation of intraoperative arteriography at a routine for vascular reconstructions. *Surg. Gynecol. Obstet.* **147**, 853–858.
10. Barnes R. W. and Garrett W. V. (1978) Intraoperative assessment of arterial reconstruction by Doppler ultrasound. *Surg. Gynecol. Obstet.* **146**, 896–900.
11. Rutter P. C., Murphy F. and Dudley H. A. F. (1980) Morphine: controlled trial of different methods of administration for postoperative pain relief. *Br. Med. J.* **280**, 12–16.
12. Gilmour D. G. and Pollock J. G. (1981) Prospective studies on the value of nasogastric aspiration in elective aortic surgery. In preparation.
13. Thompson J. E. and Talkington C. M. (1976) Carotid endarterectomy. *Ann. Surg.* **184**, 1–15.
14. Baker J. D., Gluecklich B., Watson C. W. et al. (1975) An evaluation of electroencephalographic monitoring for carotid surgery. *Surgery* **78**, 787–794.

15. Sundt T. M. (1974) Surgical therapy of occlusive vascular diseases of the brain. *Surgery Annual XI*. New York, LM Nyhus.
16. Ott D. A., Cooley D. A., Chapa L. et al. (1980) Carotid endarterectomy without temporary intraluminal shunt. *Ann. Surg.* **191**, 708–714.
17. Debakey M. E., Crawford E. S., Cooley D. A. et al. (1964) Aneurysm of abdominal aorta: analysis of results of graft replacement therapy one to eleven years after operation. *Ann. Surg.* **160**, 622–639.
18. Hildebrand H. D. and Fry P. D. (1975) Ruptured abdominal aortic aneurysm. *Surgery* **77**, 540–544.
19. Lawrie G. M., Morris G. C. J. V. and Crawford E. S. (1979) Improved results of operation for ruptured abdominal aortic aneurysms. *Surgery* **85**, 483–488.
20. Young A. E., Sandbert G. W. and Couch N. P. (1977) The reduction of mortality of abdominal aortic aneurysm resection. *Am. J. Surg.* **134**, 585–590.
21. Gardner R. J., Gardner N. L., Tarney T. J. et al. (1978) The surgical experience and a one to sixteen year follow-up of 277 abdominal aortic aneurysms. *Am. J. Surg.* **135**, 226–230.
22. Walker D. I., Bloor K., Williams G. et al. (1972) Inflammatory aneurysms of the abdominal aorta. *Br. J. Surg.* **59**, 609–714.
23. Black J., Campbell D. J., Slaney G. et al. (1978) Paper presented at the annual meeting of the Vascular Society of Great Britain and Ireland.
24. Fogarty T. J., Cranley J. J., Kranse R. J. et al. (1963) A method for extraction of arterial emboli and thrombi. *Surg. Gynecol. Obstet.* **116**, 241–244.
25. Haimovici H. (1979) Muscular renal and metabolic complications of acute arterial occlusions: myonephropathic-metabolic syndrome. *Surgery* **85**, 461–468.
26. Bergan J. J., Dean R. H., Conn J. J. R. et al. (1975) Revascularisation in treatment of mesenteric infarction. *Ann. Surg.* **182**, 430–438.
27. Ottinger L. W. (1978) The surgical management of acute occlusion of the superior mesenteric artery. *Ann. Surg.* **188**, 721–731.
28. Boley S. J., Sprayregan S., Siegelman S. S. et al. (1977) Initial results from an aggressive roentgenological and surgical approach to acute mesenteric ischaemia. *Surgery* **82**, 848–855.
29. Drury J. K. and Scullion J. E. (1980) Vascular complications of anterior dislocation of the shoulder. *Br. J. Surg.* **67**, 579–581.
30. Oosterlee J. and Dudly H. A. F. (1980) Central catheter placement by puncture of exposed subclavian vein. *Lancet* **1**, 19–20.
31. Cockett F. B. (1970) Surgery of ilio-femoral thrombosis. In: Gillespie J. A., ed., *Modern Trends in Vascular Surgery*. London, Butterworths.
32. Gruber U. F., Saldeen T., Brokop T. et al. (1980) Incidences of fatal postoperative pulmonary embolism after prophylaxis with dextran 70 and low-dose heparin: an international multicentre study. *Br. Med. J.* **1**, 69–72.
33. Cockett F. B. and Lea Thomas M. (1965) The iliac compression syndrome. *Br. J. Surg.* **52**, 816–821.
34. Ruckley C. V. (1981) The management of venous thromboembolism. *J. R. Coll. Surg. Edinb.* **26**, 120–125.
35. Elliot M. S., Immelman E. J., Jeffery P. et al. (1979) A comparative randomized trial of heparin versus streptokinase in the treatment of acute proximal venous thrombosis: an interim report of a prospective trial. *Br. J. Surg.* **66**, 838–843.
36. Reid W. and Pollock J. G. (1978) *A Surgeon's Management of Gangrene*. Tunbridge Wells, Pitman.

Chapter 21

Major Orthopaedic Trauma

J. Graham

As the result of an accident, there can be injury to many of the specific organs of the body and their associated systems, depending on the distribution and severity of the mechanical forces applied at the time. This chapter deals solely with the effect of trauma on the musculoskeletal system, although clearly, in view of the nature of the subject, this will impinge on other physiological systems. The specific effect of trauma on these others systems is dealt with in the corresponding chapters.

The function of the skeleton is three-fold.

1. It acts as the framework of the body to which muscles are attached to provide movement across joints, and within which other organs are contained.

2. As the principal store of calcium, it is important in calcium homeostasis, the control of which is exerted mainly by the endocrine system and vitamin D.

3. In certain sites it contains within its substance haemopoietic bone marrow.

These three functions are in most respects totally independent of each other except in as much as metabolic bone disease or infiltrative neoplastic conditions may reduce bone strength and contribute to failure of the supportive function under stress.

Failure of the supporting framework (fracture) leads to loss of stability with subsequent loss of function in the area of the skeleton involved. This may have a secondary effect on any contained organ.

In practical terms primary failure of the metabolic function of the skeleton does not occur. There is a massive amount of calcium and phosphate present in the bone and failure to maintain calcium homeostasis is a result of failure of the controlling mechanism for release of the element.

In similar terms failure of the haemopoietic system in bone results from other factors, such as toxins or replacement diseases.

This chapter will deal principally with the effect of major trauma in producing fractures in several areas of the skeleton. This is an acute, often catastrophic, event which may have repercussions throughout the entire body. Such events are of increasingly frequent occurrence with the extension of the motorway system and subsequent increase of the volume of speeding traffic. The motorcycle explosion over the past few years has further added to the frequency of such accidents. The continued use and abuse of drugs (including alcohol), gives a continuous supply of self-inflicted injuries such as 'high-flying' from tall buildings.

COMMON SYNDROMES AND BASIC MANAGEMENT

Major trauma frequently produces severe complicated fractures widely distributed throughout the skeleton. In many instances there is also a significant injury to the head, chest or both which significantly increases morbidity and reduces the chance of survival. An injury of the intra-abdominal structures may also be present, thus introducing a further hazard.

Confining the discussion to the context of skeletal injury alone, four major syndromes are encountered.

Blood Loss leading to Shock

This is a natural concomitant to fracture and varies with the severity and multiplicity of the fractures present. Fractures of the pelvis are particularly prone to produce extensive, and hidden, blood loss because of the rich blood supply of the cancellous bone but, more important, from injury to the extensive vascular plexus which exists on the pelvic wall for the supply of the adjoining viscera. Additional injury to other organs, particularly the liver and spleen, may add to the problem.

In simple terms management consists of the replacement of blood of appropriate volume and at the appropriate rate.

The consequences of massive blood transfusion in the correction of blood loss may lead to other problems.

Fat Embolism Syndrome

This condition is characterized by the presence of fat globules in capillaries of various organs of the body which results in secondary changes which together produce anoxia of the local tissues. The extent of the condition is greatly variable but, most commonly, most seriously affects the lungs producing not only local anoxia but interference with gaseous transfer across the alveolar membrane. The hypoxaemia produced may, in itself, cause defective function in other organs as a result of their inefficiency of function. The pathological changes may also affect the brain producing alteration of the conscious level and may impair renal function as a result of capillary damage in the kidneys. A superficial manifestation is the development of small petechial haemorrhages in the skin of the neck, shoulder and upper anterior thoracic region. Petechiae may also be present in the conjunctivae and retinae.

The aims of treatment of this complication are the maintenance of proper oxygenation by whatever means is necessary until spontaneous resolution occurs.

'Crush Syndrome'

Oliguria or anuria may result from acute renal tubular necrosis due to prolonged hypotension. It has also been described in association with the deposition of proteinous material in the renal tubules in patients with extensive or prolonged crushing of skeletal muscle. It is thought to arise from the ischaemic breakdown of muscle fibres. A similar phenomenon may occur after the restoration of circulation to a limb which has been rendered ischaemic for some period of time.

Treatment consists of the maintenance of renal function by whatever means necessary including dialysis, until spontaneous resolution occurs.

Hypercalcaemia

This phenomenon may arise in patients with Paget's disease of bone who have sustained fractures. It results from the unbalanced continued resorption of bone following immobilization, and may lead to cardiac irregularities and other problems associated with hypercalcaemia and can be controlled by the use of calcitonin.

Clearly, with every fracture there is an associated soft tissue injury which, around the fracture, may amount to a minor stretch of the periosteum or more extensively to complete disruption of the periosteum and surrounding muscles giving rise to major fracture instability. In addition, there may be significant injury to skin and any major nerves or arteries which are nearby. Certain skeletal injuries are commonly associated with specific soft tissue injuries or other skeletal injuries, and it is important to be aware of these associations since they may be missed in the confusion of the multiple injury situation.

1. Fracture of the Pelvis and Acetabulum

This may be complicated by injury to the bladder or the urethra. Although usually associated with displaced fractures of the pelvic ring, bladder rupture may occur with less severe skeletal injury if the bladder has been grossly distended at the time of injury when 'bursting' may occur.

2. Posterior Dislocation of the Hip

This may result in sciatic nerve palsy which may involve either the entire nerve or simply its lateral division. The lateral division supplies the extensor muscles of the ankle and toes. Such a nerve injury is also more common if dislocation is accompanied by a fracture of the posterior wall of the acetabulum.

3. Fracture of the Shaft of the Femur

Occasionally this is accompanied by a posterior dislocation of the hip. Such an associated injury is regularly missed since the deformity related to the fracture disguises the hip deformity related to the dislocation. Such combinations of injury may occur elsewhere and illustrate the necessity of including the joints above and below any fracture in the radiological examination of an injured limb.

4. Supracondylar Fracture of the Femur or Posterior Dislocation of the Knee

Such injuries may damage the popliteal artery.

5. Fracture of the Tibial Shaft

A frequently missed complication of such an injury is muscle ischaemia in the leg from increased pressure within muscle compartments. Tibial fractures may be associated with direct damage of the major tibial arteries which will be easily diagnosed since ischaemia of the distal part of the limb will be evident. Compartmental ischaemia is much more subtle and more difficult to diagnose, particularly if the limb is encased in a plaster cast.

Elevation of the pressure within a muscle compartment arises from continued bleeding within that compartment. Eventually the pressure is such that the blood supply to the muscles and nerves within the compartment is obstructed at the arteriolar level. As a result of the pressure gradient on descending the arterial tree, the pressure within the compartment is still insufficient to obstruct major arterial flow which can, therefore, freely supply the distal part of the limb. This lesion can be recognized by the loss of sensation in the skin areas supplied by the corresponding nerves and by paralysis and developing contracture of the involved muscles. Stretching these muscles produces pain. If the leg is exposed the tension can be noted in the muscle compartment involved. (*See also Fig.* 21.2.)

6. Anterior Dislocation of the Shoulder or Displaced Fracture of the Surgical Neck of the Humerus

Many of these injuries are complicated by palsy of the axillary nerve or brachial plexus. The axillary artery and vein are also at slight risk.

7. Fracture of the Shaft of the Humerus

In view of the close apposition of the radial nerve to the diaphysis of the humerus in the spiral groove, damage to this structure may occur.

8. Supracondylar Fracture of the Humerus

Such an injury may damage the brachial artery which in turn may produce Volkmann's ischaemia contracture of the forearm flexor muscles. It should be noted, however, that this latter condition is more likely to be produced by increased pressure within the flexor compartment of the forearm from fractures of the radius and ulna. Palsy of the median nerve associated with supracondylar fracture of the humerus is more common than brachial artery damage.

9. The 'Monteggia' Principle

In the forearm or leg a fracture of one bone *with displacement* must be associated with injury to the other bone. If no fracture is present then dislocation of one or other end of the bone must exist. Thus a displaced fracture of the proximal end of the ulna must be associated with dislocation of the head of the radius if the radius shaft remains intact. (Monteggia fracture).

10. Displaced Colles Fracture or Dislocation of the Carpal Lunate

Such injuries are not infrequently associated with a stretching injury of the median nerve.

11. Unstable Spinal Injury

Frequently such injuries result in damage to the spinal cord. This may be of particular importance in the presence of unconsciousness due to a head injury, since the force which produced the head injury may also have produced the significant injury of the cervical spine. Therefore, it is a sound policy that patients rendered unconscious as a result of head injury should have adequate X-rays taken of the cervical spine.

MEASUREMENTS AND MONITORING

The parameters which require measurement in patients with multiple injuries will clearly vary depending on the severity and extent of the injuries and any later complication. The frequency with which these measurements are made will vary during the course of the condition, being more frequent in the early unstable state after injury.

The measurements required relate to the blood loss, the fractures and the late complications.

Blood Loss

All patients will require some assessment of the circulating volume and state of shock by some or all of the following:

1. *Pulse rate.*
2. *Blood pressure.* Although this is most commonly measured by a pneumatic cuff, a more accurate assessment can be made following arterial cannulation which is of especial importance in low pressure states.
3. *Central venous pressure.* Not only is the absolute reading important but the response in extent and time to a small bolus of colloid infusion can be of great value.
4. *Urinary output.* This provides a fairly sensitive index of cardiac output and the estimation of output at hourly intervals will aid in the assessment of fluid requirements.
5. *Electrocardiograph.* This simple and unobstrusive monitoring can give valuable information on the performance of the myocardial response to infusion. It can also provide information on the previous myocardial state and, in the presence of a chest injury, may indicate myocardial damage.
6. *Blood, pH and gases.* These measurements will give a more accurate assessment of the acidotic state and allow accurate correction with bicarbonate infusion. Their estimation is mandatory in the presence of a significant chest injury.
7. *Haemoglobin.* This measurement will be of more value in the later stages of resuscitation and will give some idea of the state of haemodilution.

8. *Clotting factors.* Accurate estimation of the blood clotting mechanism will be necessary after massive blood transfusion to prevent unnecessary continued blood loss.

Injuries

1. *Fractures.* Appropriate radiographic assessment will be necessary.
2. *Chest injuries.* The importance of *sequential radiographs* at appropriate periods is stressed to be aware of developing changes. This assessment should include not only lung fields and pleural cavities, but also the size and shape of the mediastinum and heart which may also have been injured.
3. *Abdominal injuries.* Appropriate radiographs may assist in the diagnosis of ruptured bowel and increase in *sequential girth measurements* may provide evidence of intra-abdominal bleeding.
4. *Pelvic injuries.* Blood in the urine after catheterization may indicate bladder or renal injury which can be more accurately assessed by a cystogram or intravenous pyelogram, respectively.
5. *Arterial injury.* The continued presence of ischaemic changes in a limb after restoration of an adequate circulating volume and cardiac output will require investigation by arteriography.

Later Complications

1. *Fat embolism.* This condition may be suspected in the presence of hypoxaemia, a sudden drop in haemoglobin and platelet count, and radiographic changes in the lungs.
2. *Hypercalcaemia.* In patients with extensive Paget's disease, fractures and immobilization may give rise to significant elevation of the serum calcium which should be monitored regularly.
3. *'Crush' kidney.* As with other causes of renal failure the development and progression of the condition will be followed by measuring the urinary output, the blood and urine osmolality and the concentrations of electrolytes, urea and creatinine in blood and urine.

PATHOPHYSIOLOGICAL MECHANISMS

Shock

The mechanism of the development of shock is complex, with various factors interrelated. Many of the sequences are common to shock, no matter the cause, but the initial trigger following multiple injuries is blood loss. This leads to a reduction in the circulatory volume which produces a lowered cardiac output. In response to this low pressure state, the baroreceptors in the atria and pulmonary veins together with the systemic baroreceptors of the carotid sinus and the aortic arch, provide a reduced output of signals to the peripheral vessels with consequent reduction in the inhibition of vasoconstriction. The resultant vasoconstriction affects the inessential areas initially, namely the skin, muscles and splanchnic area and the normal circulation is preserved to the vital centres of the brain, heart and, for some time, the kidneys. With continued bleeding the latter circulation is also reduced by vasoconstriction, and reduction in glomerular filtration and hence urinary output is a consequence. A further result of the inhibition of the baroreceptor influence is the development of tachycardia.

Thus, in the compensated state, the clinical appearance is of sympathetic over-activity of the skin and muscles with peripheral coolness, pallor and some sweating. The systemic blood pressure is maintained and there is a tachycardia. If this condition persists, and bleeding continues, then urinary output falls when the renal circulation becomes impaired.

One other factor which assists with the vasoconstrictor compensatory mechanism is the stimulation of the chemoreceptors of the carotid body and aortic areas by the reduction in Po_2 and elevation of CO_2, consequent on 'shunting' in the pulmonary circulation.

As blood loss continues, the compensatory mechanism becomes more intense until it is fully operational, following which further reduction in blood volume leads to a decompensated state with lowered blood pressure and progressive reduction in circulation to the vital organs.

The clinical picture, at this stage, is of more serious consequence. The tachycardia continues but is accompanied by a fall in the blood pressure. The appearance of peripheral shutdown is extreme and, as the vital organs become hypoxic, they may show signs of failure. The patient becomes restless and agitated with a reduced level of consciousness. Cardiac failure may become manifest by electrocardiographic changes and, eventually, despite the low circulating volume, there is a rising central venous pressure as the myocardium is unable to cope even with this reduced load. During the period of shock there is also some evidence of the appearance of an abnormal protein which specifically depresses myocardial function and adds to the problems.

Renal shutdown becomes complete and progression of all factors leads to death.

The respiratory rate accelerates for several reasons. Hypoxia stimulates the chemoreceptors previously described to produce reflex tachypnoea which is exacerbated by the failing heart and the acidosis from tissue anoxia produces air hunger.

Metabolic changes result from the compensatory vasoconstriction which produces hypoxia of the tissues supplied. These turn to anaerobic metabolism with the production of lactic acid and the increasing acidosis which, with the passage of time, further depresses the cell function throughout the body and contributes to the eventual failure.

There comes a stage in the above sequence of events when resuscitation with replacement of fluid is of no avail and a state of irreversible shock results.

Additional factors may influence this sequence of events. The drunk patient may have a significant degree of peripheral vasodilatation as a result of alcohol which may produce a peripheral circulation which belies his clinical state, and, what is more, may contribute to inefficiency of the compensatory mechanism. In contrast the patient who has been exposed to the elements may well be grossly constricted yet have minimal blood loss.

Fat Embolism Syndrome

Fat embolism syndrome is a term used to describe a group of symptoms rather than pathology which sometimes follows long-bone fractures.

The pathological changes are not fully understood although, as the name suggests, it was originally thought that the condition was brought about entirely by the embolization of marrow fat from the fractured limb to the lung where the fat globules were filtered off in the capillaries. This did not adequately explain the development of systemic fat embolism with the discovery of fat globules in the skin, retina, kidney and brain. Accordingly it was postulated that the condition arose from alteration of the normal serum lipids with the development of maxiglobules of fat.

It is possible that both mechanisms contribute to the development of the condition.

There is certainly strong evidence that much of the fat sequestered in the lung has the fatty acid profile of marrow fat rather than the circulating plasma lipids. However, the changes in serum lipids which have been described in response to trauma do not produce larger aggregates of fatty material. There is an increase in free fatty acids and triglycerides, and β-lipoprotein has also been found to increase. These changes are attributed to catecholamine release as a result of the stress situation. It is probably these changes which also induce increased platelet stickiness with tendency to aggregation and thrombosis.

These latter changes occur both systemically and in the pulmonary circulation producing intravascular coagulation on a wide scale which will also include, within the clots, the increased fatty elements. This would account for the dramatic fall in haematocrit and platelet level in the established case.

These changes are compounded in the lung by the filtered fat globules which are broken down by lipases to constituent fatty acids. The effect in the lung of these substances, plus the intravascular coagulation, is to produce increased permeability of the pulmonary capillaries with the progressive development of interstitial oedema. Much of this effect may be mediated by serotonin release from the platelets.

Pulmonary interstitial oedema has two main effects. First, it reduces lung compliance with consequent reduction of movement of air in and out of the alveoli. Secondly, it reduces gaseous exchange across the alveolar membrane. This affects carbon dioxide transport less since it can diffuse much more rapidly than oxygen which is dramatically affected. Thus there is a severe fall in Po_2 which may give rise to secondary effects in other organs. In such organs, this hypoxia exacerbates the reduced function which may already have taken place as a result of the systemic effects of the pathological changes. Clinically, cerebral changes, with altered conscious level, may occur, the myocardium may fail, and anuria may supervene.

Alteration in Bone Metabolism

Fractures result either from the application of an abnormal force to normal bone or the application of normal force to abnormal bone. The latter is termed a pathological fracture. Obviously fractures may also result from abnormal force on abnormal bone which may explain the severity and multiplicity of fractures often found in elderly females involved in road traffic accidents. Such patients inevitably have some degree of osteoporosis as a result of deficient ovarian function after the menopause. Added to this, as many as 15% of elderly patients with fractures may have osteomalacia contributing to their osteopenic state. Failure to treat adequately with vitamin D and calcium supplements will lead to delayed healing of fractures.

Immobilization of bones, either locally by splintage or generally by rest in bed, has an important effect on the dynamic replacement of bone which is a continuing process of resorption and formation. One of the most important stimuli to bone formation is the use of a limb. This effect is probably mediated through the piezo-electric currents generated by bone deformation under the stress of use. Thus all immobilized bone becomes osteoporotic as a result of the imbalance in favour of resorption which is produced. In normal circumstances this leads to no alteration in the serum levels of calcium and phosphate. However, in active Paget's disease, there is great increase in the resorption by osteoclasts which is, in normal circumstances, balanced by a similar great increase in new bone formation (hence the raised alkaline phosphatase). In this situation, immobilization switches off new bone formation and resorption continues apace. It is therefore possible to get a significant degree of hypercalcaemia resulting from the calcium released by the rapid rate of bone resorption.

THERAPY

The two most important aspects in the management of patients with multiple injuries are:
1. Continuous assessment.
2. The allocation of priorities in treatment.
Priorities must also continuously be appraised since they may alter with changing circumstances. The usual order of priorities consists of:
Maintenance of airway and oxygenation.
Maintenance of circulatory volume.
First aid treatment of injuries.
Definitive treatment of injuries.
Only when there is control of and stability in the clinical state of the patient, is the definitive treatment of any injury considered. Such treatment may even be deferred for many days if it is felt unsafe to proceed in the presence of some other life-threatening injury. Very occasionally, exceptions to this rule may arise when the definitive treatment may be necessary to secure the stability of the circulating volume, e.g. splenectomy for uncontrolled bleeding from a splenic rupture.

Maintenance of Airway and Oxygenation

Details of these aspects are dealt with elsewhere. It must be remembered that attention to adequate oxygenation goes hand in hand with the maintenance of the circulatory volume since neither can be fully effective without the other.

Maintenance of the Circulatory Volume

There are two aspects of this part of treatment. Any blood loss must be brought under control and that which has been lost must be replaced.

I. Control of Blood Loss

The control of blood loss in the maintenance of the circulatory volume is frequently neglected in the care of the patient with multiple injuries. This is particularly true in the early management where it may be lost sight of in the general confusion of resuscitation and assessment, and it is just at this stage where it may be able to contribute most. Adequate control of blood loss means a reduced physiological compensatory mechanism and a reduced replacement requirement.

There are several ways in which blood loss can be minimized.

1. Simple pressure dressings can be applied to open wounds. This is of particular importance in the head area where scalp lacerations can bleed profusely. Such pressure dressings contribute even more during resuscitation when the rising blood pressure induces further bleeding.

2. Any obvious arterial bleeding in a wound should be secured either by an artery forceps and ligature or, in the case of a major artery, by an arterial clip.

3. Fractures should be adequately splinted to prevent excessive movement which may contribute to the blood loss. Pneumatic splints, where appropriate, have the additional benefit of applying pressure to bleeding from any wound area and yet allow the visualization of the limb circulation. They may also contribute to resuscitation by partly exanguinating the limb and thus returning to the central area blood which, in an acute situation, is not required distally. This property has been extended to the use of pneumatic trousers during routine resuscitation which, together with elevation of the leg, may provide a significant auto-transfusion.

4. The effective control of pain by suitable analgesic reduces restlessness and thus aids fracture splintage as well as general well-being.

5. In a few patients with uncontrolled blood loss, the situation can only be retrieved by definitive surgery. There is no effective conservative way of controlling intra-thoracic or intra-abdominal bleeding from major structures for which operation may be required.

II. Replacement of Blood Loss

Where significant blood loss arises following major trauma, the ideal replacement is whole blood. This will not be immediately available in view of the time required for blood grouping and cross matching even in the emergency situation. Meanwhile the lost circulatory volume should be replaced by transfusion with one or more of the recognized plasma volume expanders: plasma protein solution, plasma, dextran 70, or other synthetic plasma volume expanders such as 'Haemaccel'.

The rate of transfusion should be determined by analysis of the measurements enumerated earlier. Such a decision should not necessarily be based on a single measurement, but on a series of measurements which may indicate more clearly the state of 'shock' and its progress. As stated earlier there must be continuous assessment of the whole patient and the rate of transfusion may have to be modified in the light of changes in the vital signs.

The volume of blood (or temporary substitute) which will eventually be required can only initially be an estimate. It is an important exercise to carry out since it does give the blood bank a reasonable assessment of the requirements and also gives the clinician the expected volume of transfusion which will be required to produce a stable state. This is of extreme importance where replacement of the expected volume does not produce stability in the vital signs, a situation which should lead to a search for a further source of bleeding. It should be noted that head injuries do not produce the hypotensive state and experience has shown that the commonest source of continuing circulatory instability after transfusion of the anticipated loss is intra-abdominal bleeding.

As a simple rule of thumb, the following blood loss should be estimated for each fracture:

Tibia—0·5 litre
Femur—1 litre (these figures should be doubled if the fracture is open)
Pelvis—1–3 litres depending on the severity (this figure may be greater if there is a specific vascular complication)
Chest—0·5 litre

Other injuries from which significant blood loss may occur but for which estimation can be difficult are large scalp lacerations, severe facial fractures and intra-abdominal trauma.

It should be remembered that these estimates are for blood loss over a period of approximately 24 hours and that, although major losses occur in the first few hours, significant bleeding continues thereafter.

As previously stated, the rate of transfusion depends entirely on the continuous analysis of the various clinical measurements.

Massive blood transfusions are occasionally required in the aftermath of very severe injuries and have their own complications which are detailed elsewhere.

Correction of Metabolic Acidosis

If there has been blood loss of any significant degree the compensatory vasoconstriction of the non-essential areas will have produced a metabolic acidosis. Since this, in itself, is harmful to all cell function it is necessary to correct the defect. Initially 100 mmol bicarbonate can be given slowly intravenously: repeat measurement of the pH and base deficit will guide further therapy.

Fat Embolism

Much has been written on fat embolism and its treatment without yielding the definitive answer.

It is now universally recognized that the major part of treatment consists of the control of the respiratory failure which is the predominant clinical feature of the condition. In the severe case, this requires controlled ventilation.

Attention must also be paid to the possible failure of any other system which has been affected, such as the kidney.

There are numerous reports concerning the use of drugs in fat embolism but, although sporadic improvement has been claimed for each, the fact that no single therapy has proved universally and consistently effective speaks for itself. Part of the problem lies in the condition itself, since its relative infrequency and wide and varied spectrum of presentation makes a controlled trial difficult to construct.

It has been suggested that steroids are effective when given in large doses. In addition to their general anti-inflammatory effect they may stabilize lysosomal membranes and capillary walls, thus reducing the capillary leakage in the lungs with reduction of the interstitial oedema.

Reports concerning the use of Trasylol (aprotinin) have been encouraging but, as with others, have not withstood the test of time and widespread use.

More recently, diuretics have been advocated in view of their alleged benefit in the 'shock lung' situation. It is unlikely that their use is of benefit except where fluid overload has been superimposed on a fat embolism syndrome.

Heparin, low molecular weight dextran and clofibrate have all been used as adjuncts to the general therapeutic measures but have not been shown to be of benefit.

There is no known method of prophylaxis although, clearly, reducing the fracture manipulation to a minimum should be practised in view of the possible aetiology in terms of bone marrow fat and general response to trauma. It would be convenient to be able to identify possible susceptible individuals in such circumstances and, although work has been done along such lines, there has been no application in the clinical situation.

Metabolic Changes

I. Hypercalcaemia

Hypercalcaemia is fortunately a rare phenomenon. It should always be anticipated in patients with widespread Paget's disease who are immobilized. The immediate effects of hypercalcaemia can be controlled and the serum calcium lowered by prednisolone, 50 mg four times daily, but better long-term control of the disease reducing the hypercalcaemia can be achieved by calcitonin in a dose of 50 MRC units daily which inhibits the resorptive process.

II. Osteomalacia

If vitamin D deficiency is discovered in the elderly patient or immigrant, it should be treated vigorously to avoid delay in fracture union. A convenient regime is 50 000 units of calciferol daily for one week, then 50 00 units weekly thereafter. Calcium supplements should also be added in view of the increased utilization of calcium which will follow the promotion of ossification by the vitamin D.

Fractures

I. First aid treatment

Adequate and appropriate first aid treatment of fractures is important during the early resuscitative phase of the treatment of the patient with multiple injuries for reasons mentioned before. Open wounds should be covered with clean dressings and bandaged to reduce bacterial contamination and give some control of the bleeding. Rigid or pneumatic splints may be applied to the limbs, but in the leg these tend not to splint the femur well. A useful appliance for leg splintage is a Thomas splint with a splint ring at the top and made from radiolucent material. The leg is placed within the splint on the splint slings and immobilized by traction applied usually by a foot piece which is strapped to the foot and ankle.

After resuscitation has been completed, it may be possible to consider the definitive treatment of any fractures present. If the patient's general condition does not permit this, more efficient splintage will be required for a longer period of time. Control of fractures of the arm and the leg below the knee can be simply achieved by a well-padded plaster cast.

Femoral and pelvic fractures are more effectively controlled by traction on the limb applied through a Steinmann or Denham pin introduced into the upper tibia. This is easily performed after local anaesthetic infiltration into the area and the limb then suspended in balanced (Hamilton–Russell) traction or supported in a Thomas splint.

These forms of immobilization can be maintained for many days until the patient's condition allows definitive treatment.

II. Definitive Treatment of Fractures

1. Limb fractures

It is clearly not necessary to cover this topic in detail but simply to outline in general the current methods of fracture treatment (*Fig.* 21.1) Hopefully this will clarify a subject which more than any other is less understood and correspondingly causes more alarm in the staff of intensive therapy units. In turn this should lead to better patient care.

All fractures are treated by the same basic approach. The first question posed is whether reduction is necessary. Undisplaced fractures and some displaced fractures require no reduction. Having made this decision it is still necessary to determine whether immobilization is necessary. Clearly fractures which have been reduced from a displaced position will require immobilization. Some undisplaced fractures will also require immobilization to prevent displacement, whereas others will simply be treated by active movement with minimal rest. Into this latter category fall such fractures as those of the upper humerus and *stable* crush fractures of the lumbar vertebrae.

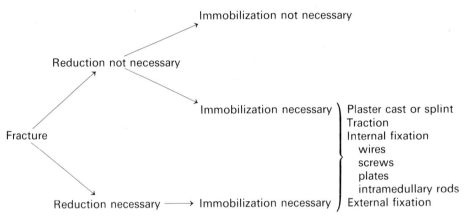

Fig. 21.1. The steps in the management of a fracture.

If immobilization is deemed to be necessary, the most appropriate form has to be selected from either plaster cast, traction, internal fixation or external fixation.

PLASTER CAST. This represents the most common method of temporary immobilization of fractures and also the most common method of external splintage in the definitive treatment. Although most still use plaster-of-Paris, newer materials have been introduced which are stronger, lighter and more waterproof, but much more expensive. These are either resin-impregnated plasters or plastic materials.

The two main problems associated with plaster immobilization of limbs in the ICU are the possible pressure damage to skin and the inability to view the leg properly.

Pressure areas occur at the margins of the cast or within the cast as a result of deformity of the surface on application. Marginal pressure can be avoided by adjustment of limb position and proper skin care. Cutting back the edges should be reduced to a minimum since this may only produce similar problems in a different area. Pressure is of particular significance over points where specific structures are vulnerable, such as the common peroneal nerve at the neck of the fibula.

Deeper problems should be anticipated in the presence of undue pain in areas at some distance from the fracture, and such symptoms should be investigated by inspection of the area through an appropriate 'window' cut in the plaster.

The difficulties associated with inability to view the limb can only be overcome by considering the possible pathology and relating this to what can be seen and other indirect signs. The most commonly encountered complications of injury which will require diagnosis will be ischaemia and infection.

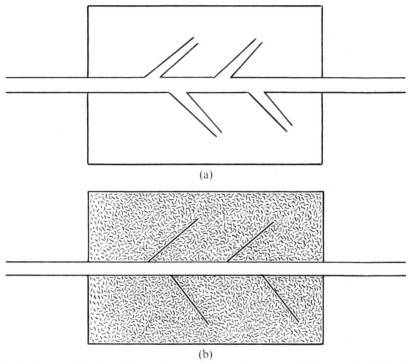

(a)

(b)

Fig. 21.2. The mechanism of muscle compartment pressure. (a) Normal circulation to muscle and distal region. (b) Increased pressure within the muscle compartment abolishes local circulation, but the circulation to distal region at the higher pressure continues.

Major vascular occlusion will be easy to diagnose by the signs of ischaemia in the exposed periphery. Muscle ischaemia due to intracompart-mental pressure will not be easy to diagnose since the toes and fingers remain fairly pink and warm (*Fig.* 21.2). It should be suspected:

a. Where limb pain is more severe than anticipated.

b. Where paralysis of fingers or toes is present especially in one direction, and associated with diminished sensation.

c. Where passive stretching of the muscles of the affected compartment produces pain.

When diagnosed the condition requires treatment by surgical decom-pression of the involved muscle compartment (fasciotomy).

The possibility of wound infection has to be considered in the presence of:

Pyrexia with no other source of infection.

Undue increasing local pain.

Increasing swelling of the exposed periphery.

Malodour from the plaster; altered blood by itself has a relatively sweet smell.

In such instances further inspection of the leg will be necessary after removal of all or part of the plaster cast.

TRACTION. Traction is a form of immobilization after fracture which is almost exclusively applied to the lower limb. The traction force can be applied either by adhesive tape (skin traction) or by pins passed through the bone (skeletal traction).

Thereafter, the force can be used to suspend the leg in slings as well as to provide traction: balanced traction sometimes referred to as Hamilton–Russell traction. The counter-traction in this instance is the patient's body weight plus the frictional resistance of the bed clothes and any increase in traction may need to be balanced by elevating the foot of the bed to increase the counter-traction.

With some fractures the limb may be placed on a sling within a Thomas splint. In this splint strong traction can be applied since the counter-traction is produced by the resistance of the splint ring in the groin: fixed traction. For convenience the splint is then suspended by some means, but it should be noted that this manoeuvre does not alter the fixed traction system.

Pressure over prominent areas is the main complication of traction and should be avoided by prophylactic skin care and, where possible, adjustment of the traction system.

More detailed knowledge and understanding of traction systems can be obtained elsewhere.

INTERNAL FIXATION. If it is decided that internal fixation of a fracture is indicated, then the most common approach is for *rigid* internal fixation using screws and/or plates or wire to provide compression across the fracture. As an alternative, an intramedullary nail of as large a calibre as possible can be introduced.

The application of compression techniques in the fixation of fractures provides *rigid* fixation and has the great advantage of the ability to dispense with the use of any external splintage in most instances. Thus there is less of an encumbrance and, more important, this allows active use of the limb (within reason) and provides easy access for inspection of the limb.

The intramedullary nail, where applicable, provides the same advantages.

EXTERNAL FIXATION. Although an old idea, in more recent years various forms of apparatus have been developed to provide an exoskeleton around a fracture to provide rigid fixation either as an alternative to internal fixation or in situations where internal fixation is contra-indicated.

No matter the type, these basically involve the insertion of two or more percutaneous pins into the bone on either side of the fracture and the incorporation of these pins into an external fixation rod. This system also provides rigid fixation with its advantages but avoids the infective and other complications associated with the insertion of metal around a fracture.

There are two situations in which fixation, either internal or external is mandatory: in the presence of a major vascular injury, any fracture needs to be firmly fixed to protect the vascular repair and allow adequate limb visualization. These conditions cannot be filled by plaster cast immobilization. Similarly, fracture fixation is necessary in the presence of extensive damage to skin and soft tissues where additional plastic surgical treatment will be necessary. In this situation, internal fixation or carefully planned external fixation will allow the plastic surgeon access for his procedure.

2. *Fractures of the pelvis*

The most important feature of pelvic fractures is their ability to produce concealed bleeding of large volume. There is no difference in the basic approach to treatment of these fractures in that undisplaced fractures need no reduction, but if instability is present immobilization will be required to prevent displacement. Displaced fractures on the other hand may require reduction and will require some form of immobilization.

In simple terms, the pelvis is a ring structure. Single fractures of the ring are stable and require no treatment (unless in the acetabulum), whereas fracture of two places in the ring produces an unstable segment. If situated anteriorly (the butterfly fracture) usually no treatment is required, but the more common lateral fracture (the fore-and-aft fracture) contains the limb in its unstable segment and treatment will be required.

Classically, the proximal displacement due to muscle pull is corrected by balanced traction of the limb to which a sling around the pelvis could be added if there was a tendency for external rotation to occur. More recently, it has been possible to apply the techniques of external fixation to unstable fractures of the pelvis and thus to provide better and firm fixation without the constricting and concealing effects of pelvic sling and leg traction.

3. *Fractures of the spine (including dislocation)*

Stable fractures of the spine do not lay the spinal cord at risk and require no treatment.

Unstable fractures, whether displaced or not, place the cord at risk and require some form of immobilization. In some instances, cord injury may already be present. If a spinal cord injury is complete, then no recovery of this is possible. Recovery can only occur after injury of the nerve roots including the cauda equina.

CERVICAL SPINE. If there is no displacement of an unstable fracture of the cervical spine, it is usually treated initially by traction, although fusion of the affected segment may be carried out later. Temporary traction can be effected by a halter apparatus beneath the chin and occiput. This is inconvenient and inefficient for long-term use and permanent traction of the neck is better provided by callipers inserted into the outer table of the skull above the ears. The direction of traction will be dictated by the injury. If such a fracture is complicated by a spinal cord injury, it will be necessary to nurse this patient on a frame or bed which allows turning without disturbing the traction. If there is no cord injury and there is no other injury to contra-indicate its use, it is very convenient to nurse such patients in the sitting position in a cardiac bed to which a gallows-type extension has been added for the traction apparatus.

If there is dislocation of the cervical spine it is usual to attempt reduction by traction as described above, failing which the dislocation may be manipulated or more likely reduced at open operation. In the event of the latter fusion is also performed. The postoperative treatment will be as described above, until it is felt safe to apply only a collar for support.

The decision on operative treatment may become more difficult if dislocation is complicated by cord injury. In this situation other factors have to be considered, in particular the severity of the injury and its level in the cord with subsequent effects and potential for recovery. Since there will always be some impairment of respiratory muscle function, the operative risk is high and must be balanced against the possible benefits which might be obtained, for example, from nerve root recovery or improvment in a particular cord lesion.

THORACOLUMBAR SPINE. Unstable but undisplaced fractures in the thoracic or lumbar spine, whether complicated by cord injury or not, are treated either in a turning frame or bed or by careful nursing in a firm ordinary bed using pillows for additional support.

Displaced fractures accompanied by dislocation but with no cord injury are likely to be treated in a similar manner.

If cord injury is present then it may be decided to carry out open reduction. In the lumbar spine this may be accompanied by internal fixation using plates and bolts and, thereafter, treatment should continue as outlined above.

SYSTEM REPLACEMENT

In the context of multiple trauma, system replacement involves amputation of a limb or more commonly its distal part, with later replacement by a prosthesis. Amputation of the leg is indicated mainly for uncorrectable ischaemia which usually results from severe and extensive damage. Crush injuries, in particular, lead to extensive soft tissue damage in addition to fracture which may make vascular repair technically impossible or may produce so much damage that restoration of the main vascular channels would be of little or no value. Extensive nerve damage, especially proximal, would lend weight to any such decision in view of the poor prognosis for recovery of reasonable function in such circumstances. Modern artificial lower limbs provide such a reasonable replacement of normal function that they provide a better alternative in such circumstances.

The attitude in the upper limb is quite different. The hand is a prehensile organ and also provides a multitude of coarse and fine functions. Even the most developed prosthesis cannot provide such movement and certainly no sensation, and a hand with severely disturbed function is usually of more use than an artificial limb. For this reason, strenuous efforts are made to preserve any damaged arm even to the extent of replantation following traumatic amputation.

Limited replacement of part of the skeleton, although fairly frequent for neoplastic disease, is uncommon following trauma and virtually confined to the femoral head. In younger patients, femoral neck fractures are treated by reduction followed by internal fixation usually with one form of nail and plate device. In the elderly such an approach produces an increasing number of failures due to the nail tending to redisplace from the osteoporotic femoral head. As a better alternative a femoral head replacement, or occasionally a total hip replacement, is preferred.

Chapter 22

Paediatrics

D. G. Young

Intensive care in paediatric practice has to take account of two main aspects in which the patient differs from the adult patient. First there are differences in the structure and physiology of the neonate from that of the adult and this fact becomes apparent on superficial inspection. The neonate has a different configuration with a large head and short limbs in relation to the adult. The more subtle physiological differences are not so obvious but are of significance in planning management. The second difference is that many of the disorders affecting the infant and child are peculiar to the young age group and are quite different from those afflicting the adult. Examples of these are coliform meningitis which affects infants within the first month of life and necrotizing enterocolitis which is relatively common in premature infants who survive other problems as a result of the development of neonatal intensive care.

The evolution of intensive care in paediatric practice has been gradual. The initial impetus came from advances in neonatal surgery with the inevitable demand for more intensive postoperative support. Atresia of the alimentary tract, with the resulting fluid and electrolyte imbalance, which often developed before diagnosis was established and the postoperative period when alimentary tract absorption was impaired stimulated detailed study of fluid, electrolytes and subsequently nutritional balance. There was then the gradual and widespread development of special care baby units in maternity hospital and, subsequently, intensive care facilities in the major or regional centres. Many of the problems in these units were related to respiratory function and have been the source of many of the developments of respiratory support.

The concept of intensive care departments for the older children followed and, taking Glasgow as an example, the intensive care department in the Children's Hospital was opened in 1971. This multidisciplinary area for eight patients serves a wide variety of patients who require intensive care. Any patient considered to need intensive care is admitted to the unit by the clinician responsible. In the 4-year period, 1977–80, the number of patients admitted was 1547. The majority of these patients (846) were under the care of the surgeons and the surgical specialty groups primarily involved were:

1. General paediatric   16·8% (of the total admitted)
2. Orthopaedic   3·2%
3. Cardiac postoperative   34·6%

The remaining 701 (45·3%) patients were admitted under the care of paediatric physicians and the following is a breakdown of the primary system or disorder which was the reason for their admission:

a. Respiratory   12·5%
b. Convulsions   7·4%
c. Cardiac   6·5%
d. Ingestion of drugs   5·8%
e. Meningitis   3·0%
f. Diabetes   2·5%
g. Septicaemia   1·7%
h. Others   5·8%

Collaborating in the care of their patients are the anaesthetic staff who are mainly involved with the respiratory problems. Unlike many adult intensive care areas, the patients remain in the care of the clinician responsible for them and who will be continuing their care when they return to the wards.

Excluded from the above list are the neonatal patients except those undergoing cardiac surgery. Within the hospital group is a neonatal surgical ward in which an area is designated for intensive care of newborns who have been referred to the regional centre for surgical care. Also physically attached and within the group, is a paediatric department in the Queen Mother's Hospital in which 'medical' infants are nursed and given the required intensive care.

The aspects of intensive care in paediatrics may, therefore, be seen to encompass a wide variety of problems. In this chapter attention will be focused on some aspects on neonatal care, fluid and electrolyte balance, nutrition and respiration followed by mention of some of the particular system problems encountered in children.

NEONATAL CARE

The newborn infant is particularly vulnerable, having to adjust from the very protected environment in the uterus to the challenges of the outside world where gas exchange, feeding and temperature control are no longer automatic but require effort and control. Added to this is the danger of injurious agents, such as bacteria, which on first acquaintance may be pathogenic whereas in the older infant, child or adult the same bacteria would simply be commensals.

The younger the patient the more important is the thermal environment in which the patient is nursed. Not only is the total surface area of an infant relatively greater but the head accounts for more than double the percentage of surface area when compared to an adult. The sick neonate is usually nursed in an incubator with maximal exposure to allow close observation and examination. The use of one of the modern types of incubator helps control the infant's immediate environment. Radiant heat loss must be countered as well as conducted and convected losses. Another useful method of conserving heat is the use of a space blanket or the specially prepared silver swaddlers in which the infant may be wrapped. These are particularly useful when transporting infants and have the added benefit that they are radiolucent. Heat loss from the infant may also be decreased by the provision of warm humidified gasses.[1] Simple expedients, such as using tube gauze to make caps for babies, also help cut down the heat loss.

The small infant, particularly the premature baby, does not tolerate interference and all interventions have some systemic effect. A fall in arterial Po_2 has been clearly demonstrated in the premature infant when subjected even to such simple procedures as taking a temperature by a thermometer. The least possible handling, with performance of only the necessary procedures to small infants, is desirable. The results published by Hughes-Davies[2] indicate that intensive care management is not appropriate for all small infants. Careful selection should identify the infant who is not going to survive without intensive care.

Nutrition of the neonate presents problems in those who have a delay in establishing normal alimentary tract function. This may be due to a congenital anomaly of the alimentary tract, such as atresia, or to inadequate peristalsis in the low-birth-weight infant in whom hypoxia may be a contributory factor. The point at which intervention becomes necessary varies with each infant. The baby of 1 kg birth weight has very limited reserves and has only approximately 10 g of fat available as an emergency source.[3] In contrast the 3-kg baby has 600 g fat and is therefore able to survive for much longer with a minimal supply of exogenous calories. Very basic requirements for infants are 50 cal/kg. This will just keep the infant alive for some time but does not allow for growth or the calories used for increased energy expenditure. The main energy demand is from respiratory effort and, where an infant is dyspnoeic and tachypnoeic, the calorie requirements may be substantially elevated. A total of 100 cal/kg is the lower level of provision for such infants and where the additional demands for calorie supply resulting from surgery or infection are taken into account, 120 cal/kg should be the aim for the neonate or young infant.

Body water constitutes a higher proportion of the paediatric patient than the adult. The neonate has a body water at birth which amounts to about 80% body weight. The extracellular compartment in the newborn is of equivalent size to the intracellular compartment, whereas in the adult the ratio is 1–2. Blood volume in the newborn is 85 ml/kg, whereas by 1 year of age this has fallen to 80 ml/kg and by 10 years old to 75 ml/kg. These differences have to be taken into account in resuscitation and replacement of fluids. It is important to maintain an adequate blood volume and to do so may require infusion of plasma or albumin to maintain the osmotic tension in the intravascular compartment.

The choice of drug dosage is important in the small patient. Perlstein et al.[4] in a study of medication in a simulated newborn intensive care area found that 8% of all doses calculated by 95 registered nurses were 10 times greater or less than ordered. Interestingly, their attempt to assess the nurses discriminatory powers as to the correctness of a prescribed dosage led to the conclusion that experienced nurses were more certain and more wrong than the inexperienced. Even with the eleven paediatricians tested the error rate was approximately 4%.

WATER AND ELECTROLYTES

Water and electrolyte balance in paediatric patients must take account of the varying demands of the patients depending on maturity and age. The kidney is the main regulator and is already functioning *in utero*. Postnatally the kidney is efficient within the range for which it is physiologically designed, i.e. the high volume but low solute load which is the normal young infant's diet. Function changes over the first year of life as the kidney develops the ability to cope with a higher solute load and relatively lower fluid intake.

Patients requiring intensive care often have fluid and electrolyte losses in excess of normal. These have to be included in the calculation of daily fluid requirements. Examples of increased fluid loss are the invisible sweat loss in the pyrexial patient, the losses from drains or fistulae, and the inability of the kidney to conserve water after the relief of an obstructive uropathy.

The basic water requirements may be summarized:

$$
\begin{array}{ll}
\text{Day} & 1\text{---}50\,\text{ml/kg} \\
& 2\text{---}100\,\text{ml/kg} \\
& 10\text{---}150\,\text{ml/kg} \\
& 15\text{---}150\text{--}180\,\text{ml/kg} \\
\text{Year} & 1\text{---}120\,\text{ml/kg} \\
& 10\text{---}75\,\text{ml/kg}
\end{array}
$$

Where an infant or child requires intravenous fluids as part of intensive care electrolyte requirements must also be met. In addition to water, sodium (4 mmol/kg) and potassium (4 mmol/kg) are necessary daily. If the duration of the intravenous therapy is to be less than 72 hours there is rarely any indication for addition of the other electrolytes, such as calcium and magnesium, or for trace elements and vitamins. It is desirable to maintain normal water and electrolyte balance rather than to be adept at correcting deviations. Addition of other elements, such as calcium, magnesium and trace elements does, however, become necessary with prolonged intravenous therapy.

The common syndromes in paediatric practice which give rise to water and electrolyte disturbances are usually the result of a combination of decreased intake and excessive loss. Gastroenteritis in infancy is a common cause of water and electrolyte imbalance and may give rise to the syndrome of hypertonic dehydration, particularly when infants continue to be fed with artificial milks containing a high sodium load. As the term implies there are two factors. First, the dehydration is due to the water loss. Secondly, the hypertonic aspect is due to the infant having been given too high a solute load for the kidneys to excrete, particularly when there is coexisting dehydration. This sodium load is retained in the extracellular compartment, drawing water from the intracellular compartment and resulting in an intracellular to extracellular imbalance with dehydration and hypertonicity. Another relatively common cause of water and electrolyte imbalance is hypertrophic pyloric stenosis. In this condition there is again a decreased intake and an increased loss by vomiting due to gastric outlet obstruction. The net result is loss of water, sodium and chloride and these infants may develop severe metabolic alkalosis with the blood pH rising to over 7·6.

In contrast, overhydration is an uncommon syndrome in paediatrics. It rarely occurs unless the infant or child is being fed by tube into the alimentary tract or intravenously. Tube feeding to the stomach or jejunum is commonly practiced in low-birth-weight infants and, whereas with normal feeding an infant will refuse an excess water load, that instilled by tube is absorbed. It is usually best to withdraw further feeding until the excess load has been cleared. On occasion medication with 2 mg/kg frusemide is beneficial in accelerating correction.

Monitoring of water and electrolyte balance by precise measurement may not be possible in the clinical situation. Useful factors in the assessment of the patient are the haematocrit, serum electrolytes, urea and osmolality, and urine electrolytes and osmolality together with a detailed history of abnormal losses. Serial weighing of the infant or child is a most valuable measurement which should always be available.

Isolated serum levels do not give an accurate guide to water and electrolyte balance because quite different pathophysiological mechanisms may give rise to the same serum sodium level. The sequence of events ultimately resulting in a decrease or increase in serum sodium are illustrated below.

1. *Cause*— Excess water intake (intravenous or nasogastric tube)

Effect— Distribution of water to extra- and intracellular compartments resulting in increase in body weight; fall in serum sodium

Inappropriate treatment— Sodium given

Result— Further extracellular expansion (increase in body weight and oedema)

2. *Cause*— Losses from gastrointestinal tract through vomiting, diarrhoea and fistula

Effect— Sodium loss; decrease in extracellular compartment with water moving into intracellular compartment (body weight static); fall in serum sodium

Treatment— Medication with sodium

Result— Redistribution of water between intracellular and extracellular compartments, i.e. sodium deficit which would be correctly treated by giving sodium

3. *Cause*— Too ill or unable to drink; water deficit

Effect— Decrease in extra- and intracellular compartment (fall in body weight); increase in serum sodium

Inappropriate treatment— Sodium deprivation, rehydration with water only

Result— Further decrease in extracellular compartment (fall in body weight)

4. *Cause*— Sodium excess (overload of saline: excess sodium bicarbonate to correct acidosis)

Effect— Increase in extracellular and decrease in intracellular compartment (body weight static); increased serum sodium level

Treatment— Increase water intake, induce diuresis

In the clinical situation indicated in examples 1 and 3, inappropriate action to correct an apparent change in serum sodium levels compounded the existing problem.

With the larger extracellular compartment in the neonate the movement of water and electrolytes is proportionately greater than in adults. It appears that the infant tolerates substantial deviations of serum electrolytes remarkably well but the intra- and extracellular volume changes which follow may contribute to deterioration in other functions such as gas exchange in the lungs. The central nervous system may be triggered into abnormal activity by the imbalance across the cell membranes and convulsions may result. The induction of fits is not infrequently triggered by an attempt to 'rehydrate' the infant too rapidly and so correct the electrolyte imbalance which has taken days to develop. Similar duration of time is necessary in achieving correction.

Therapy of water and electrolyte imbalance should be aimed first at maintaining an adequate circulatory blood volume and then correcting the extracellular and intracellular deficits more slowly. The latter take at least 72 hours for gradual return to normal but unfortunately there is no adequate simple method of checking on the rate of progress of the intracellular correction.

Acid–base studies contribute to the assessment of the sick infant. The main factor in infants which differs from adults is the larger extracellular component. Attempts to correct an acidosis with sodium bicarbonate, which is only effective in the extracellular component, require relatively larger doses. In small infants with recurrent acidosis, problems may arise due to an excess load of sodium and in these infants some of the correction may be made by the use of THAM.

NUTRITION

The paediatric patient requiring intensive care must have adequate attention given to his nutritional status, and feeding may be by the alimentary route or intravenously. The former is strongly favoured where possible as the precision required is much less than that required in intravenous feeding and complications are less frequent and less serious. Feeding by the alimentary route in the seriously ill is usually by instillation of prepared liquidized feeds through a nasogastric, nasojejunal, gastrostomy or jejunostomy tube. Intravenous feeding may be given either by peripheral line or by insertion of a central line. The former incurs more disturbance to the patient while the latter has a higher morbidity. Extensive literature has been accumulated on this subject.[5-9]

The caloric requirements of infants and children are higher than those of adults. The infant requires 120 cal/kg daily while the child requires 100 cal/kg through the remainder of the first decade of life. Adequate protein must be supplied, the infant requiring 4 g/kg while the older child only requires 2·5 g/kg unless the patient is in a severe state of catabolism. The remainder of the calorie intake may be made up of carbohydrate and fat, the latter accounting for about 40% of the total calorie intake, although the use of intravenous fat solutions is again being questioned.[10,11] The essential minerals and vitamins must be added to the dietary intake if nutritional support is to continue for more than a very brief period of time.

The patients in paediatric practice who require nutritional support are predominantly neonatal patients, but older children with extensive burns including respiratory burns, patients with complications of appendicitis and intussusception, patients with complications following major operations such as that for Hirschsprung's disease also require short-term nutritional support. This last group usually have an infective element which complicates their course and increases their calorie requirements.

With the current range of products available for intravenous feeding numerous regimes have been advocated and most have worked satisfactorily in the different centres. It is important that, before commencing intravenous feeding, hypovolaemia is corrected and as far as possible any water and electrolyte imbalance is rectified. The infant or child's acid–base status should also be assessed as a metabolic acidosis commonly accompanies starvation states. Too rapid intravenous feeding may itself induce a metabolic acidosis in a sick patient. When introducing intravenous feeding a gradual increase in calorie provision is recommended from 60 cal/kg on the first day, to 80, 100, 110 and 120 on successive days. Thereafter, this input may be satisfactory or further gradual increase in calories may be given until the infant regains his anticipated weight. A regime for a 3-kg infant giving approximately 120 cal/kg is:

1. Glucose 10%— (10 ml/h)	With addition to each 500 ml of 5 ml Solivito, 12 mmol potassium and 1·5 mmol phosphate
+2. Vamin" with glucose— (6 ml/h)	With addition to each 100 ml of 8 ml Ped-El solution and 4 mmol sodium
+3. Intralipid (soya oil) 20%— (3 ml/h)	with addition to each 100 ml of 3 ml Vitlipid

The solutions may be infused through 3-way taps close to the patient. The above regime gives an adequate intake of essential nutrients. Recently the necessity of fat solutions has become a matter for further debate but most would consider it desirable for the growing paediatric patient.

Assessment of the efficacy of the treatment can be made partly by the child's general appearance, by body weight, and by checking the haemoglobin, plasma proteins and urea, and electrolytes. Initially blood checks may be necessary daily for 2–3 days and then twice a week. Thereafter, single weekly checks are adequate unless particular complications occur. If the patient has abnormal losses, supplements have to be added to the regime and more frequent blood checks may be necessary. Additional guidance can be obtained from urine collection and estimates of the urinary loss of electrolytes, amino acids and sugar.

Nutrition for the older child differs only in that the requirements of calories, protein and minerals are slightly less than that for the young infant although still in excess of that required for adults.

RESPIRATION

The fetus *in utero* has detectable chest wall movements but, postnatally, dramatic changes occur in which the airways are cleared of fluid and the lungs expanded with air. The baby has to take over the function of exchanging oxygen and carbon dioxide from the mother. The premature infant born at 26–30 weeks has not yet developed adequate alveoli but despite this is usually able to exchange gas and may not require mechanical support but simply an increase in inspired Po_2. With longer gestation the development of the alveoli progresses, but there is a relative deficiency of surfactant and infants born after 30–35 weeks' gestation frequently develop respiratory problems. This respiratory distress syndrome may progress until the infant requires respiratory support. Radiologically these infants have the characteristic air bronchograms with very opaque lung fields. Infants born after 36 weeks gestation are much less likely to have respiratory distress syndrome but aspiration pneumonia then becomes a more common cause of hypoxia and excessive respiratory effort, so that mechanical ventilation becomes necessary. Small infants have immature control of their respiratory system and may have recurrent apnoeic attacks. Although in the majority of infants these do not seem to require respiratory support, intubation and ventilation may become necessary.

Some infants with structural congenital abnormalities require respiratory support. The most dramatic of these is congenital diaphragmatic hernia. In this condition effects of the diaphragmatic hernia have already been established in the fetus *in utero*. The passage of gut from the abdominal cavity into the chest results in interference with the outgrowth of the lung buds. This space-occupying mass in the thorax results in a severe degree of pulmonary hypoplasia on the ipsilateral side and a lesser degree of hypoplasia on the contralateral side.[12] In consequence of the combination of hypoplastic lungs and the mass of gut which is usually in the left thoracic cavity, the infant may not be able to establish spontaneous ventilation at birth. Intubation and immediate respiratory support may be necessary in resuscitating the newborn infant and, in some, ventilation will be required to continue. In others, spontaneous respiration may be established for a time, but as swallowed air distends the alimentary tract the infant shows increasing respiratory distress. It is important to maintain adequate oxygenation in these infants as hypoxia predisposes to the development of intraventricular haemorrhage which may either cause death or significant cerebral damage. Postoperatively these infants may require continued ventilation for some time until the infant is gradually able to maintain adequate gas exchange with spontaneous ventilation. During this period of ventilation there is probably considerable postnatal lung development which ultimately allows the infant to breath spontaneously. This speculation is difficult to prove at the present time, but is in accord with the clinical course.

After corrective surgery for oesophageal atresia or congenital heart disease continued mechanical ventilation is usually indicated. The act of breathing is the main form of energy expenditure in the infant, and an early decision to ventilate electively for a time postoperatively will obviate the risk of the infant becoming exhausted, with hypoxia and hypercapnoea developing.

In the older infant the principal condition for which intensive care and respiratory support is necessary is acute laryngotracheobronchitis. These infants have upper airway obstruction which may develop so rapidly that within 2 or 3 h of being apparently well the infant may develop complete respiratory obstruction. Emergency relief of the obstruction by endo-tracheal intubation may become necessary. If intubation proves technically impossible, a tracheostomy is performed. If facilities for doing this are not available the insertion of a cannula percutaneously into the trachea may be life-saving. For older children, most of the situations in which respiratory support may be necessary are similar to conditions in adults, e.g. children undergoing major cardiac surgery or patients with severe head injuries, but it is seldom necessary in paediatric patients with multiple injuries from trauma and flail chest problems are rare.

Careful monitoring of the blood gas levels in infants with respiratory problems is of particular importance. The small infant is at considerable danger from hypoxic damage if inadequate supply of oxygen is given but, unlike the older infant or adult, is also at considerable danger from excessive levels of oxygen in the arterial blood. The epidemic of retrolental fibroplasia several years ago, following the administration of excessive concentrations of oxygen to premature infants, highlighted this problem and emphasizes the importance of very careful monitoring of the oxygen tensions in the blood of neonates. An umbilical catheter or peripheral arterial cannula should be inserted so that blood samples may be obtained to measure the oxygen tension. Oxygen therapy is then adjusted appro-priately. Complications of intra-arterial cannulation can be significant in small infants. Fortunately, transcutaneous Po_2 monitors have now been developed which will yield a measurement of the tissue Po_2 continuously and with reasonable accuracy. Since the electrode is heated, the site of application should be changed every 4 h. Similar transcutaneous Pco_2 monitors are also under development.

Hypoxia in the infant has many deleterious effects. The brain is particularly susceptible to hypoxia and may suffer a significant degree of damage which is not apparent for months after the insult. The development of intraventricular cerebral haemorrhage, due to hypoxia, has been recognized for many years. Most information has come from post-mortem studies of premature infants.[13] In recent years, the use of echoencepha-lography has led to the detection of many intraventricular haemorrhages in infants which had previously passed unrecognized.[14] The full extent of this potential hazard is not yet clear. Where hypoxia occurs as part of the respiratory distress syndrome, there is also retention of carbon dioxide and the development of a 'mixed' respiratory and metabolic acidosis. Cor-rection of the acidosis by administration of bicarbonate may present the infant with an excessive sodium load, with consequent water retention and the development of oedema. Treatment is directed towards maintaining an adequate supply of oxygen and elimination of carbon dioxide. Where there is upper airway obstruction this may be achieved by intubating the infant. Commonly there is no upper airway obstruction and treatment includes the following steps.

1. Increase in inspired oxygen tension.
2. Continuous positive airway pressure.
3. Mechanical ventilation.

Increase in inspired oxygen tension is achieved with the use of a head box. The oxygen concentration in the box is measured by an oxygen meter, with the sensor placed near to the point from which the baby is breathing. The concentration is adjusted to maintain a transcutaneous oxygen level (or if arterial sampling is being performed, a Pao_2) of 50–90 mmHg. The concentration should be reduced if the level rises to over 90 mmHg on either of these measurements and so danger to the eyes is eliminated. If adequate oxygen levels are not being obtained with this regime or if there is a continual rise in the carbon dioxide tension in the blood, further treatment is necessary. A rising Pco_2, especially if rising in excess of 10 mm/h is best treated by proceeding directly to mechanical ventilation.

Continuous positive airway pressure (CPAP) can be administered by a face mask or through an endotracheal tube. The infant continues to breathe spontaneously and this method of treatment is beneficial in the infants with respiratory distress syndrome, pulmonary oedema and post-thoracotomy patients despite the theoretical danger of decreasing venous return and consequent reduction in cardiac output. A fall in pulmonary resistance has been demonstrated with CPAP[16] and the lowered oxygen cost of breathing is important in an infant approaching a critical situation.

Mechanical ventilation is necessary when the above measures have failed. In the postoperative patient it may be decided to ventilate electively. Intubation is either by the orotracheal or the nasotracheal route. There are advocates of each route. The oral route is simpler but it is more difficult to ensure that the tube is fixed securely in position. The nasal route is technically more difficult and occasionally the nasal passages will only allow the passage of an unacceptably small tube. It is easier to secure a nasotracheal tube. A tube by either route can cause problems by pressure necrosis, the oral tube occasionally eroding through the palate or, more commonly, the nasal tube causing necrosis of the septum or ala. If these dangers are appreciated they may usually be avoided by adequate nursing care.

Intubation

Prior to intubation of an infant, preoxygenation with 100% oxygen should be given by face mask and bag for 2 minutes. If intubation is not accomplished within 30 seconds, repeat oxygenation should be given prior to further attempts at intubation. It is of help to have an assistant pin the shoulders of the infant firmly onto the surface the infant is lying on. The straight blade of the laryngoscope is then inserted into the pharynx allowing the tongue to be lifted forward and the larynx visualized. The endotracheal tube should then be inserted 2 cm into the larynx and fixed in position after reoxygenating the baby.

The tubes used in infants and younger children, whether they be endotracheal or tracheostomy, are non-cuffed. As a result the hazard of mucosal necrosis and subsequent tracheal stenosis are lessened. However, repeated endotracheal intubation may cause mucosal damage in the narrow subglottic region and this can cause the secondary development of subglottic stenosis. If the necessity for intubation continues for more than 2 weeks, then tracheostomy must be considered. The care of an infant with either nasotracheal or endotracheal tube is similar. Warm humidified gases have to be supplied in the early period after the upper airways have been bypassed.[17] Secretions have to be aspirated from the tracheobronchial tract. This should be performed as a sterile procedure to avoid introducing pathogenic bacteria into the respiratory tract. With adequate humidification the secretions are maintained sufficiently liquid so that aspiration can be performed hourly. Instilling 1 ml of sterile water into the tube prior to aspirating helps liquify the secretions further and allows better clearance. Infants with copious secretions require more frequent tracheobronchial toilet. Once the infant or child has had a tracheostomy tube for a time, gradual weaning from high humidity to normal air can be achieved.

In establishing a tracheostomy the young patients do not require the same operative approach as adults. Turning a flap from the trachea to stitch to skin is undesirable in the infant as this weakens the trachea and may produce tracheal collapse which is difficult to treat. A simple transverse incision between tracheal cartilages is used to open the trachea. The lower edge of the trachea is pulled forward by a hook or pressure forceps and the tracheostomy tube inserted. A tracheostomy tube one size larger than the appropriate endotracheal tube, e.g. a 3·5-mm inside diameter for the infant who had a 3-mm endotracheal tube is used. Tying the tube in place is very important and flexing the neck before tying the tapes allows the tube to be fitted snugly. It is vital that the tube is not able to be displaced as this is very dangerous. Replacing the tube in the first 48 hours can be very difficult although later this procedure becomes easier.

Ventilation

Having instituted mechanical ventilation it is important to check that adequate gas exchange is being achieved. This can be assessed clinically by the colour and perfusion of the child, the adequacy of the chest movements and auscultation to ensure that the endotracheal or tracheostomy tube has not slipped beyond the carina to produce ventilation of one lung only. Measurement of the transcutaneous or arterial P_{O_2} and P_{CO_2} should, however, be the principal guide to adequacy of ventilation.

In addition, because of the toxic effect on the lungs of exposure to high oxygen tensions, it is important to monitor the arterial oxygen tension to reduce the pulmonary alveolar oxygen tension as soon as possible. Weaning the patient from the ventilator may present a problem. A transitional period on intermittent mandatory ventilation[17] or mandatory minute ventilation[18] may assist. Gradual extension of the time the infant is allowed on spontaneous breathing is usually successful in those with more prolonged problems. Maintenance of infants with severe respiratory failure by extracorporeal membrane-oxygenation has been carried out for limited periods of time, but further developments in this field are necessary before this becomes a practical proposition for many infants.

RENAL FAILURE

Dialysis in the young patient can be either by the peritoneal route or by haemodialysis. The former is more useful as the infant has a large peritoneal surface area which can allow a satisfactory dialysis. Haemodialysis is performed after insertion of an A–V shunt to allow access.

The patient who has relief of an obstructive uropathy may have a profuse diuresis and requires close monitoring to keep pace with losses and the inability of the kidney to function adequately for a time. Also a few patients may develop hypertension which can be sufficiently severe to induce a hypertensive encephalopathy and careful monitoring is necessary to control this until reduction of the pressure spontaneously occurs.

NERVOUS SYSTEMS

Children are susceptible to head injuries and the sequelae discussed elsewhere of raised intracranial pressure following this. Peculiar to the paediatric group are some conditions such as Reye's syndrome and in this intracranial monitoring is necessary. This can be achieved in the younger infants by percutaneous insertion of a cannula into the subdural space through the lateral aspect of the fontanelle. The cannula is then connected to a transducer to give a pressure readout or printout. Control of the intracranial pressure may be achieved by mannitol infusions and by hyperventilation but, if recurrent, craniotomy has to be considered. The various biochemical effects of the syndrome require corrections as far as possible along with the full supportive measures of an intensive care unit.

REFERENCES

1. Sulyok E., Jequier E. and Prod'hom L. S. (1973) Respiratory contribution to the thermal balance of the newborn infant under various ambient conditions. *Paediatrics* **51**, 641.
2. Hughes-Davies T. H. (1979) Conservative care of the newborn baby. *Arch. Dis. Child.* **54**, 59.
3. Cockburn F., Drillien C. M., Couthgate I. et al. (1976) *Neonatal Medicine*, p. 278. Oxford, Blackwell Scientific Publications.
4. Perlstein P. H., Callison C., White M. et al. (1979) Errors in drug computations during newborn intensive care. *Am. J. Dis. Child.* **133**, 376.
5. Dudrick S. J., Vars H. M. and Rhoads J. E. (1967) Longterm parenteral nutrition with growth in puppies and positive nitrogen balance in patients. *Surg. Forum* **18**, 356.
6. Logan R. W., Young D. G., Ross D. A. et al. (1974) Comparison of an oral and intravenous feeding regimen in the newborn. *Arch. Dis. Child.* **49**, 200.
7. Cohen I. T., Dahms B. and Hays D. M. (1977) Peripheral total parenteral nutrition employing lipid emulsion (Intralipid): complications encountered in paediatric patients. *J. Pediatr. Surg.* **12**, 837.
8. Nelson R. (1974) Minimizing systemic infection during complete parenteral alimentation of small infants. *Arch. Dis. Child.* **48**, 16.
9. Leader (1980) Parenteral nutrition in the newborn—a time for caution. *Lancet* **2**, 838.
10. Fisher G. W., Hunter K. W., Wilson S. R. et al. (1980) Diminished bacterial defences with intralipid. *Lancet* **2**, 819.
11. Levene M. L., Wigglesworth J. S. and Desai R. (1980) Pulmonary accumulation after Intralipid infusion in the preterm infant. *Lancet* **2**, 815.
12. Lewis M. A. H. and Young D. G. (1969) Ventilatory problems with congenital diaphragmatic hernia. *Anaesthesia* **24**, 571.
13. Wigglesworth J. S., Keith I. H. and Girling D. J. (1976) Hyaline membrane disease, alkali, and intraventricular haemorrhage. *Arch. Dis. Child.* **51**, 755.
14. Ziervogel M. A. (1981) Echoencephalography in neonates and infants. *Ann. Radiol. (Paris)* **24**, 25.
15. Rozkovec A. and Rithalia S. V. S. (1980) Transcutaneous oxygen monitoring. *Br. J. Clin. Equip.* **5**, 24.
16. Cogswell J. J., Hatch D. J., Kerr A. A. et al. (1975) Effects of continuous positive airway pressure on long mechanics of babies after operation for congenital heart disease. *Arch. Dis. Child.* **50**, 799.
17. Lawler P. G. P. and Dunn J. F. (1977) Intermittent mandatory ventilation. A discussion and a description of necessary modifications to the Brompton Manley ventilation. *Anaesthesia* **32**, 138.
18. Hewlett A. M., Platt A. S. and Terry V. G. (1977) Mandatory minute volume. A new concept in weaning from mechanical ventilation. *Anaesthesia* **32**, 163.

Index